HEPATITIS B RESEARCH ADVANCES

HEPATITIS B RESEARCH ADVANCES

ALICIA P. WILLIS
EDITOR

Nova Biomedical Books
New York

For permission to use material from this book please contact us:
Telephone 631-231-7269; Fax 631-231-8175
Web Site: http://www.novapublishers.com

LIBRARY OF CONGRESS CATALOGING-IN-PUBLICATION DATA

Hepatitis B research advances / Alicia P. Willis, editor.
p. ; cm.
Includes bibliographical references and index.
ISBN-13: 978-1-60021-666-4 (hardcover)
ISBN-10: 1-60021-666-8 (hardcover)
1. Hepatitis B. I. Willis, Alicia P.
[DNLM: 1. Hepatitis B. 2. Hepatitis B Vaccines. 3. Liver Neoplasms--etiology. WC 536 H53352 2007]
RC848.H44H4844 2007
616.3'623--dc22 2007013309

Published by Nova Science Publishers, Inc. ✦ New York

CONTENTS

PREFACE

Hepatitis B is a disease of the liver caused by the Hepatitis B virus (HBV), a member of the Hepadnavirus family and one of several unrelated viral species which cause viral hepatitis. It was originally known as "serum hepatitis" and has caused current epidemics in parts of Asia and Africa. Hepatitis B is recognized as endemic in China and various other parts of Asia. The proportion of the world's population currently infected with the virus is 3 to 6%, but up to a third have been exposed. Symptoms of the acute illness caused by the virus include liver inflammation, vomiting, jaundice, and rarely, death. Chronic hepatitis B may cause liver cirrhosis which may then lead to liver cancer. This book presents the latest advances in the field.

Chapter I - The birth dose of hepatitis B vaccine is needed in regions where vertical transmission of the disease is a problem. It should be given within 24 hours of birth for maximum protection. However, in some Pacific nations where mother-to-infant transmission is prevalent, births may occur outside of the formal health sector, mostly in the home. This presents a challenge for the timely administration of the vaccine. How can a birth dose be administered to mothers delivering at home and miles from health services? Should the vaccine be presented in single- or multiple-dose vials? Who should give the injection? Should there be specially designed equipment? The presentation of the vaccine can be modified to facilitate delivery of this birth dose. For instance, it can be offered in a single dose vial, using a delivery mechanism that can be administered by an untrained birth attendant. Such single-doses vials do not need a preservative such as thiomersal, another advantage when considering the needs of the newborn. There is also the potential for novel delivery systems to be developed to facilitate the administration of the birth dose such as transdermal patches.

Chapter II - Patients with chronic hepatitis B (CHB) are characterized by (1) ongoing replication of hepatitis B virus (HBV), (2) presence of HBV DNA in the sera and the liver, and (3) distorted HBV-specific immune responses. At present, there is no curative therapy for patients with CHB and antiviral drugs are used to control HBV replication and to minimize the damages of the hepatocytes. The ultimate aim of therapy is blocking or delaying the occurrence of progressive liver diseases such as liver cirrhosis and hepatocellular carcinoma. Antiviral drugs quickly reduce the amounts of the HBV in patients with CHB, however, the response is not usually sustained. A naturally-occurring defense system is essential for sustained control of viral replication. Recent studies have shown that at least two types of immune responses are detected in patients with CHB; (1) HBV-specific and (2) non HBV-specific. Circumstantial evidences indicate that HBV-specific immune responses control the replication of the HBV, whereas, non HBV-specific immune responses induce liver damages. Vaccine therapy in which vaccine containing surface antigens of the HBV are administered to CHB patients induce HBV-specific immune responses and cause reduction of HBV replication. The authors revisited the clinical experiences of two decades about usage of antiviral agents and one decade of using of vaccine therapy in CHB patients. It is getting clear that monotherapy with antiviral agent or with vaccine therapy is unlikely to stand the test of time. However, if a combination therapy of antiviral agents and immune modulators can be given in patients with CHB that may have better therapeutic outcome. More potent and newer antiviral agents have been developed by multinational drugs companies. On the contrary, many experimental data have been accumulating regarding antigen-specific immune therapy in animal model of HBV, but only few of them has been tested in patients with CHB. Recently, cell-based therapy has shown considerable optimism regarding their utility in HBV carriers. In this communication, the authors will discuss about the scopes and limitations of combination therapy with antiviral agents and antigen-specific immune therapy for treatment of CHB patients.

Chapter III - Hepatitis B is a highly contagious viral infection. It can lead to chronic carrier state and the hepatocellular carcinoma in the worst case. To prevent is better than to treat athis infection. An effective tool for prevention and control of hepatitis B infection is the vaccination. In this article, topics on the hepatitis B vaccination will be presented. The new concepts on vaccination strategies will be discussed. Also, the new advances on hepatitis B vaccinology will be presented.

Chapter IV - Hepatitis B virus (HBV) infection is endemic in many parts of sub-Saharan Africa including Nigeria. Surveillance of HBV infection markers in blood donor population is important in recognizing trends in prevalence and incidence of transfusion related infections and also provides opportunity to estimate the risk of infectious donations inadvertently entering the blood supply. In this study, a comparative evaluation of latex agglutination (LA), immunochromatographic strip (ICS), and ELISA techniques was performed in the seroepdemiological survey of hepatitis-B surface antigen (HBsAg) among blood donors in south-eastern Nigeria. A total of 1570 donors (1406 males and 164 females, aged 18-41 years old) were enrolled in the study. Serum separated from 5ml of venous blood obtained from each subject was screened using the three techniques. The prevalence rates of HBsAg were 8.0% (95% CI., 6.7-9.3%) by ELISA; 10.4%(95% CI., 8.9-11.9) by LA; and 10.3% (95% CI., 8.8-11.8%) by ICS techniques. A total of 117(8.3%, 95% CI., 6.9-9.7%) of the males and 9(5.5%,95% CI., 2.0-9.0%) of the females had HBsAg as detected by ELISA and the difference was significant (χ^2=16.02, df=1, P<0.05). The LA technique indicated that 147(10.5%, 95% CI., 8.9-12.1%) males and 16(9.8%, 95% CI., 5.2-14.4%) females had HBsAg, the difference was also significant (χ^2=7.70, df=1,P<0.05). By the ICS technique, 145(10.3%, 95% CI., 5.3-15.3%) males and 17(10.4%, 95% CI., 5.7-15.1%) females were positive for HBsAg, but the difference was not statistically significant (χ^2=0.0004, df=1, P<0.05). The highest and lowest prevalence rates of HBsAg were observed among individuals of age groups 25-29 years and >35 years respectively and the differences were statistically significant. The respective prevalence figures were 11.5%(95% CI., 8.9-14.1%) vs 2.4%(95% CI., 0.8-4.0%) (χ^2=26.18, df=3, P<0.05) by ELISA; 12.5%(95% CI.,9.8-15.2%) vs 6.3%(3.7-8.9%) (χ^2=9.67, df=3, P<0.05) by LA; and 13.6(95% CI., 10.8-16.4%) vs 4.5%(95% CI., 2.3-6.7%) (χ^2=22.9, df=3, P<0.05) by ICS. Commercial motorcyclists and those who engage in business had higher prevalence of HBsAg than the farmers and students, but differences were not statistically significant by any of the diagnostic techniques. Results showed that ELISA technique appeared to be a more useful diagnostic tool that LA and ICS techniques in the detection of HBsAg among blood donors. The 126 positive samples detected by ELISA were observed to be either positive with LA, ICS or both, showing no variation as was observed with LA and ICS results. Protection of the blood supply from virus-infected donations through effective donor selection and testing with highly sensitive technique is recommended.

Chapter V - Hepatitis virus infections are traditionally a major health problem among drug users (DUs). Several factors may favor the rapid spread of hepatitis infection in this category of patients. HBV and HCV are easily transmitted through exposure to infected blood and body fluids. DUs often prepare and use drug solutions together. Many in the DU community are infected and this provides multiple opportunities for transmission to others. Many of these patients with chronic hepatitis virus infection are not aware of their infections and this facilitates the spread of the diseases. Viral hepatitis is not inevitable for DUs. Although multiple factors have prevented the development of vaccines for hepatitis C, both hepatitis A and hepatitis B can be prevented by immunization. The purpose of this overview is to show some epidemiological data about HBV and the other bloodborne viral hepatitis among DUs, to summarize and discuss the hepatitis vaccination in this population. HBV vaccination can also prevent hepatitis D infection which in most developed countries, is almost exclusively restricted to IDUs. Data on IDUs compliance to immunisation schedules and immunological responsiveness are scarce, and in particular the response of drug users to immunisation has received little attention.

Previous studies have reported a reduced antibody response to HBV vaccine among IDUs, but factors associated with a lack of response have not yet been well identified. We try to focus most significant results achieved in successful vaccination programs as reported in scientific literature and, little, from our direct experience. We trust that results reported in this Chapter will contribute to the international efforts aimed at improving hepatitis prevention. In our opinion HBV vaccination campaigns among DUs represent a highly effective form of health education. It also makes them aware of the other forms of infection and create the ideal basis for future vaccination campaigns against HCV.

Chapter VI - Design of novel treatment options for chronic hepatitis B virus (HBV) infections is actually of particular importance, since current therapies based on IFNα and nucleoside analogues (lamivudine, adefovir) are limited by the emergence of drug–resistant mutants and the persistence of intranuclear covalently closed circular viral DNA (cccDNA) responsible for persistence of infection. Increasing number of recent data suggest that rationale therapy of hepatitis B may combine the use of antiviral drugs and immunotherapeutic approaches. In this regard, DNA-based immunization appears as a pertinent new approach, inducing rapid, potent and specific immune responses to hepadnavirus structural proteins as demonstrated in naïve chimpanzees, woodchuck and duck models. However the therapeutic DNA vaccination against chronic hepatitis B was less investigated.

The authors aim was to explore in the chronic duck HBV (DHBV) infection model, whether DNA vaccine-based immunotherapy in combination or not with an antiviral drug (adefovir, lamivudine,) treatment is able to enhance cccDNA clearance and break humoral immune tolerance in chronic DHBV carriers. We have first realized a study associating adefovir with DNA vaccine against DHBV envelope and compared herein its therapeutic efficacy with our recent study combining lamivudine with DNA vaccine against viral envelope and/or core proteins.

In adefovir-DNA study, a group of DHBV-infected ducks received adefovir treatment (weeks 6-10 p.i.) in combination or not with DNA immunization to DHBV preS/S protein (weeks 6, 9, 12 and 22). A marked drop in viremia titres (97%), reaching the limit of detection of the assay, was observed during the 4 weeks of drug administration in all adefovir-treated as compared with untreated ducks, although it was followed by a rebound of viral replication after drug withdrawal. At the end of follow-up, analysis of intrahepatic DHBV DNA revealed a more pronounced decrease in viral DNA in combination therapy group as compared with DNA or adefovir monotherapy groups suggesting a trend to an additive effect of drug and DNA vaccine. However only few animals eliminated liver viral DNA and no correlation with humoral anti-preS response restoration was observed.

In lamivudine-DNA study, lamivudine was administrated alone in combination with DNA vaccine to DHBV envelope and/or core proteins. DHBV-carrier ducks received lamivudine treatment earlier (weeks 1-8), with higher number of DNA immunizations (weeks 6,10,14,28,35), shorter overlap with DNA vaccination (2 weeks), larger amounts of plasmid and a longer follow-up in larger animal groups. A decrease in viremia titers (70%) was observed in all lamivudine-treated compared to untreated animals, although it was limited to only the first 3 weeks of lamivudine treatment and was followed by a rapid rebound in viral replication. Interestingly about 30% animals, which received DNA vaccine alone or in association with lamivudine had cccDNA levels that were at or under the lower real-time PCR detection limit and was associated for majority of them with restoration of anti-preS response.

In conclusion, our comparison of two combination therapy studies associating DNA vaccine-based immunotherapy with either adefovir or lamivudine indicates a better efficacy of the lamivudine-DNA protocol. In adefovir-DNA study, only modest effect in term of viral cccDNA clearance and seroconversion was observed, in spite of higher antiviral potency of the drug. By contrast, data obtained in lamivudine-DNA study provided a first demonstration that DNA vaccine alone and associated with drug treatment was able to induce drastic and sustained suppression of viremia and enhance viral cccDNA clearance in one third of DHBV-carriers, which was tightly associated with break of immune tolerance. Because both studies differed not only by the choice of drug but, importantly, by the design of DNA immunization protocol, thus number of factors known to determine the success of genetic vaccination such as plasmid construct, amount of plasmid DNA, number of DNA injections and immunization schedule may play an important role in better therapeutic efficacy of lamivudine-DNA study. Further investigations aiming to increase the potency of DNA vaccine–based immunotherapeutics need to be performed in animal models in view to obtain a complete and sustain recovery from chronic hepatitis B.

Chapter VII - Hepatitis B virus (HBV) is the most common cause of hepatitis world wide and a major cause of hepatitis in Nigeria of which blood transfusion has been identified as the most common means of transmission. This has led to the compulsory screening of HBV in all blood meant for transfusion, this has been done neglecting other transmission channels which may be responsible for the high infection rate in the population because despite screening of blood meant for transfusion, HBV remains a major killer in Nigeria and Sub Saharan Africa. We undertook a five year cases –control study (2000 – 2005) to determine the risk factors of HBV infection using the spot test kit and confirming with ELISA technique. A total of 2,987 patients (cases) attending various clinics in Nigeria for hepatitis related illness and 3,798 age and sex matched controls were screened for HBV virus. Of the 2,987 cases only 1,899 (63%) were positive. From the positive cases were patients who have marked their bodies with different sharp objects for the purpose of obtaining charms and have a very high relative risk of 5.5 (95%, CI). This was followed by injecting drug users with a relative risk of 3.5 (95%, CI) while the Yoruba ethnic group had the lowest relative risk of 0.7 (95%, CI). Other risk factors determined included injecting drug use, tattoo, blood transfusion, ear piercing, native surgery for splenitis, female genital mutilation, health care workers, sharing tooth brush, 6 or more sex partners, 2 to 5 sex partners, regular visit to barber shop, personal and family history of jaundice, tribal marks, and ethnicity (Yoruba, Ibo, Hausa, Ijaw and other related minorities). All these exposures posses a risk in the population, however, charms markings, tribal marks and native surgery for splenitis had very high percentages of attributable cases of 23%, 14.4% and 9.2% respectively.

Chapter VIII - Although hepatitis B virus (HBV) has been documented to cause hepatocellular carcinoma (HCC), the exact role of HBV in the development of HCC remains enigmatic. Several hypotheses have been proposed to explain the potential mechanism, including insertional mutagenesis of HBV genomes, transcriptional activators of HBV gene products such as HBx and truncated middle S mutants and chromosomal alterations. HBx and integrated preS2/S sequences increased the expression levels of C-myc. C-myc inactivation resulted in HCC cells differentiating into hepatocytes and biliary cells forming bile duct structures. Malignant transformation of hepatocytes may occur in the context of chronic liver injury, regeneration and cirrhosis. Chronic liver inflammation and hepatic regeneration induced by cellular immune responses may favor the accumulation of genetic alterations and the proliferation of oval cells. Chronic liver inflammation is the setting for the accumulation of ECM, resulting in cirrhosis. ECM remodeling plays an important role in hepatocarcinogenesis through providing the survival signals, promoting the proliferation, invasion and metastasis and blocking the differentiation and apoptosis. Both mature cells and stem cells (oval cells and bone marrow stem cells) may be the targets of hepatocarcinogenesis. Two topics about the correlation between HBV and hepatocarcinogensis are very interesting and must be identified: whether the virus or viral protein directly induces HCC, or the long-term inflammatory changes caused by chronic HBV infection play more important roles in accelerating hepatocarcinogenesis; whether HCC originates from the de-differentiation of mature cells or differentiation block of stem cells.

Chapter IX - Hepatitis B virus (HBV) infection is a global health problem and causes a wide spectrum of clinical manifestations, ranging from acute or fulminant hepatitis to various forms of chronic liver disease, including inactive carrier state, chronic hepatitis, cirrhosis and hepatocellular carcinoma (HCC). Most HBV carriers in the endemic regions acquire the virus during birth or early childhood. Liver injury associated with HBV infection is predominantly mediated through immune mediated mechanisms. The natural history of HBV carriers who are infected early in life can thus be divided into 4 dynamic phases based on the virus-host interaction. During the immune tolerance phase, serum HBV DNA levels are high and hepatitis B e antigen (HBeAg) is present. In the immune clearance phase, the majority of carriers seroconvert from HBeAg to anti-HBe. After HBeAg seroconversion, patients are usually in the integration or low replication phase, with low HBV DNA level and normal serum alanine aminotransferase activity. However, a small proportion of patients continue to have moderate level of HBV replication and active liver disease designated reactivation phase. The frequency and severity of hepatitis flares during the immune clearance and/or reactivation phase predicts progression of liver disease. In general, early HBeAg seroconversion typically confers a favorable outcome, whereas late or absent HBeAg seroconversion after multiple hepatitis flares may accelerate the progression of chronic hepatitis to cirrhosis, and therefore, has a poor clinical outcome. Other factors identified as risk factors of cirrhosis and HCC development include male gender, older age, presence of cirrhosis, family history of HCC, persistence of ALT elevations, co-infection with HCV or HDV, cigarette smoking, alcohol drinking, aflatoxin exposure, and co-morbidities of diabetes and obesity. Recently, new hepatitis B viral factors predictive of clinical outcomes have been identified. Three large-scale, population-based prospective cohort studies (7 townships in Taiwan, Haimen city in China, and Philadelphia in the US) of Asian HBV carriers aged between 25-65 years all indicated that the best predictor of adverse outcomes (cirrhosis, HCC and death from liver disease) in chronic HBV infection is the serum HBV DNA level at enrollment, independent of HBeAg status, baseline serum ALT level and other risk factors. The higher the serum HBV DNA level in the immune clearance phase, the higher the incidence of adverse outcomes over time. In addition, several hospital-based cohort or case control studies from Taiwan and Hong Kong indicated that high HBV DNA level, HBV genotype C, basal core promoter mutation and pre-S deletion are associated with increased risk of liver disease progression as well as HCC development. In conclusion, the lessons learned from the natural history of chronic HBV infection in adult HBV carriers from endemic areas can help us better define the clinical threshold as well as therapeutic endpoint of "safe" HBV DNA level (e.g. 10,000 copies or 2,000 IU/ml) for the prevention of long-term liver related complications in patients during later phases of chronic HBV infection.

Chapter X - Chronic hepatitis B virus infection is the most important cause of hepatocellular carcinoma (HCC) in Asia. Regular surveillance of HCC by ultrasound and alfa-fetoprotein can detect early HCC that may be amendable to surgical resection. However, there is still much controversy on the survival benefit and cost-effectiveness of HCC surveillance programs. Lead-time bias and length-time bias impose major difficulties in the interpretation of clinical studies. The high false positive rate of alfa-fetoprotein and large demand for ultrasound examination limit the cost-effectiveness of surveillance programs. Risk stratification of patients may direct the resource allocation in the public health perspective. On top of the clinical factors of HCC, viral factors including HBV genotypes, basal core promoter mutations and viral load are emerging as hot research areas. Chemoprevention of HCC by treatment of HBV has shown preliminary success. Incidence of HCC is reduced among responders to conventional interferon-alfa treatment on long-term follow-up. Peginterferon can potentially improve the virological response and may offer a better hope for HCC prevention. Virological suppression by nucleotide analogues particularly among cirrhotic patients can also reduce of risk of HCC.

Chapter XII - Approximately 2 billion people – one third of the world's population – have serologic evidence of past or present Hepatitis B virus (HBV) infection, and 350 million people are chronically infected. Each year over 1 million people die from HBV-related chronic liver disease. Liver transplantation is indicated in HBV-infected patients with end-stage diseases, such as, chronic encephalopathy, refractory ascites or recurrent variceal bleeding. However, in last century, liver transplantation for HBV related-liver diseases was a very controversial issue because the graft was inevitably recurrent after liver transplantation. HBV reinfection after liver transplantation results from HBV particles in circulation, or other extrahepatic sites. Significant progress has been made in the prophylaxis and treatment of recurrent hepatitis B after liver transplantation. Hepatitis B immune globulin (HBIG) was effective in reducing HBV reinfection and improving graft survival after liver transplantation. Lamivudine has also dramatically reduced the recurrence of HBV in the patient undergoing liver transplantation. Combination HBIG and lamivudine is the most effective porphylatic regimen. HBV-related liver disease is no longer a contraindication for liver transplantation. This article focuses on the mechanisms and prophylaxis of hepatitis B recurrent after liver transplantation.

Chapter XIV - The fundamental principle of radiotherapy is to destroy malignant cells while minimizing damage to normal tissues. Almost all patients who receive radiotherapy to the head and neck area develop some grade of acute mucositis, which is not only painful, but may compromise tumor control by determining decrease in dose intensity and interruptions of the treatment. The term ‘oral mucositis’ describes the adverse effect of chemotherapy or radiation induced inflammation of the oral mucosa. Symptoms of mucositis vary from pain and discomfort to an inability to tolerate food or fluids. The degree and duration of mucositis in patients receiving radiotherapy are related to radiation source, cumulative dose, dose intensity, volume of irradiated mucosa, smoking/alcohol consumption and oral hygiene conditions. To our knowledge, there is no other controlled study which has evaluated vitamin E as a single radioprotective agent in patients with head and neck tumors treated with radiation therapy alone or post-operative. For this reason, we conducted a double-blind, randomized trial with the objective to investigate the potential mucosal protection of vitamin E in irradiated patients with head and neck cancer, motivated by its simplicity of administration, no severe toxicity in conventional doses, low cost and easy availability.

Chapter XV - Although a vaccine is available for the prevention of hepatitis B virus (HBV) infection, HBV infects nearly two billion people around the world and mainly in the underdeveloped countries. The liver is the primary target of HBV. The virus infects the hepatocytes leading to the release of infectious virions and non-infectious particles into the blood. HBV infection can be either acute, which may last for several months or chronic which is a life long infection.

The immune system both innate and acquired (humoral and cell mediated) responses, play essential roles in HBV infection. It is known that neutralizing antibodies play an important role during HBV infection and can reduce the spread of infection. Cellular immune mechanisms are also important for the clearance of HBV and disease pathogenesis. The different structural forms of the hepatitis B viral proteins, can elicit different T helper cell subsets with different cytokines being produced. Cytokines are very important proteins in the defense against viral infections including HBV.

In this chapter, the authors will discuss our current knowledge of the immunology of the HBV infection and factors that make this infection more common in the underdeveloped countries, especially the middle-eastern countries. The authors will discuss in detail the essential role played by the immune system innate and acquired responses and will briefly discuss the ways of controlling HBV infection in general and in particular to this part of the world.

In: Hepatitis B Research Advances
Editor: Alicia P. Willis, pp. 1-7

ISBN: 978-1-60021-666-4

Chapter I

Birth Dose of Hepatitis B Vaccine – How Methods of Administration Affect Presentation

***C. John Clements**[*]

Centre for International Health, The Macfarlane Burnet Institute for Medical Research and Public Health Ltd, GPO Box 2284, Commercial Road, Melbourne, VIC 3004 Australia

Abstract

The birth dose of hepatitis B vaccine is needed in regions where vertical transmission of the disease is a problem. It should be given within 24 hours of birth for maximum protection. However, in some Pacific nations where mother-to-infant transmission is prevalent, births may occur outside of the formal health sector, mostly in the home. This presents a challenge for the timely administration of the vaccine. How can a birth dose be administered to mothers delivering at home and miles from health services? Should the vaccine be presented in single- or multiple-dose vials? Who should give the injection? Should there be specially designed equipment? The presentation of the vaccine can be modified to facilitate delivery of this birth dose. For instance, it can be offered in a single dose vial, using a delivery mechanism that can be administered by an untrained birth attendant. Such single-doses vials do not need a preservative such as thiomersal, another advantage when considering the needs of the newborn. There is also the potential for novel delivery systems to be developed to facilitate the administration of the birth dose such as transdermal patches.

[*] Correspondence concerning this article should be addressed to Dr. C. John Clements, MD, Associate Professor, Centre for International Health, The Macfarlane Burnet Institute for Medical Research and Public Health Ltd, GPO Box 2284, Commercial Road, Melbourne, VIC 3004 Australia. Tel (office): +613.9282.2199; Fax: +613.9282.2144; Email: john@clem.com.au.

Introduction

Hepatitis B vaccines were developed and marketed in the 1980s from a desire to reduce the burden of disease from the infection. The initial price of the product was around US$100 for a course of three doses. The first vaccines were plasma-derived and were used in industrialized countries for adults at high risk such as health care workers and renal dialysis patients. As the price came down, public health strategists began to see the potential for using the vaccine on a wide scale to reduce the burden of disease across whole populations. The preferred way was to introduce mass vaccination of infants, thus preventing acquisition of infection from their infected mothers (vertical transmission), or from infected siblings and peers (horizontal transmission). Global recommendations were in favour of one of two strategies. The first was in areas where vertical transmission was not occurring and the risk of infection was outside of the newborn period. Such infants could be given three doses of vaccine at the same time as the three doses of triple antigen (DTP) at approximately 6, 10 and 14 weeks of age.

The second strategy was designed to prevent vertical transmission by immunizing with the first dose as near to the time of birth as possible. If left too late after birth, the vaccine's protective effect was reduced. In addition, some industrialized countries also used human immunoglobulin (HIG).

This two-pronged policy was widely adopted and implemented. Those areas where vertical transmission was not a problem were able to introduce the vaccine alongside triple antigen with little difficulty. However, some of the practical implications of the policy against vertical transmission were not dealt with at the global or national level. How could a birth dose be administered to mothers delivering at home and miles from health services? Should the vaccine be presented in single- or multiple-dose vials? Who should give the injection? Should there be specially designed equipment? How could the presentation of the vaccine be modified to facilitate delivery of the birth dose?

Implication of the Epidemiology of Hepatitis B Infection

In countries with a high prevalence of chronic hepatitis B infection, a high proportion is infected during infancy or childhood. 25-50% of chronic infections in such countries are caused by "vertical" mother-to-infant transmission at the time of birth. Administration of hepatitis B (HepB) vaccine as soon as possible after birth, preferably within 24 hours, is crucial to preventing vertical transmission [1]. Failure to administer it in a timely manner will reduce the impact of immunization. The highest documented prevalence of hepatitis B carrier rates are in Africa, Asia and some Pacific Island Countries [2].

Not withstanding clear policies from the World Health Organization (WHO) about the importance of administering the first dose within 24 hours of delivery [3], the practical implications of this for home births have been incompletely worked out. In a real sense, HepB is the first infant vaccine whose delivery at birth is critical – even though two vaccines already in widespread use are recommended to be given at birth – BCG and oral polio vaccine, in reality they are oftentimes given days or weeks later.

Place of Delivery

A review of hepatitis B immunization in the Western Pacific [4] confirmed that countries where the majority of deliveries were in health facilities were able to achieve high coverage rates with the birth dose. Such countries included Singapore and Malaysia. But the majority of births in countries such as Papua New Guinea and much of Indo-China were conducted at home without trained assistance. These countries had low coverage of the birth dose of HBV. Vaccine needs to be available at community level in such countries, as births are predominantly in the home. This requires that they be given outside of the health centre, outside of routine immunization sessions, and with no or minimal reliance on the cold chain.

Personnel

There are three scenarios that can play out for the birth dose, and these have a bearing on which personnel administer the vaccine:

a) Deliveries requiring the first dose of vaccine to be given at the same time as DTP-1, around six weeks of age. This is not strictly a "birth dose" but a "first dose". The regular immunization staff will administer this dose.
b) Deliveries in hospitals, clinics and health centres when the birth dose must be given within 48 hours. In this case, the trained nurse or midwife will likely administer the vaccine. It can be given within moments of birth, at roughly the same time as the oxytocin.
c) Deliveries at home when the birth dose must be given within 24 hours. Community midwives may attend home deliveries, or, in more remote rural areas, no trained staff may be available. In this case a traditional birth attendant (TBA) will probably attend.

For scenarios "a" and "b", no special arrangements are needed to administer the first dose. Staff will be trained already in administering injectable vaccines. But for home births (scenario c), attending personnel will probably not be trained in such techniques, and indeed may be prohibited from doing so by the law of the country. A presentation that can be given by an untrained attendant is therefore highly desirable.

Mono-Dose vs. Multi-Dose Presentation

In general, the cost per dose of vaccine decreases as the number of doses in the vial increases. Thus a ten- or twenty-dose vial is much lower cost than a mono-dose vial. But for the birth dose, it is very unlikely that twenty or even ten babies will all be born within a short time of each other. The wastage rate will be very high if more than two doses are provided per vial. In general, then, a compromise has been reached and the vaccine is provided in two-dose vials.

Syringe or Not

A presentation that can be administered by needle and syringe for health facility deliveries makes sense. Training of staff and equipment are all in favour of this. Indeed, it makes good economic sense to use a multidose vial, thereby reducing the cost-per-dose of the vaccine. But a home delivery by an untrained person needs another approach. While even conventional mono-dose preparations administered with needle and syringe allow for outreach beyond the cold chain, newer technologies can make it easier. Uniject™ is a non-reusable plastic pouch with a needle directly attached, containing a single-dose of drug or vaccine. The device was developed by the Program for Appropriate Technology in Health (PATH). In Indonesia, the use of Uniject™ by village midwives to deliver the first dose of HepB was associated with increased coverage [5,6]. Studies of Uniject™ have generally reported high user-preference attributed to ease of use and speed of injection, as well as economic benefits such as reduced wastage and simplified logistics. Uniject also evoked less fear within the family of the vaccine recipient. [7-10]. While the potential barriers to using the Uniject™ include higher cost and the need for licensure of the product in a given country, this single-dose delivery system has none the less been found to be economically worthwhile [6]. Many other needle-free technologies are being investigated including the use of powdered vaccine and the application of skin patches impregnated with vaccine.

The Need for a Preservative

Many hepatitis B vaccines are manufactured with thiomersal as a preservative. Indeed, a preservative is essential for safety reasons for multi-dose presentations - where vaccine vial caps are punctured more than once during use there is a risk of introducing potentially fatal contamination.

Discussion

While there was initial concern that it may be harmful, there is now widespread scientific acceptance that thiomersal is a safe preservative for use in vaccines administered to infants

[11]. But for a number of reasons, very low birth weight premature infants may be at increased risk from thiomersal-containing vaccines [12]. It is very difficult to undertake ethical studies that demonstrate the actual amounts of ethyl mercury (the active mercury component of thiomersal) in the blood of newborns. Pichichero et al [13] conclude that thiomersal in routine vaccines poses extremely little risk to full term infants, and recommend caution regarding administering thiomersal-containing vaccines at birth to premature or very low birth-weight infants.

A study in 2000 measured the exposure of mercury after HepB vaccine in preterm infants [14]. It showed that preterm infants had greater than 10-fold higher mean mercury levels at the baseline reading compared with term infants, although this difference was not statistically significant. Preterm infants may not be able to metabolize mercury as well because of immature livers that are not able to synthesize the metal-binding protein metallothionein [15]. After vaccination, they had 5 times higher mercury levels compared with term infants (this was statistically significant). Another factor that may contribute to higher mercury levels is the reduced body mass of pre-term babies. There is clearly an incomplete understanding of the metabolism of mercury in general and ethyl mercury in particularly around the time of birth.

The question remains incompletely answered whether the infant birth dose of thiomersal-containing HepB vaccine is a risk for the newborn. Currently most HepB vaccines available for developing countries contain thiomersal, even if they are mono-dose preparations. WHO is now promoting animal model studies to evaluate this aspect [16]. The incompletely quantified risk to the fetus, the premature infant and the low birth weight infant suggest it would be better to avoid this preservative in these groups until more data are assembled about the preservative's safety in these special groups. HepB vaccine is the only preservative-containing multidose vaccine to be offered at birth. Eventually it should be possible to avoid altogether HepB vaccine presentations that contain thiomersal for the birth dose. This has been achieved in the United States already by the use of mono-dose preparations that are thiomersal-free. Developing countries could achieve the same if the birth dose was a mono-dose preparation. Changing to a thiomersal-free presentation would require expensive re-licensing procedures. To date the international community has not been sufficiently encouraging towards manufacturers (mostly in developing countries) to switch to thiomersal-free lines for part of their production.

Conclusion

There are a number of challenges posed by the need to deliver a timely dose of HepB vaccine for mothers delivering at home and miles from health services. The presentation of the vaccine can be modified to facilitate delivery of this birth dose. While there are undoubted cost advantages in using a multi-dose presentation, safety considerations suggest that thiomersal should not be used as a preservative until there is more reassurance about its safety in the pre-term and low birth weight infants (a significant proportion of births in developing countries). The knock-on effect of this is that presentations for use in home deliveries should be mono-dose vials that do not need a preservative. For instance, it has been shown to be particularly useful to have one-shot disposable injection devices such as Uniject™ filled with thiomersal-free vaccine. Such devices can be used safely by relatively untrained staff. However, the economics of vaccine production would make this an expensive decision to implement.

Further research is needed to ensure the safety of the use of thiomersal in the newborn period. Human ingenuity is certain to come up with ever more methods of delivering vaccines without the use of needles and syringes. Such alternative methods of vaccine delivery will need to be tested as to their usefulness in administering the birth dose at home by relatively untrained birth attendants. HepB vaccine needs to be among the most heat-stable vaccines as it is required for use outside cold chain. Further research that leads to improved heat stability properties would be welcome.

References

[1] Maynard JE, Kane MA, Hadler SC. Global control of hepatitis B through vaccination: role of hepatitis B vaccine in the Expanded Programme on Immunization. *Rev Infect Dis* 1989;11 (suppl. 3):S574–8.

[2] Kao JH, Chen DS. Global control of hepatitis B virus infection. *Lancet Infect Dis* 2002 Jul;2(7):395-403.

[3] Core information for the development of immunization policy. Department of Vaccines and Biologicals. World Health Organization, Geneva, 2002. WHO/V&B/02.28. http://www.who.int/vaccines-documents/DocsPDF02/www557.pdf viewed on 27 December 2006.

[4] Clements CJ, Baoping Yang, Crouch A, Hippgrave D, Mansoor O, Nelson CB, Treleaven S, van Konkelenberg R, Wiersma S. Using hepatitis B control to improve immunization services in the Western Pacific Region. *Vaccine* 24 (2006) 1975-1982.

[5] Achieving universal childhood immunization with Hepatitis B vaccine: policy and cost-effectiveness issues, prepared for the Ministry of health of Indonesia, PATH, April 1996.

[6] Levin CE, Nelson CM, Widjaya A, Moniaga V, Anwar C. The cost of home delivery of a birth dose of hepatitis B vaccine in a prefilled syringe in Indonesia. *Bull World Health Organ* 2005; 83:456-461.

[7] Sutanto A, Suarnawa IM, Stewart T, SoewarsoTI. Home delivery of heat-stable vaccines in Indonesia: outreach immunization with prefilled, single-use injection devices. *Bull World Health Organ* 1999, 77(2):119-126.

[8] Soewarso TI, Widjaya A, Saleh A. Early integrated efforts for maternal and child survival. Ministry of Health of Indonesia in cooperation with the Program for Appropriate Technology in Health (PATH), 1996.

[9] Widjaya A; Saleh A, Purwanto H, Anwar C. Improving the safety and effectiveness of hepatitis B immunization in Indonesia through Uniject introduction in DI Yogyakarta, East Java and West Nusa Tenggara Provinces, August 2000-July 2001. Ministry of Health of Indonesia in cooperation with the Program for Appropriate Technology in Health (PATH), 2002.

[10] Quiroga R et al. A prefilled injection device for outreach tetanus immunization by Bolivian traditional birth attendants. *Rev Panam Salud Publica/Pan Am J Public Health*, 1998,4(1).

[11] Clements CJ, McIntyre PB. When science is not enough – a risk/benefit profile of thiomersal-containing vaccines. *Expert Opinion on Drug Safety* 2006, Jan;5(1):17-29.

[12] Clements CJ. The evidence for the safety of thiomersal in newborn and infant vaccines. *Vaccine* 2004; 22 (15-16),1854-1861.

[13] Pichichero ME, Cernichiari E, Lopreiato J, Treanor J. Mercury concentrations and metabolism in infants receiving vaccines containing thiomersal: a descriptive study. Lancet 2002; 360: 1737-41.

[14] Stajich GV, Lopez GP, Harry SW, Sexson WR. Iatrogenic exposure to mercury after hepatitis B vaccination in preterm infants. *J. Pediatr.* 2000:136, 679-81.47

[15] Yoshida M, Ohata H, Yamauchi Y, Seki Y, Sagi M, Yamazaki K et al. Age-dependent changes in metallothionein levels in liver and kidney of the Japanese. Biol Trace Elem Res 1998; 65: 167-73.

[16] Thiomersal: neuro-behavioural studies in animal models. *Wkly Epidem Record* 2005; 80:3-7. http://www.who.int/wer/2005/en/wer8001.pdf viewed 27 December 2006.

In: Hepatitis B Research Advances
Editor: Alicia P. Willis, pp. 9-20
ISBN: 978-1-60021-666-4

Chapter II

REVISITING THE MONOTHERAPY WITH ANTIVIRAL DRUG IN PATIENTS WITH CHRONIC HEPATITIS B: ETHICAL AND SCIENTIFIC BASIS OF COMBINATION THERAPY AND THEIR APPLICATION IN CLINICS

Fazle Akbar**, *Osamu Yoshida and Morikazu Onji
Department of Gastroenterology and Metabology,
Ehime University Graduate School of Medicine, Ehime, Japan

ABSTRACT

Patients with chronic hepatitis B (CHB) are characterized by (1) ongoing replication of hepatitis B virus (HBV), (2) presence of HBV DNA in the sera and the liver, and (3) distorted HBV-specific immune responses. At present, there is no curative therapy for patients with CHB and antiviral drugs are used to control HBV replication and to minimize the damages of the hepatocytes. The ultimate aim of therapy is blocking or delaying the occurrence of progressive liver diseases such as liver cirrhosis and hepatocellular carcinoma. Antiviral drugs quickly reduce the amounts of the HBV in patients with CHB, however, the response is not usually sustained. A naturally-occurring defense system is essential for sustained control of viral replication. Recent studies have shown that at least two types of immune responses are detected in patients with CHB; (1) HBV-specific and (2) non HBV-specific. Circumstantial evidences indicate that HBV-specific immune responses control the replication of the HBV, whereas, non HBV-

* Correspondence concerning this article should be addressed to Dr. Sk. Md. Fazle Akbar, MD, Ph. D., Department of Gastroenterology and Metabology, Ehime University Graduate School of Medicine, Ehime, Japan, Shitsukawa 454, Toon City, Ehime 791-0295, Japan. Telephone: 81 89 960-5308; Fax: 81 89 960 5310; E. mail: akbar@m.ehime-u.ac.jp.

specific immune responses induce liver damages. Vaccine therapy in which vaccine containing surface antigens of the HBV are administered to CHB patients induce HBV-specific immune responses and cause reduction of HBV replication. We revisited the clinical experiences of two decades about usage of antiviral agents and one decade of using of vaccine therapy in CHB patients. It is getting clear that monotherapy with antiviral agent or with vaccine therapy is unlikely to stand the test of time. However, if a combination therapy of antiviral agents and immune modulators can be given in patients with CHB that may have better therapeutic outcome. More potent and newer antiviral agents have been developed by multinational drugs companies. On the contrary, many experimental data have been accumulating regarding antigen-specific immune therapy in animal model of HBV, but only few of them has been tested in patients with CHB. Recently, cell-based therapy has shown considerable optimism regarding their utility in HBV carriers. In this communication, we will discuss about the scopes and limitations of combination therapy with antiviral agents and antigen-specific immune therapy for treatment of CHB patients.

INTRODUCTION

The hepatitis B virus (HBV), a prototype member of the family *Hepadnaviridue*, is an enveloped DNA virus. After the entry of the HBV in human, the virus is attached to appropriate hepatocyte receptors, which still remains unknown. The virion is internalized and uncoated in the cytosol. Most of the molecular and cellular events regarding this are not completely understood. The HBV genome translocates to the nucleus, where it is converted into a double-stranded covalently closed circular DNA (cccDNA) molecule, following completion of the shorter positive (+)-strand and repair of the nick in the negative (–)-DNA strand. In this form, cccDNA serves as the template for viral transcript synthesis by host RNA polymerase. Recently, viral kinetic studies have indicated that the half life of the virus is different in the sera and in the hepatocytes. It is about a day in the sera, but the half-life of the HBV in infected cells is much longer and variable, ranging from 10 to 100 days [1].

HBV is transmitted following perinatal, percutaneous and sexual exposure, but also by contact with open cuts and sores, as may occur between children in hyperendemic areas. HBV can cause both acute as well as chronic infection. Also, in some cases, a life threatening fulminant hepatitis may develop. Following HBV infection, the risk of becoming a chronic carrier of HBV mostly depends on the age of the subjects. This exceeds 90% in newborns of hepatitis B e antigen-positive mothers, ranges between 25% and 30% in infants and very young children, but in adults this risk is only between 5% and 10%. In addition to age, HBV-related factors such as HBV genotype and host-related factors such as immune status of the hosts may also influence the pathogenesis of HBV infection [2].

According to the World Health Organization estimate, two billion people worldwide have serological evidence of past or present HBV infection with the HBV. Among these, about 350-400 million are chronically infected with the virus. If hepatitis B surface antigen (HBsAg) is detected in the sera for more than 6 months after initial infection, the person is regarded as chronic HBV carrier. Also, these patients harbor replicating HBV, HBV DNA in the liver and the sera and different types of HBV-related antigens and antibodies in the liver and the sera [3].

Most chronic HBV carriers harbor the HBV from their birth or during neonatal or perinatal period. However, features suggestive of hepatitis are not found in these subjects until they become adult. In addition, some HBV carriers never develop hepatitis during their life time. Chronic HBV carriers without any feature of liver injury are regarded as inactive HBV carriers. On the other hand, some HBV carriers develop features of hepatitis usually during their twenties or thirties. The extent of liver damages can be assessed by various methods, but estimation of alanine aminotransferase is widely used for this purpose around the world. Patients harboring HBV for more than 6 months with increased serum levels of alanine aminotrasferase are regarded as patients with chronic hepatitis B (CHB). Patients with CHB exhibit exacerbation and remission of liver diseases and many of them develop progressive liver diseases such as liver cirrhosis and hepatocellular carcinoma.

The existence of million of chronic HBV carriers represents a major global public health problem. All chronic HBV carriers (irrespective of their HBV load and liver damages) are permanent and living sources of the HBV and they are practically responsible for transmission of the HBV to healthy persons. Although inactive HBV carriers do not develop features of progressive liver damages, they may show signs and symptoms of liver damages any time. Most importantly, patients with CHB are at major risk of development progressive liver diseases such as liver cirrhosis and hepatocellular carcinoma. Taken together, therapy of chronic HBV infection especially that of patients with CHB is a major challenge of contemporary virology, hepatology and immunology.

HBV is a non cytopathic virus and there is no evidence that HBV can directly destroy the hepatocytes. The immune responses of the hosts are extremely important for both control of the virus as well as for induction and maintenance of liver damages. HBV-specific immune responses are strong, polyclonal and multispecific in HBV-infected patients who clear the virus after acute infection (resolved acute hepatitis B). Sustained HBV-specific immune responses are also detected in these subjects for several years or for whole life. Both HBV-specific cellular and humoral immune responses are detected in these subjects. These patients become negative for HBV DNA and HBsAg in the sera, although very low levels of HBV may be detected in the liver for prolonged period. These patients exhibit antibody to HBsAg (anti-HBs) and are protected from future HBV infection. However, if these subjects become immune suppressed, replication of HBV may recur in these subjects.

On the other hand, HBV-specific immune responses are either undetectable or weak and narrowly-focused in chronic HBV carriers (Both inactive HBV carriers and patients with CHB). Although these patients exhibit weak HBV-specific immune responses, non HBV-specific immune responses are not diminished in these patients. Rather, these are highly pronounced in some patients with CHB. Taken together, both the magnitude of immune responses and the nature of immune responses (HBV-specific and non HBV-specific immune responses) critically determine whether one will resolve the HBV infection after an acute infection or will run an inactive course of chronic HBV infection or will develop chronic HBV infection as well as liver damages [4,5].

Based on this observation, we assumed that management of a complex disease like CHB would require comprehensive therapeutic approaches in which both antiviral agents and immune modulators are required. The viral load should be decreased by antiviral agents and a condition similar to naturally-occurring defense system (immune responses) should be induced by immune modulators in patients with CHB. The rationale for combination therapy and design of interventional strategy will be discussed in this review.

Present Treatment Options for Chronic HBV Carriers

Chronic HBV carriers can be broadly divided into two categories; (1) inactive HBV carrier without any features of clinical evidence of liver injuries and (2) patients with CHB with signs and symptoms of liver damages. At present, treatment is not recommended for inactive HBV carriers. Inactive HBV carriers harbor HBV and express HBV-related antigens including HBsAg. In spite of harboring HBV and their antigens, they do not show features of liver damages. However, they are permanent reservoir of the HBV and transmit the virus to healthy individuals. From the public health view point, inactive HBV carriers are more dangerous than patients with CHB because most of these persons are unaware that they are HBV carriers. This is especially important in developing countries of Asia and Africa, where, the health care delivery system is poorly developed and people are not normally screened for HBV. Treatment is not recommended for inactive HBV carriers because currently-available antiviral drugs are not effective in these patients.

Treatment is now recommended for only patients with CHB and antiviral drugs are given when they are in immune modulatory phase [6]. This indicates that antiviral drugs are only effective if host immune responses to HBV exist. It is not clear what should be proper levels of alanine aminotrasferase for getting better therapeutic efficacy of antiviral drugs in patients with CHB. In general, the levels of alanine aminotrasferase should be 2-5 times of the upper limit of normal to have potent therapeutic effects of antiviral drugs, however, this is not strictly followed by clinicians. Before 20 years, only a single licensed drug, interferon alfa was available for using in these patients. A 4- to 6-month course of interferon resulted in a sustained loss of hepatitis B e antigen and non detectable HBV DNA in approximately 30% of patients. However, complete eradication of HBV DNA was not seen due to usage of interferon. In addition, the rate of HBsAg seronegativity and seroconversion to anti-HBs was seldom seen due to interferon therapy. Interferon has also been used for prolonged period in CHB patients. The treatment option of CHB patients dramatically changed over the past 10 years. At present, two formulations of interferon and three oral nucleoside agents are available for treatment of CHB patients. Qualitative improvements have been made in new form of interferon. In addition to these three nucleoside analogs, new drugs have been available for treatment of CHB patients. Monitoring of efficacy of therapy has been improved due to availability of various commercial tests for serum HBV DNA. The more sensitive polymerase chain reaction assays can detect 50 HBV genomic copies/ml or less. Taken together, newer drugs and improved viral assessing techniques have led to development of evidence-based treatment guidelines for the management of CHB [7]. Studies have shown that all types of nucleoside analogs are capable of reduction of HBV quickly and patients with CHB treated with these drugs show delayed progression to HCC. Usage of interferon has been limited due to its poorer tolerability, high cost, need for subcutaneous injection, and a potential to precipitate immunological flares and liver failure in patients with advanced liver disease. Although nucleoside analogs are extremely well tolerated, disadvantages to their use include a high rate of relapse on withdrawal, frequent need for prolonged or maintenance therapy, relatively high expense, and drug resistance when used as monotherapy. Increased virological response has been demonstrated with an increasing duration of therapy, but this has also been associated with increasing rates of viral resistance. This outcome requires the use of another nucleoside analog that has antiviral activity against both the wild-type and drug-resistant HBV. Some nucleoside analogs have been started recently and more time will be required to develop insights about their antiviral potentialities and adverse effects. Especially, long term follow up of these patients is required to have proper insights about their broader usage [8]. In addition to antiviral agents, various immune modulators such as cytokines and growth modulators have been used in patients with CHC as pilot studies. The efficacy of these immune modulators is questionable because few randomized controlled trials have been done with these agents [9].

Control of HBV Replication and Liver Damages in Resolved Acute Hepatitis B

Eradication of the HBV from HBV-infected persons is an unachievable goal due to complexicity of the life cycle of HBV. The virus is integrated into host genome and produce cccDNA that do not replicate, but act as template for replication. The virus is detected mainly in the sera and the liver. The half life of the HBV in the sera (about 24 hours) and the liver (10-100 days) is different. Most antiviral agents so far have been unable to prevent the replenishment of the cccDNA pool from genomic HBV DNA recycled from the cytoplasm, or to effect efficient clearance of cccDNA-containing hepatocytes. Based on these observations, the goal of therapy of chronic HBV infection is to suppress HBV replication and induce reduced damages of the liver so that progressive liver diseases can be arrested or blocked. However, persistent suppression of the HBV in chronic HBV carriers is achieved in only few patients with CHB and in most of these cases treatment with nucleoside analogs must be done for prolonged period. This contrasts with the control of HBV replication in patients with resolved acute hepatitis B, who usually control HBV replication and liver damages without any antiviral agents. After an acute infection, high levels of HBV replication are detected in patients with resolved acute hepatitis. Also, moderate to severe levels of liver damages are also seen in these subjects. HBV is also integrated in the liver in patients with acute hepatitis B and cccDNA are also detected in their liver. However, naturally-occurring immune responses against the HBV develop in these patients and these control the further replenishment of the HBV in these subjects, although many of these subjects harbor the HBV for the rest of their life [10].

Lessons Learnt from the Natural Course of HBV Infection: Strategy for Therapeutic Maneuver

Presence of millions of chronic HBV carriers without any evidence of liver injury indicates that the virus by itself is not cytopathic for the infected hosts. Moreover, considerable numbers of subjects infected by the HBV during neonatal or prenatal period usually do not show any feature of liver diseases either in their whole life or until they become adult. On the other hand, some HBV-infected patients develop necroinflammatory liver diseases of various degrees. Some recent studies have unveiled that inactive HBV carriers exhibit features of liver damages if they become immune suppressed. As mentioned before, no single HBV-related or host-related unique factors may be accountable for development of liver damages in chronic HBV carriers.

As the HBV is unable to cause liver damage directly, their indirect role has been suspected by several investigators during the last three decades. The studies have shown very interesting role of immune systems in HBV control and liver damages. Patients who clear the HBV after an acute infection usually exhibit strong, polyclonal and multi-specific immune responses against various HBV-related antigens. Interestingly, these responses persist even after the HBV is controlled and hepatitis is resolved. On the other hand, HBV-specific immune responses are weak, monoclonal and limited in patients who do not control the HBV. Moreover, these responses wane with time. But, most of these studies could not assess the kinetics of immune responses of CHB patients or resolved acute hepatitis B patients serially.

During the last one decade, several elegant information were accumulated regarding control of the HBV because a murine model of HBV, HBV transgenic mice (HBV-Tg) become available from mid'1980s. Chisari and his group provided evidences to counter some conventional concept about viral clearance in chronic HBV infection using HBV-Tg. They showed that destruction of HBV-infected hepatocytes is not essential for control of the HBV because HBV can be destroyed and their replication can be well controlled by a non cytopathic mechanism in which various cytokines play pivotal roles [11,12].

In a second series of studies conducted by Bertoletti and his group supported the concept of noncytopathic control pathway of HBV replication in patients with CHB. They showed that both HBV-specific and non HBV-specific immune responses are induced due to infection with HBV. Also, their study unveiled that HBV-specific immune responses are beneficial for the host because that can control replication of the HBV without inducing massive damages of the liver. On the other hand, antigen non-specific immune responses cause destruction of the hepatocytes, but those are incapable of controlling HBV replication. In addition, non HBV-specific immune responses are related to damages of the hepatocytes [13,14]

Engineering Therapeutic Approaches against Chronic HBV Infection

Considering various scientific constrains, the target of therapy of chronic HBV infection may be to establish a condition similar to resolved acute hepatitis B in which HBV replication and liver damages can be controlled to significant degrees so that complications of chronic hepatitis can be minimized.

As it is assumed that HBV-specific immunity can reduce HBV replication without damage of hepatocytes, one of the therapeutic approaches may be to induce HBV-specific immunity in patients with CHB. However, induction of non HBV-specific immunity must be controlled in these patients.

Induction and Maintenance of HBV-Specific Immunity in Chronic HBV Carriers: Experience from HBV-Tg

Chronic HBV carriers harbor the HBV and all of them also express abundant amounts of HBsAg in the sera and the liver, In spite of having HBsAg in all HBV carriers, HBsAg-specific immune responses are either undetectable or inadequate in these subjects. These are seen in patients with CHB and also in murine model of chronic HBV carrier state, HBV-Tg. The apparent inability of HBV carriers to respond to HBsAg has mainly been accounted to neonatal tolerance because most HBV carriers are infected by the HBV during neonatal or perinatal periods when the immune systems are immature. A concept of neonatal tolerance has originally been proposed by Burnett and his colleagues during early 1950s [15]. Accordingly, almost no attempts have been taken to overcome immunological tolerance in chronic HBV carriers.

A fundamental breakthrough came in this field when Matzinger and her groups challenged the concept of neonatal tolerance. They showed that impaired immune responses of neonates are not due to neonatal tolerance, rather neonates can not induce proper immune responses due to defective functions of antigen-presenting dendritic cells (DC), a professional antigen-presenting cell [16]. However, the studies of Matzinger et al. have not been done with HBV. To assess the relevance of these findings in chronic HBV carriers, we used a line of HBV-Tg that express HBV DNA, HBsAg, HBeAg, and Dane particles in the sera. HBV-Tg have been expressing HBsAg from 17 days of their gestation and high levels of HBsAg were detected in their sera throughout their life. Apparently, HBV-Tg are tolerant to the stimulation of HBsAg and they do not produce anti-HBs and HBsAg-specific lymphocytes in vitro and in vivo. Further studies revealed that there T cells and B cells of these mice had no functional defects, rather spleen DCs of HBV-Tg are incapable of performing their functions as potent antigen-presenting cells [17]. To provide further support to our hypothesis that impaired functional capacities of DC may be relevant to impaired HBV-specific immunity in HBV-Tg, we showed that stimulation of DCs of HBV-Tg in situ by various immune modulators was related to induction of HBsAg-specific cellular and humoral immunity [18]. Finally, we showed that activation endogenous DC of HBV-Tg by a vaccine containing HBsAg induced anti-HBs in 25-50% of these mice. Administration of vaccine containing HBsAg (vaccine therapy) also induced HBsAg-specific cellular immune responses and caused reduced HBV replication in the sera and the liver. A tempting question came forward regarding the role of vaccine therapy in HBV-Tg; why endogenous HBsAg was unable to induce HBsAg-specific immune responses in HBV-Tg, but administration of vaccine containing HBsAg induced HBsAg-specific immunity in HBV-Tg. Studies from various laboratories showed that the importance of danger signal for induction of immune responses in these conditions [19].

Antigen-Specific Therapy (Vaccine Therapy) in Patients with CHB

In 1994, Pol et al. reported that administration of HB vaccine in CHB patients have antiviral and immune modulatory functions. During the last one decade, several investigators have used HB vaccine in CHB patients. Initially, vaccine was administered for three times, however, subsequently different investigators have used vaccine for 3-12 times. We vaccinated CHB patients with HB vaccine for 12 times. Different types of vaccine have also been injected to CHB patients. Different types of criteria have been used for evaluation of response. Vaccine therapy is safe in patients with CHB. However, there is controversy about their efficacy. In some studies, potent therapeutic efficacy of vaccine therapy has been reported, whereas, no significant efficacy has been found in others [20-24]. Although several potent antiviral agents are used in patients with CHB, the limitations of these drugs are now almost clear. Antiviral drugs reduce HBV replication in almost all patients, but sustained responses are seen in some patients only. The exact mechanism underlying this is not clear at this moment. In this respect, Boni et al. [25] have shown that treatment with nucleoside analogs results in revival of immune responses in CHB patients. Two factors may be important in this regard. The first, nucleoside analogs may have some direct immune modulatory potentials, however, little has been explored about this. The next, due to reduced HBV replication by nucleoside analogs, patients with CHB may regain their responsiveness to immune systems.

Similarly, pilot studies about vaccine therapy have shown that the therapeutic efficacy of vaccine therapy is better in patients with low viral load. Similar phenomenon has also been found in patients with cancers. Now, cancer patients are treated by different types of immune therapy, however, the response is relatively better in patients with low cancer burden. A combination of surgery and ablation therapy with immune therapy has also been proposed for treating cancer patients [26].

Ethical and Scientific Basis of Combination Therapy against Chronic HBV Infection

The limitations of antiviral agents and immune modulators for treating CHB are getting clear. It is true that newer and more potent antiviral agents will be marketed so that the emergence of HBV mutants, breakthrough of HBV, and breakthrough hepatitis will be diminished in future. In the context of vaccine therapy, cell-based vaccine has been developed for treating chronic HBV carriers. Now, several investigators including we have developed next generation vaccine, in which DCs have been loaded with antigens. DC-based vaccines have shown potent therapeutic efficacy in HBV-Tg [27].

Based on present realities, it seems that a combination therapy of antiviral agents and immune modulators in patients with CHB may be an effective therapeutic approach. The immune modulation should be done by antigen-specific immune therapy. Some pilot studies have shown that combination therapy of antiviral agents and immune modulators is a better therapeutic option than monotherapy with either of the agents [28]. In the context of combination therapy, it will be important to ascertain about the protocol of combination therapy. There may be two patterns of combination therapy. In one, antiviral agents may be given prior to vaccine therapy. In another, vaccine therapy can be given first and then the patients can be given antiviral agents. Also both antiviral agents and the vaccine can be administered together. At present, data about combination therapy is available from the clinical trials of some pilot studies only. In one study, we provided lamivudine to patients with CHB and after 3 months the patients were given vaccine therapy for 12 times. After one year of treatment, HBV negativity and rate of seroconversion to anti-HBe were significantly higher in patients with combination therapy than patients that received lamivudine monotherapy [29]. However, other combinations of antiviral agents and immune modulators should be tested in patients with CHB.

A Long Term Motive of Combination Therapy

At present, only patients with CHB are treated by antiviral drugs and this is only well-accepted method of therapy of chronic HBV infection. HBV carriers those do not exhibit features of liver damages are not recommended for treatment. There are about 300 million inactive HBV carriers and they are not given any treatment at present. It is not true that inactive HBV carriers do not need treatment, but commercial-available antiviral drugs are inefficient in these subjects. However, inactive HBV carriers may develop features of liver diseases, especially HCC during their life time. These patients are treated when they develop features of liver damages. It is not ethical to induce liver injury in inactive HBV carriers for the sake of treatment. However, HBV-specific immune responses may be induced in inactive HBV carriers by administration of vaccine or antigen-pulsed DCs if randomized clinical trials reproducibly show that these therapies do not cause liver damages.

Another area of application of combination therapy may be in patients with liver transplantation with HBV background. Liver transplantation is the final tool of saving life of several HBV-infected patients. However, reactivation of HBV is seen in many liver transplanted patients. These patients are now given hepatitis B immunoglobulin (HBIG) for control of reactivation. Also, many of these patients are treated with antiviral agents. In lieu of HBIG, many of these patients have been treated with vaccine containing HBsAg and other surface antigens of the HBV [30,31]. However, the outcome is not still satisfactory. In this context, combination therapy may be an alternate choice of therapy of these patients. These patients may be treated with antiviral agents followed by vaccine therapy.

Conclusion

Antiviral drugs are recommended for patients with CHB with active viral replication and having features of liver damages. Liver damage is a sign of ongoing immune response of the host to the HBV. Patients with inactive HBV carriers are not given antiviral drugs because in the absence of immune responses against the HBV, commercially-available antiviral drugs are not effective.

Polyclonal immune modulators like cytokines have shown limited utility in CHB patients. Recent studies have shown that antigen-specific immune therapy may be effective in CHB patients. This is because control of HBV replication and liver damages can be attained by antigen-specific immune responses. However, monotherapy with vaccine therapy, the most widely used immune therapy, has shown limited efficacy. In this context, combination therapy of antiviral agents and immune therapy may be a practical choice for treatment of CHB patients. Indeed, combination therapy is getting popular for treatment of cancer patients. These include resection of cancer by surgery, ablation by other method, followed by immune therapy such as epitope-based or peptide-based or cell-based vaccine. The ultimate purpose of combination therapy in CHB patients is to reduce HBV load and thus to prepare a working ground for functioning of immune therapy. Clinical trials have shown that immune therapy is safe for patients with CHB. These are also effective in some patients with CHB. Antiviral drugs have been used by the hepatologists for several years. The scope and limitations of these drugs are also well known. Taken together, this may the proper time to start treatment of CHB patients with combination of antiviral drugs and immune modulators. We have only mentioned about HBsAg-based vaccine as immune therapeutic agent for treating patients with CHB, but other HBV-related antigens-based vaccine can also be used for this purpose. Hepatitis B core antigen (HBcAg)-based vaccine can also be used for this purpose and it is expected that this type of vaccine will have more potent antiviral potentially than HBsAg-based vaccine. However, clinical trial could not be materialized with HBcAg due to unavailability of human consumable HBcAg. In addition to antigen-based vaccine, peptide-based vaccine may also be used for this purpose. Finally, cell-based vaccine will be another tempting candidate for this type of therapeutic approach. Indeed, we have conducted a clinical trial of DC-based vaccine in HB vaccine nonresponders and interestingly all HB vaccine nonresponders developed anti-HBs due to a single injection of HBsAg-pulsed DC, although these vaccine nonresponders never developed anti-HBs due to administration of traditional vaccine for 6-9 times. The safety of HBsAg-pulsed DC has also been confirmed in patients with CHB and Chen et al. from China have shown that HBsAg-pulsed DCs also have potent antiviral potential.

In conclusion, various data about therapy of CHB patients indicate the inherent limitation of antiviral agents for treatment of CHB patients. Although antigen-specific immune therapy is in its infancy, a combination of antiviral and immune therapy may be effective in CHB patients. The next is to develop the strategies of therapy and clinical protocols of combination therapy. Chronic HBV infection, which is global in nature, can be controlled by comprehensive approaches of hepatologists, virologists and immunologists.

References

[1] Karayiannis, P. Hepatitis B virus: old, new and future approaches to antiviral therapy (2003). *J Antimicrob Chemther*, *51*, 761-785.

[2] Fattovich, G. (2003) Natural history and prognosis of hepatitis B. *Semin Liver Dis*, *23*, 47-58.

[3] Hilleman, M.R. (2003) Critical overview and outlook: pathogenesis, prevention, and treatment of hepatitis and hepatocarcinoma caused by hepatitis B virus. *Vaccine, 21*, 4626-4649.

[4] Rehermann, B. (2003) Immune responses to hepatitis B virus infection. *Semin Liver Dis*, *23*, 21–37.

[5] Milich, D.R.; Sallberg, M.; Maruyama, T. (1995) The humoral immune response in acute and chronic hepatitis B virus infection. *Springer Semin Immunopathol, 17*,149-166

[6] Xu, X.W & Chen, Y.G. (2006) Current therapy with nucleoside/nucleotide analogs forpatients with chronic hepatitis B. *Hepatobiliary Pancreat Dis Int, 5*, 350-359.

[7] Zoulim, F. (2006) Entacavir: a new therapeutic option for chronic hepatitis B. *J Clin Virol, 36*, 8-12.

[8] Fung, S,K, & Lok, A.S. (2005) Update of viral hepatitis in 2004. *Curr Opin Gastroenterol, 21*, 300-307.

[9] Sprengers, D & Janssen, H.L. (2005) Immunomodulatory therapy for chronic hepatitis B virus infection. *Fundam Clin Pharmacol, 19*,17-26.

[10] Chisari, F.V. & Ferrari, C. (1995) Hepatitis B virus immunopathogenesis. *Annu Rev Immunol, 13*, 29-60.

[11] Guidotti, L.G. & Chisari, F.V. (2001) Noncytolytic control of viral infections by the innate and adaptive immune response. *Annu Rev Immunol, 19*, 65-91.

[12] Guidotti, L.G.; Rochford, R.; Chung, J.; Shapiro, M.; Purcell, R.; Chisari, F.V. (1999) Viral clearance without destruction of infected cells during acute HBV infection. *Science, 284*, 825-829.

[13] Bertoletti, A. & Maini, M.K. (2000) Protection or damage: a dual role for the virus-specific cytotoxic T lymphocyte response in hepatitis B and C infection? *Curr Opin Microbiol, 3*, 387-392.

[14] Maini, M.K.; Boni, C., Lee, C.K.; Larrubia, J.R.; Reignat, S.; Ogg, G.S.; King, A.S.; Herberg, J.; Gilson, R.; Alisa, A.; Williams, R.; Vergani, D.; Naoumov, N.V. ; Ferrari, C.; Bertoletti, A. (2000) The role of virus-specific CD8(+) cells in liver damage and viral control during persistent hepatitis B virus infection. *J Exp Med, 191*, 1269-1280.

[15] Burnett, F.M.; Stone, J.D.; Edey, M. (1950) The failure of antibody production in the chick embryo. *Aust J Exp Biol Med Sci*, 28, 291-297.

[16] Matzinger, P. (1994) Tolerance, danger and extended family. *Annu Rev Immunol 1994*, 991-1045.

[17] Akbar, S.M.; Onji, M..; Inaba, K.; Yamamura, KI.; Ohta, Y. (1993) Low responsiveness of hepatitis B virus transgenic mice in antibody response to T-cell-dependent antigen: Defect in antigen presenting activity of dendritic cells. *Immunology, 78*, 468-473.

[18] Akbar, S.M.; Inaba, K.; Onji, M. (1996) Upregulation of MHC class II antigen on dendritic cells from hepatitis B virus transgenic mice by interferon-gamma: abrogation of immune response defect to a T-cell-dependent antigen. *Immunology 87*, 519-527.

[19] Akbar, S.M.; Kajino, K.; Tanimoto, K.; Michitaka, K.; Horiike, N.; Onji M. (1997) Placebo-controlled trials of vaccination with hepatitis B virus surface antigen in hepatitis B virus transgenic mice. *J Hepatol, 26*: 131-137.

[20] Pol, S.; Driss, F.; Michel, M.L.; Nalpas, B.; Berthelot, P.; Brechot, C. (1994) Specific vaccine therapy in chronic hepatitis B infection. *Lancet, 344*, 342.

[21] Wen, Y. M.; Wu, X. H.; Hu, D. C.; Zhang, Q. P.; Guo, S.Q. (1995) Hepatitis B vaccine and anti-HBs complex as approach for vaccine therapy. *Lancet 345*, 575.

[22] Pol, S.; Nalpas, B.; Driss, F.; Michel, M. L.; Tiollais, P.; Denis, J.; Brechot, C.; and a multicenter stud group. (2001) Efficacy and limitations of a; specific immunotherapy in chronic hepatitis B. *J Hepatol*, *34*, 917.

[23] Senturk, H.; Tabak, F.; Akdogan, M.; Erdem, L.; Mert, A.; Ozaras, R.; Sander, E.; Ozbay, G.; Badur, S. (2002) Therapeutic vaccination in chronic hepatitis B. *J Gastroenterol Hepatol*, *17*: 72-76.

[24] Yalcin, K.; Acar, M.; Degertekin, H. (2003) Specific hepatitis B vaccine therapy in inactive HBsAg carriers: a randomized controlled trial. *Infection*, *31*, 221.

[25] Boni, C.; Bertoletti, A.; Penna, A.; Cavalli, A.; Pilli, M.; Urbani, S.; Scognamiglio, P.; Boheme, R.; Panebianco, R.; Fiaccadori, F.; Ferrari C. (1998) Lamivudine treatment can restore T cell responsiveness in chronic hepatitis B. *J Clin Invest*, *102*: 968-975.

[26] Akbar, S.M.; Abe, M.; Yoshida, O.; Murakami, H.; Onji, M. Dendritic cell-based therapy as a multidisciplinary approach to cancer treatment: present limitations and future scopes. (2006) Curr Med Chem, 13, 3113-3119.

[27] Akbar, S.M.; Furukawa, S.; Hasebe, A.; Horiike, N.; Michitaka, K.; Onji M. (2004) Production and efficacy of a dendritic cell-based therapeutic vaccine for murine chronic hepatitis B virus carrier. *Int J Mol Med*, 14, 295-299.

[28] Ren, F.; Hino, K.; Yamaguchi, Y.; Funatsuki, K.; Hayashi, A.; Ishiko, H.; Furutani, M.; Yamasaki, T.; Korenaga, K.; Yamashita, S.; Konishi, T.; Okita, K. (2003) Cytokine-dependent anti-viral role of CD4-positive T cells in therapeutic vaccination against chronic hepatitis B viral infection. *J Med Virol*, *71*, 376.

[29] Horiike, N.; Akbar, S.M.; Michitaka, K.; Joukou, K.; Yamamoto, K.; Kojima, N.; Hiasa, Y.; Abe, M.; Onji, M. (2005) In vivo immunization by vaccine therapy following virus suppression by lamivudine: a novel approach for treating patients with chronic hepatitis B. *J Clin Virol, 32*: 156-161

[30] Sanchez-Fueyo, A.; Rimola, A.; Grande, L.; Costa, J.; Mas, A.; Navasa, M.; Cirera. J.; Sanchez-Tapias, J.M.; Rodes, J. (2000) Hepatitis B immunoglobulin discontinuation followed by hepatitis B virus vaccination: A new strategy in the prophylaxis of hepatitis B virus recurrence after liver transplantation. *Hepatology*, *31*: 496-501.

[31] Angelico, M.; Di Paolo, D.; Trinito, M.O.; Petrolati, A.; Araco, A.; Zazza, S.; Lionetti, R.; Casciani, C.U.; Tisone, G. (2002). Failure of a reinforced triple course of hepatitis B vaccination in patients transplanted for HBV-related cirrhosis. *Hepatology, 35*, 176-181.

In: Hepatitis B Research Advances
Editor: Alicia P. Willis, pp. 21-33

ISBN: 978-1-60021-666-4

Chapter III

RECENT TOPICS FOR HEPATITIS B VACCINATION

Viroj Wiwanitkit
Department of Laboratory Medicine, Faculty of Medicine, Chulalongkorn University, Bangkok, Thailand

ABSTRACT

Hepatitis B is a highly contagious viral infection. It can lead to chronic carrier state and the hepatocellular carcinoma in the worst case. To prevent is better than to treat athis infection. An effective tool for prevention and control of hepatitis B infection is the vaccination. In this article, topics on the hepatitis B vaccination will be presented. The new concepts on vaccination strategies will be discussed. Also, the new advances on hepatitis B vaccinology will be presented.

INTRODUCTION

Hepatitis B virus (HBV) infection is a worldwide viral infection. The main mode of transmission is via blood contact. This infection is highly endemic in many developing countries. The infection is highly prevalent in Asia, Africa, southern Europe and Latin America. In addition, it becomes an important problem for medical personnel. Hospital staff and all other human or veterinary health care workers, including laboratory, research, emergency service, or cleaning personnel are exposed to the risk of occupational infection following accidental exposure to blood or body fluids (BBF) contaminated with this virus [1].

Hepatitis B is a highly contagious viral infection and can lead to chronic carrier state and the hepatocellular carcinoma in the worst case. Around 450 million people worldwide are chronically infected with hepatitis B virus and are therefore at risk of developing chronic liver disease. To prevent is better than to treat this infection. Since 1985, the number of reported cases has declined as a direct result of universal immunization of neonates, vaccination of at-risk populations, lifestyle or behavioral changes in high-risk groups, refinements in the screening of blood donors, and the use of virally inactivated or genetically engineered products in patients with bleeding disorders [2]. At present, vaccination is an effective preventive measure for this disease. HBV vaccination has effectively reduced the acute and chronic infection rates as well as related complications in vaccinated children [3]. The incidence of hepatocellular carcinoma in children has been reduced to approximately 25% of the incidence before the vaccination program, and fulminant hepatitis in children has also been reduced after universal hepatitis B vaccination [3].

In this article, the topics on the hepatitis B vaccination will be presented. The new concepts on vaccination strategies will be discussed. Also, the new advances on hepatitis B vaccinology will be presented.

History of Hepatitis B Vaccine

Although the HBV was discovered about 40 years ago (1967) the hepatitis B vaccine is still new [4-6]. The development of the hepatitis B vaccine started in the late 1970's. At first, progressively sophisticated assays for hepatitis antigens and antibodies have been applied to the study of viral hepatitis epidemiology and biochemical-biophysical characterization of the agents [7]. On early phase, knowledge learned from such studies has been exploited to develop a prototype non-infectious but immunogenic hepatitis B vaccine using hepatitis B surface antigen (HBsAg) purified in large quantities from chronic HBsAg carriers [7]. Briefly, HBsAg was purified from human plasma by gel chromatography, isopyknic centrifugation, and zonal centrifugation [8]. Up to 65 % of the starting antigen was recovered at the end of the purification process. One dose of vaccine (1 ml) has a titre in HBsAg of 1/4 in countercurrent electrophoresis and a protein amount of 2-10 micron/ml [9]. In the early trial, treatment with formaldehyde concentrations up to 0.1% for inactivation of residual infectivity did not significantly reduce antigenicity in vitro and immunogenicity in guinea pigs [8]. The vaccine was also highly potent, inducing antibody in grivet monkeys and chimpanzees [10]. In human trials, the results, 2 years after immunization, suggested that the vaccine was protective against hepatitis B infection in high-risk hemodialysis settings [11]. Preliminary studies with an inactivated hepatitis B vaccine similarly prepared, but with aluminum hydroxide as adjuvant, indicate that such a preparation induces a more rapid and stronger anti-HBs response [11].

In the early 1980's, the first vaccine for hepatitis B was available in the USA [12]. However, there are many limitations for the human-derived hepatitis B vaccine.

The preparation of hepatitis B vaccine from a human source is restricted by the available supply of infected human plasma and by the need to apply stringent processes that purify the antigen and render it free of infectious HBV and other possible living agents that might be present in the plasma [13]. Therefore, the progression of the vaccine to recombinant vaccine started. Human hepatitis B vaccine from recombinant yeast is one of the first launched recombinant hepatitis B vaccines. Such vaccines would be free of the potential safety problems associated with plasma source material and could assure the continued supply of uniform HBsAg for vaccine use [14]. This vaccine was developed from recombinant yeast (*Saccharomyces cerevisiae*) cell culture [13]. With the present advances in biotechnology, recombinant DNA vaccines have been produced in prokaryotic and eukaryotic cells, notably in yeast [15]. The yeast-derived recombinant vaccine has proved safe and effective in extensive clinical trials, eliciting antibodies of equal quantity and quality of specificity to those elicited by plasma-derived vaccine [15].

Besides the attempts in the USA and Europe, there is also much hepatitis B vaccine research and many developments from other countries. For the endemic countries, investigation of HBV vaccine development in China was almost simultaneous with the same kind of work in the international community [16]. It seems that vaccination with the HBV vaccine in China has been successful and has obtained great achievements in the prevention and therapy of HB. Integration of the hepatitis B vaccine into newborn vaccination programmes on a worldwide basis represents a major step in the effort to eliminate this infectious disease and its complications [4]. Knowledge about the virus and the infection it causes led to the development of first, a plasma-derived vaccine and later a recombinant vaccine for the prevention of the infection [4]. However, there are still aspects of the hepatitis B vaccine which could be improved: three doses are needed for a full course of vaccination (which is sometimes difficult to achieve because of poor compliance or difficult logistic situations in some regions), there is a comparably high rate of non-responders to the vaccine (about 5% in adults) and, finally, it is possible that there are strains of HBV showing mutations of HBsAg which could escape the immunity induced by present vaccines [17]. To overcome these problems is the goal of the present hepatitis B vaccine development [17].

Types of Hepatitis B Vaccine

At present, hepatitis B vaccine is produced by a recombinant technique. There are many manufacturers that produce recombinant hepatitis B vaccine. RECOMBIVAX HB (Merck Sharpe & Dohme Ltd) is a good example of recombinant hepatitis B vaccine. It is produced based on *S. cerevisiae* and is indicated for vaccination against infection caused by all known subtypes of HBV [18]. Engerix-B (Smith Kline Biologicals) is another recombinant hepatitis B vaccine and has the same indication as RECOMBIVAX HB [19]. It is produced from genetically engineered yeast (*S. cerevisiae*) [19]. Intramuscular has excellent immunogenicity in healthy neonates and infants, children, adolescents and adults, with seroprotection rates of 85-100% seen approximately, 1 month after the final dose of vaccine [19]. There was a study by Hammond et al. conducted on the immunogenicity of these two yeast recombinant vaccines with different doses [RECOMBIVAX HB vs. Engerix-B] [20]. According to this report, the 95% confidence interval showed an overlap of the means of the GMT for both vaccine groups, and there was no significant difference in immunogenicity of these two vaccines [20]. Rustgi et al. performed another randomized trial to compare the safety and immunogenicity of Engerix-B administered intramuscularly (IM) at 0, 1, 2, and 12 months with RECOMBIVAX HB 10 micrograms administered IM at 0, 1, and 6 months in healthy adults [21]. According to this work, seroprotect rates were similar between the vaccination groups approximately 1 year after administration of the initial dose [21].

Recently, the oral hepatitis B vaccine was proposed. In 2006, oral hepatitis B vaccine formulation was prepared by successful encapsulation of an immunogenic peptide representing residues 127-145 of the immunodominant B-cell epitope of HBsAg in poly(D,L-lactide co-glycolide) (PLG) microparticles [22]. Single oral immunization of mice with BCEM led to the significant induction of specific serum IgG and IgM anti-HB antibodies [22]. After the termination of antibody induction, the orally immunized mice were infected with HBsAg, which resulted in the rapid production of antibodies against HBsAg as a result of secondary immune response [22].

Reported Side Effects of Hepatitis B Vaccination

Safety is a considerable factor for every vaccination. Side effects of vaccine must be closely monitored. Side effects of hepatitis B vaccine are also reported [23-24]. Immune response is believed to be the important factor leading to the side effect. The hypersensitivity type 3 is the possible main cause. Systemic lupus erythematosus (SLE) is an important adverse effect resulting from vaccination against hepatitis B [25-29]. During the past two decades, increasing numbers of reports regarding possible autoimmune side effects of vaccination have been published. However, the existing data does not link the vaccines and the autoimmune phenomena observed in a causal relationship, nevertheless a temporal connection has been described [30]. Hepatitis B vaccine might also be followed by other rheumatic conditions including rheumatoid arthritis and might trigger the onset of underlying inflammatory or autoimmune rheumatic diseases [31]. However, a causal relationship between hepatitis B vaccination and the observed rheumatic manifestations cannot be easily established [31].

Severe acute hepatitis B is another described side effect of hepatitis B vaccination [32-33]. The exact cause of this finding has not yet clarified. Neurological defects are also reported as adverse effects of hepatitis B vaccine. Many cases of multiple sclerosis following hepatitis B vaccination are reported [34-36]. The possibility that hepatitis B vaccine may cause or exacerbate multiple sclerosis stems from several case reports of onset or recurrence of symptoms of central nervous system demyelination shortly following vaccination [34-37]. The question is raised whether infectious agents or vaccines are involved in the pathogenesis or induced worsening of multiple sclerosis [38]. The possibility of activating autoantigen-specific T cells by pathogens or vaccines is raised [38]. According to a recent work, the multivariate relative risk of multiple sclerosis associated with exposure to the hepatitis B vaccine at any time before the onset of the disease was 0.9 and the relative risk associated with hepatitis B vaccination within two years before the onset of the disease was 0.7 [36]. In conclusion, there is only weak, nonspecific evidence to support the biological plausibility of an association between hepatitis B vaccine and multiple sclerosis [34-37]. In addition, epidemiological studies have found that hepatitis B vaccine does not increase the risk of developing multiple sclerosis or cause exacerbations [34-36]. Ascherio et al. conducted a nested case-control study in two large cohorts of nurses in the USA [36].

Expanded Programme for Immunization for Hepatitis B Vaccination

The first three priorities for hepatitis B immunization strategies in order of importance are: a) routine infant vaccination, b) prevention of perinatal HBV transmission and c) catch-up vaccination for older age groups. The infant vaccination is the focused plan for almost all countries. WHO documented that HBV infection is a vaccine preventable infection. Expanded Programme for Immunization (EPI) for hepatitis B vaccination was set. The implementation of the EPI has had a dramatic impact on HBV infection in many endemic countries. Since 1992, hepatitis B vaccine has been an integrated part of Thailand's EPI. According to a recent study of Poovorawan et al. for evaluation of the success of EPI in Thailand, the coverage rate of hepatitis B vaccination after its inclusion into the EPI 71.2-94.3% and only 0.7% of the children born after the implementation of this the novel EPI strategy were HBV carriers [39]. In Malaysia, the implementation of the EPI in 1989 has had a dramatic impact on hepatitis B virus (HBV) infection in school children [40]. The school children vaccinated under EPI had a 0.4% HBsAg carrier rate, which was significantly lower than school children vaccinated on a voluntary basis (HBsAg carrier rate 1.3%) and non-vaccinated school children (HBsAg carrier rate 2.7%), suggesting that HBV vaccination of infants was the most effective measure in preventing vertical transmission of HBV in the hyperendemic region [40]. In the Gambia, high vaccine coverage was achieved with EPI [41].

Table 1. Schedule for Hepatitis B Vaccination

Dose	Schedule
First	at birth
Second	2 months
Third	6 months

* For the general population: first injection - at any given time, second injection - at least 1 month after the first dose, third injection - 6 months after the first dose.

Prevention of Perinatal HBV Transmission

Vertical transmission of HBV is another important mode of infection. The infection by the hepatitis viruses, when appearing during pregnancy, could result in damage to the infant [42]. HBV infection, for which prevalence varies according to areas, is injurious when the mother is a chronic HBsAg carrier [42]. Risk consists of the neonate's contamination during labor, and if contaminated, the neonate becomes a chronic carrier in 80 to 90% of cases [42]. The high prevalence of HBsAg and hepatitis B e antigen (HBeAg) in pregnant women is considered to be the most important factor contributing to the high carrier rate of HBsAg in some populations [43]. The hepatitis B vaccination is a method for control of vertical transmission.

Van Steenbergen et al. said that tracing and immunizing susceptible contacts of women screened as HBsAg-positive, should be an integral component of any country's HBV control program [44]. Briefly, women at high risk for hepatitis B should be screened, including during pregnancy, by testing for hepatitis B core antibody [45]. Those at low risk should be screened by testing for HbsAg [45]. Susceptible high-risk women should be vaccinated; pregnancy is not a contraindication [45]. Administration of hepatitis B immune globulin and vaccine to newborns is effective in preventing transmission from a hepatitis B-infected mother [45].

HBV Vaccination for the Elderly

For the non - endemic countries, the elderly are a vulnerable group of HBV infection. However, the infection is usually mild. Since the response rate to hepatitis B vaccination decreases with age, developing vaccines with greater immunogenicity is crucial [46]. The role of prophylaxis vaccination in the elderly is limited. The therapeutic vaccination is more frequently used. Since most of hepatitis B infection in the elderly are in the form of chronic carrier. The hepatitis B vaccination decreases serum HBV-DNA levels in the majority of patients with chronic HBV infection and sustained clearance can be achieved in some patients [47]. Combination of interferon-alpha with hepatitis B vaccine is effective for the vaccine failures and may increase sustained response compared to interferon-alpha alone; however, the mechanism of action is yet to be explained [47].

HBV Vaccination in HIV infected Patients

Co-infection between HBV and HIV is common since these two viruses share the common mode of transmission. Pathologically, HIV magnifies HBV viremia and the risk of HBV reactivation, chronic active HBV infection, cirrhosis, and death [48]. Because of these concerns, hepatitis B vaccination is also recommended for all HIV-positive persons lacking prior immunity. However, immune reactivity to hepatitis B vaccines is frequently suboptimal in terms of patients' rate of response, antibody titer, and durability [48]. Relatively high CD4+ T-cell counts (> or =500/mm3) and low levels of HIV viremia (<1,000 RNA genome copies/mL plasma) are necessary to ensure adequate hepatitis B vaccine response [48]. Revaccination should be instituted if post vaccination titers of antibodies to HbsAg are <10 mIU/mL (<10 IU/L) [48].

Winnock et al. performed an interesting study to gain insight into the attitude towards HBV and its vaccination in HIV seropositive patients [49]. According to this work, the main reasons for not prescribing HBV vaccine more often were forgetting, difficulty to identify subjects at risk and being afraid of post-vaccinal complications [49]. Therefore, there is no doubt about the usefulness of hepatitis B vaccination in HIV-infected patients. For HIV-infected with additional immunosuppressive pathology, this recommendation can also be applied. Ahuja et al. found that hepatitis B vaccination should be offered to all HIV-infected end stage renal disease (ESRD) patients because over half of the patients with HIV and ESRD can develop protection. [50].

However, an important problem of hepatitis B vaccination in HIV patient is that the HIV patients are usually vaccine hyporesponsive. CPG 7909, a synthetic oligodeoxynucleotide containing immunostimulatory CpG motifs, is a new adjuvant to hepatitis B vaccine that is reported to enhance the effectiveness of vaccination in HIV-infected cases [51]. Addition of CPG 7909 achieves rapid, higher, and sustained HBV seroprotection and increases HBV-specific T helper cell response to HBV vaccine in HIV-infected subjects [51].

HBV Vaccination in the Patients Requiring Hemodialysis

Ever since the first outbreaks of hepatitis in hemodialysis units in the late 1960s, a number of hepatotropic viruses transmitted by blood and other body fluids have been identified [52]. HBV was the first significant hepatotropic virus to be identified in hemodialysis centers [52]. HBV infection has been effectively controlled by active vaccination, screening of blood donors, the use of erythropoietin, and segregation of HBV carriers [52]. Hepatitis B vaccination is recommended for the hemodialytic cases [53-54]. Miller et al. suggested that hepatitis B vaccine had a significant protective effect against acquiring HBV infection in chronic hemodialysis patients, and efforts should be expanded to increase the use of hepatitis B vaccine in this patient population [55]. They found that the risk for HBV infection was 70% lower in vaccinated patients [55]. However, the problems of vaccination are reported. The main problem is the low response, which is believed to relate to host-related and immunization-related causes [53]. Various possibilities to improve the vaccine performance through appropriate dosage and schedule, as well as immunopotentiating procedures are reported [53]. Oddone et al. performed an interesting study to assess the cost effectiveness of hepatitis B vaccine in predialysis patients in 1993 [56]. They found that additional HBV infection could be prevented by immunizing predialysis patients, but the cost is high [56]. They concluded that decisions concerning vaccination policy should be influenced by local prevalence of HBV infection [56].

HBV Vaccination for the Traveler

Long distance journeys are more and more frequent [57]. In certain instances, one shall consider vaccination against hepatitis B [57-59]. Routine childhood vaccinations may need to be accelerated for young infants traveling before the standard primary vaccine series can be completed [59]. Since last minute protection of hepatitis B vaccine can be expected, full dosage is required [60-61]. However, many travelers depart within weeks of planning their trip (too late to complete the accelerated 0, 1, 2 month regimen for hepatitis B), and a majority of those traveling depart without being vaccinated [62]. Although extended-stay travelers are at high risk for hepatitis B, short-stay travelers also are at risk [62]. Connor et al. found that most US travelers to hepatitis B endemic regions did not secure pre-travel health advice, and most had not received three doses of hepatitis B vaccine [60]. Substantial shares are candidates for hepatitis B vaccination based on their domestic activities, and/or face hepatitis B risks during travel [60]. A new accelerated, 3-dose regimen on a 0,7 and 21-day schedule suggest that excellent, rapid, and long-term protection might be conferred [62].

HBV Vaccination for Health Care Workers

Health care workers are a population at risk for HBV infection via blood and blood product contact [63]. The outcomes following infection can be significant in terms of both health and employment [64]. It is for these reasons that effective preventative health care is the goal of occupational health practitioners [64]. It therefore is critical for health care workers to encourage the development and assessment of effective preventive and control strategies, including the design and use of safe devices, targeted interventions based on occupation-specific hazards, and surveillance and analysis of exposures in the health care setting [65]. Hepatitis B vaccination is a good preventative for the health care worker. Mihaly et al. said that vaccination was an effective tool in hepatitis B prevention [66]. They noted that every effort had to be made to promote hepatitis B immunity to all health care workers and strictly follow hygienic preventive measures [66]. However, Jefferson et al. performed a metanalysis and found that plasma-derived vaccines appeared to be efficacious and safe for use in high-risk health-care workers, such as the staff of renal dialysis and transplant units [67]. They also found that there was some uncertainty concerning the effectiveness of the vaccine in lower risk health-care workers, although the trend is towards benefit [67]. Chen and Gluud performed another metanalysis to assess the beneficial and harmful effects of hepatitis B vaccination in health-care workers [68]. They found that the intramuscular route with 20 microgram recombinant vaccine was significantly more effective compared with the intradermal route with 2 microgram recombinant vaccine as was the standard schedule compared with a rapid schedule and deltoid intramuscular injection compared with the gluteal intramuscular injection [68]. However, they noted that it was unclear if booster vaccination of non-responders offers higher anti-HBs seroconversion and hepatitis B vaccine prevented the infection of hepatitis B mutants in health-care workers [68]. In addition to the general health care worker, health science students form a high-risk group for infection with blood-borne pathogens, including HBV [69]. Wiwanitkit found that more than 40% of the pre-clinical students did not know their HBV status and fewer than 50% had been vaccinated against the virus [69]. Wiwanitkit proposed that those students entering medical schools for the first time clearly need to be better educated about hepatitis B and to be encouraged to be vaccinated before they begin any clinical practices [69].

Although hepatitis B vaccination is accepted as being useful for health care workers, the cost effectiveness of universal vaccination is still doubtful [67,70]. Pre-selection is considered. Many strategies including interviewing and serological screening are proposed [71]. The decisions must be based on the epidemiological data and the cost effectiveness analysis for each setting.

VACCINE ESCAPE MUTANT: A NEW PROBLEM OF HEPATITIS B VACCINATION

Vaccine escape mutant is a new problem of hepatitis B vaccination. The HBV has evolved a unique life cycle resulting in the production of enormous viral loads during active replication without actually directly killing the infected cell [72]. Because the virus uses reverse transcription to copy its DNA genome, mutant viral genomes are frequently found [72]. Particular selection pressures, both endogenous (host immune clearance) and exogenous (vaccines and antivirals), readily select out these escape mutants [72]. Cooreman et al. proposed that most escape mutations that influence HBsAg recognition by anti-HBs antibodies were located in the second 'a' determinant loop [73]. Notably, HBsAg with an arginine replacement for glycine at amino acid 145 is considered the quintessential immune escape mutant because it has been isolated consistently in clinical samples of HBIg-treated individuals and vaccinated infants of chronically infected mothers [73]. Cooreman et al. proposed that vaccine- and hepatitis B immune globulin might induce escape mutations of HbsAg [73]. Finding of the new recombinant vaccine to overcome the problem of vaccine escape mutant becomes a new focus on hepatitis B vaccinology. In 1999, Ogata et al. first reported their successful licensed recombinant hepatitis B vaccines that could protect chimpanzees against infection with the prototype surface gene mutant of HBV [74]. Several trials on other new vaccines are presently ongoing.

REFERENCES

[1] Tarantola A, Abiteboul D, Rachline A. Infection risks following accidental exposure to blood or body fluids in health care workers: a review of pathogens transmitted in published cases. *Am J Infect Control.* 2006 Aug;34(6):367-75.

[2] Hollinger FB, Lau DT. Hepatitis B: the pathway to recovery through treatment. *Gastroenterol Clin North Am.* 2006 Jun;35(2):425-61, x.

[3] Chang MH. Impact of hepatitis B vaccination on hepatitis B disease and nucleic acid testing in high-prevalence populations. *J Clin Virol.* 2006 May;36 Suppl 1:S45-50

[4] Yap SF. Hepatitis B: review of development from the discovery of the "Australia Antigen" to end of the twentieth Century. *Malays J Pathol.* 2004 Jun;26(1):1-12.

[5] Percell RH. Hepatitis B: a scientific success story (almost). *Prog Clin Biol Res.* 1985;182:11-43.

[6] Blumberg BS. The discovery of the hepatitis B virus and the invention of the vaccine: a scientific memoir. *J Gastroenterol Hepatol.* 2002 Dec;17 Suppl:S502-

[7] Katkov WN. Hepatitis vaccines. *Med Clin North Am.* 1996 Sep;80(5):1189-200.

[8] Stamm B, Gerlich W, Thomssen R. Experiments for the development of a hepatitis B vaccine: immunogenicity of HBsAg in guinea pigs (author's transl)]. *Med Microbiol Immunol (Berl).* 1979 May 15;167(2):83-97.

[9] Barin F, Andre M, Goudeau A, Coursaget P, Maupas P. Large scale purification of hepatitis B surface antigen (HBsAg). *Ann Microbiol (Paris).* 1978 Jul;129B(1):87-100.

[10] Buynak EB, Roehm RR, Tytell AA, Bertland AU 2nd, Lampson GP, Hilleman MR. Development and chimpanzee testing of a vaccine against human hepatitis B. *Proc Soc Exp Biol Med.* 1976 Apr;151(4):694-700.
[11] Maupas P, Goudeau A, Coursaget P, Drucker J, Bagros P. Hepatitis B vaccine: efficacy in high-risk settings, a two-year study. *Intervirology.* 1978;10(3):196-208.
[12] Dienstag JL, Purcell RH. Recent advances in the identification of hepatitis viruses. *Postgrad Med J.* 1977 Jul;53(621):364-73.
[13] McAleer WJ, Buynak EB, Maigetter RZ, Wampler DE, Miller WJ, Hilleman MR. Human hepatitis B vaccine from recombinant yeast. *Nature.* 1984 Jan 12-18;307(5947):178-80.
[14] Gerin JL, Purcell RH. New approaches to hepatitis B vaccines. *Prog Clin Biol Res.* 1983;143:369-77.
[15] Zuckerman AJ. Novel hepatitis B vaccines. *J Infect.* 1986 Jul;13 Suppl A:61-71.
[16] Tao Q, Feng B. Prevention and therapy of hepatitis B. *Chin Med J (Engl).* 1999 Oct;112(10):942-6.
[17] Jilg W. Novel hepatitis B vaccines. *Vaccine.* 1998 Nov;16 Suppl:S65-8.
[18] Venters C, Graham W, Cassidy W. Recombivax-HB: perspectives past, present and future. *Expert Rev Vaccines.* 2004 Apr;3(2):119-29.
[19] Keating GM, Noble S. Recombinant hepatitis B vaccine (Engerix-B): a review of its immunogenicity and protective efficacy against hepatitis B. *Drugs.* 2003;63(10):1021-51.
[20] Hammond GW, Parker J, Mimms L, Tate R, Sekla L, Minuk G. Comparison of immunogenicity of two yeast-derived recombinant hepatitis B vaccines. *Vaccine.* 1991 Feb;9(2):97-100.
[21] Rustgi VK, Schleupner CJ, Krause DS. Comparative study of the immunogenicity and safety of Engerix-B administered at 0, 1, 2 and 12 months and Recombivax HB administered at 0, 1, and 6 months in healthy adults. *Vaccine.* 1995 Dec;13(17):1665-8.
[22] Rajkannan R, Dhanaraju MD, Gopinath D, Selvaraj D, Jayakumar R. Development of hepatitis B oral vaccine using B-cell epitope loaded PLG microparticles. *Vaccine.* 2006 Jun 12;24(24):5149-57.
[23] Carmeli Y, Oren R. Hepatitis B vaccine side-effect. *Lancet.* 1993 Jan 23;341(8839):250-1.
[24] Fields HA, Mahoney FJ, Margolis HS. Safety of hepatitis B vaccine. *Science.* 1996 May 3;272(5262):633-4.
[25] Tudela P, Marti S, Bonal J. Systemic lupus erythematosus and vaccination against hepatitis B. *Nephron.* 1992;62(2):236.
[26] Guiserix J. Systemic lupus erythematosus following hepatitis B vaccine. *Nephron.* 1996;74(2):441.
[27] Maillefert JF, Tavernier C, Sibilia J, Vignon E. Exacerbation of systemic lupus erythematosus after hepatitis B vaccination: comment on the article by Battafarano et al and the letter by Senecal et al. *Arthritis Rheum.* 2000 Feb;43(2):468-9.
[28] Senecal JL, Bertrand C, Coutlee F. Severe exacerbation of systemic lupus erythematosus after hepatitis B vaccination and importance of pneumococcal

vaccination in patients with autosplenectomy: comment on the article by Battafarano et al. *Arthritis Rheum*. 1999 Jun;42(6):1307-8.

[29] Fineschi S. Can recombinant anti-hepatitis B vaccine be a cause of systemic lupus erythematosus? *Lupus*. 2001;10(11):830.

[30] Aron-Maor A, Shoenfeld Y. Vaccination and systemic lupus erythematosus: the bidirectional dilemmas. *Lupus*. 2001;10(3):237-40.

[31] Maillefert JF, Sibilia J, Toussirot E, Vignon E, Eschard JP, Lorcerie B, Juvin R, Parchin-Geneste N, Piroth C, Wendling D, Kuntz JL, Tavernier C, Gaudin P. Rheumatic disorders developed after hepatitis B vaccination. *Rheumatology (Oxford)*. 1999 Oct;38(10):978-83.

[32] Ballinger AB, Clark ML. Severe acute hepatitis B infection after vaccination. *Lancet*. 1994 Nov 5;344(8932):1292.

[33] Lilic D, Ghosh SK. Liver dysfunction and DNA antibodies after hepatitis B vaccination. *Lancet*. 1994 Nov 5;344(8932):1292-3

[34] Salleras L, Bruguera M, Prat A. Hepatitis B vaccine and multiple sclerosis: an unproved association. *Med Clin (Barc)*. 2006 Apr 22;126(15):581-8.

[35] DeStefano F, Verstraeten T, Chen RT. Hepatitis B vaccine and risk of multiple sclerosis. *Expert Rev Vaccines*. 2002 Dec;1(4):461-6.

[36] Ascherio A, Zhang SM, Hernan MA, Olek MJ, Coplan PM, Brodovicz K, Walker AM. Hepatitis B vaccination and the risk of multiple sclerosis. *N Engl J Med*. 2001 Feb 1;344(5):327-32.

[37] Demicheli V, Rivetti A, Di Pietrantonj C, Clements CJ, Jefferson T. Hepatitis B vaccination and multiple sclerosis: evidence from a systematic review. *J Viral Hepat*. 2003 Sep;10(5):343-4.

[38] Zipp F, Wandinger KP. Current concepts on vaccinations in multiple sclerosis. *Nervenarzt*. 2001 Oct;72(10):802-6.

[39] Poovorawan Y, Theamboonlers A, Vimolket T, Sinlaparatsamee S, Chaiear K, Siraprapasiri T, Khwanjaipanich S, Owatanapanich S, Hirsch P, Chunsuttiwat S. Impact of hepatitis B immunisation as part of the EPI. *Vaccine*. 2000 Nov 22;19(7-8):943-9.

[40] Ng KP, Saw TL, Baki A, Rozainah K, Pang KW, Ramanathan M. Impact of the Expanded Program of Immunization against hepatitis B infection in school children in Malaysia. *Med Microbiol Immunol (Berl)*. 2005 May;194(3):163-8.

[41] Viviani S, Mendy M, Jack AD, Hall AJ, Montesano R, Whittle HC. EPI vaccines-induced antibody prevalence in 8-9 year-olds in The Gambia. *Trop Med Int Health*. 2004 Oct;9(10):1044-9.

[42] Ranger-Rogez S, Alain S, Denis F. Hepatitis viruses: mother to child transmission. *Pathol Biol (Paris)*. 2002 Nov;50(9):568-75.

[43] Vranckx R, Alisjahbana A, Meheus A. Hepatitis B virus vaccination and antenatal transmission of HBV markers to neonates. *J Viral Hepat*. 1999 Mar;6(2):135-9.

[44] van Steenbergen JE, Baayen D, Peerbooms PG, Coutinho RA, Van Den Hoek A. Much gained by integrating contact tracing and vaccination in the hepatitis B antenatal screening program in Amsterdam, 1992-1999. *J Hepatol*. 2004 Jun;40(6):979-85.

[45] Culpepper L. Preventing hepatitis B: focus on women and their families. *J Am Board Fam Pract.* 1993 Sep-Oct;6(5):483-91.
[46] Marcus EL, Tur-Kaspa R. Viral hepatitis in older adults. *J Am Geriatr Soc.* 1997 Jun;45(6):755-63.
[47] Senturk H, Tabak F, Akdogan M, Erdem L, Mert A, Ozaras R, Sander E, Ozbay G, Badur S. Therapeutic vaccination in chronic hepatitis B. *J Gastroenterol Hepatol.* 2002 Jan;17(1):72-6.
[48] Laurence JC. Hepatitis A and B immunizations of individuals infected with human immunodeficiency virus. *Am J Med.* 2005 Oct;118 Suppl 10A:75S-83S.
[49] Winnock M, Neau D, Castera L, Viot J, Lacoste D, Pellegrin JL, Dupon M, Jutand MA, Colombani F, Dabis F; Groupe d'Epidemiologie Clinique du SIDA en Aquitaine. Hepatitis B vaccination in HIV-infected patients: a survey of physicians and patients participating in the Aquitaine cohort. *Gastroenterol Clin Biol.* 2006 Feb;30(2):189-95.
[50] Ahuja TS, Kumar S, Mansoury H, Rodriguez H, Kuo YF. Hepatitis B vaccination in human immunodeficiency virus-infected adults receiving hemodialysis. *Kidney Int.* 2005 Mar;67(3):1136-41.
[51] Cooper CL, Davis HL, Angel JB, Morris ML, Elfer SM, Seguin I, Krieg AM, Cameron DW. CPG 7909 adjuvant improves hepatitis B virus vaccine seroprotection in antiretroviral-treated HIV-infected adults. *AIDS.* 2005 Sep 23;19(14):1473-9.
[52] Tang S, Lai KN. Chronic viral hepatitis in hemodialysis patients. *Hemodial Int.* 2005 Apr;9(2):169-79.
[53] Rapicetta M. Hepatitis B vaccination in dialysis centres: advantages and limits. *Nephron.* 1992;61(3):284-6.
[54] Davis JP. Experience with hepatitis A and B vaccines. *Am J Med.* 2005 Oct;118 Suppl 10A:7S-15S.
[55] Miller ER, Alter MJ, Tokars JI. Protective effect of hepatitis B vaccine in chronic hemodialysis patients. *Am J Kidney Dis.* 1999 Feb;33(2):356-60.
[56] Oddone EZ, Cowper PA, Hamilton JD, Feussner JR. A cost-effectiveness analysis of hepatitis B vaccine in predialysis patients. *Health Serv Res.* 1993 Apr;28(1):97-121.
[57] Van Laethem Y. Vaccinations for the traveler. J Pharm Belg. 2002 Nov-Dec;57(6):130-4.
[58] Marchou B, Picot N, Massip P. Vaccinations of the traveller. *Ann Med Interne (Paris).* 1998 Oct;149(6):332-9.
[59] Mackell SM. Vaccinations for the pediatric traveler. *Clin Infect Dis.* 2003 Dec 1;37(11):1508-16.
[60] Connor BA, Jacobs RJ, Meyerhoff AS. Hepatitis B risks and immunization coverage among American travelers. *J Travel Med.* 2006 Sep-Oct;13(5):273-80.
[61] Birkenfeld G. Last minute vaccinations. MMW Fortschr Med. 2006 Jun 29;148(26):24-6.
[62] Keystone JS. Travel-related hepatitis B: risk factors and prevention using an accelerated vaccination schedule. *Am J Med.* 2005 Oct;118 Suppl 10A:63S-68S.
[63] Occupational transmission of hepatitis B. *Plast Surg Nurs.* 2003 Winter;23(4):160-3.
[64] Murphy E. Hepatitis B, vaccination and healthcare workers. *Occup Med (Lond).* 2000 Aug;50(6):383-6.

[65] Lanphear BP. Transmission and control of bloodborne viral hepatitis in health care workers. *Occup Med.* 1997 Oct-Dec;12(4):717-30.

[66] Mihaly I, Nagy E, Ibranyi E, Majoros I, Lukacs A. Effect of vaccination on the risk of hepatitis B infection in hospital personnel. *Orv Hetil.* 1996 Mar 31;137(13):681-5.

[67] Jefferson T, Demicheli V, Deeks J, MacMillan A, Sassi F, Pratt M. Vaccines for preventing hepatitis B in health-care workers. *Cochrane Database Syst Rev.* 2000;(2):CD000100.

[68] Chen W, Gluud C. Vaccines for preventing hepatitis B in health-care workers. *Cochrane Database Syst Rev.* 2005 Oct 19;(4):CD000100.

[69] Wiwanitkit V. How medical students in their pre-clinical year perceive their own hepatitis-B-virus status: the results of a study in a Thai medical school. *Ann Trop Med Parasitol.* 2002 Sep;96(6):627-30.

[70] Lohiya G, Lohiya S, Caires S, Reesal MR. Occupational exposure to hepatitis B virus. Analysis of indications for hepatitis B vaccine. *J Occup Med.* 1984 Mar;26(3):189-96.

[71] Perrillo RP. Screening of health care workers before hepatitis B vaccination: more questions than answers. *Ann Intern Med.* 1985 Nov;103(5):793-5.

[72] Locarnini S, McMillan J, Bartholomeusz A. The hepatitis B virus and common mutants. *Semin Liver Dis.* 2003 Feb;23(1):5-20.

[73] Cooreman MP, Leroux-Roels G, Paulij WP. Vaccine- and hepatitis B immune globulin-induced escape mutations of hepatitis B virus surface antigen. *J Biomed Sci.* 2001 May-Jun;8(3):237-47.

[74] Ogata N, Cote PJ, Zanetti AR, Miller RH, Shapiro M, Gerin J, Purcell RH. Licensed recombinant hepatitis B vaccines protect chimpanzees against infection with the prototype surface gene mutant of hepatitis B virus. *Hepatology.* 1999 Sep;30(3):779-86.

In: Hepatitis B Research Advances
Editor: Alicia P. Willis, pp. 35-57
ISBN: 978-1-60021-666-4

Chapter IV

A Comparative Evaluation of Latex Agglutination, Immunochromatographic Strip and ELISA Techniques in the Seroepdemiological Survey of Hepatitis-B Surface Antigen Among Blood Donors in Southeastern Nigeria

***O. Ogbu*[1] *and C. J. Uneke*[2]**

[1]Department of Applied Microbiology, Faculty of Applied and Natural Sciences, Ebonyi State University, PMB 053 Abakaliki, Nigeria
[2]Department of Medical Microbiology, Faculty of Clinical Medicine, Ebonyi State University, PMB 053 Abakaliki, Nigeria

Abstract

Hepatitis B virus (HBV) infection is endemic in many parts of sub-Saharan Africa including Nigeria. Surveillance of HBV infection markers in blood donor population is important in recognizing trends in prevalence and incidence of transfusion related infections and also provides opportunity to estimate the risk of infectious donations inadvertently entering the blood supply. In this study, a comparative evaluation of latex agglutination (LA), immunochromatographic strip (ICS), and ELISA techniques was performed in the seroepdemiological survey of hepatitis-B surface antigen (HBsAg) among blood donors in south-eastern Nigeria. A total of 1570 donors (1406 males and 164 females, aged 18-41 years old) were enrolled in the study. Serum separated from 5ml of venous blood obtained from each subject was screened using the three techniques. The prevalence rates of HBsAg were 8.0% (95% CI., 6.7-9.3%) by ELISA; 10.4%(95% CI., 8.9-11.9) by LA; and 10.3% (95% CI., 8.8-11.8%) by ICS techniques. A total of 117(8.3%, 95% CI., 6.9-9.7%) of the males and 9(5.5%,95% CI., 2.0-9.0%) of the females had HBsAg as detected by ELISA and the difference was significant (χ^2=16.02, df=1, $P<0.05$). The LA technique indicated that 147(10.5%, 95% CI., 8.9-12.1%) males and 16(9.8%, 95% CI., 5.2-14.4%) females had HBsAg, the difference was also significant ($\chi^2=7.70$, df=1,$P<0.05$). By the ICS technique, 145(10.3%, 95% CI., 5.3-15.3%) males and 17(10.4%, 95% CI., 5.7-15.1%) females were positive for HBsAg, but the difference was not statistically significant ($\chi^2=0.0004$, df=1, $P<0.05$). The highest and lowest prevalence rates of HBsAg were observed among individuals of age groups 25-29 years and >35 years respectively and the differences were statistically significant. The respective prevalence figures were 11.5%(95% CI., 8.9-14.1%) vs 2.4%(95% CI., 0.8-4.0%) ($\chi^2=26.18$, df=3, $P<0.05$) by ELISA; 12.5%(95% CI.,9.8-15.2%) vs 6.3%(3.7-8.9%) ($\chi^2=9.67$, df=3, $P<0.05$) by LA; and 13.6(95% CI., 10.8-16.4%) vs 4.5%(95% CI., 2.3-6.7%) ($\chi^2=22.9$, df=3, $P<0.05$) by ICS. Commercial motorcyclists and those who engage in business had higher prevalence of HBsAg than the farmers and students, but differences were not statistically significant by any of the diagnostic techniques. Results showed that ELISA technique appeared to be a more useful diagnostic tool that LA and ICS techniques in the detection of HBsAg among blood donors. The 126 positive samples detected by ELISA were observed to be either positive with LA, ICS or both, showing no variation as was observed with LA and ICS results. Protection of the blood supply from virus-infected donations through effective donor selection and testing with highly sensitive technique is recommended.

INTRODUCTION

Hepatitis B virus (HBV) is the most common cause of serious liver infection in the world. It is estimated that worldwide more than two billion people have been infected by HBV and 350 million people have chronic infection [1]. The virus causes transient and chronic infections of the liver. Transient infections may produce serious illness, and approximately 0.5% terminate with fatal, fulminant hepatitis while chronic infections may also have serious consequences: nearly 25% terminate in untreatable liver cancer [2]. Worldwide deaths from liver cancer caused by HBV infection probably exceed one million per year [3,4]. The clinical presentation Hepatitis B ranges from subclinical hepatitis to symptomatic hepatitis and, in rare instances, fulminant hepatitis [5]. Long-term complications of hepatitis B include cirrhosis and hepatocellular carcinoma [6]. Hepatitis B infection has thus assumed an important public health problem due to its chronic serious sequelae. It has been estimated that at the most, 33% of the infected subjects have evidence of clinical hepatitis [7], and depending on the age of infection, up to one third of infected patients become chronic carriers of hepatitis B surface antigen (HBs Ag) [7]. Chronic carriers have a higher incidence of and mortality due to hepatocellular carcinoma and cirrhosis [8]. Perinatal or childhood infection is associated with few or no symptoms, but it has a high risk of becoming chronic [5].

HBV is a Hepadna virus. It is an extremely resistant strain capable of withstanding extreme temperatures and humidity. It can survive when stored for 15 years at -20°C, for 24 months at -80°C, for 6 months at room temperatures, and for 7 days at 44°C [3]. The discovery in 1965 of Australia antigen, now referred to as hepatitis B surface antigen (HBsAg), and its subsequent association with hepatitis B virus led to the development of sensitive, specific markers of HBV infection [9-12]. During acute and chronic HBV infection, HBsAg is produced in excess amounts, circulating in blood as both 22-nm spherical and tubular particles. HBsAg can be identified in serum 30-60 days after exposure to HBV and persists for variable periods depending on the resolution of the infection. Antibody to HBsAg (anti-HBs) develops after a resolved infection and is responsible for long-term immunity [13]. Anti-HBc develops in both resolved acute infections and chronic HBV infections and persists indefinitely [14]. Immunoglobulin M (IgM) anti-HBc appears early in infection and persists for greater than or equal to 6 months and it is a reliable marker of acute HBV infection [15].

The HBV is highly contagious and relatively easy to transmit from one infected individual to another. According to report by the Centre for Disease Control and Prevention (CDC) [16], transmission of HBV occurs via percutaneous or permucosal routes, and infective blood or body fluids can be introduced at birth, through sexual contact or by contaminated needles. Infection can also occur in settings of continuous close personal contact (such as in households or among persons in institutions for the developmentally disabled), presumably via inapparent or unnoticed contact of infective secretions with skin lesions or mucosal surfaces. Furthermore the report indicated that persons at increased risk of acquiring HBV infection include members of the following groups: a) parenteral drug users, b) heterosexual men and women and homosexual men with multiple partners, c) household contacts and sexual partners of HBV carriers, d) infants born to HBV-infected mothers, e) patients and staff in custodial institutions for the developmentally disabled, f) recipients of certain plasma-derived products (including patients with congenital coagulation defects), g) hemodialysis patients, h) health and public-safety workers who have contact with blood, and i) persons born in areas of high HBV endemicity and their children [16].

The HBV carrier rate variation is 1-20% worldwide and this variation is related to differences in the mode of transmission and age at infection [17]. The prevalence of the disease in different geographical areas has been characterized as low, intermediate and high prevalence areas. The low-prevalence areas (rate of 0.1-2%) include Canada, western Europe, Australia, and New Zealand and in these areas of low prevalence, sexual and percutaneous transmission during adulthood are the main modes of transmission. The intermediate-prevalence areas (rate of 3-5%) include eastern and northern Europe, Japan, the Mediterranean basin, the Middle East, Latin and South America, and central Asia and in these areas of intermediate prevalence, sexual and percutaneous transmission and transmission during delivery are the major routes. The High-prevalence areas (rate of 10-20%) include China, Indonesia, sub-Saharan Africa, the Pacific islands, and Southeast Asia and here, the predominant mode of transmission is perinatal, and the disease is transmitted during early childhood vertically from the mother to the infant [17].

The safety of blood products is one of the major issues in the area of transfusion medicine. Transmission of hepatitis B virus (HBV) infection through donated blood is reportedly very common particularly in the developing world including the sub-Saharan Africa. The prevalence of hepatitis B virus chronic carriage in sub-Saharan Africa ranges between 3% and 22% in blood donors [18-20]. Typically, more than 50% of blood donors and blood recipients have had natural exposure to HBV, and the need for hepatitis B surface antigen screening of blood donations has often been considered of secondary importance because many donors are not infectious and many recipients are not susceptible [19]. At present, the World Health Organization (WHO) estimates that no more than 50% of the blood supply in sub-Saharan Africa is screened for HBsAg and this low rate of screening is due to lack of perceived utility, lack of funds, or both [21]. Furthermore, no systematic study of donor and recipient populations has been undertaken that could provide the basic data to estimate the transfusion-related risk of HBV infection in high-prevalence areas of Africa.

In spite of availability of sensitive screening assay for detection of hepatitis B virus surface antigen (HBsAg), occasional cases of post-transfusion hepatitis B virus infection (PTH) are common [22] . Possible explanations for false negative results in commercial assays have been postulated [23]. Blood donors infected with HBsAg mutants and those circulating low level of viral protein may escape detection by screening assay and therefore, may affect the safety of blood supply [24]. Another explanation is that virus variants yield sequences that are not recognized by the antibodies employed in the assays [25]. There are variants in other parts of the genome that down regulate the production of HBsAg [26]. Occasionally, a superinfection with hepatitis C virus (HCV) may induce clearance of hepatitis B. This could be due to the dominant role of HCV in eliciting an immune response [27]. Antibodies to hepatitis B core (HBc) antigen are marker of acute, chronic, or resolved HBV infection and remain detectable for life. These can be present in the absence of both HBsAg and anti-HBs antibodies, during the convalescent period following acute hepatitis B before the appearance of anti-HBs antibodies, or in patients who resolved infection but lost detectable anti-HBs antibodies. Anti-HBc is therefore detected in anyone who has been infected with HBV [28]. It has been demonstrated that some HBsAg negative individuals and those positives for anti-HBc continue to replicate HBV [29,30]. These findings suggest that recovery from acute hepatitis B virus infection may not result in complete virus elimination, but rather the immune system keeps the virus at a very low level. A positive correlation has been shown between anti-HBc titre and detection of HBV-DNA in serum samples of HBsAg negative individual [31].

It is pertinent to state that the increase in awareness of the potential risk of transfusion-transmitted HBV infection has led to the policy of screening all blood donations for HBV surface antigen (HBsAg) since in many urban settings including the sub-Saharan Africa. It was generally accepted that the disappearance of HBsAg indicates the clearance of HBV. Meanwhile, reports abound on positive findings for HBV DNA in the liver and blood of HBsAg-negative individuals positive for antibodies against HBV core antigen (anti-HBc) and/or HBsAg (anti-HBs) [32-39]. The reactivation of apparently cured HBV infection has been described under chemotherapy or immunomodulating therapy after renal and bone marrow transplantation, and in some of these cases a reverse seroconversion from anti-HBs to HBsAg has been observed [40-43]. Thus the residual risk of posttransfusion HBV infection is well established [44,45], and It has been shown that blood donations of HBsAg- and anti-HBs–negative but anti-HBc–positive HBV carriers can cause posttransfusion hepati-tis B [46,47]. Furthermore, it has been suggested that anti-HBc screening of blood donations might prevent HBV transmission from HBsAg-negative blood donors and that donors positive for anti-HBs as well should be considered noninfectious for HBV [48].

Nigeria is classified among the group of countries highly endemic for HBV infection. About 75% of the Nigerian population is reportedly likely to have been ex-posed to HBV at one time or the other in their life [49]. There is a high level of occurrence of blood demanding health conditions in many parts of sub-Saharan Africa. In Nigeria the increase in road accidents, pregnancy-related hemorrhage, armed robbery attacks, and violent events, increase the possibility of the transmission of HBV (and other blood-borne pathogens) through contaminated blood as reported by United Nations System in Nigeria [50]. Information is very scarce on the prevalence of HBsAg among healthy blood donors in Nigeria. As a result of this dearth of information, guidelines, and other adequate information on the preventive and control measures are essentially lacking in many settings in Nigeria. Our objective therefore was to determine the prevalence of HBsAg infection among voluntary blood donors by comparing three different HBsAg serological assays. The implication of findings with respect to increase in the risk of transfusion-transmitted HBV infection in the south-eastern Nigeria are discussed in this chapter. This is with the view to establishing effective guidelines on the prevention and control of HBV infection in Nigeria and other parts of the world with similar setting.

Materials and Methods

Study Area

This investigation was conducted in Ebonyi State, south-eastern Nigeria. The six largest hospitals in the various parts of the State were used for the study. The hospitals included the Federal Medical Centre (FMC), Abakaliki, Ebonyi State University Teaching Hospital (EBSUTH), Abakaliki, St. Vincent Hospital (SVH) Ndubia, Mile Four Hospital (MFH), Abakaliki, Mater Misericoidae Hospital (MMH), Afikpo, and Presbyterian Joint Hospital (PJH), Uburu. The study was conducted from February 2004 to January 2005. The vegetation characteristic is that of the tropical rain forest with an average annual rainfall of about 1,600mm and an average atmospheric temperature of 30°C. There are two distinct seasons, the wet and the dry seasons, the former takes place between April and October, while the latter occurs from November to March.

Ethical Considerations

The study protocol was approved by the Department of Applied Microbiology, Ebonyi State University, Abakaliki and from the Ethical/Medical Advisory Committees of all the six hospitals used for the study. The approval was on the agreement that patient anonymity must be maintained, good laboratory practice/quality control ensured, and that every finding would be treated with utmost confidentiality and for the purpose of this research only. All work was performed according to the international guidelines for human experimentation in clinical research [51,52].

Study Population/Sampling Technique

A total of 1570 apparently healthy individuals who visited the six major hospitals in the state within the study period for blood donation were considered for the study. The number of individuals included 338 at FMC, Abakaliki; 386 at EBSUTH, Abakaliki; 245 at SVH, Ndubia; 180 at MFH, Abakaliki; 225 at MMH, Afikpo; and 196 at PJH, Uburu. Subjects were made up of a total of 1406 males and 164 females, aged 18-41 years old. Before inclusion into the study population, each donor's HIV-serostatus was determined. This was the number one pre-requisite for blood donation at the hospitals. Hence the 1570 individuals enrolled were HIV-negative. The donors included commercial blood donors who offer a unit of blood for a fee paid by the contracted hospital vendor, replacement blood donors who were family members or relations of recipients of blood, and volunteer blood donors who were well-meaning members of the society who offered themselves for free, non-remunerated, non-directed blood donation. All donors were verbally notified prior to sample collection and their informed consent was duly obtained. About 5mls of blood sample was obtained by venepuncture from each patient, serum separated and stored at $-20^{o}C$ until assayed for HBsAg. For the purpose of the research, no personal identifiers (names, ID number, address, etc) were used on the blood sample of the participants. Instead bar-coded numbers were used to ensure anonymity of the donors, to facilitate laboratory procedures and minimise the chances of errors during the handling of the blood specimens. The sex of each patient was recorded while age and occupation were obtained by interview.

Laboratory Analysis

The HBsAg screening was performed using three distinct types of serological assays. These were the Latex agglutination (LA) kit (Cal-Tech Diagnostics, West San Bernardino Road, Covina, CA 91722, USA), the Rapid immunochromatographic strip (ICS) test (Diaspot Rapid Diagnostics Pondok Kelapa 13450, Jakarta Indonesia), and the HBsAg Enzyme-linked immunosorbent assay (ELISA) (DIALAB HBsAg Diagnostics, Panikengasse 3-5, A-1163 Vienna, Austria). All the tests were performed according to the diagnostic kit manufacturers' instructions to determine the HBsAg seropostivity or otherwise of each serum sample.

Statistical Analysis

Differences in proportion were evaluated using the chi-square test. Statistical significant was achieved if $P < 0.05$.

RESULTS

Of the total of 1570 donors (1406 males and 164 females, aged 18-41 years old) enrolled in the study, the prevalence rates of HBsAg were 8.0% (95% CI., 6.7-9.3%) by ELISA;

10.4%(95% CI., 8.9-11.9) by LA; and 10.3% (95% CI., 8.8-11.8%) by ICS techniques (Table 1). A total of 117(8.3%, 95% CI., 6.9-9.7%) of the males and 9(5.5%,95% CI., 2.0-9.0%) of the females had HBsAg as detected by ELISA and the difference was significant (χ^2=16.02, df=1,P<0.05). The LA technique indicated that 147(10.5%, 95% CI.,8.9-12.1%) males and 16(9.8%, 95% CI., 5.2-14.4%) females had HBsAg, the difference was also significant (χ^2=7.70, df=1,P<0.05). By the ICS technique, 145(10.3%, 95% CI., 5.3-15.3%) males and 17(10.4%, 95% CI., 5.7-15.1%) females were positive for HBsAg, but the difference was not statistically significant (χ^2=0.0004, df=1,P<0.05) (Table 1).

Table 1. Summary of the prevalence of HBsAg among blood donors using ELISA, latex agglutination (LA) and Immunocromatographic strip (ICS) techniques in Ebonyi State, Southeastern Nigeria

Parameter	No. Examined	ELISA No. (%) Positive	95% CI	LA No. (%) Positive	95% CI	ICS No. (%) Positive	95% CI
Sex							
Male	1406	117(8.3)	6.9-9.7	147(10.5)	8.9-12.1	145(10.3)	5.3-15.3
Female	164	9(5.5)	2.0-9.0	16(9.8)	5.2-14.4	17(10.4)	5.7-15.1
Total	1570	126(8.0)	6.7 -9.3	163(10.4)	8.9-11.9	162(10.3)	8.8-11.8
Age(yrs)							
<24	294	18(6.1)	3.4-8.8	28(9.5)	6.1-12.9	23(7.8)	4.7 -10.9
25-29	582	67(11.5)	8.9-14.1	73(12.5)	9.8-15.2	79(13.6)	10.8-16.4
30-35	359	33(9.2)	6.2-12.2	41(11.4)	8.1-14.7	45(12.5)	9.1-15.9
>35	335	8(2.4)	0.8-4.0	21(6.3)	3.7-8.9	15(4.5)	2.3-6.7
Total	1570	126(8.0)	6.7-9.3	163(10.4)	8.9-11.9	162(10.3)	8.8-11.8
Occupation							
Farmers	209	12(5.7)	2.6-8.8	15(7.2)	3.7-10.7	14(6.7)	3.3-10.1
Business	345	28(8.1)	5.2-11.0	33(9.6)	6.5-12.7	38(11.8)	8.4-15.2
Motocyclists	570	55(9.6)	7.2-12.0	69(12.1)	9.4-14.8	67(11.8)	9.2-14.4
Students	446	31(7.0)	4.6-9.4 4	6(10.3)	7.5-13.1	43(9.6)	6.9-12.3
Total	1570	126(8.0)	6.7-9.3	163(10.4)	8.9-11.9	162(10.3)	8.8-11.8
Hospital							
FMC	338	31(9.2)	6.1-12.3	37(10.9)	7.6-14.2	39(11.5)	8.1-14.9
EBSUTH	386	33(8.5)	5.7-11.3	44(11.4)	8.2-14.6	41(10.6)	7.5-13.7
SVH	245	18(7.3)	6.4-10.6	23(9.4)	5.7-13.1	19(7.8)	4.4-11.2
MFH	180	9(5.0)	1.8-8.2	14(7.7)	3.8-11.6	13(7.2)	3.4-11.0
MMH	225	24(10.7)	6.6-14.7	30(13.3)	8.9-17.7	33(14.7)	10.1-19.3
PJH	196	11(5.6)	2.4- 8.8	15(7.7)	4.0-11.4	13(7.2)	3.6-10.8
Total	1570	126(8.0)	6.7-9.3	163(10.4)	8.9-11.9	162(10.3)	8.8-11.8

The highest and lowest prevalence rates of HBsAg were observed among individuals of age groups 25-29 years and >35 years respectively and the differences were statistically significant. The respective prevalence figures were 11.5%(95% CI., 8.9-14.1%) vs 2.4%(95% CI., 0.8-4.0%) (χ^2=26.18, df=3, P<0.05) by ELISA; 12.5%(95% CI.,9.8-15.2%) vs 6.3%(3.7-8.9%) (χ^2=9.67, df=3, P<0.05) by LA; and 13.6(95% CI., 10.8-16.4%) vs

4.5%(95% CI., 2.3-6.7%) (χ^2=22.9, df=3, P<0.05) by ICS (Table 1). Commercial motorists and those who engage in trading/business had higher prevalence of HBsAg than the farmers and students, but differences were not statistically significant by any of the diagnostic techniques. Highest prevalence rates of HBsAg were recorded at MMH, Afikpo; FMC, Abakaliki; and EBSUTH, Abakaliki; while the least prevalence rate was recorded at the MFH, Abakaliki (Table 1). Results showed that ELISA technique appeared to be a more useful diagnostic tool that LA and ICS techniques in the detection of HBsAg among blood donors. The 126 positive samples detected by ELISA were observed to be either positive with LA, ICS or both, showing no variation as was observed with LA and ICS results.

Discussion

The discovery that HBV and other viral infections could be transmitted by blood transfusion has long heightened public concern about blood safety. Transfusion-transmitted hepatitis B virus (TT-HBV) infections, when analysed in detail provide information about the nature and relative frequency of the sources of infectious donations. These cases are therefore used to inform blood safety strategies.

Accurate estimates of the risks of transfusion-transmitted viral infections are needed in order to monitor the safety of the blood supply and evaluate the yield and cost effectiveness of new techniques of screening and alternatives to allogeneic transfusion. However, the greatest threat to the safety of the blood supply is the donation of blood by seronegative donors during the infectious window period when the donors are undergoing seroconversion. Such people represent new, or incident infections. Estimating rates of seroconversion, or incidence, requires the ability to track large numbers of donors at multiple centers. When rates of seroconversion are combined with estimates of the probability that blood was donated during the donor window period, the residual risks of transmitting infectious disease can be calculated [53].

There is continuous enhancement of measures to protect the blood supply from the possibility of TT-HBV infection. Donor selection criteria and precautionary exclusions have been introduced to protect against clinical and theoretical risks. In addition, improvements in laboratory testing have reduced the risk of transfusion-transmitted infection [54]. Mathematical models have been developed for this purpose, including the incidence/window period model [55-58], which estimates "residual risk" per million donations. Residual risk is the chance that an infected donation will escape detection because of the laboratory test 's window period [55,56] (i.e.,the time between first infection and when the viral load becomes detectable by the test). These models which have been used in the developed countries are yet to be applied in the developing world particularly in the sub-Saharan Africa, largely because of the paucity of information on the seroepidemiology of viral infections including HBV. This information is important for determining the safety of blood transfusion and for accurately communicating known risks versus benefits of blood transfusion as a clinical intervention.

Protection of the blood supply from virus-infected donations has reached a very high level in developed countries due to effective donor selection and testing with the latest techniques, which have resulted in the current very low risk of transfusion-transmitted infections in the affluent nations. Unfortunately the risk of transfusion-transmitted infections is relatively high in the sub-Saharan Africa. The frequency of an infectious donation entering the blood supply is usually due to the window period, assay failures and human and technical errors in testing and processing. It is clear that the guidelines for blood screening developed in and adopted by the affluent, low-prevalence countries are essentially unsuitable for resource-poor, high-prevalence countries. Improving blood safety necessitates conceptual changes, taking into consideration resources, assay technology, epidemiology, and blood-banking operations.

Prevalence of Hepatitis B Surface Antigen among Blood Donors

The classification of high endemicity for HBV has been defined as HBsAg greater than 7% in an adult population [59]. The HBsAg seropositivity determined in this investigation (8.0% by ELISA; 10.4% by LA; 10.3% by ICS) confirmed that the south-eastern Nigeria is endemic for HBV infection. In a number of previous reports among blood donors in various regions of Nigeria, a consistently high prevalence rates of HBsAg were recorded, including 14.3% obtained in Jos [60], 4.98% in Port-Harcourt [61], 11.0% in Benin [62], 21.3% in Ibadan [63] and 22.0% Maiduguri [64]. Our results were in conformity with earlier reports from community and hospital based studies in some other parts of Nigeria, which showed high prevalence of HBsAg ranging from 7.4-26% [65]. This is comparable to the prevalence rates ranging from 8.2% to 14.7% observed in Ghana, West Africa [21] and in other parts of sub-Saharan Africa such as Ougadougou, Burkina Faso (14.3%) [66], Dar es Salaam, Tanzania (8.8%) [67], Peltier, Djibouti (10.4%) [68], Kinshasa, Congo Democratic Republic (9.2%) [69], Nouakchott, Mauritania (20.3%) [70], Maputo, Mozambique (18.6%) [71] and Addis Ababa, Ethiopia (11.0%) [72].

The prevalence rates of HBsAg among blood donors in the present study and in other parts of sub-Saharan Africa were relatively higher than those obtained from some developing countries in Asia including Oman (2.8%) [73], Kuwait (1.1%) [74], Pakistan (2.0%) [75], Mongolia (8.0%) [76] and Saudi Arabia (1.9%) [77]. The very high prevalence of HBsAg among blood donors in Nigeria and other African countries clearly demonstrates that the risk of transfusion-transmitted HBV infection is very high in the continent. This is completely unlike what obtains in developed countries where blood supply is the safest it has ever been and the risk of transfusion-transmitted viral infections including HBV is extremely low due to a combination of donor education, donor screening, and new laboratory test procedures [53,78,79]. In the United States for instance, a combination of more sensitive third-generation tests (reversed passive hemagglutination and radioimmunoassay (RIA)) for HBsAg screening and exclusive use of non-paid donors reduced the rate of post-transfusion hepatitis B to 0.3%-0.9%/transfusion recipient by as early as the mid-1970s [80], and in 2001, the prevalence of HBsAg among blood donors was as low as 0.077% [81].

Due to endemicity of infections causing anemia, malnutrition, and surgical and obstetrical emergencies associated with blood loss in the sub-Saharan Africa, the demand for blood transfusion services is high . However, blood safety remains an issue of major concern in transfusion medicine in this part of the globe because national blood transfusion services and policies, appropriate infrastructure, trained personnel and financial resources are inadequate. This is aggravated by the pre-dominance of family and replacement, rather than regular benevolent, non-remunerated donors and lack of comprehensive and systematic screening of donated blood for transfusion-transmissible agents other than HIV [60-66]. A large number of blood transfusion centers in sub-Saharan Africa, screen donor blood for HIV alone. Other main transfusion transmissible infections such as Hepatitis B and C, malaria, and syphilis are not routinely screened [66-68,82]. As a result, some of the blood being transfused is likely to contain unscreened pathogens.

In this present study, significantly higher prevalence rates of HBsAg were observed in the males than the females by the ELISA and LA diagnostic techniques. A similar result was obtained in a related study among blood donors in Dar es Salaam, Tanzania [67]. In Nigeria the prevalence of viral hepatitis is reportedly higher in the male than the females [83,84], presumably due to the multiple sexual partnerships and promiscuity which are habits occurring with higher frequency among males than females [50], and also due to the higher frequency of exposure to infected blood and blood products by the males as a result of occupation and social behaviours [85]. It is well established that exacerbations of chronic HBV infection are observed more often in men than in women. Although the reason for this sex difference is not clear, the higher frequency of exacerbations in men may account, in part, for the higher incidence of HBV-related cirrhosis and hepatocellular carcinoma among men [2-4]. This may also explain in part why individuals of the 25-35 years age category were significantly more likely to be HBsAg positive as observed in this study and that conducted in Jos, Central Nigeria [60]. Furthermore, majority of the donors in this study who were commercial motorcyclists fall in this age category and it is well established that individuals in this kind of occupation have high frequency of multiple sexual partners including commercial sex workers [50]. This is also similar to the findings in Dar es Salaam, Tanzania [67]. Age may thus be considered as a major factor in the epidemiology of HBV infection because in the general population, most of acute HBV infections occur among young adults, although about one third of patients acquire chronic infections through perinatal and early childhood exposures [3,4]. The prevalence increases with age and the age at infection primarily determines the rate of progression from acute infection to chronic infection, which is approximately 90% in the perinatal period, 20-50% in children aged 1-5 years, and less than 5% in adults [7].

Screening of HBV Infection: Detection of Hepatitis B Virus Surface Antigen

Although the prevalence of HBsAg among the blood donors in this study could be considered as high, the possibility of underestimation of the prevalence may not be ruled out completely. The diagnostic techniques used in this study to identify HBV infected donors through the detection of HBsAg are known to be reasonably reliable. However, several circumstances which can lead to HBV infectious donations entering the blood supply have been identified [78], these include; (i) collection of donations during the infectious 'window period' following infection when tests in use are unable to detect the infection; (ii) donations testing falsely negative due to test sensitivities less than 100%; (iii) donations falsely issued as negative due to an error in sampling, testing, recording of test results, or removal of positive donations; (iv) donations collected from individuals with fluctuating or waning levels of hepatitis B surface antigen (HBsAg) during later stages of HBV carriage. Furthermore it has been demonstrated that transmission by blood components negative for HBsAg can still occur during chronic stages of infection (i.c. "occult" HBV infection, OHB). OHB is defined as the presence of HBV DNA in blood or liver tissues in patients negative for HBsAg, with or without any HBV antibodies [86]. Because of limitations in current blood screening practices, OHB is an overlooked source of HBV transmission. This problem is compounded by the fact that in most developing countries particularly in Africa, screening of HBV in blood donors is limited to HBsAg testing.

In this study, the detection of HBsAg via ELISA, latex agglutination and immunochromatographic strip was used to demonstrate HBV infection. These are the most common diagnostic procedures used to demonstrate the presence of HBV infection in Nigeria and other sub-Saharan African countries. Our findings appeared to suggest that ELISA assay is more valuable. In an earlier study in Ghana, findings clearly indicated that latex agglutination and dipstick assays have insufficient sensitivity and that ELISA assays have higher sensitivity and thus a more valuable HBsAg diagnostic tool [21]. However, latex agglutination and dipstick assays are both used in developing countries because of their low cost and flexibility to screen few samples without waste. It is important to note that sera containing HBsAg are now known to contain additional antigenic specificities unrelated to the determinants present on the surface antigen. The first of these is the core antigen, so termed because of its close association with the inner component of the 42 nm particle [87]. This particle is believed to represent the hepatitis B virus of man. Core antigen may be detected after removal of the outer surface antigen coat either by direct serological examination or indirectly by assay of an integral DNA-dependent DNA polymerase activity [88]. A third precipitating antigen in some sera containing the surface antigen, was recognized and designated 'e' [89]. The presence of the e antigen appears to correlate with the replication of hepatitis B virus in the host and, in general terms, with varying degrees of liver damage [90]. Thus if anti-HBc testing and sensitive HBV nucleic acid amplification testing (NAT) for routine screening are not prescribed, HBV viraemia might remain unrecognized. Thus, an HBsAg seronegative result does not rule out the presence of HBV infection.

Antibody to hepatitis B core antigen (anti-HBc) for instance is one of the earliest serological markers during hepatitis B virus (HBV) infection and is generally present during acute, convalescent, and chronic phases of the disease [91,92]. Anti-HBc usually persists for many years after infection and may be the only marker of previous exposure, since anti-body to hepatitis B surface antigen (anti-HBs) may wane with time [93]. In many developed countries, tests for anti-HBc have been widely used for screening blood donors, since epidemiological studies have shown that anti-HBc could serve as a surrogate marker for non-A, non-B hepatitis [94,95]. Several investigators have observed low-level anti-HBc test results near the assay cutoff in healthy blood donors testing negative for hepatitis B surface antigen (HBsAg) and have suggested that most of these results were due to poor specificity of the current, commercial immunoassays [96-98]. The implication of this from the present study is that there is a substantial residual risk of posttransfusion HBV infection in this part of the globe, although this has not been quantified in many endemic areas of the sub-Saharan including Nigeria.

The residual risk of posttransfusion HBV infection has however been calculated in the United States and Germany on the basis of HBV incidence data and the duration of the early window period until HBsAg becomes detectable to be 1:63 000 and less than 1:100 000 blood donations, respectively [45,53]. Since it has been shown that blood donations of HBsAg- and anti-HBs–negative but anti-HBc–positive HBV carriers can cause posttransfusion hepati-tis B [46,47], it was suggested that anti-HBc screening of blood donations might prevent HBV transmission from HBsAg-negative blood donors and that donors positive for anti-HBs as well should be considered noninfectious for HBV [48]. The feasibility of routine polymerase chain reaction (PCR) screening of blood donations in a blood bank setting has been shown [99], but this is undoubtedly beyond the reach of developing countries. The implementation of NAT for screening of blood donors warrants consideration. The NAT technology has substantially lowered the risk of transfusion-transmitted HBV infection but at an additional cost to the health-care system, because the cost-effectiveness of whole-blood NAT is poor [100]. The testing cost would need to decrease significantly to bring the cost-effectiveness in line with most other accepted medical practices especially in developing countries. There is need for each country to develop its blood screening strategy based on HBV endemicity, yields of infectious units detected by different serologic/NAT screening methods, and cost effectiveness of test methods in ensuring blood safety. This is very vital in reducing transfusion-transmitted HBV infection. In Brazil for instance a case was reported of a blood donor had her sample tested for HBsAg and anti-HBc, which resulted negative. At the second donation the sample demonstrated to be seropositive for anti-HBc, anti-HBs and seronegative for HBsAg. The first stored sample was tested for the presence of HBV DNA. Two fragments could be identified in the genomic region corresponding to HBV core and precore. Only one individual was involved in the transfusion of hemo-derivatives originating from the processing of this bag, and was seropositive for HBsAg, HBeAg and anti-HBc markers and seronegative for the anti-HBe and anti-HBs markers [101]. This case illustrates the possibility of the occurrence of HBV transmission from blood bank donors seronegative for HBsAg and anti-HBc. This fact could be associated with the possibility of the donor to be in the pre-seroconversion phase of a recent infection, when the levels of HBsAg present in the circulation are below the limits of detection. The implementation of molecular tests such as the NAT or higher sensitivity HBsAg assays could further reduce the risk of HBV transmission via blood transfusion.

Comparison data on seroconversion panels using HBsAg assays of varying sensitivities and pooled- or single-sample NAT, along with viral load estimates corresponding to HBsAg assay detection limits, have provided information on the theoretical benefits of NAT relative to HBsAg [102]. Model-derived estimates have generally been predictive of the yields of DNA-positive, HBsAg-negative window period blood units detected in a number of studies from Europe, Asia, and the US [86,100,103-107]. Studies indicate that the added benefit of pooled-sample NAT is relatively small in areas of low endemicity, with greater yields in areas highly endemic for HBV. Single-sample NAT would offer more significant early window period closure and could prevent a moderate number of residual HBV transmissions not detected by HBsAg assays; however, no fully automated single-sample HBV NAT systems are currently available. Even single-sample HBV NAT may not substitute for anti-HBc screening, as indicated by studies of donors with isolated anti-HBc who have extremely low DNA levels undetectable by standard single-sample NAT and who have been associated with transfusion-transmitted HBV [102]. Moreover, HBsAg testing may still be needed even in the setting of combined anti-HBc and NAT screening. HBsAg-positive units from donors in the chronic stage of infection may contain very low or intermittently detectable DNA levels that single-sample NAT would miss. Although such donors are usually anti-HBc reactive and would be interdicted by anti-HBc screening, some lack anti-HBc. Extensive parallel testing will be needed to determine whether single-sample NAT in combination with anti-HBc might be sufficient to detect all the infectious donors currently interdicted by HBsAg testing [102]. In countries that do not screen for anti-HBc, HBsAg testing would be the only means of detecting donations from chronically infected individuals with low/intermittently detectable DNA, since even single-donor NAT would not identify these potentially infectious blood units. In the future, the current fully automated HBsAg assays may incorporate significant sensitivity improvements, and automated single-sample HBV NAT may become a reality.

It is already well established that by introduction of NAT, the diagnostic window period can be reduced significantly. This is of major importance in the context of screening blood and plasma. With more sensitive HBsAg assays, the serologic window period is approximately 45 days and with single-donation NAT, it is possible to reduce the window period by another 25 days [100]. However, to increase capacity and reduce cost, NAT are performed in the donor screening setting on minipools of 16-24 samples that might provide relatively little benefit over HBsAG testing, particularly since newer, more sensitive HBsAG assays have been introduced [108]. Additionally, there may be problems with samples, particularly from patients with HBe antigen-negative chronic hepatitis B, who may have low serum/plasma levels of HBV DNA, even below the detection limit of a highly sensitive NAT [109]. Hence for developing countries the use of HBsAg enzyme immunoassays appear to be most ideal for screening blood donors.

Public Health Considerations

Since blood transfusion is an important part of modern medicine, the safety of blood and blood products remains a global issue. Although many countries screen all blood donations for a number of infectious agents, a significant proportion of the world's blood supply particularly in the developing countries is either unscreened or poorly screened, with the resultant risk to recipients of transfusion transmitted HBV infection. The substantial risk of transfusion transmitted HBV infection in many developing countries is a consequence of poorly developed healthcare systems and limited resources. In these countries, the safety of the blood supply is compromised frequently, either because of lack of resources with which to purchase screening assays, or because of acute blood shortages and insufficient time to screen blood prior to transfusion [110]. As part of public health interventional measures, the transmission of HBV can be minimized by the screening of donors prior to donation, exclusion of high-risk donors, followed by the in-vitro screening of donations for HBsAg

(+anti-HBc in some countries) prior to transfusion. Infection control measures in health-care settings including safe injection practices and proper sterilization techniques of medical instruments and education of barbers about the significance of sterilization of their instruments may reduce the burden of HBV infection particularly in low income settings with high HBV endemicity [111]. There is also an urgent need of developing locally relevant guidelines for counseling and management of HBsAg positive blood donors. It is important to encourage and actively support the introduction of appropriate screening programmes which can be based upon simple assay formats, such as agglutination, rather than the favoured but more complex enzyme immunoassays which are more expensive, require specific equipment and support, and take longer to perform [110]. Such approaches will help reduce greatly the transfusion transmission of HBV. However, since the residual risk of posttransfusion infection resides essentially in chronic infections with low viral load and HBsAg level, to ensure blood safety, HBsAg testing will require highly sensitive assays which would enable the identification of donors carrying low viral and antigen loads. Current enzyme immmunoassays (EIAs), but not rapid tests, appear adequately sensitive [21]. Policy for checking the collected blood unit by 3 tests for anti-HBc, anti-HBsAg and HBsAg should be reconsidered in favor of HBV-DNA testing by polymerase chain reaction, to possibly achieve the zero risk goal of transfusion transmitted HBV infection in settings that can afford this [112]. Accurate assessment of transfusion-transmitted HBV infection which necessitates knowledge about donation histories and person-years at risk is very essential in order to establish comprehensive frameworks for monitoring blood donations and infectious disease markers which remains a key to monitoring blood safety [113].

For policy development on screening for HBV infection in blood donors, it would be useful to assess the relative contribution of transfusion-transmitted HBV infection from HBsAg-negative donations which occur in the acute phase of infection during the seronegative window period, or during chronic stages of infection (i.c. "occult" HBV infection, OHB). New screening policy should be evaluated on the basis of available data or newly designed studies. While anti-HBc screening can climinate residual risk of occult HBV transmission by transfusion in low-endemic areas, it would not be practical in most parts of the world where the prevalence of anti-HBc is >10% as too many otherwise healthy donors will be ineligible [86]. On the contrary, nucleic acid amplification test (NAT) or new HBsAg tests of enhanced sensitivity would be effective in the screening of blood donors for OHB in highly endemic countries.

Persons at risk of exposure to HBV, who are shown or judged likely to be susceptible, should receive hepatitis B vaccine [114]. Ideally, hepatitis B vaccine should be provided to such persons before they engage in behaviors, occupations, or treatments that place them at risk of infection. Prophylactic treatment (hepatitis B immune globulin and hepatitis B vaccine) to prevent HBV infection after exposure to HBV should be provided for infants born to HBsAg-positive mothers, persons with accidental percutaneous or permucosal exposure to HBsAg-positive blood, sexual partners of an HBsAg-positive person, and infants less than 12 months of age whose primary care giver has acute hepatitis B [114]. Hepatitis B vaccine should also be given to all susceptible household contacts of HBV carriers.

CONCLUSION AND FUTURE PROSPECTS

Available facts have indicated that HBV infection is wide spread in sub Sahara Africa including Nigeria and the rate will continue to increase due to some factors peculiar to the sub region. One major factor is the inadequate blood screening techniques employed in pretransfusion screening of blood. The most commonly used assays for screening blood before transfusion in the sub region can only detect HBsAg which does not rule out the presence of the virus in the blood. Therefore to transfuse HBV-free blood, there is a dire need to employ more sensitive assay for screening blood from all sources. Such assays must be able to detect antibody against anti HBV core antigen, HBV e-antigens, and the viral nucleic acid, as well as HBV DNA. This approach will definitely reduce the present of endemicity in the sub region to the barest minimum. The absence of a well-organised blood banking system in most parts of the sub-Saharan Africa constitutes an overwhelming challenge in transfusion medicine. Many hospitals essentially lack blood banks. Furthermore, there appears to be no programme in place that encourages well-meaning citizens to participate in voluntary, non-remunerated blood donation. Sources of blood for transfusion in many hospitals in these countries are usually from relatives of patients and are usually requested in emergency situations. This type of approach does not allow proper screening of blood before transfusion especially during emergency, even when sensitive techniques are available.

It is therefore pertinent for developing countries to embark on total over-haul of existing blood donation and blood banking system. There is need to evolve policies that would encourage and ensure the development of blood banks, educating citizenry on the importance of blood donation and to enlighten them about the realities of transfusion transmitted pathogens including HBV infection. In most parts of the developing world, certain cultural and behavioural practices have increased the risk of blood borne viruses, such as the use of unsterilized sharps for tribal marks, circumcision, and for traditional surgical operation. The practice of unprotected sex and the use of same injection needles by intravenous drug users are also increasing the risk of blood borne viral infection including HBV. As part of public health measures, interventional efforts therefore should target populations at highest risk of HBV infection including the commercial blood donors in order to minimize the rate of HBV infection.

The control of HBV infection remains a serious challenge in the developing world and the danger imposed by up to 360 million chronic carriers necessitates the exploitation of various sources of possible treatment of the infection including herbal medicines. Africa is enriched with herbal bio-resources which can be exploited for use in reducing the viral load among infected individuals as is the case in China [115,116]. A number of publications have indicated the potency of herbal medicine for the treatment of HBV infection [115-119]. There are however many unpublished claims of successful treatments of HBV infection with tropical medicinal plants in many parts of Africa including Nigeria. There is therefore the need to verify these claims, scientifically, because little formal assessment of the clinical effectiveness of these treatments has been conducted. Studies are highly needed to evaluate the clinical evidence of the effectiveness of these herbal medicines in the treatment of HBV infection. Break through in this area will be of immense value to the world.

References

[1] Drosten C, Nippraschk T, Manegold C, Meisel H, Brixner V, Roth WK, Apedjinou A, Gunther S. Prevalence of hepatitis B virus DNA in anti-HBC-positive/HBsAg-negative sera correlates with HCV but not HIV serostatus. *J Clin Virol* 2004; *29*: 59-68.

[2] Beasley R. Hepatitis B virus: the major etiology of hepatocellular carcinoma. *Cancer* 1988; 61:1942–1956.

[3] Evans AA, London W T. Epidemiology of hepatitis B, p. 107–114. In A. J. Zuckerman and H. C. Thomas (ed.), *Viral hepatitis*. Harcourt Brace & Co., Ltd., London, United Kingdom. 1998

[4] Parkin, DM, Pisani, P Ferlay. J. Estimates of the worldwide incidence of 25 major cancers in 1990. *Int J Cancer*. 1999; 80:827–841.

[5] Chan HLY, Lok ASF. Hepatitis B in adult-a clinical perspective. *Clin Liver* Dis 1999; 3(2): 291-307.

[6] Mahoney FJ, Long SS, Pickering LK: Hepatitis B virus. In: *Principles and Practice of Pediatric Infectious Diseases*. 1997: 1194-202.

[7] McMahon BJ, Alward WLM, Hall DB, Heyward WL, Bender TR, Francis DP, Maynard JE. Acute hepatitis B virus infection: relation of age to the clinical expression of disease and subsequent development of the carrier state. J *Infect Dis* 1985; 151: 599–603.

[8] Beasley RP, Heang LY, Lin CC, Chien CS,. Hepatocellular carcinoma and hepatitis B virus. A prospective study of 22,707 men in Taiwan. *Lancet* 1981; 318: 1129–1133.

[9] Blumberg BS, Alter HJ, Visnick S. A "new" antigen in leukemia sera. *JAMA* 1965;191:541-6.

[10] Blumberg BS, Gerstley BJS, Hungerford DA, London WT, Sutnick AI. A serum antigen (Australia antigen) in Down's syndrome, leukemia, and hepatitis. *Ann Intern Med* 1967;66:924-31.

[11] Prince AM. An antigen detected in the blood during the incubation period of serum hepatitis. *Proc Nat Acad Sci* 1968;60:814-21.

[12] Giles JP, McCollum RW, Berndtson LW Jr, Krugman S. Viral hepatitis -- relation of Australia/SH antigen to the Willowbrook MS-2 strain. *N Engl J Med* 1969;281:119-21.

[13] Holland PV, Alter HJ. The clinical significance of hepatitis B virus antigens and antibodies. *Med Cl No Amer* 1975;59:849-55.

[14] Hoofnagle JH, Gerety RJ, Barker LF. Antibody to hepatitis B core antigen. *Am J Med* Sci 1975;270:179-87.

[15] Chau KH, Hargie MP, Decker RH, Mushahwar IS, Overby LR. Serodiagnosis of recent hepatitis B infection by IgM class anti-HBc. *Hepatology* 1983;3:142-9.

[16] CDC. Public Health Service Inter-Agency Guidelines for Screening Donors of Blood, Plasma, Organs, Tissues, and Semen for Evidence. *MMWR* 1991; 40(RR-4): 1-17.

[17] Pyrsopoulos NT. Hepatitis B. *e-Medicine*. 2006

[18] Saha V, John TJ, Dhamodaran S, Carman RH. Highly sensitive screening tests for hepatitis B surface antigen in transfusion centres of developing countries. *Br Med J.* 1988;297:646-647.

[19] Ndumbe PM, Nyouma E. Transmission of hepatitis B virus by blood transfusion in Yaounde, Cameroon. *Br Med J.* 1990;301:523-524.

[20] Sarkodie F, Adarkwa M, Candotti D, Acheampong JW, Allain JP. Screening for viral markers by EIA in volunteer and replacement donors in Kumasi, Ghana. *Vox Sang.* 2001;80:142-147.

[21] Allain JP, Candotti D, Soldan K, Sarkodie F, Phelps B, Giachetti C, Shyamala V, Yeboah F, Anokwa M, Owusu-Ofori S, Opare-Sem O. The risk of hepatitis B virus infection by transfusion in Kumasi, *Ghana Blood.* 2003;101(6):2419-25.

[22] Saraswat S, Banerjee K, Chaudhury N, Mahant T, Khandekar P, Gupta RK, *et a*l. Post-transfusion hepatitis type B following multiple transfusions of HBsAg-negative blood. *J Hepatol* 1996; *25* : 639-43.

[23] Behzad-Behbahani A, Mafi-Nejad A, Tabei SZ, Lankarani KB, Torab A, Moaddeb A. Anti-HBc & HBV-DNA detection in blood donors negative for hepatitis B virus surface antigen in reducing risk of transfusion associated HBV infection. *Indian J Med Res*. 2006 Jan;123(1):37-42.

[24] Jongerius JM, Wester M, Cuypers HT, van Oostendorp WR, Lelie PN, van der Poel CL, *et a*l. New hepatitis B virus mutant form in a blood donor that is undetectable in several hepatitis B surface antigen screening assays. *Transfusion* 1998; *38* : 56-9.

[25] Carman WF. The clinical significance of surface antigen variants of hepatitis B virus. *J Viral Hepat* 1997; 4 (Suppl 1) : 11-20.

[26] Carman WF, Mimms LT. Pre-S/S gene variants of hepatitis B virus. In: Rizzetto M, Purcell RH, Gerin JL, Verne G, editors. *Viral hepatitis and liver diseas*e. Torino, Italy: Edizioni Minerva Medica; 1997 p. 108-15.

[27] Tsai S, Liaw Y, Yeh C, Chu CM, Kuo GC. Cellular immune responses in patients with dual infection of hepatitis B and C viruses: dominant role of hepatitis C virus. *Hepatology* 1995; *21* : 908-12.

[28] Lee WM. Hepatitis B virus infection. *N Engl J Med* 1997; *337* : 1733-45.

[29] Ben Ayed M, Triki H, Cointe D, Karray H, Masmoudi MA, Dellagi K, *et a*l. The isolated presence of anti-HBc antibodies: prevalence and interpretation based on the results of viral DNA research and anti-HBs antibodies measurement after vaccination. *Ann Biol Clin (Paris)* 2001; *59* : 53-60.

[30] Gomes SA, Yoshida CF, Niel C. Detection of hepatitis B virus DNA in hepatitis B surface antigen-negative serum by polymerase chain reaction: evaluation of different primer pairs and conditions. *Acta Virol* 1996; *40* : 133-8.

[31] Iizuka H, Ohmura K, Ishijima A, Satoh K, Tanaka T, Tsuda F, *et a*l. Correlation between anti-HBc titers and HBV DNA in blood units without detectable HBsAg. *Vox Sang* 1992; *63* : 107-11.

[32] Brechot C, Degos F, Lugassy C, et al. Hepatitis B virus DNA in patients with chronic liver disease and negative tests for hepatitis B surface antigen. *N Engl J Med.* 1985;312:270-276.

[33] Marcellin P, Martinot-Peignoux M, Loriot MA, et al. Persistence of hepatitis B virus DNA demon-strated by polymerase chain reaction in serum and liver after loss of HBsAg induced by antiviral therapy. *Ann Intern Med.* 1990;112:227-228.

[34] Kaneko S, Miller RH, Di Bisceglie AM, Feinstone SM, Hoofnagle JH, Purcell RH. Detection of hepatitis B virus DNA in serum by polymerase chain reaction. Application for clinical diagnosis. *Gastroenterology*. 1990;99:799-804.

[35] Loriot MA, Marcellin P, Bismuth E, et al. Demonstration of hepatitis B virus DNAby polymerase chain reaction in the serum and the liver after spontaneous or therapeutically induced HBeAg to anti-HBe or HBsAg to anti-HBs seroconversion in patients with chronic hepatitis B. *Hepatology*. 1992;15:32-36.

[36] Paterlini P, Driss F, Nalpas B, et al. Persistence of hepatitis B and hepatitis C viral genomes in primary liver cancers from HBsAg-negative patients: a study of a low-endemic area. *Hepatology*. 1993;17:20-29.

[37] Gomes SA, Yoshida CF, Niel C. Detection of hepatitis B virus DNA in hepatitis B surface antigen negative serum by polymerase chain reaction: evaluation of different primer pairs and conditions. *Acta Virol*. 1996;40:133-138.

[38] Hennig H, Dennin RH, Haase D, Kirchner H. [HBV-DNA positive findings in HBsAg negative blood donors and patients]. *Beitr Infusionsther Transfusionsmed*. 1997;34:26-30.

[39] Yotsuyanagi H, Yasuda K, Iino S, et al. Persistent viremia after recovery from self-limited acute hepatitis B. *Hepatology*. 1998;27:1377-1382.

[40] Marusawa H, Imoto S, Ueda Y, Chiba T. Reactivation of latently infected hepatitis B virus in a leukemia patient with antibodies to hepatitis B core antigen. *J Gastroenterol*. 2001;36:633-636.

[41] Marcellin P, Giostra E, Martinot-Peignoux M, et al. Redevelopment of hepatitis B surface antigen after renal transplantation. *Gastroenterology*. 1991;100:1432-1434.

[42] Dhedin N, Douvin C, Kuentz M, et al. Reverse seroconversion of hepatitis B after allogeneic bone marrow transplantation: a retrospective study of 37 patients with pretransplant anti-HBs and anti-HBc. *Transplantation*. 1998;66:616-619.

[43] Nordbo SA, Skaug K, Holter E, Waage A, Brinch L. Reactivation of hepatitis B virus infection in an anti-HBc and anti-HBs positive patient after allogeneic bone marrow transplantation. *Eur J Haematol*. 2000;65:86-87.

[44] Gonzalez M, Regine V, Piccinini V, Vulcano F, Giampaolo A, Hassan HJ. Residual risk of transfusion-transmitted human immunodeficiency virus, hepatitis C virus, and hepatitis B virus infections in Italy. *Transfusion*. 2005 Oct;45(10):1670-5.

[45] Glu¨ ck D. [Risk of HIV, HCV, and HBV transmission by blood products. Current data 1997 and 1998—study on the epidemiology of HIV and hepatitis in blood donors in Germany]. *Infusion-sther Transfusionsmed*. 1999;26:335-338.

[46] Larsen J, Hetland G, Skaug K. Posttransfusion hepatitis B transmitted by blood from a hepatitis B surface antigen-negative hepatitis B virus carrier. *Transfusion*. 1990;30:431-432.

[47] Norder H, Hammas B, Larsen J, Skaug K, Magnius LO. Detection of HBV DNA by PCR in serum from an HBsAg negative blood donor implicated in cases of post-transfusion hepatitis B. *Arch Virol Suppl*. 1992;4:116-118.

[48] Mosley JW, Stevens CE, Aach RD, et al. Donor screening for antibody to hepatitis B core antigen and hepatitis B virus infection in transfusion recipients. *Transfusion*. 1995;35:5-12.

[49] Sirisena ND, Njoku MO, Idoko JA, Isamade E, Barau C, Jelpe D, Zamani A, Otowo S 2002. Carriage rate of hepatitis-B surface antigen (HbsAG) in an urban community in Jos, Plateau State, Nigeria. *Nig Postgrad Med* J 9: 7-10.

[50] UNSN 2001. Nigerian Common Country Assessment, World Health Organization, Geneva, 563 pp.

[51] World Medical Association Declaration of Helsinki. Ethical principles for medical research involving human subjects. World Medical Association, 2000 (http://www.wma.net/e/policy/b3.htm) (Accessed 15/6/2006).

[52] International ethical guidelines for biomedical research involving human subjects. Geneva, Council for International Organizations of Medical Sciences (CIOMS), 2002.

[53] Schreiber GB, Busch MP, Kleinman SH, Korelitz JJ. The risk of transfusion-transmitted viral infections. The Retrovirus Epidemiology Donor Study. *N Engl J Med.* 1996;334(26):1685-90.

[54] Chiavetta JA, Escobar M, Newman A, He Y, Driezen P, Deeks S, Hone DE, O'Brien SF, Sher G. Incidence and estimated rates of residual risk for HIV, hepatitis C, hepatitis B and human T-cell lymphotropic viruses in blood donors in Canada, 1990-2000. *CMAJ.* 2003;169(8):767-73

[55] Pillonel J,Laperche S,Saura C,Desenclos JC,Couroucé AM.Trends in residual risk of transfusion-transmitted viral infections in France between 1992 and 2000. *Transfusion* 2002;42:980-8.

[56] Kleinman SH,Busch MP.The risks of transfusion-transmitted infection:direct estimation and mathematical modelling.*Baillieres Best Pract Res Clin Haematol* 2000;13:631-49.

[57] Müller-Breitkreutz K.Results of viral marker screening of unpaid blood donations and probability of window period donations in 1997. EPFA Working Group of Quality Assurance.Vox Sang 2000;78:149-57.

[58] Seed CR,Cheng A,Ismay SL,Bolton WV,Kiely P,Cobain TJ,et al.Assessing the accuracy of three viral risk models in predicting the outcome of implementing HIV and HCV NAT donor screening in Australia and the implications for future HBV NAT. *Transfusion* 2002;42:1365-72.

[59] Hodges M, Sanders E, Aitken C 1998. Seroprevalence of hepatitis markers: HAV, HBV, HCV, and HBV amongst primary school children in Freetown Sierra Leone. *W Afr J Med* 17:3-7.

[60] Uneke CJ, Ogbu O, Inyama PU, Anyanwu GI, Njoku MO, Idoko JH. *Prevalence of hepatitis-B surface antigen among blood donors and human immunodeficiency virus-infected patients* in Jos, Nigeria. Mem Inst Oswaldo Cruz. 2005 Feb;100(1):13-6. Epub 2005 Apr 12.

[61] Ejele OA, Ojule AC. The prevalence of hepatitis B surface antigen (HBsAg) among prospective blood donors and patients in Port Harcourt, *Nigeria Niger J Med.* 2004 Oct-Dec;13(4):336-8.

[62] Oronsaye FE, Oronsaye JI. Prevalence of HIV-positives and hepatitis B surface antigen-positives among donors in the University of Benin Teaching Hospital, *Nigeria Trop Doct.* 2004 Jul;34(3):159-60

[63] Otegbayo JA, Fasola FA, Abja A. Prevalence of hepatitis B surface and e antigens, risk factors for viral acquisition and serum transaminase among blood donors in Ibadan, *Nigeria Trop Gastroenterol.* 2003 Oct-Dec;24(4):196-7.

[64] Harry TO, Bajani MD, Moses AE. East Afr Med J. Hepatitis B virus infection among blood donors and pregnant women in Maiduguri, Nigeria 1994 Sep;71(9):596-7

[65] Ekpo M, Sasegbon H, Oyewole F 1995. HIV and HBV serostatus of non- intravenous drug users in Lagos, Nigeria. *Nig Med J* 29: 35-36.

[66] Collenberg E, Ouedraogo T, Ganame J, Fickenscher H, Kynast-Wolf G, Becher H, Kouyate B, Krausslich HG, Sangare L, Tebit DM. Seroprevalence of six different viruses among pregnant women and blood donors in rural and urban Burkina Faso: A comparative analysis. *J Med Virol.* 2006 May;78(5):683-92.

[67] Matee MI, Magesa PM, Lyamuya EF. Seroprevalence of human immunodeficiency virus, hepatitis B and C viruses and syphilis infections among blood donors at the Muhimbili National Hospital in Dar es Salaam, Tanzania. *BMC Public Health.* 2006 Jan 30;6:21.

[68] Dray X, Dray-Spira R, Bronstein JA, Mattera D. [Prevalences of HIV, hepatitis B and hepatitis C in blood donors in the Republic of Djibouti][Article in French] *Med Trop (Mars).* 2005;65(1):39-42.

[69] Mbendi Nlombi C, Longo-Mbenza B, Mbendi Nsukini S, Muyembe Tamfum JJ, Situakibanza Nanituma H, Vangu Ngoma D. [Prevalence of HIV and HBs antigen in blood donors. Residual risk of contamination in blood recipients in East Kinshasa, Democratic Republic of the Congo] [Article in French] *Med Trop (Mars).* 2001;61(2):139-42.

[70] Lo BB, Meymouna M, Boulahi MA, Tew M, Sow A, Ba A, Sow MB. [Prevalence of serum markers of hepatitis B and C virus in blood donors of Nouakchott, Mauritania][Article in French] *Bull Soc Pathol Exot.* 1999 May;92(2):83-4.

[71] Perez O, Lastre M, Miyar R, Valdemar Meneses L. [Prevalence of HBSAG in blood donors and patients at the central hospital of Maputo, Mozambique, 1985][Article in Spanish] *Rev Cubana Med Trop.* 1989 Sep-Dec;41(3):355-61.

[72] Tsega E, Mengesha B, Nordenfelt E, Hansson BG, Lindberg J. Prevalence of hepatitis B virus markers among Ethiopian blood donors: is HBsAg screening necessary? *Trop Geogr Med.* 1987 Oct;39(4):336-40.

[73] Kaminski G, Alnaqdy A, Al-Belushi I, Nograles J, Al-Dhahry SH. Evidence of occult hepatitis B virus infection among Omani blood donors: a preliminary study. *Med Princ Pract.* 2006;15(5):368-72.

[74] Ameen R, Sanad N, Al-Shemmari S, Siddique I, Chowdhury RI, Al-Hamdan S, Al-Bashir A. Prevalence of viral markers among first-time Arab blood donors in Kuwait *Transfusion.* 2005 Dec;45(12):1973-80.

[75] Akhtar S, Younus M, Adil S, Hassan F, Jafri SH. Epidemiologic study of chronic hepatitis B virus infection in male volunteer blood donors in Karachi, *Pakistan BMC Gastroenterol.* 2005 Aug 8;5:26

[76] Tsatsralt-Od B, Takahashi M, Nishizawa T, Inoue J, Ulaankhuu D, Okamoto H. High prevalence of hepatitis B, C and delta virus infections among blood donors in Mongolia *Arch Virol.* 2005 Dec;150(12):2513-28. Epub 2005 Jul 14

[77] Panhotra BR, Al-Bahrani A, Ul-Hassan Z. Epidemiology of antibody to hepatitis B core antigen screening among blood donors in Eastern Saudi Arabia. Need to replace the test by HBV DNA testing. *Saudi Med J.* 2005 Feb;26(2):270-3.

[78] Soldan K, Davison K, Dow B. Estimates of the frequency of HBV, HCV, and HIV infectious donations entering the blood supply in the United Kingdom, 1996 to 2003 *Euro Surveill.* 2005 Feb;10(2):17-9

[79] Glynn SA, Kleinman SH, Schreiber GB, Busch MP, Wright DJ, Smith JW, Nass CC, Williams AE. Trends in incidence and prevalence of major transfusion-transmissible viral infections in US blood donors, 1991 to 1996. Retrovirus Epidemiology Donor Study (REDS) *JAMA*. 2000 Jul 12;284(2):229-35

[80] Alter HJ, Purcell RH, Holland PV, Feinstone SM, Morrow AG, Moritsugu Y. Clinical and serological analysis of transfusion-associated hepatitis. *Lancet* 1975;2:838-41.

[81] Zou S, Dodd RY, Stramer SL, Strong DM; Tissue Safety Study Group. Probability of viremia with HBV, HCV, HIV, and HTLV among tissue donors in the United States. *N Engl J Med.* 2004 Aug 19;351(8):751-9.

[82] Uneke CJ, Ogbu O, Nwojiji V (2006) Potential risk of induced malaria by blood transfusion in South-eastern Nigeria. *MJM 9:*8-13

[83] Halim N K D, Offor E, Ajayi O I. Epidemiologic study of the seroprevalence of hepatitis-B surface antigen (HBsAg) and HIV-1, in blood donors. *Nig J Clin pract* 1992; 2:42-5.

[84] Baba MM, Gashau W, Hassan AW, Detection of hepatitis-B surface antigenaemia in patients mirth and without the manifestations of AIDS in Maiduguri, Nigeria. *Nig Postgrad Med J* 1998; 5:125-8.

[85] Mutimer D J, Olomu A, Skidmore S, Olomu N, Ratcliffe D. Viral hepatitis in Nigeria - sickle cell disease and commercial blood donors. *Q J Med* 1994;87:407-11.

[86] Liu CJ, Chen DS, Chen PJ. Epidemiology of HBV infection in Asian blood donors: emphasis on occult HBV infection and the role of NAT *J Clin Virol.* 2006 May;36 Suppl 1:S33-44

[87] Dane, D. S., Cameron, C. H., and Briggs, M. (1970). Virus-like particles in serum of patients with Australia-antigen- associated hepatitis. *Lancet*, 1, 695-698.

[88] Kaplan, P. M., Greenman, R. L., Gerin, J. L., Purcell, R. H., and Robinson, W. S. (1973). DNA polymerase associated with human hepatitis B antigen. *Journal of Virology*, 12, 995-1005.

[89] Magnius, L. O., and Espmark, J. A. (1972). New specificities in Australia antigen positive sera distinct from the Le Bouvier determinants. *Journal of Immuno-logy*, 109, 1017-1021.

[90] Nielsen, J. O., Dietrichson, O., and Juhl, E. (1974). Incidence and meaning of the 'e' determinant among hepatitis-B-antigen positive patients with acute and chronic liver diseases. *Lancet*, 2, 913-915.

[91] Hoofnagle, J. H., R. J. Gerety, and L. F. Barker. 1973. Antibody to hepatitis-B-virus core in man. *Lancet* ii:869-873.

[92] Szmuness, W., J. H. Hoofnagle, C. E. Stevens, and A. M. Prince. 1976. Antibody against the hepatitis type B core antigen. *Am. J. Epidemiol.* 104:256-262.

[93] Seeff, L. B., G. W. Beebe, J. H. Hoofnagle, J. E. Normal, Z. Buskell-Bales, J. G. Waggoner, N. Kaplowitz, R. S. Koff, J. T. Petrini, E. R. Schiff, J. Shorey, and M. M. Stanley. 1987. A serological follow up of the 1942 epidemic of post vaccination hepatitis in the United States Army. *N. Engl. J. Med.* 316:965-970.

[94] Koziol, D., P. V. Holland, D. W. Alling, J. C. Melpolder, R. E. Solomon, R. E. Purcell, L. M. Hudson, F. J. Shoup, H. Krakauer, and H. J. Alter. 1986. Antibody to hepatitis B core antigen as a paradoxical marker for non-A, non-B hepatitis agents in donated blood. *Ann. Intern. Med.* 104:488-495.

[95] Stevens, C. E., R. D. Aach, F. B. Hollinger, J. W. Mosley, W. Szmuness, R. Kahn, J. Werch, and V. Edwards. 1984. Hepatitis B virus antibody in blood donors and the occurrence of non-A, non-B hepatitis in transfusion recipients. An analysis of the transfusion-transmitted viruses study. *Ann. Intern. Med.* 101: 733-738.

[96] Caspari, G., H. J. Beyer, G. Elbert, K. Koerner, P. Muss, F. W. Schunter, A. Uy, W. Gerlich, R. Thomssen, and H. Schmitt. 1989. Unsatisfactory specificities and sensitivities of six enzyme immunoassays for antibodies to hepatitis B core antigen. *J. Clin. Microbiol.* 27:2067-2072.

[97] Chau, K. H., E. H. Chun, R. H. Decker, and J. P. Brodsky. In F. B. Hollinger, S. M. Lemon, and H. S. Margolis (ed.), *Inter-national symposium on hepatitis and liver disease-1990*. The Williams & Wilkins Co., Baltimore.

[98] Schmidt, P. J., G. F. Leparc, and C. T. Samia. 1988. Comparison of assay for anti-HBc in blood donors. *Transfusion* 28:389- 391.

[99] Roth WK, Weber M, Seifried E. Feasibility and efficacy of routine PCR screening of blood donations for hepatitis C virus, hepatitis B virus, and HIV-1 in a blood-bank setting. *Lancet.* 1999;353:359-363.

[100] Jackson BR, Busch MP, Stramer SL, AuBuchon JP. The cost-effectiveness of NAT for HIV, HCV, and HBV in whole-blood donations. *Transfusion.* 2003 Jun;43(6):721-9

[101] Almeida RP, Cardoso DD. Detection of HBV DNA by nested-PCR in a HBsAg and anti-HBc negative blood bank donor. *J Clin Virol.* 2006 Jul;36(3):231-4. Epub 2006 Mar 29

[102] Kuhns MC, Busch MP. New strategies for blood donor screening for hepatitis B virus: nucleic acid testing versus immunoassay methods. *Mol Diagn Ther.* 2006;10(2):77-91.

[103] Gonzalez R, Echevarria JM, Avellon A, Barea L, Castro E. Acute hepatitis B virus window-period blood donations detected by individual-donation nucleic acid testing: a report on the first two cases found and interdicted in Spain. *Transfusion.* 2006;46(7):1138-42

[104] Offergeld R, Faensen D, Ritter S, Hamouda O. Human immunodeficiency virus, hepatitis C and hepatitis B infections among blood donors in Germany 2000-2002: risk of virus transmission and the impact of nucleic acid amplification testing. *Euro Surveill.* 2005;10(2):8-11.

[105] Busch MP. Should HBV DNA NAT replace HBsAg and/or anti-HBc screening of blood donors? *Transfus Clin Biol.* 2004;11(1):26-32

[106] Roth WK, Weber M, Petersen D, Drosten C, Buhr S, Sireis W, Weichert W, Hedges D, Seifried E. NAT for HBV and anti-HBc testing increase blood safety. *Transfusion.* 2002;42(7):869-75

[107] Ohnuma H, Tanaka T, Yoshikawa A, Murokawa H, Minegishi K, Yamanaka R, Lizuka HY, Miyamoto M, Satoh S, Nakahira S, Tomono T, Murozuka T, Takeda Y, Doi Y, Mine H, Yokoyama S, Hirose T, Nishioka K; Japanese Red Cross NAT Screening Research Group. The first large-scale nucleic acid amplification testing (NAT) of donated blood using multiplex reagent for simultaneous detection of HBV, HCV, and HIV-1 and significance of NAT for HBV. *Microbiol Immunol.* 2001;45(9):667-72.

[108] Tabor E, Epstein JS. NAT screening of blood and plasma donations: evolution of technology and regulatory policy. *Transfusio*n 2002; 42: 1230-1237

[109] Kessler HH, Preininger S, Stelzl E et al. Identificaion of different states of hepatitis B virus infection with a quantitative PCR assay. *Clin Diagn Lab Immunol* 2000; 7: 298-300.

[110] Kitchen A. Hepatitis B and blood safety Vaccine. 1998 Nov;16 Suppl:S34-7.

[111] Akhtar S, Younus M, Adil S, Hassan F, Jafri SH Epidemiologic study of chronic hepatitis B virus infection in male volunteer blood donors in Karachi, Pakistan *BMC Gastroenterol.* 2005;5:26

[112] Panhotra BR, Al-Bahrani A, Ul-Hassan Z. Epidemiology of antibody to hepatitis B core antigen screening among blood donors in Eastern Saudi Arabia. Need to replace the test by HBV DNA testing. *Saudi Med J.* 2005;26(2):270-3

[113] Wang B, Schreiber GB, Glynn SA, Kleinman S, Wright DJ, Murphy EL, Busch MP; Retrovirus Epidemiology Donor Study. Does prevalence of transfusion-transmissible viral infection reflect corresponding incidence in United States blood donors? *Transfusion.* 2005;45(7):1089-96

[114] CDC. Protection against viral hepatitis: recommendations of the Immunization Practices Advisory Committee (ACIP). *MMWR* 1990;39(No. RR-2).

[115] McCulloch M, Broffman M, Gao J, Colford JM Jr. Chinese herbal medicine and interferon in the treatment of chronic hepatitis B: a meta-analysis of randomized, controlled trials. *Am J Public Health.* 2002;92(10):1619-28.

[116] Liu J, McIntosh H, Lin H. Chinese medicinal herbs for chronic hepatitis B: a systematic review. *Liver.* 2001;21(4):280-6.

[117] Liu J, Lin H,McIntosh H. Genus Phyllanthus for chronic hepatitis B virus infection: a systematic review. *J Viral Hepat.* 2001;8(5):358-66.

[118] Liu JP, McIntosh H, Lin H. Chinese medicinal herbs for chronic hepatitis B Cochrane Database. *Syst Rev.* 2001;(1):CD001940.

[119] Liu JP, McIntosh H, Lin H. Chinese medicinal herbs for asymptomatic carriers of hepatitis B virus infection Cochrane Database. *Syst Rev.* 2001;(2):CD002231.

In: Hepatitis B Research Advances
Editor: Alicia P. Willis, pp. 59-76
ISBN: 978-1-60021-666-4

Chapter V

HEPATITIS B VIRUS AND OTHER BLOOD-BORNE VIRAL HEPATITIS INFECTIONS AMONG DRUG USERS: THE ROLE OF VACCINATION

***Fabio Lugoboni*[1], *Gianluca Quaglio*[1], *Sabrina Migliozzi*[2] and *Paolo Mezzelani*[1]**

[1]Medical Unit for Addictive Disorders, Department of Internal Medicine, University of Verona, Policlinico GB Rossi, 37134 Verona, Italy

[2]Addiction Treatment Clinic, Local Health District # 22, 37026 Bussolengo (VR), Italy

ABSTRACT

Hepatitis virus infections are traditionally a major health problem among drug users (DUs). Several factors may favor the rapid spread of hepatitis infection in this category of patients. HBV and HCV are easily transmitted through exposure to infected blood and body fluids. DUs often prepare and use drug solutions together. Many in the DU community are infected and this provides multiple opportunities for transmission to others. Many of these patients with chronic hepatitis virus infection are not aware of their infections and this facilitates the spread of the diseases. Viral hepatitis is not inevitable for DUs. Although multiple factors have prevented the development of vaccines for hepatitis C, both hepatitis A and hepatitis B can be prevented by immunization. The purpose of this overview is to show some epidemiological data about HBV and the other bloodborne viral hepatitis among DUs, to summarize and discuss the hepatitis vaccination in this population. HBV vaccination can also prevent hepatitis D infection which in most developed countries, is almost exclusively restricted to IDUs. Data on IDUs compliance to immunisation schedules and immunological responsiveness are scarce, and in particular the response of drug users to immunisation has received little attention.

Previous studies have reported a reduced antibody response to HBV vaccine among IDUs, but factors associated with a lack of response have not yet been well identified. We try to focus most significant results achieved in successful vaccination programs as reported in scientific literature and, little, from our direct experience. We trust that results reported in this Chapter will contribute to the international efforts aimed at improving hepatitis prevention. In our opinion HBV vaccination campaigns among DUs represent a highly effective form of health education. It also makes them aware of the other forms of infection and create the ideal basis for future vaccination campaigns against HCV.

INTRODUCTION

Hepatitis virus infections have long been a major health problem among persons who use illicit psychoactive drugs. Drug users (DUs) and particularly, injecting drug users (IDUs), are at increased risk for infection with at least four different hepatitis viruses: hepatitis A virus (HAV), hepatitis B virus (HBV), hepatitis C virus (HCV), and hepatitis D virus (HDV) [1-3]. We want to summarize briefly highlights of non-B hepatitis among Dus.

Injection of illicit drug is the most important risk factor for HCV infection in developed countries, with a mean prevalence among IDUs of 79% in the USA, 80% in western Europe and up to 92% in eastern Europe. Over the last two decades, there have been large increases in the numbers of non-injecting users of heroin in several countries, including the U.S. and Europe. Hepatitis C virus infection represents actually the leading cause of chronic liver disease in developed countries. There are an estimated 150 million chronic HCV carriers throughout the world, with an estimated 5 million in western Europe and 4 million in the USA. The World Health Organization estimates that the global prevalence of HCV infection ranges from 0.1% to 5% in different countries, with an average of 3% [4-14]. There are multiple reasons for the increased risks. HCV can be easily transmitted through exposure to infected blood, far less to body fluids. Thus multi-person use ("sharing") of drug preparation equipment and drug injection equipment can lead to rapid transmission of HCV among IDUs. The sharing of equipment for intranasal use of cocaine and of pipes for smoking crack cocaine may also lead to transmission of these viruses [15-20].

Hepatitis A is an acute, usually self-limiting infection of the liver caused by HAV. HAV infection occurs throughout the world, affecting 1.5 million people annually. Oral-fecal is the most common mode of transmission, with parenteral, transfusions, sexual (expecially by anal intercourse) and vertical transimmion occurring less frequently. HAV infection is highly correlated with poor social and economic conditions. Outbreaks have been reported among IDUs for many years and have occurred in the U.S. and Europe. Approximately 40 to 50% of IDUs in northern Europe are anti-HAV positive. Cross-sectional serologic surveys have shown IDUs to have higher anti-HAV seroprevalence than the general U.S. population. There are several reasons IDUs are at higher risk for HAV infection compared to the general population. Poor standards of living and unsafe sexual behaviors are strong risk factors leading to transmission. Contamination of drug solutions is believed to be the most common mode of transmission among IDUs, but needle sharing and blood-to-blood transmission have been suggested as possible patterns of transmission. HAV can also be potentially spread among DUs by contamination from rectally carried drugs. Various injected drugs have been associated with HAV outbreaks, including heroin, amphetamines and cocaine. HAV has been reported in cases of drug use not involving injection [21-28].

The World Health Organization has stated that, in developed countries, hepatitis A vaccination should be considered for specific high-risk populations such as injecting DUs. The Advisory Committee on Immunization Practices of the Centers for Disease Control and Prevention recommends hepatitis A vaccination for injecting DUs. Hepatitis A superimposed on chronic liver diseases is associated with more severe disease, including fulminant hepatic failure and a higher fatality rate. Hepatitis A thus poses a particular threat to injecting DUs because the high prevalence of HCV in this group. IDUs can be vaccinated in long-term vaccination programs [29-32].

HDV is a defective RNA virus that requires the presence of hepatitis B surface antigen (HBs-Ag) from HBV for HDV packaging and transmission. In Europe and in the U.S., HDV infection has virtually disappeared in transfusion subjects, remaining mainly confined to IDUs [33-34]. IDUs are currently the largest source of HDV infection in the Western world. Outbreaks of HBV-HDV coinfection have been reported most frequently among IDUs; [35-37].

HDV can be acquired either by co-infection with HBV or by superinfection of chronic HBs-Ag carriers. HDV coinfection can cause fulminant hepatitis more frequently than HBV infection alone while HDV supeinfection involves mostly serious chronic liver disease. Because HDV replication requires coinfection with HBV, immunoprophylaxis for HDV infection can be successfully achieved by vaccination against HBV. However, because no effective vaccine specific for HDV has been developed, there is currently no vaccine to protect carriers of HBs-Ag against superinfection [38,39].

HBV is transmitted primarily through parenteral and sexual exposure to HBs-Ag positive blood or other body fluids. Blood and body fluids typically contain high concentrations of the virus, making HBV transmission relatively efficient. HBV carriers may have acute hepatitis B or chronic infection. HBV may be transmitted not only through sharing of the needles and syringes for injecting drugs, but also through the cookers, cottons and rinse water used in the preparation of the drugs. HBV is a sexual transmitted disease and sexual route is a very common source of infection by percutaneous and mucosal exposure to blood or other body fluids of an infected person. HBV is transmitted also perinatally. Clinical manifestations of acute HBV can be severe and serious complications (i.e. cirrhosis and liver cancer) are more likely to develop in chronically infected persons. In the United States, approximately 1.2 million persons have chronic HBV infection and are sources for HBV transmission to others [1-3]. Death related to acute HBV occurs in approximately 1% of patients; DUs present a higher rate of fulminant, letal hepatitis probably related to the exposure to factors potentiating hepatic damage with acute HBV like alcohol, methamphetamine, acetaminophen [40]; HDV coinfection is another relevant factor of increased risk of fulminant hepatitis among IDUs.

In Europe, from 20% to 60% of IDUs are seropositive for HBV. IDUs are a very large proportion of all persons diagnosed with HBV in Europe, from 40–70% of all cases [41]. In the U. S., it is estimated that IDUs comprise 17% of all the new cases of hepatitis B. Among younger IDUs, HBV seroprevalence is about 25%, while for adult IDUs it is often more than 80%, compared with about 5% in the general U.S. population [42-44]. In 1999, after more than a decade of decline, the incidence of hepatitis B among men aged over 19 and among women aged 40 or over, has increased in the U.S. The most common risk factors among adults continue to be multiple sex partners, male with male sex, and injecting drug use [45]. High HBV prevalence among IDUs has been reported in several other countries with low endemic levels for HBV [46,47].

Below are briefly reported some epidemiologic data about DUs and HBV infection:

- The prevalence of HBV infection among DUs attending a methadone maintenance treatment (MMT) in Geneva (CH) showed great different rate between older DUs (80.5%) vs. younger DUs (20.1%); the incidence rate was 2.1% per person-year of follow-up [48].
- 70.1% the prevalence of anti-HBc in a cohort of IDUs enrolled in a syringe/needle exchange in Malmo (S); no seroconversion for HIV but 11.7 seroconversions/100 year at risk for HBV were observed [49].
- 49.7% the prevalence of anti-HBc in a cohortof IDUs attending a MMT in Wellington (NZ); 1,8% the presence of anti-HBc of previous vaccination [50].
- 42.5% tested positive for exposure to HBV among street-recruited IDUs from Buenos Aires (AR) [51].
- Among IDUs from Rio de Janeiro (BR), HBV seems to be more closely associated with unsafe sex, whereas HCV is positively correlated with high risk injecting behaviour [52].
- High rate of HCV (66%) but low rate of HBV (17%) in a cross-sectional survey of clients attending 21 specialist addiction treatment clinics in greater Dublin. Targeted vaccination for IDUs against HBV has shown more successful than previously reported in Ireland [53].
- Sera were tested positive for sntibodies against HBc (40.2%), against HCV (60.9%9 and against HIV (4.7%) in a large cohort of IDUs from Munich (D) [54].
- In a large cohort study among IDUs performed in Switzerland 53.3% were HBV positive and 41.2% were HAV positive. Authors illustrate the need for improving vaccination against HBV and HAV in IDUs [55].
- 55.2% tested positive for exposure to HBV among street-recruited IDUs from Tbilisi, Georgia [56].
- 46.5% tested positive for exposure to HBV among a large cohort of IDUs attending 16 addiction treatment clinics in NE of Italy [57].
- 24% tested positive for exposure to HBV in a cohort of cocaine and heroin HCV negative DUs; evidence for primarily role due to sexual behaviour; Providence, RI (USA) [58].
- New York City: DUs never-injectors infected with HBV and HIV appear to have become infected mainly through sexual transmission, whereas former injectors appear to have become infected with HCV and HIV mainly through injecting risk and with HBV through both injecting and sexual risk [59].

A vaccine against HBV was developed in 1982, and the first official recommendations for its use in high risk populations were published the same year. Nevertheless, only 10-25 percent of IDUs reported being offered vaccination in U.S. and Europe, and outbreaks of hepatitis B among this population continue to occur [1-5].

More recently also a combined anti-HAV and anti-HBV vaccine containing 720 ELISA units of HAV antigen obtained from formaldehyde-inactivated HAV and 20 mcg of recombinant HBV surface antigen (HbsAg), has been available since 1996.

Immunogenicity and Safety of HBV Vaccine

Although protective serum titer of anti-HBs (≥10 mIU/ml) develops in 95-99% of young adult in the overall population who receive a series of three doses, suboptimal responses (58%-77%) have been reported among IDUs, particularly when short protocols (0-1-2 months) are used [60-62]. Dysfunction of cell-mediated immunity, alcohol use, polydrug abuse, multiple bacterial infections, smoking, HCV positivity, and malnutrition are possible explanations of the lower immune response to anti-HBV vaccination in IDUs. The reduced rate of seroconversion has led many to administer 1-3 booster doses of the vaccine instead of the standard protocol [63,64]. In individuals with chronic hepatitis C infection, a very frequent condition among IDUs, a larger dosage of vaccine antigen (40-80 μg) or multiple exposures to vaccine antigen over a short interval may be useful [65]. HBV vaccination proved safe and is uninfluential for longstanding chronic hepatitis C.

No adverse reactions after vaccination among IDUs have been reported, similar to the general population. Pre-immunization testing may be cost effective among IDUs, where the expected prevalence of prior infection exceeds 30%. IDUs, particularly those known to be infected with HIV and/or HCV, should be subject to post-immunization testing for anti-HBs. Aggressive patient education regarding modes of HBV transmission should be provided to those who do not respond to the vaccination [66-68].

Although the presence of the antibody to hepatitis B core antigen (anti-HBc) in the absence of other HBV markers is uncommon in the general population (prevalence, 0.1%-2%) this condition is much more common among IDUs, where it can be over 30% [68,69].

The response to HBV vaccine in isolated anti-HBc carriers appears to vary greatly. It can range from a primary response, defined as ≥10 sample ratio units (SRU) of anti-HBs 1 month after the third dose of vaccine, to a booster or secondary response, defined as development of ≥50 SRU of anti-HBs after one dose of vaccine. In the case of an occult HBV carrier state, the subject could be infected with very low levels of HBV with HBV-DNA integrated in the host DNA. In this case the response to the vaccine should be a lack of anti-HBs production. In patients where the condition of isolated anti-HBc is a consequence of the reduction of anti-HBs levels, immune response should be secondary.

In studies where isolated anti-HBc subjects were vaccinated for HBV, generally there was a primary response [61,70,71]. Follow-up studies of IDUs with anti-HBc and no other markers showed resistance to HBV re-infection, indicating that these patients do not require vaccination [68]. The most likely explanation is that these patients have occult liver disease or are false positives. In some studies investigating serum samples positive only for anti-HBc (by either RIA or EIA), PCR analysis has shown between 25% and 45% to be positive for HBV-DNA [70,72]. Since there is no practical means for predicting the response to vaccination among IDUs with isolated anti-HBc, the most practical approach could be to provide HBV vaccination and then evaluate their response to the vaccination [68,71].

Factors Associated with Low Coverage of HBV Vaccination Among IDUs

It has been difficult to achieve high levels of hepatitis B vaccination among IDUs. The low coverage for HBV vaccination may be attributed to a combination of factors:

- economic and social barriers, such as homelessness, poverty, unemployment, lack of health insurance or lack of public health infrastructure that reduce access to medical care for IDUs [73];
- the absence of targeted healthcare programs to provide hepatitis B vaccination for this risk group [74,75];
- the low number of health workers with the required training and experience to carry out vaccination among IDUs [76]. Family practitioners may have a key role, because they often know the patient and their social circumstances. However, they may not have the necessary time (or compensation) to offer vaccination and they frequently see this as a public health task;
- the lack of awareness among IDUs about the risk of hepatitis [73];
- many healthcare workers have negative attitudes toward IDUs, assuming that these patients are “incurable” and “unmotivated” [77].

Venues Which Could Provide HBV Immunization for IDUs

Given the high risk of HBV infection, a lower post-vaccination seroprotection rate, and difficulties in follow-up with IDUs, it is important to administer the vaccination whenever possible. Places where IDUs meet could act as venues for efforts to increase vaccination. Several studies have shown that IDUs miss a number of opportunities for HBV vaccination. If vaccination were available at all these sites, many IDUs could receive vaccination.

- Methadone maintenance clinics and other drug treatment programs that require frequent attendance could provide vaccination services. Several studies have demonstrated the feasibility of administering HBV vaccine in these facilities, with a high completion rate. HBV vaccination programs should be integrated into the regular functioning of drug abuse treatment centers [61,62,78].
- The U.S. CDC recommends HBV vaccination in juvenile and adult correctional facilities, where a high percentage of DUs are present [79].
- CDC also recommends that all patients seeking treatment for sexually transmitted diseases should be vaccinated [80]. It has been shown that STD clinics can integrate vaccination into their routine work [81].
- HBV immunization can be successfully carried out in on-site syringe exchange services [82,83].

- Other venues that could provide immunization are emergency departments [77]. Previous reports suggest that emergency departments can be used for screening for sexually transmitted diseases and HIV [84]; HBV immunization could be an extension of such a program [76].

Note, however, that there could be problems in reaching IDUs prior to exposure to HBV and in maintaining vaccination schedules at some of these sites.

Considerations and Recommendations

The goal of hepatitis B vaccination programs is to achieve the highest possible rate of complete vaccination coverage. Considering the particular characteristics of IDUs, we believe the following recommendations should be stressed:

- the inability to ensure high rates of completion should not preclude the initiation of vaccination. Protective levels of antibody develop in 30% to 55% of adults following a single dose of vaccine and in 75% after 2 doses. Therefore a percentage of IDUs who have not completed the vaccination series are probably protected against HBV infection, although long term protection cannot be ensured without complete vaccination [85];
- in some countries, the lack of reimbursement is a major barrier to hepatitis B vaccination. Providing additional funding would overcome a major barrier to vaccinating IDUs [4];
- it is not necessary to add doses or restart the series if the interval between doses is longer than recommended, and there is no harm in receiving more than three doses [2];
- hepatitis B vaccination, is recommended as soon as possible after the start of illicit drug use, because approximately 50 to 70% of IDUs are infected within 5 years of initiating injecting drugs [3];
- implementation of needle-exchange programs is recommended [74]. The prescription of sterile syringes to IDUs by physicians is also a prevention-and-treatment strategy [73];
- a combination of street outreach and financial incentives, as used for other treatments [86], may provide a significant contribution [82];
- because many hepatitis infections, especially those caused by HCV, are asymptomatic and knowledge of infection status seems to be associated with behavior which is less risky for others, greater efforts should be made to increase the access of IDUs to hepatitis screening [76];
- if chronic infection is diagnosed, referring IDUs to counseling and treatment services, and referral of the IDUs' household contacts and sex partners to preventive services is recommended.

Hepatitis A Vaccine

Approximately 40 to 50% of IDUs in northern Europe are anti-HAV positive. Cross-sectional serologic surveys have shown IDUs to have higher anti-HAV seroprevalence than the general U.S. population [29]. Nonetheless, it should be noted that in some developed countries the HAV prevalence among IDUs is not different than that of the population in general [32]. In a recent study, HAV viremia persisted for an average of 79 days after the liver enzyme peak. In addition, HAV-RNA was detected several days before IgM antibodies to HAV were detected [87]. These results indicate that adults with HAV infection are viremic for as long as 30 days before the onset of symptoms and that the duration of viremia may be longer than previously described, suggesting that the opportunity for transmission may be greater than previously suspected [87,88].

The infection is usually self limiting, but typically produce fever, malaise, anorexia, nausea and abdominal discomfort; the severity of disease and mortality increases in older age groups. Complications of HAV infection can include fulminant hepatitis. The World Health Organization has recommended, in developed countries, HAV vaccination for specific high-risk populations such as DUs [29,67]. Vaccination is raccomended also in order to prevent superinfection in HCV positive subjects, which can be severe. Several inactivated and attenuated hepatitis A vaccines have been developed and evaluated in human clinical trials and in primate models but only inactivated vaccines have been evaluated for efficacy in controlled clinical trials; the vaccines currently licensed in the United States are inactivated vaccines. Commercially available inactivated hepatitis A vaccines have been extensively studied in persons of all ages. The majority of these studies demonstrate nearly a 100% seroconversion rate after a primary vaccination course in both adults and children.

HAV vaccination of IDUs can be carried out as a short-term measure to control outbreaks. Such a locally implemented approach, however, cannot entirely prevent future outbreaks in this mobile population.

A two-dose schedule is recommended for HAV vaccine, with the second dose 6-18 months after the first. The vaccine should be administrated intramuscolary into the deltoid muscle.

Pre-vaccination testing is not recommended for the vaccination of adolescent users of illegal drugs but might be warranted for adults [89]. The vaccine is considered to be very safe [90]. Seroconversion is defined as the achievement of anti-HAV levels of $\geq$20 mIU/ml, as determined by enzyme-linked immunosorbent assay, in previously seronegative vaccinees [91].

Inactivated hepatitis A virus vaccines are highly immunogenic in the general population; neutralizing antibodies are present in more than 94% of vaccinees one month after the first dose has been given, and essentially all recipients have a response after the second dose [90,91]. The only study which analyzed seroconversion among DUs reported high immunogenicity [31]. However, although all DUs proved seropositive after the second dose, the seroconversion rate after the first dose was much lower than in healthy subjects, with seroconversion percentages after 2 and 6 months of 37% and 44% respectively [31]. In the general population, the timing of the booster dose is not critical; efficient boosting occurs even when the two doses are 24 months or more apart [91]. In IDUs the second dose must be administered after a short time, preferably a 0-6 month schedule rather than a 0-12 month schedule, in order to reduce the unprotected period [31,92].

The final geometric mean titer (GMT) of anti-HAV among IDUs observed in this study was lower than that observed in the healthy subjects [67,31]. Similar results have emerged in subjects with chronic liver disease [93]. It is possible that the presence of other liver diseases also leads to a low antibody titer in IDUs, as occurs after vaccination against HBV. The lower GMT could affect the kinetics of antibody titers among IDUs, and the protection conferred by vaccination may be less durable in these patients. The persistence of anti-HAV titers, the duration of protection, and the possible need for additional vaccine booster doses should be addressed in future research [31].

Hepatitis A vaccination in IDUs generally induces a satisfactory immunoresponse, but patients should be tested to determine antibody response following vaccination. The evaluation of efficacy and immunogenicity of higher doses or alternative schedules of HAV vaccine in IDUs is needed in the future [31].

Combination Hepatitis A–Hepatitis B Vaccine

In addition to the monovalent vaccines against hepatitis A and B, a combined vaccine containing HBs-Ag and HAV-Ag is available. This vaccine appears to be both as safe and as effective as individual vaccines for the two viruses separately [94,95]. The 1-ml dose is given in a three-dose schedule at 0, 1, and 6 months .

Recently the combined vaccine was administered to 38 Italian DUs. The vaccine was well tolerated. Antibody response was evaluated at month 8, in 34 subjects. All had satisfactory responses for HAV and 33 subjects (97%) did for HBV. The vaccine, studied for the first time in IDUs, proved to be safe and immunogenic. Anti-HAV response was 1272 mIU/ml and 1726 mIU/ml for anti-HBV, however, and these titers are lower than those reported in literature for the general population. The study suggests that IDUs who are HAV/HBV-negative could be vaccinated with the combined vaccine [96]. The combined vaccine may not give sufficient protection if the course is not completed, a not unlikely scenario with IDUs. Booster vaccination to patients without satisfactory response could be an answer, as in other patient categories [95,96].

All of Authors of this chapter have been working as staff members in vaccination campaigns among DUs. We have tried to point out from our own experience the essential matters to mind for safe, successful vaccination programs in such hard-to-reach population. Remember that:

- Good addiction therapy means good adherence to vaccination programs.
- Vaccination programs with minor drop-out come out to be those administrated directly by addiction treatment clinics (ATC) personnel. In, our experience, this is the first of all issues.
- ATC which vaccinate less are also those who have worse adherence in vaccination programs.

- Vaccine boosters are no longer made to patients who have documentated seroconversion even if anti-HBs titre, through time, get lost.
- Main issue is no longer to quantify anti-HBs titre, but is there is any seroconversion or not; on that purpose it is mainly important to follow the vaccine schedule in estabilished times (0,1,6 months) with a serum control at the end; possible a booster dose in lack of response.
- Short schedule (0,1,2 months) even allowing to limit drot-out, come out to be less immunogenic comparing with usual one (0,1,6 months).
- DUs are less responsive both in immunogenicity and reactogenicity than general population.
- It is not worth it to vaccinate carriers of isolated anti-HBc: those subjects usually will not develop a new hepatitis B and are generally not responsive to boosters.
- Self-reported HBV infection status and immunization status in IDUs have proved to be unreliable and 52% claiming to be vaccinated were tested susceptible to HBV; some clinician invite to adopt a "Don't ask, vaccinate" vaccination policy for IDUs [76]; we believe that a good data collecting can be easier, less expensive and more correct.
- It should be remembered that HIV positive subjects have more difficult seroconversion to anti-HBs.
- Carriers of HCV chronic hepatitis could respond worse to HBV vaccination.
- A combined vaccine (HAV and HBV) can give better results than monovalent ones both in adherence and seroconversion rate.
- Prevent HBV and HAV among DUs can really limit the spread in general population.
- Italy was the fist developed country starting since 1991 with universal vaccination against HBV in newborn and teen-agers. Data about an effective role of universal vaccination in young DUs are not available in scientific literature. In an on-going study universal vaccination has proving to be immunogenic and really effective in a cohort of young DUs attending an ATC in NE of Italy (personal unpublished data).
- Schedule in use for HAV vaccination has been studied for travelers who need quick protection. When valuated among DUs it proved to be far less immunogenic and reactogenic than general population. Titer after seroconversion (whilst HBV vaccination) is relevant: when it is under 20 mUI/ml subject loose protection. Our personal opinion is that the former schedule (0, 1, 6 month) of the old vaccine (720 units of antigen) was more effective than new one. This can be a further reason for using combined vaccine (HAV and HBV).
- Finally, we believe that a successful vaccination campaign among DUs can be effective towards HIV spread. In a ATC near Verona (I), an HBV vaccination program was offered to 185 HBV and HIV negative IDUs attending drug treatments; 159 accepted, 26 declined. Both groups were followed over time and tested at list twice for HIV with a mean of 5.3 tests over 3460 person-months for the vaccination group and a mean of 3.5 tests in 638 person-months for non-vaccination group. 93% of the HBV vaccination group successfully completed the schedule; none of this group seroconverted for HIV during the follow-up, compared to 3 of the non-

vaccination group (5.6/100 person-years at risk; $p<.02$ by exact binomial test). 5 HBV seroconversions occurred in non-vaccination group, none in the other group. The excellent adherence to the vaccination schedule (that means more counseling contacts, more tests) maybe has led to lower risk behaviour (personal, unpublished data).

Vaccines for other Hepatitis Viruses: HCV and HDV

Hepatitis C Virus

HCV was discovered about in 1989. Since then, the epidemiology of HCV has undergone important changes, at least in industrialized countries. After the introduction of blood screening procedures in the early 1990s, transmission through transfusion of blood products has become a rare event. At present, the injection of illegal drugs is the most important risk factor for HCV infection in industrialized countries. HCV is usually the first blood-borne virus IDUs acquire [67,96,97].

In Europe, HCV prevalence in IDUs is extremely high, with a mean prevalence of 80% in Western Europe [7], and up to 92% in Eastern Europe [13]. Ninety per cent of cases of HCV infection in the EU involved injecting drug use [4]. In the US cross-sectional studies of DUs have reported prevalence rates ranging from 50% to more than 90% [97], with a mean prevalence of 79%, compared with a prevalence of 5% in the general U,S. population. It is estimated that 60% of the new cases of HCV in the US involve injecting drug use [4].

One study of DUs showed an interesting relationship between vaccination for hepatitis B and HCV serostatus. In this study, HBV seropositivity was strongly associated with HCV seropositivity. However, DUs who had been vaccinated for HBV were no more likely to be HCV seropositive than DUs who were HBV negative. HBV vaccination does not provide biological protection against HCV; however, vaccinating DUs against HBV may help to create a stronger pro-health attitude among DUs, leading to a reduction in HCV risk behavior [57].

Development of a vaccine for HCV has been delayed by numerous obstacles, including the lack of a suitable animal model, a high degree of genomic diversity, and the inability to grow large amounts of virus in vitro [98]. Consequently, prevention of HCV infection by other means will continue to be an indispensable strategy for the foreseeable future [99].

Conclusion

The health consequences of the higher prevalence of hepatitis virus infection among DUs extend beyond individual DUs to their sexual partners, households and communities as a whole.

Groups at high risk for HBV and/or HAV infection such as DUs will need special attention over the coming two decades, until vaccinated birth cohorts have reached the high-risk age.

Further studies Are required to clarify situations correlated with a lower immune response to vaccinations in DUs and for a vaccine schedule giving better immune protection. This is particulary needed for HAV vaccination among DUs: for this data are really scarce.

Coordinated hepatitis vaccination programs aimed at DUs could also provide infrastructure for future HIV and HCV vaccine initiatives when effective vaccines become available. It would indeed be paradoxical if, given the lengthy period of waiting for vaccines for HIV and HCV, coverage of DUs was poor due to lack of experience in the implementation of vaccine programs among at risk populations.

The ability of DUs to improve their health, reducing the risk of acquiring or transmitting hepatitis and other blood-borne diseases, is directly related to the quality of the prevention and care services they receive. Improving HAV and HBV vaccination programs for DUs is an important next step.

REFERENCES

[1] Centers for Diseases Control and Prevention. Inactivated hepatitis B vaccine. *MMWR Morb Mortal Wkly Rep* 1982; 31: 317-318.

[2] Rich, JD; Ching, CG; Lally, MA; Gaitanis, MM; Schwartzapfel, B; Charuvastra, A; Beckwith, CG; Flanigan, TP. A review of the case for hepatitis B vaccination of high-risk adults. *Am J Med* 2003; 114: 316–318.

[3] Centers for Disease Control and Prevention. Hepatitis B vaccination among high-risk adolescents and adults—San Diego, California, 1998–2001. *MMWR Morb Mortal Wkly Rep* 2002; 51: 618–621.

[4] Centers for Diseases Control and Prevention. Viral hepatitis and injecting drug users. *MMWR Morb Mortal Wkly Rep* 2002; http://www.cdc.gov/idu.

[5] European Monitoring Centre for Drugs and Drug Addiction (EMCDDA). *Annual report 2003: the state of the drugs problem in the European Union and Norway.* Lisbon: EMCDDA 2003; 24-28.

[6] Trépo, C & Pradat, P. Hepatitis C virus infection in Western Europe. *J Hepatol* 1999; 31:80-3.

[7] Gombas, W; Fischer, G; Jagsch, R. Prevalence and distribution of hepatitis C subtypes in patients with opioid dependence. *Eur Add Res* 2000; 6: 198-204.

[8] Diaz, T; Des Jarlais, DC; Vlahov, D. Factors associated with prevalent hepatitis C: differences among young adult injection drug users in lower and upper Manhattan, New York City. *Am J Public Health* 2001; 91: 23–30.

[9] Murrill, CS; Weeks, H; Castrucci, BC. Age-specific seroprevalence of HIV, hepatitis B virus, and hepatitis C virus infection among injection drug users admitted to drug treatment in 6 US cities. *Am J Public Health* 2002; 92: 385–387.

[10] Asselah, T; Bernuau, J; Marcellin, P. Prevalence of hepatitis C virus infection in patients hospitalized for hepatitis A. *Ann Intern Med* 1999; 130: 451.

[11] Guadagnino, V; Stroffolini, T; Rapicetta, M. Prevalence, risk factors, and genotype distribution of hepatitis C virus infection in the general population: a community-based survey in southern Italy. *Hepatol* 1997; 26: 1006-11.

[12] Edlin, BR; Kresina, TF; Raymond, DB. Overcoming barriers to prevention, care, and treatment of hepatitis C in illicit drug users. *Clin Infect Dis* 2005; 40: S276-285.

[13] Naoumov NV. Hepatitis C virus infection in Eastern Europe. *J Hepatol* 1999; 31: 84-87.

[14] Devi, KhS; Brajachand, N; Singh, HL; Singh, YM. Co-infection by human immunodeficiency virus, hepatitis B and hepatitis C virus in injecting drug users. *J Commun Dis* 2005; 37:73-7.

[15] Bellentani, S; Pozzato, G; Saccoccio, G. Clinical course and risk factors of hepatitis C virus related liver disease in the general population: report from the Dionysos Study. *Gut* 1999; 44: 874-80.

[16] Quaglio, GL; Lugoboni, F; Pajusco, B; Sarti, M; Talamini, G; Mezzelani, P; Des Jarlais, DC; GICS. Hepatitis C virus infection: prevalence, predictor variablees and preventive opportunities among drug users in Italy. *J Viral Hepat* 2003; 10:394-400

[17] Santana Rodriguez, OE; Male Gil, ML; Hernandez Santana, JF; Liminana Canal, JM, Martin Sanchez, AM. Prevalence of serological markers of HBV, HDV, HCV and HIV in non-injecting drug users compared to injection drug users in Gran Canaria, Spain. *Eur J Epidemiol* 1998; 14:555-61.

[18] van den Hoek, JAR ; van Haastrecht, HJA ; Goudsmit, J ; de Wolf, F ; Coutinho, RA. Prevalence, incidence, and risk factors of hepatitis C virus infection among drug users in Amsterdam. *J Infect Dis* 1990; 162:823-6.

[19] Gyarmathy, VA; Neaigus, A; Miller, M; Friedman, SR; Des Jarlais, DC. Risk correlates of prevalent HIV, hepatitis B virus, and hepatitis C virus infections among noninjecting heroin users. *J Acquir Immune Defic Syndr* 2002; 30:448-56.

[20] Winstock, AR; Anderson, CM; Sheridan, J. National survey of HIV and hepatitis testing and vaccination services provided by drug and alcohol agencies in Australia. *Med J Aust* 2006; 184:560-2.

[21] Cuthbert, JA. Hepatitis A: old and new. *Clin Microb Rev* 2001; 14: 38-58.

[22] Granerød, J & Crowcroft, N. Hepatitis A epidemiology in England and Wales. *Eurosurveillance Weekly* 2002; 6: 50.

[23] Crowcroft NS. Hepatitis A virus infections in injecting drug users. *Commun Dis Public Health* 2003; 6: 82-84.

[24] Hutin, YJ; Bell, BP; Marshall, KL. Identifying target groups for a potential vaccination program during a hepatitis A communitywide outbreak. *Am J Public Health* 1999; 89: 918-921.

[25] Hutin, YJ, Sabin, KM; Hutwagner, LC. Multiple modes of hepatitis A virus transmission among methamphetamine users. *Am J Epidemiol* 2000; 152: 186-192.

[26] Perrett, K; Granerød, J; Crowcroft, N; Carlisle, R. Changing epidemiology of hepatitis A: should we be doing more to vaccinate injecting drug users? *Commun Dis Public Health* 2003; 6: 97-100.

[27] Villano, SA; Nelson, KE; Vlahov, D; Purcell, RH; Saah, AJ; Thomas, DL. Hepatitis A among homosexual men and injection drug users: more evidence for vaccination. *Clin Infect Dis* 1997; 25: 726-728.

[28] van Steenbergen, JE; Tjon, G; van den Hoek, A; Koek, A; Coutinho, RA; Bruisten, SM. Two years' prospective collection of molecular and epidemiological data shows

limited spread of hepatitis A virus outside risk groups in Amsterdam, 2000-2002. *J Infect Dis* 2004; 189: 471-482.

[29] WHO. Hepatitis A vaccines. WHO position paper. *Weekly Epidemiol Rec* 2000; 5: 38-44.

[30] Vento, S; Garofano, T; Renzini, C. Fulminant hepatitis associated with hepatitis A virus superinfection in patients with chronic hepatitis C. *N Engl J Med* 1998; 338: 286-290.

[31] Quaglio, GL; Pajusco, B; Civitelli, P; Migliozzi, S; Des Jarlais, DC; Romano, L; Lechi, A; Mezzelani, P; Lugoboni F. Immunogenicity, reactogenicity and adherence with hepatitis A vaccination among drug users. *Drug Alcohol Depend* 2004; 74: 85-88.

[32] Lugoboni, F; Quaglio, GL; Pajusco, B; Foroni, M; Blengio, G; Talamini, G; Mezzelani, P; Des Jarlais, DC. Prevalence of hepatitis A among drug users in north-eastern Italy. *Eur J Public Health* 2005; 15: 464-6.

[33] Rosina, F; Saracco, G; Rizzetto, M. Risk of post-transfusion infection with the hepatitis delta virus. A multicenter study. *N Engl J* Med 1985; 312: 1488-1491.

[34] Polish, LB; Gallagher, M; Fields, HA; Hadler, SC. Delta hepatitis: molecular biology and clinical and epidemiological features. *Clin Microbiol Rev* 1993; 6: 211-229.

[35] Gaeta, GB; Stroffolini, T; Chiaramente, M. Chronic hepatitis D: a vanishing disease? An italian multicenter study. *Hepatol* 2000; 32: 824-827.

[36] Poovorawan, Y; Chatchatee, P; Chongsrisawat, V. Epidemiology and prophylaxis of viral hepatitis: a global prospective. *J Gastroenterol Hepatol* 2002; 17: 155-166.

[37] Caredda, F; Rossi, E; D'Arminio Manforte, A; Farci, P; Lavorini, C. An outbreak of delta agent among a group of drug addicts and their close contacts. *J Infect Dis* 1984; 149: 286-287.

[38] Lettau, LA ; McCarthy, JG ; Smith, MH. Outbreak of severe hepatitis due to delta and hepatitis B viruses in parenteral drug abusers and their contacts. *N Engl J Med* 1987; 317: 1256-1262.

[39] Farci, P. Delta hepatitis: an update. *J Hepatol* 2003; 39: S212-219.

[40] Garfein, RS; Bower, WA; Loney, CM; Hutin, YJ; Xia, GL; Jawanda, J; Groom, AV; Nainan, OV; Murphy, JS; Bell, BP. Factors associated with fulminant liver failure during an outbreak among injection drug users with acute hepatitis B. *Hepatol* 2004; 40:790-2.

[41] O'Donovan, D; Cooke, RP; Joce, R; Eastbury, A; Waite, J; Stene-Johansen, K. An outbreak of hepatitis A amongst injecting drug users. *Epidemiol Infect* 2001; 127: 469-473.

[42] Centers for Disease Control and Prevention. Achievements in public health: hepatitis B vaccination—United States, 1982–2002. *MMWR Morb Mortal Wkly Rep* 2002; 51: 549–563.

[43] Centers for Disease Control and Prevention. Hepatitis B vaccination for injection drug users-Pierce County, Washington, 2000. *MMWR Morb Mortal Wkly Rep* 2001; 50: 388–399.

[44] Edeh, J & Spalding, P. Screening for HIV, HBV, and HCV markers among drug users in treatment in rural south-east England. *J Public Health Med* 2000;22:531-9.

[45] Centers for Disease Control and Prevention. Incidence of acute hepatitis B-United States, 1990-2002. *MMWR Morb Mortal Wkly Rep* 2004; 52: 1252–1254.

[46] Roy, E; Haley, N; Lemire, N; Boivin, JF; Leclerc, P; Vincelette, J. Hepatitis B virus infection among street youths in Montreal. *CMAJ* 1999; 161: 689-693.

[47] Maher, L; Chant, K; Jalaludin, B; Sargent, P. Risk behaviours and antibody hepatitis B and C prevalence among injecting drug users in south-western Sydney, Australia. *J Gastroenterol Hepatol* 2004; 19: 1114-1120.

[48] Broers, B; Junet, C; Bourquin, M; Deglon, JJ; Perrin, L; Hischel B. Prevalence and incidence rate of HIV, HBV and HCV among drug users on methadone maintenance treatment in Geneva between 1988 and 1995. *AIDS* 1998; 12: 2059-66.

[49] Mansson, AS; Moestrup, T; Nordenfelt, E; Widell, A. Continued transmission of hepatitis B and C viruses, but no transmission of human immunodeficiency virus among intravenous drug users partecipating in a syringe/needle exchange program. *Scand J Infect Dis* 2000; 32: 253-8.

[50] Carter, H; Robinson, G; Hanlon, C; Hailwood, C; Massarotto, A. Prevalence of hepatitis B and hepatitis C ia a methadone clinic population : implication for hepatitis B vaccination. *N Z Med J* 2001; 114: 324-6.

[51] Weissenbacher, M; Rossi, D; Radulich, G; Sosa-Estefani, S; Vila, M; Vivas, E; Avila, MM; Cuchi, P; Rey, J; Peralta, LM. High seroprevalence of bloodborne viruses among street-recruited injection drug users from Buenos Aires, Argentina. *Clin Infect Dis* 2003; 37: 348-52.

[52] Oliveira, ML ; Bastos, FI ; Telles, PR ; Yoshida, CF ; Schwartzmayer, HG ; Paetzold, U ; Pauli, G ; Schreier, E. Prevalence ahd risk factors for HBV, HCV and HDV infections among injecting drug users from Rio de Janeiro, Brazil. *Braz J Med Biol Res* 1999; 32: 1107-14.

[53] Grogan, L; Tiernan, M; Geogeghan, N; Smyth, B; Keenan, E. Bloodborne virus infections among drug users in Ireland: a retrospective cross-sectional survey of screening, prevalence, incidence and hepatitis B immunization uptake. *Ir J Med Sci* 2005; 174: 14-20.

[54] Backmund, M; Meyer, K; Schuetz, C; Reimer, J. Factors associated with exposure to hepatitis B virus in injection drug users. *Drug Alcohol Depend* 2006; 84: 154-9.

[55] Gerlich, M; Gschwend, P; Uchtenhagen, A; Kramer, A; Rehm, J. Prevalence of hepatitis B and HIV infections and vaccination rates in patients entering the heroin-assisted treatment in Switzerland between 1994-2002. *Eur J Epidemiol* 2006; 21:545-9.

[56] Shapatava, E; Nelson, KE; Tsertsvadze, T; del Rio C. Risk behaviour and HIV, hepatitis B and hepatitis C seroprevalence among injection drug users in Georgia. *Drug Alcohol Depend* 2006; 82: 35-8.

[57] Quaglio, GL; Lugoboni, F; Pajusco, B; Sarti, M; Talamini, G; Lechi, A; Mezzelani, P; Des Jarlais, DC. Factors associated with hepatitis C virus infection in injection and noninjection drug users in Italy. *Clin Infect Dis* 2003; 37:33-40.

[58] Rich, JD; Anderson, BJ; Schwartzapfel, B; Stein, MD. Sexual risk for hepatitis B virus among hepatitis C virus-negative heroin and cocaine users. *Epidemiol Infect* 2006; 143: 478-84.

[59] Gyarmathy, VA ; Neaigus, A ; Miller, M ; Friedman, SR ; Des Jarlais, DC. Risk correlates of prevalent HIV, hepatitis B virus and hepatitis C virus infections among noninjecting heroin users. *J Acquir Immune Defic Syndr* 2002; 30:448-56.

[60] Lum, PJ; Ochoa, KO; Hahn, JA; Shafer, KP; Evans, JL; Moss, AR. Hepatitis B virus. Immunization among young injection drug users in San Francisco, Calif: The UFO Study. *Am J Public Health* 2003; 93: 919-923.

[61] Quaglio, GL; Talamini, G; Lugoboni, F; Lechi, A; Venturini, L; GICS, Des Jarlais, DC; Mezzelani, P. Compliance with hepatitis B vaccination in 1175 heroin users and risk factors associated with lack of vaccine response. *Addiction* 2002; 97: 985-992.

[62] Lugoboni, F; Migliozzi, S; Schiesari, F; Pauletto, N; Bovo, GL; Mezzelani, P. Immunoresponse to hepatitis B vaccination and adherence campaign among injecting drug users. *Vaccine* 1997; 15: 1014-1016.

[63] Lugoboni, F; Migliozzi, S; Mezzelani, P; Pajusco, B; Ceravolo, R; Quaglio, GL. Progressive decrease of Hepatitis B in a cohort of drug users followed over a period of 15 years: the impact of anti-HBV vaccination. *Scand J Infect Dis* 2004; 36: 131-133.

[64] Quaglio, GL ; Lugoboni, F ; Pajusco, B ; Sarti, M ; Mezzelani, P. Managerial considerations in implementing hepatitis B vaccination programs among drug-using cohorts. *Addiction* 2002; 97: 1613-1614.

[65] Idilman, R; De Maria, N; Colantoni, A; Nadir, A; Van Thiel, DH. The effect of high dose and short interval HBV vaccination in individuals with chronic hepatitis C. *Am J Gastroenterol* 2002; 97: 435-439.

[66] van Houdt, R; Sonder, GJ; Dukers, NH; Bovee, LP; van den Hoek, A; Coutinho, RA, Briusten, SM. Impact of a targeted hepatitis B vaccination program in Amsterdam, The Netherlandas. *Vaccine* 2006; 12; [Epub ahead of print].

[67] Lemon, SM & Thomas, DL. Vaccines to prevent viral hepatitis. *N Engl J Med* 1997; 33: 196–204.

[68] Quaglio, GL; Lugoboni, F; Vento, S; Lechi, A; Accordini, A; Bossi, C; Faccini, M; mezzelani, P. Isolated presence of antibody to hepatitis b core antigen in injection drug users: do they need to be vaccinated? *Clin Infect Dis* 2001; 32: E143-144.

[69] Gandhi, RT; Wurcel, A; Lee, H. Isolated Antibody to Hepatitis B Core Antigen in Human Immunodeficiency Virus Type-1–Infected Individuals. *Clin Infect Dis* 2003; 36: 1602–1605.

[70] Silva, AE ; McMahon, BJ ; Parkinson, AJ ; Sjogren, MH ; Hoofnagle, JH ; Di Bisceglie, AM. Hepatitis B virus DNA in persons with isolated antibody to hepatitis B core antigen who subsequently received hepatitis B vaccine. *Clin Infect Dis* 1998; 26: 895-897.

[71] Minniti, F; Baldo, V; Trivello, R. Response to HBV vaccine in relation to anti-HCV and anti-HBc positivity: a study in intravenous drug addicts. *Vaccine* 1999; 17: 3083-3085.

[72] Torbenson, M ; Kannangai, R ; Astemborski, J ; Strathdee, SA ; Vlahov, D ; Thomas, DL. High Prevalence of Occult Hepatitis B in Baltimore injection drug users. *Hepathol* 2004; 39: 51–57.

[73] Rich, JD; McKenzie, M; Macalino, GE. A syringe prescription program to prevent infectious disease and improve health of injection drug users. *J Urban Health* 2004; 81: 112-134.

[74] François, G; Hallauer, J; Van Damme, P. Hepatitis B vaccination: how to reach risk groups. *Vaccine* 2002; 21: 1–4.

[75] Kuo, I; Sherman, SG; Thomas, DL; Strathdee, SA. Hepatitis B virus infection and vaccination among young injection and non-injection drug users: missed opportunities to prevent infection. *Drug Alcohol Depend* 2004; 73: 69–78.

[76] Kuo, I; Mudrick, DW; Strathdee, SA; Thomas, DL; Sherman, SG. Poor validity of self-reported hepatitis B virus infection and vaccination status among young drug users. *Clin Infect Dis* 2004; 38: 587–590.

[77] Knowlton, AR; Hoover, DR; Chung, SE. Access to medical care and service utilization among injection drug users with HIV/AIDS. *Drug Alcohol Depend* 2001; 64: 55–62.

[78] Quaglio, GL; Lugoboni, F; Mezzelani, P. HBV vaccination should be performed in service centres for drug users: an Italian experience. *J Public Health* 2004; 26: 320.

[79] Weinbaum, C; Lyerla, R; Margolis, HS. Prevention and control of infections with hepatitis viruses in correctional settings. Centers for Disease Control and Prevention. *MMWR Mortal Wkly Rep* 2003; 52: 1–36.

[80] Centers for Disease Control and Prevention. Sexually transmitted diseases treatment guidelines 2002. *MMWR Morb Mortal Wkly Rep* 2002; 51: 1–78.

[81] van Steenbergen JE. Working group vaccination high-risk groups hepatitis B for the Netherlands. Results of an enhanced-outreach programme of hepatitis B vaccination in the Netherlands (1998-2000) among men who have sex with men, hard drug users, sex workers and heterosexual persons with multiple partners. *J Hepatol* 2002; 37: 507-513.

[82] Des Jarlais, DC ; Fisher, DG ; Newman, JC. Providing hepatitis B vaccination to injection drug users: referral to health clinics vs on-site vaccination at a syringe exchange program. *Am J Public Health* 2001; 91: 1791-1792.

[83] Altice, FL; Bruce, RD; Walton, MR; Buitrago, MI. Adherence to hepatitis B virus vaccination at syringe exchange sites. *J Urban Health* 2005; 82: 151-61.

[84] Rothman, RE; Ketlogetswe, KS; Dolan, T; Wyer, PC; Kelen, GD. Preventive care in the emergency department: should emergency departments conduct routine HIV screening? A systematic review. *Acad Emerg Med* 2003; 10: 278–285.

[85] Goldstein, ST; Alter, MJ; Williams, IT. Incidence and risk factors for acute hepatitis B in the United States, 1982–1998: implications for vaccination programs. *J Infect Dis* 2002; 185: 713–719.

[86] Tulsky, JP ; Hahn, JA ; Long, HL. Can the poor adhere? Incentives for adherence to TB prevention in homeless adults. *Int J Tuberc Lung Dis* 2004; 8: 83-91.

[87] Bower, WA; Nainan, OV; Han, X; Margolis, H. Duration of viremia in hepatitis A virus infection. *J Infect Dis* 2000; 182: 12–17.

[88] Crowcroft, NS. Hepatitis A virus infections in injecting drug users. *Commun Dis Public Health* 2003; 6: 82-84.

[89] Centers for Disease Control. Prevention of hepatitis A through active or passive immunization: recommendations of the Advisory Committee on Immunization Practices (ACIP). *MMWR Morb Mortal Wkly Rep* 1999; 48: 1-37.

[90] Craig, AS & Schaffner, W. Prevention of hepatitis A with the hepatitis A vaccine. *N Engl J Med* 2004; 350: 476-481.

[91] Andre, F; Van Damme, P; Safary, A; Banatvala, J. Inactivated hepatitis A vaccine: immunogenicity, efficacy, safety and review of official recommendations for use. *Expert Rev Vaccines* 2002; 1: 9-23.

[92] Lugoboni, F; Quaglio, GL; Residori, M; Mecenero, V; Mezzelani, P. Hepatitis A virus vaccination among injecting drug users: do we have to change the vaccination schedule? *Clin Infect Dis* 2000; 31: 847-848.

[93] Keeffe, EB; Iwarson, S; McMahon, BJ. Safety and immunogenicity of hepatitis in patients with chronic liver disease. *Hepatol* 1998; 27: 881–886.

[94] Joines, RW; Blatter, M; Abraham, B. A prospective, randomized, comparative US trial of a combination hepatitis A and B vaccine (Twinrix®) with corresponding monovalent vaccines (Havrix® and Engerix-B®) in adults. *Vaccine* 2001; 19: 4710–4719.

[95] Wolters, B; Junge, U; Dziuba, S; Roggendorf, M. Immunogenicity of combined hepatitis A and B vaccine in elderly persons. *Vaccine* 2003; 21: 3623–3628.

[96] Mathei, C; Buntinx, F; van Damme, P. Seroprevalence of hepatitis C markers among intravenous drug users in western European countries: a systematic review. *J Viral Hepat* 2002; 9: 157-173.

[97] Chou, R; Clark, EC; Helfand, M; U.S. Preventive Services Task Force. Screening for hepatitis C virus infection: a review of the evidence for the U.S. Preventive Services Task Force. *Ann Intern Med* 2004; 140: 465-479.

[98] Berzofsky, JA; Ahlers, JD; Janik, J. Progress on new vaccine strategies against chronic viral infections. *J Clin Invest* 2004; 114: 450-462.

[99] Kew, M; Francois, G; Lavanchy, D. Prevention of hepatitis C virus infection. *J Viral Hepat* 2004, 11: 198–205.

In: Hepatitis B Research Advances
Editor: Alicia P. Willis, pp. 77-97
ISBN: 978-1-60021-666-4

Chapter VI

IMMUNOTHERAPEUTIC EFFICACY OF DNA VACCINE ALONE AND COMBINED WITH ANTIVIRAL DRUGS IN THE CHRONIC DUCK HEPATITIS B VIRUS INFECTION MODEL

Alexandre Thermet[1,2], Thierry Buronfosse[1,2,3], Franck Le Guerhier[1,2], Pierre Pradat[4], Christian Trepo[1,2,4], Fabien Zoulim[1,2,4] and Lucyna Cova[1,2*]

[1]INSERM, Unit 871, Lyon F-69424, France
[2]Université Lyon 1, IFR62, Lyon F-69008, France
[3]Ecole Nationale Vétérinaire, Marcy l'Etoile F-69280, France
[4]Department of Hepatology, Hotel-Dieu, Lyon F-69002, France

ABSTRACT

Design of novel treatment options for chronic hepatitis B virus (HBV) infections is actually of particular importance, since current therapies based on IFNα and nucleoside analogues (lamivudine, adefovir) are limited by the emergence of drug–resistant mutants and the persistence of intranuclear covalently closed circular viral DNA (cccDNA) responsible for persistence of infection. Increasing number of recent data suggest that rationale therapy of hepatitis B may combine the use of antiviral drugs and immunotherapeutic approaches. In this regard, DNA-based immunization appears as a pertinent new approach, inducing rapid, potent and specific immune responses to hepadnavirus structural proteins as demonstrated in naïve chimpanzees, woodchuck and

* Correspondence concerning this article should be addressed to Lucyna Cova, Mailing address: INSERM, U871, 151 Cours Albert Thomas, 69003 Lyon, France. Phone: (33) 4 72 68 19 81; Fax: (33) 4 72 68 19 71; E-mail address: cova@lyon.inserm.fr.

duck models. However the therapeutic DNA vaccination against chronic hepatitis B was less investigated.

Our aim was to explore in the chronic duck HBV (DHBV) infection model, whether DNA vaccine-based immunotherapy in combination or not with an antiviral drug (adefovir, lamivudine,) treatment is able to enhance cccDNA clearance and break humoral immune tolerance in chronic DHBV carriers. We have first realized a study associating adefovir with DNA vaccine against DHBV envelope and compared herein its therapeutic efficacy with our recent study combining lamivudine with DNA vaccine against viral envelope and/or core proteins.

In adefovir-DNA study, a group of DHBV-infected ducks received adefovir treatment (weeks 6-10 p.i.) in combination or not with DNA immunization to DHBV preS/S protein (weeks 6, 9, 12 and 22). A marked drop in viremia titres (97%), reaching the limit of detection of the assay, was observed during the 4 weeks of drug administration in all adefovir-treated as compared with untreated ducks, although it was followed by a rebound of viral replication after drug withdrawal. At the end of follow-up, analysis of intrahepatic DHBV DNA revealed a more pronounced decrease in viral DNA in combination therapy group as compared with DNA or adefovir monotherapy groups suggesting a trend to an additive effect of drug and DNA vaccine. However only few animals eliminated liver viral DNA and no correlation with humoral anti-preS response restoration was observed.

In lamivudine-DNA study, lamivudine was administrated alone in combination with DNA vaccine to DHBV envelope and/or core proteins. DHBV-carrier ducks received lamivudine treatment earlier (weeks 1-8), with higher number of DNA immunizations (weeks 6,10,14,28,35), shorter overlap with DNA vaccination (2 weeks), larger amounts of plasmid and a longer follow-up in larger animal groups. A decrease in viremia titers (70%) was observed in all lamivudine-treated compared to untreated animals, although it was limited to only the first 3 weeks of lamivudine treatment and was followed by a rapid rebound in viral replication. Interestingly about 30% animals, which received DNA vaccine alone or in association with lamivudine had cccDNA levels that were at or under the lower real-time PCR detection limit and was associated for majority of them with restoration of anti-preS response.

In conclusion, our comparison of two combination therapy studies associating DNA vaccine-based immunotherapy with either adefovir or lamivudine indicates a better efficacy of the lamivudine-DNA protocol. In adefovir-DNA study, only modest effect in term of viral cccDNA clearance and seroconversion was observed, in spite of higher antiviral potency of the drug. By contrast, data obtained in lamivudine-DNA study provided a first demonstration that DNA vaccine alone and associated with drug treatment was able to induce drastic and sustained suppression of viremia and enhance viral cccDNA clearance in one third of DHBV-carriers, which was tightly associated with break of immune tolerance. Because both studies differed not only by the choice of drug but, importantly, by the design of DNA immunization protocol, thus number of factors known to determine the success of genetic vaccination such as plasmid construct, amount of plasmid DNA, number of DNA injections and immunization schedule may play an important role in better therapeutic efficacy of lamivudine-DNA study. Further investigations aiming to increase the potency of DNA vaccine–based immunotherapeutics need to be performed in animal models in view to obtain a complete and sustain recovery from chronic hepatitis B.

Keywords: Hepatitis B, duck HBV (DHBV), hepatitis B; lamivudine; adefovir; DNA vaccine; combination therapy; immunotherapy; closed circular viral DNA (cccDNA); animal model.

INTRODUCTION

Chronic hepatitis B virus (HBV) infection remains a major public health problem with 350 million virus carriers who are of a high risk of cirrhosis and hepatocellular carcinoma [7]. HBV-infected patients are currently treated with interferon (IFN)-α and nucleotide analogues such as lamivudine, adefovir or entacavir. Lamivudine (2',3'-dideoxy-3'-thiacytidine or 3-TC) is a potent and the most widely anti-HBV drug actually used, known to induce a rapid decline in viral load by 3-5 log10copies/ml after a year therapy [30]. However, long-term lamivudine therapy led to the emergence of drug-resistant mutants, which results in viral breakthrough. [15,30,47]. Adefovir dipivoxil (PMEA), a recently developed antiviral compound appeared initially of particular interest since it inhibited both wild-type and lamivudine-resistant HBV mutants, however a long-term adefovir treatment also results in drug-resistance [2,33,43,47]. Thus, the efficacy of current treatments is limited by the emergence of drug–resistant mutants and the persistence of covalently closed circular viral DNA (cccDNA) in the nucleus of infected cells, which is responsible for viral relapse after treatment withdrawal [2,39,45,47].

Interestingly, studies in lamivudine-treated chronic HBV-carrier patients clearly demonstrated that the marked reduction in viremia during antiviral treatment is followed by a break of T cell nonresponsiveness resulting in the transient restoration of HBV-specific CD4+ T cell activity followed, by cytotoxic T cell activity and the CD8+ T cell proliferation [3-5]. Therefore, a concept of combination therapy has been proposed that is based on association of nucleoside analogues treatment, able to transiently restore antiviral immune responses, with immune therapeutics aiming to stimulate these responses in a sustained manner [5].

Recent studies have investigated such combination therapies in the chronic woodchuck HBV (WHV)-carrier woodchucks and showed that the association of clevudine (L-FMAU) treatment with WHsAg alum-adjuvanted vaccine led to the inhibition of chronic hepatitis and delay in onset of hepatocellular carcinoma [14]. These promising results have been strengthened by a recent clinical study in HBV carriers showing a benefit of lamivudine combination with HBsAg vaccine in terms of serum HBV DNA negativity and absence of variants emergence as compared with lamivudine monotherapy treated patients group [13].

Within the actual immunotherapeutic strategies, DNA-based vaccine appears as a pertinent new approach, inducing rapid, strong and specific immune responses to HBV, WHV and DHBV structural proteins in naïve animals as documented by several studies [9,11,22,27,34,35,36,40,42,44]. However, the therapeutic DNA vaccination against chronic HBV infection was less investigated. The ability of a DNA vaccine to HBV envelope to decrease viral replication was demonstrated in the transgenic mouse lineage, E36 [23,28], although viral cccDNA clearance cannot be analyzed in this model. The DNA vaccine-based therapy of chronic DHBV-carrier ducks resulted in variable efficacy. We have previously reported that DNA immunization of carriers with plasmid expressing viral large envelope protein induced a marked decrease in DHBV replication, although the number of animals included in that study was small and no correlation with a break of humoral immune tolerance was observed [34]. Treatment of DHBV-carrier ducks with combination of entecavir (ETV) with DNA vaccine to virus envelope and core showed a potent antiviral effect of ETV, although DNA vaccination alone or combined with ETV have not resulted in reduction of viral replication [10].

We report here the results of two independent studies conducted in our laboratory which allowed us to compare the efficacy and safety of such chemo-immunotherapy associating either DNA vaccine with adefovir [18] or lamivudine [41]. We have chosen the DHBV-infected duck model for these studies, since it is a pivotal model for evaluation of novel anti-HBV approaches and appreciation of their impact on intranuclear cccDNA clearance [1,8,19,26]. The comparison of both studies has highlighted the importance of different factors such as choice of drug, plasmid constructs, amount of plasmid DNA and therapeutic protocol design, in the antiviral efficacy of such DNA-vaccine-based immunotherapies.

MATERIALS AND METHODS

Drug

The 9-(2-phosphomethoxyethyl) adenine (adefovir (PMEA), a generous gift of Gilead Sciences, and the β-L(-)-2',3'-dideoxy-3'thia-cytidine (3TC, lamivudine), generously provided by J. Rhodes (GlaxoSmithKline), were dissolved in phosphate buffered saline (pH 7.2).

Plasmid Expression Vectors

DHBV large envelope (preS/S) and core (C) genes were previously cloned in pCI vector under the control of CMV promoter and are referred to pCI-preS/S [34] and pCI-C [40] respectively. Plasmids were purified by Endotoxin-Free Giga prep (Qiagen, Hilden, Germany). The ability of these plasmids constructs to express DHBV large envelope and core protein has been previously demonstrated [34,40] and was re-confirmed before their use in immunotherapeutic protocols.

Animals

DHBV-carrier Pekin ducks (*Anas domesticus*) ducks were obtained by intravenous inoculation of 3-day-old ducklings with a viremic serum pool ($2x10^8$ viral genome equivalent (vge)/animal) as previously described [8,16]. Ducks were housed at the facilities of the National Veterinary School of Lyon (ENVL, Marcy l'Etoile, France) Animal experimentation was performed in accordance with guidelines for animal care of the ethics committee of ENVL.

Table 1. Summary of protocols and effects on intrahepatic viral DNA clearance of two DNA vaccine-based immunotherapeutic studies

(A) Adefovir-DNA vaccine study

Treatment	Group	Adefovir	Plasmid DNA immunization	Undetectable[b] DHBV DNA	cccDNA[c] clearance
Controls	1	-	pCI or none	1/7 (0)	NT
DNA Monotherapy	2	-	pCI-preS/S	1/5 (1)	NT
Adefovir Monotherapy	3	+	none	0/5 (0)	NT
Combination Therapy	4	+	pCI-preS/S	2/5 (1)	NT

(B) Lamivudine-DNA vaccine study

Treatment	Group	Lamivudine	Plasmid DNA immunization	Undetectable[b] DHBV DNA	cccDNA[c] clearance
Controls	1	-	pCI or none	1/5	0/5 (0)
DNA Monotherapy	2	-	pCI-preS/S	0/4	0/4 (0)
	3		pCI-preS/S & pCI-C	2/4	1/4 (1)
	4		pCI-C	3/7	3/7 (2)
Lamivudine Monotherapy	5	+	pCI or none	0/7	0/7 (1)
Combination Therapy	6	+	pCI-preS/S	4/8	3/8 (3)
	7		pCI-preS/S & pCI-C	2/3	2/3 (0)
	8		pCI-C	0/4	0/4 (0)

[a]DHBV-carrier ducks were assigned into following groups: controls (untreated or empty vector-treated); DNA vaccine monotherapy with plasmids encoding either viral envelope (pCI-preS/S) and/or core (pCI-C); antiviral drug (adefovir or lamivudine) monotherapy; combination therapy with antiviral drug and DNA vaccine as detailed in Materials and Methods.

[b]number of ducks presenting undetectable liver DHBV DNA/number of treated ducks as assessed by Southern blot analysis of autopsy liver samples at the end of follow-up;

[c]cccDNA clearance was defined as cccDNA levels at or below real-time PCR detection limit (0.04 ccc-DHBV DNA copies/cell);

number of animals which seroconverted is indicated in parentheses. NT- not tested.

Therapeutic Protocols

In adefovir-DNA protocol DHBV-carrier ducks were assigned into four groups (6-9 animals/group) (Table 1): group 1 (untreated or empty vector-treated controls), group 2 (DNA monotherapy with pCI-preS/S), group 3 (adefovir monotherapy), group 4 (combination therapy with adefovir and pCI-preS/S) (Table 1A). Adefovir administration started at week 6 post-hatch at 15 mg/kg per day, via intraperitoneal (i.p.) route as previously described [32], and was followed by drug administration for 5 days/week during 4 consecutive weeks. DNA immunization began at week 6 p.i. and was followed by 3 boosts (weeks 9, 12 and 22) (Figure 1). Ducks received a total of 150 μg of pCI-preS/S or pCI plasmid/animal/boost at three injection sites as described in detail previously [34].

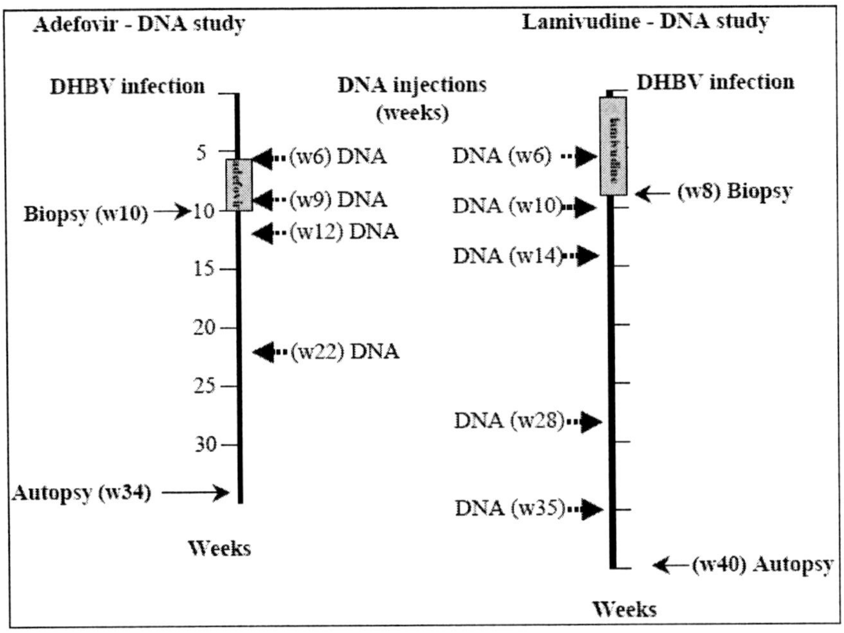

Figure 1. Design of therapeutic protocols for adefovir-DNA and lamivudine-DNA studies. DHBV-carriers ducks were obtained by i.v. inoculation of 3-day old ducklings with viremic DHBV serum pool. The antiviral treatment (grey bar) consisted in either adefovir or lamivudine administration, which was associated or not with DNA-based immunizations against DHBV envelope and/or capsid proteins (dotted arrows) at different weeks p.i. as specified in brackets (w). Arrows symbolize biopsy and autopsy.

In lamivudine-DNA protocol, chronically infected ducks were randomly assigned into 8 groups (6-9 animals/group): group 1 (untreated or empty vector-treated controls), groups 2-4 (DNA monotherapy with pCI-preS/S or pCI-preS/S and pCI-C or pCI-C respectively), group 5 (lamivudine monotherapy), groups 6-8 (combination therapy with lamivudine and pCI-preS/S or pCI-preS/S and pCI-C or pCI-C respectively) as detailed in Table 1B. Lamivudine was administrated (groups 5-8) at 25 mg/kg/day via i.p. route during 5 consecutive days of the 1st week post infection (p.i.) and thereafter 3 times/week during 7 following weeks. DNA immunization consisted in multiple intramuscular (i.m.) injections of 300 μg endotoxin-free plasmid DNA per animal (weeks 6, 10, 14, 28, 35) as described [34,35,40] (Figure 1).

In both protocols blood samples were collected three times a week during the first 5 weeks p.i. and once a week thereafter until the end of the of follow-up i.e. week 34 and 40 for adefovir-DNA and lamivudine-DNA protocols respectively. Monitoring of animal weight was performed throughout the entire follow-up.

Duck Liver Biopsy and Autopsy

Liver biopsies were performed under general anaesthesia with 15 mg/kg of tiletamin and 15 mg/kg of zolazepam (Zoletil; Virbac, Carros, France) at the end of each antiviral treatment *i.e.* at week 10th and 8th p.i. for adefovir-DNA and lamivudine-DNA study respectively in randomly selected 2 or 3 ducks from different groups. At week 40 and 34 respectively all animals from adefovir-DNA and lamivudine-DNA study were euthanized by pentobarbital injection (Dolethal; Vetoquinol, Lure, France).

ELISA Analysis of Anti-PreS Response

The humoral anti-preS response of ducks was determined in a direct ELISA using the recombinant preS protein as detailed previously [6,35]. The end-point titres were taken as the reciprocal of the highest serum dilution which gave an OD_{405} above the mean signal of 2 replicates of control sera [6,35].

Analysis of Viremia

Viremia was assessed by serum DHBV DNA detection using a previously described dot blot hybridization assay [8]. Filters were scanned by PhosphorImager (Amersham Pharmacia Biotech) and counted by the ImageQuant software as described [8]. The limit of DHBV DNA detection was 0.5 pg.

Analysis of Intrahepatic Viral DNA

Total viral DNA was extracted from biopsy or autopsy liver samples according to procedures previously described [8,18]. In addition, a specific extraction of non-protein bound cccDNA was performed as described [17,18]. Ten micrograms of total DNA or cccDNA preparation were then subjected to electrophoresis through 0.9% agarose gel, transferred by blotting to a nylon membrane (Hybond N^+, Amersham Pharmacia Biotech), and viral DNA was detected by hybridization with a radiolabelled probe followed autoradiography as described previously [8].

Quantification of Liver cccDNA by Real-Time PCR

The selective quantification of intrahepatic DHBV cccDNA was similar to that previously described by Werle-Lapostolle *et al.* [45] for HBV cccDNA quantification. Briefly, selective primers for DHBV cccDNA amplification (targeted to opposite sides of the single-stranded gap region of relaxed circular DHBV DNA) were designed using Oligo 5 software (MedProbe, Olso, Norway). To enhance specificity of cccDNA detection, Plasmide-safe DNase (Epicentre, Madison, WI) was used, which efficiently degraded single stranded and relaxed circular forms of viral DNA prior to PCR, but not cccDNA [45]. Thus, 500 ng of extracted DNA were digested for 1 hour at 37°C in a 20 μl volume containing 2.5 mM ATP, 1X Plasmid-safe DNase reaction buffer, and 2 units of Plasmid-safe DNase, followed by subsequent DNase inactivation at 70°C for 30 minutes. Real-time PCR was performed in a Light Cycler (Roche, Grenoble, France) using 4 μl of this reaction volume in the presence of 0.5 mM of the following primers used for amplification: forward 5'-GCTGCTTGCCAAGGTATC-3' (cccDS1 nt 2554-1572) and reverse primer 5'-CCCTGTGTAGTCTGCCAG-3' (cccDAS1 nt 2826-2845) and 0.2 μM and 0.4 μM of 3'-labelled fluorescein probe DHBV FL and 5'-labelled Red 640 DHBV LC probe respectively (TibMolBiol, Berlin, Germany), whose sequences were described elsewhere [31]. Amplification of 272 bp cccDNA product occurred after denaturation at 95°C for 10 minutes, followed by 45 cycles of denaturation at 95°C for 10 seconds, fluorescence acquisition at 58°C for 3 seconds, annealing for 10 seconds at 61°C and extension at 72°C for 15 seconds. All samples were analyzed in duplicate. GAPDH gene amplification, used for normalization, was performed on extracted DNA as previously described [31,38]. Detection limit was estimated as $4x10^{-2}$ copies of cccDNA per cell, after spiking of intrahepatic DNA from DHBV-negative duck livers with serial dilutions of plasmid containing DHBV monomer used as quantification standards.

Histological Analysis of Liver Samples

Three micrometers thickness formalin-fixed liver tissue sections were stained with hematoxylin-eosin-safran (HES) stain and examined, under code, with a light microscope.

Statistical Analysis

Mann-Whitney tests were used to compare the efficiency of therapies on viremia. The Bliss Independence model was used to determine the potential additive effect of the adefovir-DNA combination therapy [12]. The association between DNA vaccination and cccDNA clearance or between cccDNA clearance and seroconversion was analyzed using the Fisher exact test. The $p<0.05$ was considered as statistically significant.

RESULTS

Decrease in Viremia During Antiviral Drug Administration

In the adefovir-DNA study, a marked drop in viremia titres (97%), reaching the limit of detection of the assay, was observed during the 4 weeks of drug administration in all adefovir-treated as compared with untreated ducks (group 3, adefovir monotherapy and group 4, combination therapy) (see Figure 2). However, the rebound of viremia was observed in almost all animals each week during the 2 days off treatment. The long-term follow-up showed low and fluctuating viremia in the control groups (group1, empty vector-treated and untreated). In DNA monotherapy group 2, the viremia fluctuated with the titres comparable to that of controls (group 1), during the first 27 weeks of follow-up, although at week 29, an important drop in viremia titers was observed which was transient and was followed by a rebound at week 30. Interestingly the median serum DHBV DNA in the combination therapy group, which received DNA vaccine and adefovir, was the lowest compared with other groups, and was maintained until the end of follow-up *i.e.* week 34 without additional DNA boosts. Analysis of individual viremia titres showed that several animals have undetectable viremia and this contributed to the lower mean viremia titres in this group. However the differences observed in the viremia medians (Figure 2), did not reach statistical significance.

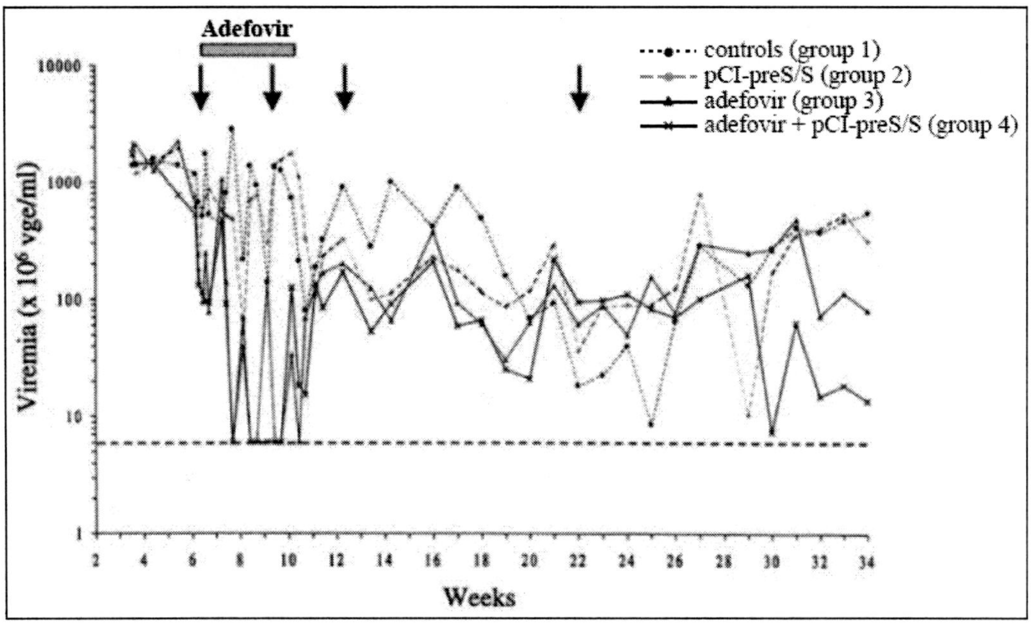

Figure 2. Effect of adefovir-DNA therapy on viremia. Viremia was monitored throughout the study period i.e. 34 weeks by DHBV DNA quantification using a dot-blot hybridization assay. The median viremia levels for each group (1-4) are plotted on the graph (logarithmic scale). Grey bar represents the adefovir treatment period (weeks 6-10 p.i.). Arrows indicate DNA injections at weeks 6, 9, 12 and 22. The cut-off of the assay is indicated by a dotted line. This figure was published by Le Guerhier et al. [18], Copyright Elsevier 2007.

In the lamivudine-DNA study, a marked decrease in viremia was observed in all drug-treated (groups 5-8) compared to untreated (groups 1-4) animals, although it was limited to only the first 3 out of 8 weeks of lamivudine treatment (Figure 3). Analysis of median viremia levels during following weeks showed a decrease and fluctuations, which were observed without significant differences between duck groups (Figure 3 and data not shown). However the review of individual viremia levels revealed that a total of 11 out of 30 animals, which received specific DNA immunization in association or not with lamivudine presented undetectable viremia starting from the 4th DNA immunization and up to the end of follow up (week 40) (data not shown).

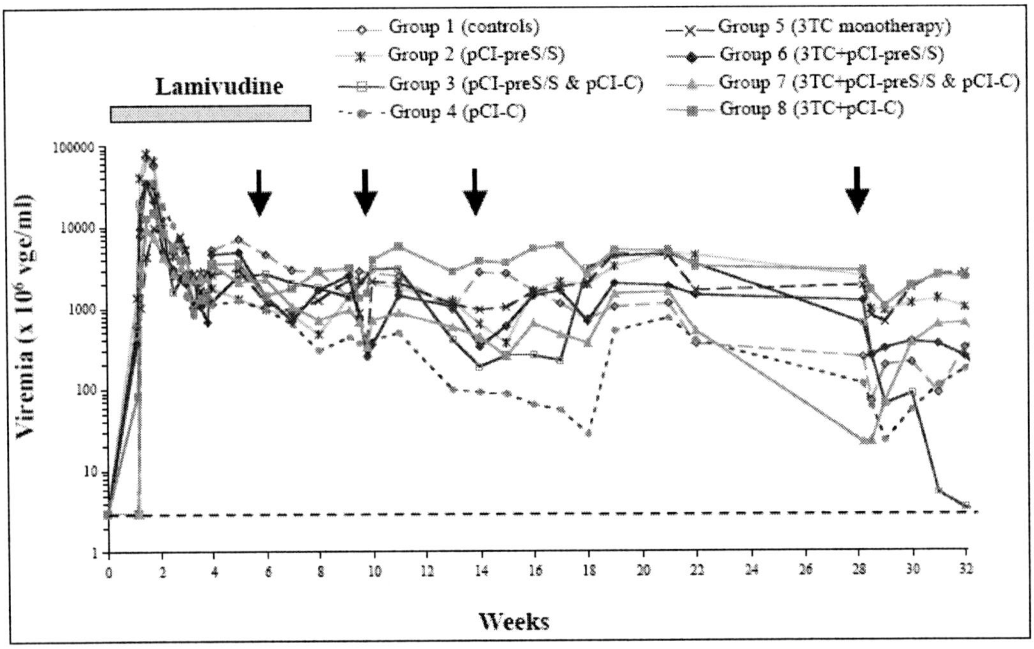

Figure 3. Effect of lamivudine-DNA therapy on viremia. Follow-up of viremia during weeks 1-32 is represented. Viremia was monitored using a dot-blot hybridization assay. The median viremia levels for each group (1-8) are plotted on the graph (logarithmic scale). Grey bar represents the lamivudine (3TC) treatment period (weeks 1-8 p.i.). Arrows indicate DNA injections at weeks 6, 10, 14, 28 and 35. The cut-off of the assay is indicated by a dotted line.

The comparison of antiviral effect of adefovir versus lamivudine suggests a more potent antiviral efficacy of adefovir on viremia, which reached undetectable levels during the drug administration period and the better efficacy of a combination therapy associating adefovir with DNA vaccine. However in both studies the drop in viremia following DNA vaccine immunotherapy alone or in association with antiviral drug treatment did not reach a statistical significance. This may be due to the large individual variations in viremia within each duck group, which included as well non-responders with high viremia titers and responders animals with low or undetectable viremia.

Impact of DNA-Based Immunotherapy on Intrahepatic Viral Replication

At the end of adefovir and lamivudine treatment (week 10 and 8 respectively), randomly selected biopsy specimens (2-3 ducks) have been performed to assess the impact of antiviral drug treatment on intrahepatic viral replication. However, Southern blot analysis of these liver biopsies revealed high amounts of intrahepatic DHBV DNA replicative intermediates, including cccDNA, in ducks from different groups with or without DNA immunization irrespectively of antiviral drug (lamivudine or adefovir) and therapeutic protocol used (data not shown).

In the adefovir-DNA study, analysis of autopsy liver samples at the end of the follow-up (week 34) showed the presence of viral DNA replicative intermediates for all controls (group 1), except one duck consistently with the absence of detectable viremia in this animal. In DNA monotherapy (group 2), 1 out of 5 ducks had undetectable viral DNA and another one presented a dramatic decrease but no clearance of viral replication (Table 1A and data not shown). No DHBV DNA clearance was observed in 5 out of 5 adefovir monotherapy-treated (group 3). By contrast within the combination therapy (group 4), 2 out of 5 ducks had undetectable DHBV DNA in their livers (Table 1A) consistent with their undetectable viremia during the 4 last follow-up weeks. PhosphorImager quantification of Southern blots revealed a greater than 51% decrease in intrahepatic DHBV DNA in the combination therapy treated group, whereas adefovir or DNA monotherapy alone decreased viral DNA by 14 and 38%, respectively, compared to controls, suggesting a trend to an additive effect of both protocols in the decrease in intrahepatic viral replication levels (51% inhibition instead of 47% expected) (data not shown). However the impact of DNA therapy alone or in combination with adefovir on DHBV DNA clearance did not reach a statistical significance.

In the lamivudine-DNA study, a similar analysis of autopsy liver samples (week 40) revealed viral DNA presence in 4 out of 5 controls (group 1). Amongst animals on DNA monotherapy (groups 2-4) viral DNA clearance was observed in a total of 5 out of 15 (30%) ducks : 2/4 (50%) receiving co-immunization against envelope and core (group 3) and 3/7 (43%) immunized against core alone (group 4) (Table 1B). Interestingly none of 7 ducks on lamivudine monotherapy (group 5) eliminated DHBV DNA. By contrast, a total of 6 of 15 (40%) ducks on combination therapy (groups 6-8) presented undetectable viral DNA. Within those, 4 of 8 (50%) ducks which were on combination of lamivudine with DNA vaccine against envelope (group 6) showed undetectable viral DNA, including cccDNA, compared to 0 of 7 on lamivudine monotherapy (group 5), suggesting a trend for a beneficial effect of such combination that was just above significance (p=0.07) (Table 1B). This benefit became significant if groups 6 and 7 receiving lamivudine and DNA immunization against envelope alone and in co-immunization against core protein were pooled together, since 6 out of 11 (55%) animals responded to therapy having undetectable liver DHBV DNA compared to 0 out of 7 on lamivudine monotherapy (p=0.038). PhosphorImager quantification of Southern blots revealed no significant difference between different treatment groups 2-8 as compared with the controls and this may be related to the relatively low mean DHBV DNA levels in the controls and individual variations in DHBV DNA each treatment group, which included as well animals with high and undetectable viral DNA (data not shown).

Collectively these results suggest a better efficacy of lamivudine-DNA study since higher percentage of DHBV-carriers presented undetectable liver DHBV DNA in Southern blot analysis as compared with adefovir-DNA study.

Clearance of cccDNA Following DNA-Based Immunotherapy

In the adefovir-DNA study the Southern blot analysis following a specific cccDNA extraction confirmed undetectable cccDNA in only 4 liver samples: 2 belonging to DNA combination therapy group, 1 to DNA monotherapy and 1 to controls (Table 1A and data not shown).

In the lamivudine-DNA study we searched for persistence of residual cccDNA by a real-time PCR in liver samples showing undetectable DHBV DNA in Southern blot analysis. Out of 12 liver samples presenting undetectable cccDNA in Southern blotting, 3 presented detectable cccDNA levels between 0.2–0.7 ccc-DHBV DNA copies/cell, including a control animal (group 1), receiving empty vector immunization (Table 1B and data not shown). Importantly, a total of 9 out of 30 (30%) ducks on DNA monotherapy (groups 2-4) and combination therapy (groups 6-8), showed cccDNA levels at or under the lowed detection limit of real-time PCR (0.04 ccc-DHBV DNA copies/cell) *i.e.* at least 1000-fold lower as compared with the controls or lamivudine monotherapy treated ducks, which had about 35 to 45 (mean 40) cccDNA copies/cell (Table 1B and data not shown). These results were reproducibly observed in three independent experiments. Therefore, DNA vaccine-based immunotherapy alone and combined with lamivudine resulted in a sustained suppression of DHBV replication in about one third of carriers.

Correlation between Virus Clearance and Restoration of Huomoral Immune Responses

Before use of pCI-preS/S and pCI-C plasmids for therapeutic DNA vaccination of chronic DHBV-carriers ducks, using either adefovir-DNA or lamivudine-DNA protocol, we have first tested their ability to induce anti-preS and anti-C humoral response in naïve ducks. Significant and specific anti-preS and anti-C antibody response that reached a plateau level after 2nd DNA boost was observed in naïves animals immunized either with preS/S or with pCI-C respectively. No difference was found in magnitude and kinetics of anti-preS response following pCI-preS/S immunization alone or in association with pCI-C plasmid (data not shown).

Next, we investigated whether humoral immune tolerance could be broken in DHBV carriers by a DNA vaccine and whether it could be correlated with viral cccDNA clearance. In the adefovir-DNA study only 2 out of 10 (20%) DHBV-carriers which received DNA mono- or combination therapy mounted a detectable anti-preS response. The presence of anti-preS antibodies was associated with low or undetectable levels of intrahepatic DHBV DNA (Table 1A and data not shown). However, anti-preS antibodies were undetectable in two other animals, one belonging to DNA monotherapy and another one to combination therapy group, which had either cleared or had dramatically lowered liver DHBV DNA (data not shown). Thus no clear correlation could be established between DHBV DNA clearance following DNA vaccine based immunotherapy and induction or restoration of anti-preS response in adefovir-DNA study.

This contrasts with the results observed in the lamivudine-DNA study. No anti-preS antibody response was detected in untreated or empty vector-immunized controls (group 1), including one duck having undetectable viral DNA in Southern blotting but clearly detectable in real-time PCR (data not shown). Only 1 of 7 ducks within lamivudine monotherapy group 5, mounted anti-preS response, although the seroconversion in this duck receiving lamivudine and empty-pCI vector immunization was not associated with serum and liver DHBV DNA clearance (Table 1B and data not shown). Interestingly, seroconversion to anti-preS was observed in 6 out of 9 (66%) ducks which cleared cccDNA as assessed by real-time PCR. Within these 6 animals, 3 belonged to combination therapy (group 6) and 3 to DNA monotherapy (groups 3-4) (Table 1B). As illustrated in Figure 4 for one representative duck (no 175) from combination therapy group 6, the seroconversion to anti-preS was observed after the 1st DNA boost.

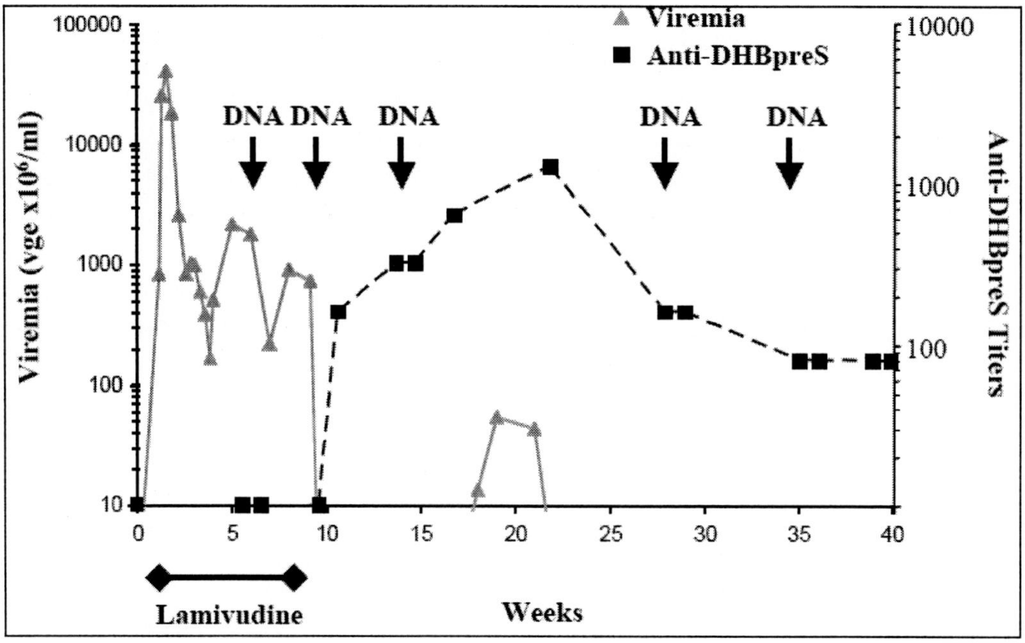

Figure 4. Individual evolution of viremia in correlation with seroconversion during DHBV infection clearance. Evolution of viremia and anti-preS humoral response (logarithmic scale) for one duck (no 175, group 6) belonging to lamivudine-DNA study. This DHBV-carrier duck received combination therapy associating lamivudine with pCI-preS/S plasmid and cleared cccDNA in its liver as assessed by real-time PCR (see also Table 1B). The anti-preS titers, determined by a direct ELISA test, and viremia were monitored throughout the study. Black arrows show DNA injections. Black bar represents the lamivudine treatment period.

Therefore, in lamivudine-DNA study the seroconversion to anti-preS was observed in 6 out of 9 (66%) ducks with cccDNA clearance, compared to seroconversion of only 1 out of

28 (3.6%) ducks without clearance whatever treatment group ($p<0.001$), suggesting a significant correlation between viral cccDNA clearance and restoration of humoral response in these animals.

Absence of Adverse Effects of Therapy

In both adefovir-DNA and lamivudine-DNA studies no significant variations in animal weight were observed indicating that treatments were well-tolerated. Several death occurred within follow-up, although they were accidental and occurred within all animal groups whatever the protocol used. Liver histology analysis showed occasional presence of steatosis, amyloidosis and mild to moderate inflammatory infiltrates in duck livers without marked differences between different treatment groups from both studies (data not shown).

Discussion

We investigated here whether DNA vaccine-based immunotherapy in combination or not with an antiviral drug (adefovir, lamivudine) treatment is able to enhance cccDNA clearance and break humoral immune tolerance in chronic DHBV-carriers. We have first realized a study associating adefovir with DNA vaccine against DHBV envelope [18] and compared herein its therapeutic efficacy with our recent study combining lamivudine with DNA vaccine against viral envelope and/or core proteins [41]. We report herein a better efficacy of lamivudine-DNA study since DNA vaccine alone and after treatment with lamivudine was able to eliminate viremia and intrahepatic cccDNA in about 30% of carriers, which was tightly correlated with the restoration of specific humoral immune responses. This is of particular interest, since in term of antiviral efficacy lamivudine was less potent as compared with adefovir. Thus, in adefovir-DNA study the viremia analysis showed the potent antiviral effect of adefovir during the 4 weeks of drug administration consistent with the observations of Nicoll et al. [32]. In addition, adefovir-treated DHBV-carrier ducks exhibited undetectable viremia levels during the drug administration period. This contrasts with the lamivudine-DNA study in which the drop of viremia was less pronounced and viremia remained detectable during the entire antiviral treatment. However, despite a marked decrease in viremia peak, adefovir or lamivudine treatments have not significantly decreased liver DHBV replication as assessed by biopsies examination from randomly chosen animals at the end of drug treatment. In addition, the decrease in viremia was transient and was followed by a rebound after drug cessation in all animals as well from lamivudine monotherapy as adefovir monotherapy groups. This is not surprising, since in both studies at the end follow-up (week 34 and 40), the intrahepatic viral cccDNA form responsible for chronicity of infection was still detectable in all ducks from adefovir or lamivudine monotherapy groups respectively. Thus, neither adefovir nor lamivudine alone had exhibited a sustained antiviral pressure during the 4 or 8 weeks respectively of drug administration in this model.

By contrast, the analysis of DHBV DNA in autopsy liver samples revealed that DNA vaccine-based immunotherapy alone and combined with antiviral drug treatment was able in both studies to considerable decrease and even eliminate the replicative DHBV DNA intermediates, including the cccDNA. Thus in adefovir-DNA study, 3 out of 10 animals (30%) which received DNA vaccine alone or combined with adefovir had undetectable viral DNA in their livers, including the cccDNA. In addition, combination therapy with adefovir led to a more pronounced decrease (51%) in the total intrahepatic viral load as compared with DNA monotherapy (38%). In spite of relatively small number of animals in this study, Bliss independence analysis [12] suggested a trend to an additive antiviral effect of therapy combining adefovir with DNA immunization against the hepadnaviral envelope protein [18]. In the lamivudine-DNA study we have also observed that elimination of replicative DHBV DNA intermediates occurred in DNA vaccine-treated groups only and was more pronounced in animals on combination (40%) as compared with those on DNA monotherapy (30%), suggesting a benefit of antiviral drug association with DNA vaccine, although this effect was relatively modest and did not reach statistical significance. It is of interest to note that if groups receiving lamivudine and DNA vaccine against envelope alone and in co-immunization against core were pooled together a significant benefit of combination therapy compared to lamivudine monotherapy was observed, suggesting a role of DNA immunization against envelope protein in therapeutic efficiency of such combination therapy.

In recent years it become increasingly apparent that intranuclear hepadnaviral cccDNA pool plays a crucial role in persistence and reactivation of viral replication as documented by studies in animal models and in chronically infected patients [1,19,25,29,45,47]. Another important issue of our studies was therefore the search for residual cccDNA presence in ducks, which apparently resolved infection following DNA mono- or combination therapy. To address this issue we designed a highly sensitive quantitative real-time PCR for DHBV cccDNA detection similar to the assay recently developed for human HBV cccDNA quantification [45]. We have not analyzed by this assay the presence of residual cccDNA in duck livers from adefovir-DNA study, since all but 3 liver samples presented detectable cccDNA in Southern blot analysis. However, analysis of 12 duck livers from lamivudine study presenting undetectable DHBV DNA in Southern blotting, revealed that 9 (30%) of carriers receiving DNA vaccine alone or combined with lamivudine had cccDNA levels that were at or under the lower limit of detection (0.04 cccDNA copies/cell) of this assay. By contrast no cccDNA clearance was observed in lamivudine monotherapy-treated animals presenting about 40 cccDNA copies/cell, consistently with reported estimates of cccDNA copy number from 30 to 50/cell in chronically DHBV-infected duck livers [1]. Whether the residual cccDNA, which was undetectable by us using the real-time PCR, may act as a template for viral replication or alternatively may be inert and non replicative, as suggested recently in a study analyzing cccDNA in ducks that resolved transient DHBV infection [19], remains an open question which deserves further investigations. In this regard our data are promising, since the viremia and cccDNA remained undetectable at week 40 in 30% of ducks indicating already no rebound in viral replication during the 5 weeks following immunotherapy cessation.

The optimal DNA vaccine-based immunotherapy would break immunologic tolerance in virus carriers. In the adefovir-DNA study, the analysis of the anti-preS response in chronically infected ducks on DNA mono-or combination therapy showed no clear correlation between antibody response and viral clearance. By contrast, in the lamivudine-

DNA study viral elimination was tightly associated with seroconversion, since 66% of ducks that cleared serum and liver DHBV DNA, including the cccDNA pool undetectable by real-time PCR, developed an anti-preS response compared to only 3% of ducks which seroconverted without viral elimination. These data indicate a significant correlation between viral cccDNA clearance following DNA-based immunotherapy and restoration or activation of specific humoral responses. This is an important finding of our study, since data accumulated in HBV-transgenic mice [23,28] and in patients [24,46] showed the ability of DNA vaccine to decrease intrahepatic hepadnaviral replication and to break immune tolerance, although the correlation with cccDNA clearance has not yet been demonstrated. However, in the lamivudine-DNA study not all carriers, which cleared viral replication, have mounted a detectable anti-preS response. This can be related to the immune complexes presence in serum of these animals, which masked circulating anti-preS antibodies and hampered their detection in our ELISA test. In both adefovir and lamivudine-DNA studies we were unable to analyze the role of T cell response in viral clearance, since the tools for duck cellular response analysis are still lacking and need to be developped. The ongoing characterization of these responses and in particular recent development by us of duck IFN-γ RNA monitoring [31], should allow a better understanding of immunity modulation during DHBV infection clearance.

It is important to note that DNA vaccine–based immunotherapy in association with adefovir or lamivudine was safe and well tolerated. Thus, in spite of accidental deaths which occurred during these long-term studies, liver histology revealed occasional presence of changes, which are frequently observed in DHBV-infected adult Pekin ducks [34], in animals from both adefovir and lamivudine-DNA study regardless of treatment group.

Altogether our results indicate a better therapeutic efficacy of the lamivudine-DNA protocol as compared with adefovir-DNA protocol in which only modest effect in term of viral cccDNA clearance and seroconversion was observed in spite of higher antiviral efficacy of the drug. Foster et al. [10] investigated entacavir (ETV) treatment combination with DNA vaccination to DHBV envelope and core and showed a potent antiviral effect of ETV on serum and liver viral DNA, however DNA vaccine was ineffective in reduction or clearance of viral cccDNA. The above-mentioned studies differed not only by the choice of antiviral drug but, importantly, by the design of DNA immunization protocol, which may play a key role in the better efficacy of DNA-lamivudine study. Thus, the lamivudine-DNA differs by a number of factors from adefovir-DNA protocol such as: i/ larger amounts of plasmid DNA (300 versus 150 μgDNA/animal/boost), ii/ higher number of DNA boosts (7 versus 5) including two delayed boosts (weeks 28, 35) versus one (week 22), iii/ and longer DNA immunization schedule. In both studies the same pCI-preS/S plasmid was used for immunization against viral envelope, although in the lamivudine-DNA study we have added core as an additional target for DNA vaccine, since genetic immunization against DHBV core has been recently set up by us and demonstrated to induce potent and specific humoral responses in naïve ducks [41]. Moreover, the schedule of combination therapy and in particular drug-DNA immunizations overlap was different in both studies as illustrated in Figure 1. Finally, a larger number of animals and a longer follow-up period allowed us to appreciate a sustained antiviral effect of DNA-vaccine based immunotherapy in the lamivudine-DNA study.

In conclusion, we have analyzed two pre-clinical combination therapy studies associating a DNA vaccine with two different antiviral drugs in the chronic DHBV infection model. We showed a higher potency of lamivudine-DNA protocol, conducted in a large group of chronic DHBV-carriers ducks, which provided a first demonstration that DNA vaccine-based immunotherapy alone and associated with antiviral drug treatment was able to induce drastic and sustained suppression of viremia and to enhance intrahepatic viral cccDNA clearance in one third of carriers, which, importantly, was tightly correlated with restoration of specific humoral responses. A number of factors known to determine the success of genetic vaccination such as plasmid construct, amounts of plasmid DNA delivered, number of DNA injections and immunization schedule [20] may play an important role in better therapeutic efficacy of lamivudine-DNA protocol described herein as compared with studies previously published by us and others [10,18,34]. The development of a therapeutic DNA vaccine has been recently accelerated with first clinical trials showing its safety and ability to activate T-cell responses in some HBV infected patients [24,46]. Further studies aiming to increase the potency of DNA vaccine–based immunotherapeutics need to be performed in animal models in view to obtain a complete and sustain recovery from chronic hepatitis B. In this view, genetic immunization with plasmid constructs encoding hepadnaviral proteins and gamma interferon has been recently demonstrated as particularly effective in immune responses stimulation [37,44] suggesting a therapeutic potential of such novel DNA vaccine that deserves further exploration in woodchuck and duck models of chronic hepatitis B.

ACKNOWLEDGEMENTS

We are grateful to Craig S. Gibbs (Gilead Sciences) to provide us with adefovir and to John Rhodes (GlaxoSmithKline) to provide us with lamivudine. This work was supported by grant from ARC and GlaxoSmithKline, AT was recipient of a fellowship from Mérieux Foundation and ARC. The authors are grateful to Catherine Jamard, for expert assistance with animals.

REFERENCES

[1] Addison, WR; Walters, KA; Wong, WWS; Wilson, JS; Madej, D; Jewell, LD; Tyrrell, DL. Half-life of the Duck Hepatitis B Virus covalently closed circular DNA pool *in vivo* following inhibition of viral replication. *J Virol*, 2002, 76, 6356-6363.

[2] Angus, PR; Vaughan, S; Xiong, H; Yang, W; Delaney, C; Gibbs, C; Brosgart, C; Colledge, D; Edwards, R; Ayres, A; Bartholomeusz, A; Locarnini, S. Resistance to adefovir dipivoxil therapy associated with the selection of a novel mutation in the HBV polymerase. *Gastroenterology*, 2003,125, 292-297.

[3] Boni, C; Bertoletti, A; Penna, A; Cavalli, A; Pilli, M; Urbani, S; Scognamiglio, P; Boehme, R; Panebianco, R; Fiaccadori, F; Ferrari, C. Lamivudine treatment can restore T cell responsiveness in chronic hepatitis B. *J Clin Invest*, 1998,102, 968-975.

[4] Boni C; Penna A; Ogg GS; Bertoletti A; Pilli M; Cavallo C; Cavalli, A; Urbani, S; Boehme, R; Panebianco, R; Fiaccadori, F; Ferrari, C. Lamivudine treatment can overcome cytotoxic T-cell hyporesponsiveness in chronic hepatitis B: new perspectives for immune therapy. *Hepatology*, 2001, 33, 963-971.

[5] Boni C; Penna A; Bertoletti A; Lamonaca V; Rapti I; Missale G; Pilli, M; Urbani, S; Cavalli, A; Cerioni, S; Panebianco, R; Jenkins, J; Ferrari, C. Transient restoration of anti-viral T cell responses induced by lamivudine therapy in chronic hepatitis B. *J Hepatol* 2003, 39, 595-605.

[6] Chassot, S; Lambert, V; Kay, A; Godinot, C; Trépo, C; Cova, L. Identification of major antigenic domains of duck hepatitis B virus pre-S protein by peptide scanning. *Virology* 1994, 200, 72-78.

[7] Chisari, FV. Rous-Whipple Award Lecture. Viruses, immunity, and cancer: lessons from hepatitis B. *Am J Pathol*, 2000, 156, 1117-1132.

[8] Cova, L; Zoulim, F. Duck hepatitis B virus model in the study of hepatitis B virus. *Methods Mol Med*, 2004, 96, 261-268.

[9] Davis, HL; McCluskie, MJ; Gerin, JL; Purcell, RH. DNA vaccine for hepatitis B: evidence for immunogenicity in chimpanzees and comparison with other vaccines. *Proc Natl Acad Sci USA*, 1996, 93, 7213-7218.

[10] Foster, WK; Miller, D; Marion, PL; Colonno, RJ; Kotlarski, I; Jilbert, AR. Entecavir therapy combined with DNA vaccination for persistent duck hepatitis B virus infection. *Antimicrob Agents Chemother*, 2003, 47, 2624-2635.

[11] Garcia-Navarro, R; Blanco-Urgoiti, B; Berraondo, P; Sanchez de la Rosa, R; Vales, A; Hervas-Stubbs, S; Lasarte, JJ; Borras, F; Ruiz, J; Prieto, J. Protection against woodchuck hepatitis virus (WHV) infection by gene gun co-immunization with WHV core and interleukin-12. *J Virol*, 2001, 75, 9068-9076.

[12] Greco, WR; Bravo, G; Parsons, JC. The search for synergy: a critical review from a response surface perspective. *Pharmacol Rev*, 1995, 47 (2), 331-385.

[13] Horiike, N; Fazle Akbar, SM; Michitaka, K; Joukou, K; Yamamoto, K; Kojima, N; Hiasa, Y; Abe, M; Onji, M. *In vivo* immunization by vaccine therapy following virus suppression by lamivudine: a novel approach for treating patients with chronic hepatitis B. *J Clin Virol*, 2005, 32, 156-161.

[14] Korba, BE; Cote, PJ; Menne, S; Toshkov, I; Baldwin, BH; Wells, FV; Tennant, BC; Gerin, JL. Clevudine therapy with vaccine inhibits progression of chronic hepatitis and delays onset of hepatocellular carcinoma in chronic woodchuck hepatitis virus infection. *Antivir Ther*, 2004, 9, 937-52

[15] Lai, CL; Dienstag, J; Schiff, E; Leung, NW; Atkins, M; Hunt, C; Brown, N; Woessner, M; Boehme, R; Condreay, L. Prevalence and clinical correlates of YMDD variants during lamivudine therapy for patients with chronic hepatitis B. *Clin Infect Dis*, 2003, 36, 687-696.

[16] Le Guerhier, F; Pichoud, C; Guerret, S; Chevallier, M; Jamard, C; Hantz, O; Li, XY; Chen, SH; King, I; Trepo, C; Cheng, YC; Zoulim, F. Characterization of the antiviral effect of 2',3'-dideoxy-2', 3'-didehydro-beta-L-5-fluorocytidine in the duck hepatitis B virus infection model. *Antimicrob Agents Chemother*, 2000, 44, 111-122.

[17] Le Guerhier, F; Pichoud, C; Jamard, C; Guerret, S; Chevallier, M; Peyrol, S; Hantz, O; King, I; Trepo, C; Cheng, YC; Zoulim, F. Antiviral activity of beta-L-2',3'-dideoxy-2',3'-didehydro-5-fluorocytidine in woodchucks chronically infected with woodchuck hepatitis virus. *Antimicrob Agents Chemother*, 2001, 45, 1065-1077.

[18] Le Guerhier, F; Thermet, A; Guerret, S; Chevallier, M; Jamard, C; Gibbs, CS; Trepo, C; Cova, L; Zoulim, F. Antiviral effect of adefovir in combination with a DNA vaccine in the duck hepatitis B virus infection model. *J Hepatol*, 2003, 38, 328-334, *Copyright Elsevier 2007.*

[19] Le Mire, MF; Miller, DS; Foster, WK; Burrell, CJ; Jilbert, A. Covalently closed circular DNA is the predominant form of duck hepatitis B virus DNA that persists following transient infection. *J Virol*, 2005, 79, 12242-12252.

[20] Leitner, WW; Ying, H; Restifo, NP. DNA and RNA-based vaccines: principles, progress and prospects. *Vaccine*, 2000, 18, 765-777.

[21] Leung, NW; Lai, CL; Chang, TT; Guan, R; Lee, CM; Ng, KY; Lim, SG; Wu, PC; Dent, JC; Edmundson, S; Condreay, LD; Chien, RN. Extended lamivudine treatment in patients with chronic hepatitis B enhances hepatitis B e antigen seroconversion rates: results after 3 years of therapy. *Hepatology*, 2001, 33, 1527-1532.

[22] Lu, MJ; Hilken, G; Kruppenbacher, J; Kemper, T; Schirmbeck, R; Reimann, J; Roggendorf, M. Immunization of woodchucks with plasmids expressing woodchuck hepatitis virus (WHV) core antigen and surface antigen suppresses WHV infection. *J Virol*, 1999, 73, 281-289.

[23] Mancini, M; Hadchouel, M; Davis, HL; Whalen, RG; Tiollais, P; Michel, ML. DNA-mediated immunization in a transgenic mouse model of the hepatitis B surface antigen chronic carrier state. *Proc Natl Acad Sci USA*, 1996, 93, 12496-12501.

[24] Mancini-Bourgine, M; Fontaine, H; Scott-Algara, D; Pol, S; Brechot, C; Michel, ML. Induction or expansion of T-cell responses by a hepatitis B DNA vaccine administered to chronic HBV carriers. *Hepatology*, 2004, 40, 874-882.

[25] Mason, WS; Cullen, J; Moraleda, G; Saputelli, J; Aldrich, CE; Miller, DS; Tennant, B; Frick, L; Averett, D; Condreay, LD; Jilbert, AR. Lamivudine therapy of WHV-infected woodchucks. *Virology*, 1998, 245, 18-32.

[26] Mason, WS; Cullen, J; Saputelli, J; Wu, TT; Liu, C; London, WT; Lustbader, E; Schaffer, P; O'Connell, AP; Fourel, I; *et al.* Characterization of the antiviral effects of 2'-carbodeoxyguanosine in ducks chronically infected with duck hepatitis B virus. *Hepatology* 1994, 19, 398-411.

[27] Michel, ML; Davis, HL; Schleef, M; Mancini, M; Tiollais, P; Whalen, RG. DNA-mediated immunization to the hepatitis B surface antigen in mice: aspects of the humoral response mimic hepatitis B viral infection in humans. *Proc Natl Acad Sci USA*, 1995, 92, 5307-5311.

[28] Michel ML. Towards immunotherapy for chronic hepatitis B virus infections. *Vaccine*, 2002, 19, 83-88.

[29] Moraleda, G; Saputelli, J; Adrich, CE; Averett, D; Condreay, L; Mason, WS. Lack of effect of antiviral therapy in nondividing hepatocyte cultures on the closed circular DNA of woodchuck hepatitis virus. *J Virol*, 1997, 71, 9392-9399.

[30] Nafa, S; Ahmed, S; Tavan, D; Pichoud, C; Berby, F; Stuyver, L; Johnson, M; Merle, P; Abidi, H; Trepo, C; Zoulim, F. Early detection of viral resistance by determination of hepatitis B virus polymerase mutations in patients treated by lamivudine for chronic hepatitis B. *Hepatology*, 2000, 32, 1078-1088.
[31] Narayan, R; Buronfosse, T; Schultz, U; Chevallier-Gueyron, P; Guerre, S; Chevalier, M; Saade, F; Ndeboko, B; Trepo, C; Zoulim, F; Cova, L. Rise in interferon gamma expression during resolution of Duck Hepatitis B Virus infection. *J Gen Virol*, 2006, 87, 3225-3232.
[32] Nicoll, AJ; Colledge, DL; Toole, JJ; Angus, W; Smallwood, R A; Locarnini, SA.. Inhibition of duck hepatitis B virus replication by 9-(2-phosphonylmethoxyethyl)adenine, an acyclic phosphonate nucleoside analogue. *Antimicrob. Agents Chemother*. 1998, 42**,** 3130-3135.
[33] Perrillo, R; Schiff, E; Yoshida, E; Statler, A; Hirsch, K; Wright, T; Gutfreund, K; Lamy, P; Murray A. Adefovir dipivoxil for the treatment of lamivudine-resistant hepatitis B mutants. *Hepatology*, 2000, 32(1),129-134.
[34] Rollier, C; Sunyach, C; Barraud, L; Madani, N; Jamard, C; Trepo, C; Cova, L. Protective and therapeutic effect of DNA-based immunization against hepadnavirus large envelope protein. *Gastroenterology*, 1999, 116, 658-665.
[35] Rollier, C; Charollois, C; Jamard, C; Tepo, C; Cova, L. Early life humoral response of ducks to DNA immunization against hepadnavirus large envelope protein. *Vaccine*, 2000, 18, 3091-3096.
[36] Rollier, C; Charollois, C; Jamard, C; Tepo, C; Cova, L. Maternally transferred antibodies from DNA-immunized avians protect offspring against hepadnavirus infection. *J Virol*, 2000, 74, 4908-4911
[37] Saade, F; Buronfosse, T; Narayan, R; Schultz, U; Zoulim, F; Trepo, C; Cova, L. Codelivery of cytokines genes DNA vaccine to ducks hepatitis B virus improves its therapeutic efficacy. *J Clin Virol*, 2006, 36, S31.
[38] Seigneres, B; Martin, P; Werle, B; Schorr, O; Jamard, C; Rimsky, L; Trepo, C; Zoulim, F. Effects of pyrimidine and purine analog combinations in the duck hepatitis B virus infection model. *Antimicrob Agents Chemother*, 2003, 47, 1842-1852.
[39] Tenney, DJ; Levine, SM; Rose, RE; Walsh, AW; Weinheimer, SP; Discotto, L; Plym, M; Pokornowski, K; Yu, CF; Angus, P; Ayres, A; Bartholomeusz, A; Sievert, W; Thompson, G; Warner, N; Locarnini, S; Colonno, RJ. Clinical emergence of entecavir-resistant hepatitis B virus requires additional substitutions in virus already resistant to Lamivudine. *Antimicrob Agents Chemother*, 2004, 48, 3498-3507.
[40] Thermet, A; Robaczewska, M; Rollier, C; Hantz, O; Trepo, C; Deleage, G; Cova, L. Identification of antigenic regions of duck hepatitis B virus core protein with antibodies elicited by DNA immunization and chronic infection. *J Virol*, 2004, 78, 1945-1953.
[41] Thermet, A; Buronfosse, T; Werle-Lapostolle, W; Chevallier, M; Pradat, P; Trepo, C; Zoulim, F; Cova, L. Immunization with DNA vaccine alone and after treatment with lamivudine breaks humoral immune tolerance and enhances cccDNA clearance in the ducks model of chronic hepatitis B virus infection. *submitted*
[42] Triyatni, M; Jilbert, AR; Qiao, M; Miller, DS; Burrell, CJ. Protective efficacy of DNA vaccines against duck hepatitis B virus infection. *J Virol*, 1998, 1, 84-94.

[43] Villeneuve, JP; Durantel, D; Durantel, S; Westland, C; Xiong, S; Brosgart, CL; Gibbs, CS; Parvaz, P; Werle, B; Trepo, C; Zoulim, F. Selection of a hepatitis B virus strain resistant to adefovir in a liver transplantation patient. *J Hepatol*, 2003, 39, 1085-1089.
[44] Wang, J; Gujar, SA; Cova, L; Michalak, TI. Bicistronic woodchuck hepatitis virus core and gamma interferon DNA vaccine can protect from hepatitis but does not elicit sterilizing antiviral immunity. *J Virol*, 2007, 2, 903-916.
[45] Werle-Lapostolle, B; Bowden, S; Locarnini, S; Wursthorn, K; Petersen, J; Lau, G; Trepo, C; Marcellin, P; Goodman, Z; Delaney, WE; Xiong, S; Brosgart, CL; Chen, SS; Gibbs, CS; Zoulim, F. Persistence of cccDNA during the natural history of chronic hepatitis B and decline during adefovir dipivoxil therapy. *Gastroenterology*, 2004, 126, 1750-1758.
[46] Yang, SH; Lee, CG; Park, SH; Im, SJ; Kim, YM; Son, JM; Wang, JS; Yoon, SK; Song, MK; Ambrozaitis, A; Kharchenko, N; Yun, YD; Kim, CM; Kim, CY; Lee, SH; Kim, BM; Kim, WB; Sung, YC. Correlation of antiviral T-cell responses with suppression of viral rebound in chronic hepatitis B carriers: a proof-of-concept study. *Gene Ther*, 2006, 13, 1110-1117.
[47] Zoulim F. Antiviral therapy of chronic hepatitis B: can we clear the virus and prevent drug resistance? *Antivir Chem Chemother*, 2004, 15, 299-305.

In: Hepatitis B Research Advances
Editor: Alicia P. Willis, pp. 99-111
ISBN: 978-1-60021-666-4

Chapter VII

RISK FACTORS OF HEPATITIS B VIRUS IN SUBURBAN AND RURAL AREAS OF NIGERIA

L.E. Okoror[1,*], O.I. Okoror[1], P.I. Umolu[1], A. Enaigbe[1], F. Aisabokhale[2], D. Akpome[3], H.A. Obiazi, I.B.A. Momodu[5] and J.T. Erimafa

[1]Department of Microbiology, Ambrose Alli University, PMB 14, Ekpoma, Edo State, Nigeria
[2]Department of Hematology, College of Medicine, Ambrose Alli University, Ekpoma, Edo State, Nigeria
[3]Department of Mathematics and Statistics, Ambrose Alli University, Ekpoma, Nigeria
[4]Irrua Specialist Teaching Hospital Irrua Edo State, Nigeria
[5]Department of Computer Science, Ambrose Alli University, Ekpoma, Nigeria

ABSTRACT

Hepatitis B virus (HBV) is the most common cause of hepatitis world wide and a major cause of hepatitis in Nigeria of which blood transfusion has been identified as the most common means of transmission. This has led to the compulsory screening of HBV in all blood meant for transfusion, this has been done neglecting other transmission channels which may be responsible for the high infection rate in the population because despite screening of blood meant for transfusion, HBV remains a major killer in Nigeria and Sub Saharan Africa. We undertook a five year cases –control study (2000 – 2005) to determine the risk factors of HBV infection using the spot test kit and confirming with ELISA technique. A total of 2,987 patients (cases) attending various clinics in Nigeria for hepatitis related illness and 3,798 age and sex matched controls were screened for HBV virus. Of the 2,987 cases only 1,899 (63%) were positive. From the positive cases were patients who have marked their bodies with different sharp objects for the purpose

* Correspondence concerning this article should be addressed to L.E. Okoror. email: Larison86@yahoo.com.

of obtaining charms and have a very high relative risk of 5.5 (95%, CI). This was followed by injecting drug users with a relative risk of 3.5 (95%, CI) while the Yoruba ethnic group had the lowest relative risk of 0.7 (95%, CI). Other risk factors determined included injecting drug use, tattoo, blood transfusion, ear piercing, native surgery for splenitis, female genital mutilation, health care workers, sharing tooth brush, 6 or more sex partners, 2 to 5 sex partners, regular visit to barber shop, personal and family history of jaundice, tribal marks, and ethnicity (Yoruba, Ibo, Hausa, Ijaw and other related minorities). All these exposures posses a risk in the population, however, charms markings, tribal marks and native surgery for splenitis had very high percentages of attributable cases of 23%, 14.4% and 9.2% respectively.

INTRODUCTION

Hepatitis B virus (HBV) is a small circular DNA virus within the family of six viruses that cause hepatitis, it was first characterized in 1965. HBV contain a neucleocapsid and an envelope. HBV neucleocapsid relatively small and incomplete double stranded 3.4KB DNA genome, viral polymerase and core protein. Its envelope is compose of viral surface protein enclosed by a lipid membrane derived from the host cells [1,2]. In the serum of infected patients, there are both mature virion with viral DNA and subviral particles without viral DNA [3,4]. Sub viral particles are overwhelmingly in excess to infectious particles [3,4].

The life cycle is believed to begin when the virus attaches to the host cell membrane via its envelope proteins. Then the viral membrane fuses with the host cell membrane and the viral genome is released into the cell [5,6]. After the viral genome reaches the nucleus, the viral polymerase converts the double stranded (ds DNA) into covalently closed circle DNA (cccDNA). The synthesis is believed to be the template for further propagation of pre – genomic RNA, which directs the synthesis of viral DNA and mRNA that encodes all viral protein [2,7,8]. HBV viral particles are assembled in the cytosol following encapsidation of pre-genomic RNA, which is then degraded during reverse transcription of pre-genomic RNA into complimentary strand of DNA [9]. HBV surface protein are initially synthesized and polymerized in the rough endoplasmic reticulum (RER). These proteins are transported to the post ER and pre-Golgi compartments where budding of the neucleocapsid follows [10]. The assembled HBV virions and sub-viral particles are transported to the Golgis for further modification of its proteins into glycans in the surface proteins, and then secreted out the host cell to finish the life cycle [11]. HBV replication in the host cell are highly elucidated but the early stage of infection are still uncertain. DNA sequence of HBV have revealed the existence of 8 viral genotypes A-H and these varies in geographic distribution. Genotype A is primarily found in North America, northern Europe, India and Africa. Genotype B and c are common in Asia; genotype D is southern Europe, the Middle East and India; genotype E in west Africa and south Africa; genotype F in south and central America; genotype G in Europe and United States [12]. Genotype H was recently identified in individuals from Central America and California. Several genotypes may be involved in severity of the disease but the relationship between genotypes and the risk of developing hepatocellular carcinoma have not been established [13]. In China and Japan researcher have found more sever liver diseases to be associated with genotype C.than compared with genotype B [12], other studies have shown no such association [14,15]. There is some evidence that show HBeAg seroconversion occurs at younger age among individuals with genotype B [13,15,16]. Genotype D has been associated with anti-HBe-positive hepatitis B infection in the Mediterranean region [17]. Mutation has been responsible for the development of several genotypes and severity in infections.

HBV has a reported mutation rate of over 10 times of other DNA viruses. These mutations can occur naturally and due to pressure from antiviral drugs [13]. There are five clinically relevant HBV types: wild- type HBV, precore mutants, core promoter mutants, tyrosine-methionine-aspartate-aspartate (YMDD) mutants induced by lamuvidine treatment, and asparagines to threonine (rtN236T) mutants recently identified in with idefovir treatment. In a study carried out in the United States, the precore variant of HBV was rarely found in association with genotype A, but it was found in almost 50% of those with genotype C and in less than 70% of individuals with genotype D. Those with precore mutants and core promoter mutations have higher HBV DNA levels in serum than those without these variants. It is observed that flares in chronic HBV infections have been associated with increase in concentration of precore mutations in proportion with wild-type HBV [13]. Worldwide, 350million people are chronically infected with HBV; it complications includes fibrous, cirrhosis and hepatocellular carcinoma, and infecting between 0.5 and 1 million people each year (foundation for live research). However, safe and efficient vaccines are available to protect against HBV [22]. Although in rural and semi urban areas the infection still thrives [23]. Despite the existence of hepatitis B vaccination hepatitis B virus (HBV) is still a cause of significant morbidity and mortality worldwide. It is encouraging that majority of patients do recover from the infection, however, those that progress to chronic state is at risk of development of complications such as hepatocellular carcinoma, cirrhosis and liver failure [13]. Primary HBV infection in susceptible individuals can be either asymptomatic or symptomatic, the latter often the case, especially in young individuals; but rarely fulminant hepatitis can develop during the acute phase. Most primary infections are self-limited with clearance of virus by the immune system. However, an estimated 3% to 5% adults and up to 95% children develop chronic HBV infection. Persistence infection can also be either symptomatic or asymptomatic; those with elevated liver chemistry and abnormal biopsies are termed as having chronic hepatitis B and those with normal studies are termed chronic carriers [13]. Long term infection increases the risk of developing cirrhosis and HCC.

In 1997, the World Health Organisation estimated that about 3% of the world's population had been infected with another hepatitis agent – hepatitis C virus (HCV).In parts of Africa the prevalence could be as high as 10%. Other high prevalence area include America and Asia. More than 170 million chronic carriers worldwide are at risk of developing liver cirrhosis, liver cancer or both. Over 4 million HCV positive live in the United States where about 4,000 deaths each year can be attributed to HCV related liver failure or hepatocellular carcinoma; HCV infection account for 30%ofliver transplant performed in the United States [19].

Hepatitis is a disease of the liver often caused by viruses. Hepattitis means inflammation of the liver. There are different kinds of hepatitis caused by different hepatitis viruses. In each case, the virus once inside the body, begins to live in the liver cells, interferes with cells normal activities and then uses the cell to make new viruses. The disease hepatitis is characterized by high rate of viral persistence and the potential to develop and of ever worsening chronic liver disease ranging from chronic hepatitis and occasionally hepatocellular carcinoma [31].

Types of hepatitis includes hepatitis D caused by hepatitis D virus which only occurs when a patient has HBV. Hepatitis E which is similar to hepatitis A is acute. Hepatitis F appears to produce hepatitis similar to hepatitis C but scientists are not certain if it is a separate virus. Hepatitis G is a newly identified virus that is probably transmitted in a similar fashion of hepatitis C.

These blood borne viruses present serious illness health risks for recipients of blood transfusion. In a study in Brazil in 1995, a total of 2,678 serum samples were collected from 2583 blood donours and the prevalence rate among the blood donours reached 9.3% and 1% respectively for HBV and HCV; 0.75% were positive for HBV surface antigen and 9.2% for anti hepatitis B core antigen and 65% of the HIV positive patients were positive for HBV while 54.1% were positive for HCV which confirms co-occurrence of both viruses (HBV and HCV). [20].

A study in the United States screened between 1985 and 1990 antibodies to HAV and HCV, HBV was excluded and the rate of new HCV infection had declined by more than 50% over the period lowering the risk of HCV seroconversion to 1.5% per unit transfused blood [21].

Risk factors for HBV had been known over the years to include injecting drug use, tattoos, ear piercing and religious scarification because most of the researches were carried out in developed world where this factor are predominant. In Sub Saharan Africa, other risk factors still remains unidentified and were included in this study. Despite screening of blood for transfusion by transfusion centres the infection in Nigeria is not on the decline [22,23].

Hepatitis B virus has been reported to posse a serious occupational risk to health workers [24]. The infection has been traced to the degree of contact with blood or blood related materials in the work place [25]. Serologic studies conducted in low HBV prevalence countries during the 1970s demonstrated that health care workers had a prevalence of HBV infection up to 10 times higher compared to the general population [15]. Because of the high risk of HBV infection in healthcare workers, routine preexposure vaccination of healthcare workers against hepatitis B and the use of universal precautions to avoid exposure of blood and other potentially infectious body fluids have been recommend in many countries since the vaccine became available since the 1980s. In the United States, regulations issued by the Occupational Health and Safety Administration have increased compliance with this recommendations [25]. In Nigeria such regulations are scarcely available and healthcare workers scarcely undergo routine vaccination. The principles and mode of transmission in healthcare settings are- 1) direct percutaneous inoculation of blood or body fluids containing HBV via needlestick or other injuries from other sharp objects 2) direct inoculation of blood or body fluids containing onto mucous membranes, cutaneous scratches, abrasions, burns or other lesions, and 3) indirect inoculation of HBV from environmental surfaces contaminated blood or body fluids onto mucous membranes cutaneous scrarches, abrasions, burns or other lesions. Blood contains the highest HBV titres and it is the most important vehicle of transmission in the healthcare settings. HBV is relatively stable at room temperature and remaining viable for at least 7 days on environmental surfaces at room temperature [25].

Although hepatitis b surface antigen (Hbsag) have been detected in a wide variety of other body fluids including breast milk, bile, cerebrospinal fluids, faeces, nasopharyngeal washings, saliva, semens, sweat and synovial fluids, the concentration of Hbsag in body fluids is can be up to 100 to 1000 –folds higher than the concentration of HBV particles. Therefore, most body fluids are not effective vehicles of transmission of HBV because they contain low concentration of infectious HBV despite the presence of hbsag.

In 1992, the World Health Assembly endorsed the recommendation issued by the Global Advisory Group of EPI (Expanded Programme on Immunization) that HBV vaccines be integrated into the national immunization programs of countries with a hepatitis B carrier prevalence of 8% of greater by 1995 and in all countries by 1997 [32]. Tremendous progress have been made thereafter. Despite all this precautions, the infection is not on the is not on the decline in low socio-economic areas and hence have a source of public health problem which has led to this study which looked at the factors necessary for the transmission of this infection and most probably how they can be curtailed.

MATERIALS AND METHODS

Intravenous blood samples were collected from 2,987 suspected cases of hepatitis and 3,798 age and sex matched controls. The blood samples were collected aseptically into sterile vacutaniers. The blood samples were immediately centrifuged (hetituch) at 3,000 rpm for 5 minutes and the sera collected into sterile vials and test carried out immediately. The spot test was carried out using the spot test kit and the test carried out as directed by the manufacturer (ACON) and the confirmatory test was done using the ELISA technique. And Immunocomb ELISA kit was used which is said to be the most sensitive by a survey of the health care workers in the population studied. All cases and control in this study agreed to be part of this study subject to anonymity. Cases and controls were interviewed using a well structured questionnaire concerning their personal, past medical, family, occupational history along with specific questions on potential risk factors which included injecting drug use, recipient of blood or blood products, tattoos, ear piercing, native surgery for splenitis, number of sexual partners and sexual orientation, tribal marks, marking of charms, sharing toothbrushes, visit to barber shops, ethnicity and female genital mutilation (to include when it was carried out as those that had their carried out at birth were excluded from the study). Health care workers were defined as paid employees with exposure to patients or their body fluids [34]. Interviews were conducted from 1999 to 2005 with cases match controls interviewed at similar times.

Relative risk (RR) were calculated as approximated by odd ratios, were derived by two methods. Epi Info version 3.3.4 was used for the calculation of univariate relative risks as the data base. Unconditional logistic regression analysis was conducted with HBV positivity as the dependent variable and other factors in the questionnaire as independent variables using the SPSS package version 11. Multiple regression analysis was also carried out and adjustments were made for all variables associated with HBV infection.

Table 1. Univariate relative risk for hepatitis B virus infection

Exposure	Cases	Control	Relative risk(95% CI)	P value
Injecting drug	20	19	3.6	0.437
Tattoos	18	10	1.1	0.189
Blood transfusion	256	252	1.0	0.849
Ear piercing	208	234	1.2	0.416
Native surgery for splenitis	238	356	1.4	0.998
Healthcare workers	86	120	1.3	0.981
Sharing tooth brush	163	164	1.4	0.936
6or more sex partners	161	178	1.2	0.920
2 to 5 sex partners	203	206	1.0	0.921
Visiting barber shop	200	239	1.8	0.335
Personal history of jaundice	35	58	1.7	0.002
Family history of jaundice	83	106	1.8	0.921
Tribal marks	354	456	1.5	0.981
Marks of charms	444	734	5.5	1.000
Yoruba ethnic group	221	300	2.1	0.920
Ibo ethnic group	262	274	0.7	0.951
Ijaw ethnic group	165	204	1.8	0.335
Hausa ethnic group	70	108	1.5	0.435

Table 2. Adjusted relative risk of selected exposure for HBV infection after exclusion of all cases with tribal marks, marking of charms and ethnicity

Exposures	Cases	Control	Relative risk
Injecting drug use	10	19	3.1
Tattoos	4	10	0.7
Blood transfusion	96	222	0.9
Visiting barber shop	100	200	1.3
Ear piercing	92	102	1.1
Spleenitis	146	324	1.3
Health care workers	40	105	1.1
Sharing tooth brush	62	144	1.2
6or more sex partners	55	144	1.0
2or more sex partners	66	206	0.8
Personal history of jaundice	23	58	1.6
Family history of jaundice	49	106	1.7

Table 3. Estimated attributable cases of HBV

Exposure	Attributable risk	Attributable cases (%)
Injecting drug use	11.3	15(0.6)
Tattoos	1.3	10(0.3)
Blood transfusion	1.0	126(6.1)
Spleenitis	2.7	178(9.2)
Health care workers	1.8	55(2.5)
Sharing tooth brushes	1.8	82(3.9)
Mark of charms	26.8	228(23)
Tribal marks	2.3	367(14.4)

RESULTS

Of the 2,987cases, 1,710 were males (mean age 32.5 years) and females 1277 (mean age 31 years). And of the 3,798 controls, 1905 were males (mean age 33.1) and females were 1893 (mean age 31.7). The prevalence in the general population was 0.28. And of the 2,987 cases 1899 (63.58%) were positive for HBV. Table 1 shows the Univariate relative risks for exposure variables while table 2 shows multivariate relative risks for significant exposures variables after exclusion of cases of ethnicity since all the cases belong to at least one ethnic group. All cases show independent risk even after exclusion of ethnic groups after adjusting for other risk factors. There were insufficient health workers to analyse for each of the risk for each sub- group of health workers but nurses were predominant in both cases and control. We carefully eliminated any chance of multivariation in the study by choosing cases and control with only one exposure as seen in the questionnaire. Table 3 shows the estimated attributable number of HBV infection for significant association in the 2,987 cases in the population identified during our study.

DISCUSSION

Our study reveals marking of charms as one of the most likely route for transmission of over 23% of HBV infection in Nigeria. Although ethnic behaviour could also be factors of transmission of the infection because after removal of the various tribes there was a sharp drop in their general risk. Though the risk factor for HBV was high in this study with injecting drug use, as has been reported [33,34]. There was no enough cases and control to adjudge injecting drug use as high risk in Nigeria as injecting drug use is not too popular in Nigeria. Since the large extent of the population are people of low economic earners who could not afford to buy drugs and only the rich could afford drugs and such people most of the time do not present themselves for screening or studies of this nature. And / or most of the rich people who could afford drugs normally seek medical care abroad. This does not however, rule out injecting drug use as a means of HBV transmission. The difference between table 1 and 2 shows that all samples screened belong to any of the excluded groups and ethnicity could also be a factor in the transmission of HBV infection. Such reasons such as ethnic behavioral pattern or generic reasons could be a reason why ethnicity so much influenced the result obtained. However, even after removal of ethnic groups the exposures still varies independently but the change in their risk factor and p values shows there was an association in table 1. In Nigeria more of the females wear tattoos, at least most of the case and controls (70%) were females with a history of having traveled or lived abroad.

Despite the fact that HBV is been screened in blood and blood products meant for transmission, the infection is still on the high side of increase and this could be as a result of the HIV / AIDS pandemic which have brought down immunity. It is possible that some of the patients could be positive although were not screened for HIV. Another reason could be the sharp practices indulged in by some blood banks in the country. Another reason could also be that most transmission channels have been neglected over the years and so much emphasis placed on blood transfusion. Though this other channels of transmission which were included in this study will be difficult to control, since they are personal behaviour, but increase in awareness campaign on the risk of this exposure especially in the rural areas could help stem down the infection rate. Such exposures which were included in this study includes marking of charms, native surgery for splenitis, female genital mutilation, visit to barber shop, sharing of tooth brushes, tribal marks and ethnicity. However, from this study, blood transfusions still a vehicle for transmission of HBV in Nigeria.

Ear piercing which contributed to about 0.5% of HBV transmission in Nigeria with a risk factor of 1.2 is seen as multiple ear piercing as only those with multiple ear piercing were used in the study as those with one ear pierced were assumed to have done that from birth at a time when blood capillaries has not been fully formed around the ear. And recently ear piercing at juvenile and adulthood have become very popular especially among the females as it is not encouraging in Africa for males to wear ear rings; however those males with a history of having traveled or lived abroad and those who prefer Western orientation still pierce their ears. Multiple ear piercing becomes a means of transmission of HBV since most of the ear piercing are done from homes and hair dressing saloons where little or no attention is given to hygiene and aseptic conditions. However, Neal *et. al.,* [34] reported that in a study in Trent region (UK) that there was no independent association with ear piercing when they studied HCV. The difference in both studies may have been necessitated by the fact that the UK is more advanced than Nigeria and have more awareness than Nigeria as per HBV and HCV infections, though Neal *et. al.,* [34] studied HCV which prevalence may not be as high as that of HBV but the two viruses have similar mode of transmission since they are both blood borne viruses.

Native surgery for treatment of splenitis in Nigeria is one of the surest way of contacting HBV infection in Nigeria accounting for 9.2% of infection of transmission of HBV a very high attributable risk. It is clear that most of the surgery carried out by the natives are usually carried out without recourse for aseptic conditions as most native surgeons has no means of sterilizing their equipments and may just clean them before using on a fresh patient and the patients themselves ignorantly agree to partake in the surgery. Most of this practice still take place in both the rural and sub-urban areas of the country. And even among the semi educated ones as they often believe that splenitis is not a hospital disease. Hence in rural and sub- urban areas of Nigeria, native surgery is still very popular.

Health care workers especially nurses and laboratory staffs are presumed to be at risk literarily. Since the nurses are the first to come in contact with the patients and the laboratory staffs collect blood samples and carry out test for HBV on the blood samples hence further putting them at risk. In the rural areas most of the patients are been attended to by nurses because of non availability of trained doctors in the various primary health care centres and this further put them at risk which explains why in this study, there was no enough numbers of health care workers as only a cross section of health care workers were available for screening in rural and semi urban areas. However, the attributable risk remains an all time high with attributable risk of 2.5% and relative risk of 1.3. This study suggests a possible increase in the risk to health care workers. This is against the back drop of the fact that other service providers in the health industry in the rural areas were not available for screening. Hence further work needs to be carried out in this regard. There is also the possibility of health care workers transmitting the virus to their patients if not detected early and treated.

Despite the screening of blood meant for transfusion, blood transfusion still remains a vehicle for transmission of HBV with a relative risk of 1.0 is still on the high side and this might probably be due to lack of confirmatory test as is been practiced in Nigeria today. It is possible that some of the spot test kits used may not be very reliable. Sharp practices by private blood banks may also be a factor for the risk noticed. This study then suggests that all blood meant for transfusion be screened and followed by a confirmatory test. All blood obtained from commercial or private blood banks should be re-screened in the hospital before been used for transfusion.

Sexual behaviour was also identified as very high risk even as HBV has not been classified as a STD disease. This was noticed when the higher the number of sexual partners the higher the relative risk for HBV. We do not suggest that the infection be classified as a STD since there could be other transmission risk during sex or kissing. There could be cuts which could bring about blood exchange and hence transmit HBV.

Another major risk is in those visiting barber shops since they represent about 6.1% of total risk. Cuts during barbing are suggested as a means of transmission of HBV. As has been identified for other infections like HIV/AIDS. Barbing equipments should be disinfected before and after each hair cut as this posses a serious public health problem.

Though not enough data were collected from those with personal and family history of jaundice, there was still an association in both cases. As HBV could be transmitted easily in closely knitted population. And jaundice happens to be one of the major symptoms of HBV. Personal history could point to a recurrent infection most probably due to a reduction of immunity or environmental factor.

There was a significant association with injecting drug users and tattoos systems which crept into Nigeria from the Western World and the Americas. Though we did not have enough cases and control to completely say they posse significant risk to the population at large. But tattooing is fast becoming popular in Nigeria.

Sharing tooth brush a system which is still been practiced as a show of love in the population gave a significant association. Broken capillaries during brushing could help transmit small amount of the virus but whether the amount of virus involved is infection dose still remains a further research.

Tribal marks and charm markings are practices which are peculiar to this part of the world. It is customary that children and certain juveniles are giving marks on their faces of which numbers and size depends on their tribes or ethnic groups. This however had a significant association as was evidenced by very high relative risk. Most of these marks are usually administered by natives with crude equipments without adequate disinfection. In most cases the same equipments are used for different people and this is responsible for the high risk posed by tribal marks. Cases with charm markings however has the highest relative risk which point to the fact these practices which continue to thrive is sure to be a means of transmission of the infection. Charm markings are very popular in this part of the world even among the elites. More than half the population still visits native doctors for spiritual protection where these charms are administered by various markings carried out with all manner of sharp objects. These objects are never disinfected and even the people do not bother to ask whether the sharp objects are disinfected of not.

Ethnicity play a very important role in the transmission of HBV ascertain ethnic norms encourage the infection. The Ibo ethnic group did not show any significant association with HBV while the Yoruba ethnic group reveal a very high risk of 2.1. The Yorubas and the Hausa ethnic groups are mostly associated with tribal marks which are also a very high risk factor. The Ibos have not been known to wear very large tribal marks from the questionnaire administered. The Ijaws and the Hausas also pose a high risk which would have been occasioned by certain life styles specific to their tribes.

There have been few case-control studies in other parts of the world which found association with injecting drug users, tattooing and blood transfusion which also had association in this study, but it is very difficult to compare both result because of different recruitment policies and different population studied. However the recruitment policy in this study was similar to those of Neal, *et. al.,* [34] but the populations were completely different and did not give any bases for comparison. Since most of the factors used in this study were not included in the study by Neal *et. al.,* [34].

A major limitation is in the response as only those with symptoms of HBV ranging from jaundice and fever. Only those cases that tested positive to HBV were interviewed and the controls had no such history hence it is possible that cases would have responded more truthfully than controls. Even some control may have hidden some information as it took sometime to convince the controls and even some cases to be part of the study. This bias was taken care of by making sure that matched controls were available for most of the factors and those whose controls were very far apart or not similar were eliminated from the study.

Vaccination has proved a sure way of preventing the infection, since it has been recommended that countries with prevalence at 8% include HBV vaccination in their national vaccination program. The proportion of WHO member states having universal infants or childhood hepatitis B vaccination program were 126 (66%) of 191 in 2001 and 151 (79%) of 192 in 2003 [29]. An estimated 32% of children below age 1 around the world were vaccinated fully with 3-dose hepatitis B vaccination series in 2001 [29]. Despite all these reported high compliance of WHO directive all over the world the infection still remain unabated in rural Nigeria. And this raise questions like how aware are the people about HBV vaccination since most of the people still visit native mid wives for child delivery and never have access to vaccination centres. Another question is how many of the rural people are very much aware of the risk involved in most to of factors stated in this study as very high risk. As a very high proportion of Nigerians whether rural or urban dwellers are still very much involved in charms markings all over their bodies without recourse to aseptic conditions. Even the scaring of tattoos have also increased the transmission of HBV in Nigeria, this has crept into Nigeria without the Hepatitis B virus has been reported to posse a serious occupational risk to health workers [27]. The infection has been traced to the degree of contact with blood or blood related materials in the work place [28]. Serologic studies conducted in low HBV prevalence countries during the 1970s demonstrated that health care workers had a prevalence of HBV infection up to 10 times higher compared to the general population [30]. Because of the high risk of HBV infection in healthcare workers, routine preexposure vaccination of healthcare workers against hepatitis B and the use of universal precautions to avoid exposure of blood and other potentially infectious body fluids have been recommend in many countries since the vaccine became available since the 1980s. In the United States, regulations issued by the Occupational Health and Safety Administration have increased compliance with this recommendations [27]. In Nigeria such regulations are scarcely available and healthcare workers scarcely undergo routine vaccination. The principles and mode of transmission in healthcare settings are- 1) direct percutaneous inoculation of blood or body fluids containing HBV via needlestick or other injuries from other sharp objects 2) direct inoculation of blood or body fluids containing onto mucous membranes, cutaneous scratches, abrasions, burns or other lesions, and 3) indirect inoculation of HBV from environmental surfaces contaminated blood or body fluids onto mucous membranes cutaneous scrarches, abrasions, burns or other lesions [26]. Blood contains the highest HBV titres and it is the most important vehicle of transmission in the healthcare settings. HBV is relatively stable at room temperature and remaining viable for at least 7 days on environmental surfaces at room temperature [30,31]. Although hepatitis b surface antigen (Hbsag) have been detected in a wide variety of other body fluids including breast milk, bile, cerebrospinal fluids, faeces, nasopharyngeal washings, saliva, semens, sweat and synovial fluids, the concentration of Hbsag in body fluids is can be up to 100 to 1000 –folds higher than the concentration of HBV particles. Therefore, most body fluids are not effective vehicles of transmission of HBV because they contain low concentration of infectious HBV despite the presence of hbsag.

Know how for asceptic tattoing which has also made both the rural and urban areas vulnerable. So in order for the vaccination efforts of the WHO to succeed in eradication of HBV there must be a reduction of most of the practices considered as high risk in this study. The only way to achieve this, is through massive awareness campaign in the general population and the rural areas in particular. Such campaign must be done in the language of the people for such a campaign to be successful.

REFERENCES

[1] Seeger C and Manson WS. Hepatitis B virus Biology. *Microbiology and Molecular Biology Reviews*. 2000. 64 (1:) 51-68.

[2] Manson WS and Seeger C. Hepadnavirus-molecular biology and pathogenesis. *Curr. Trop. Microbiol. Immunol.* 1991. 168. 1.

[3] Stibbe W and Gerlich WH. Structural relationship between minor and major protein of hepatitis B surface antigen. *J. virol.* 1983. 46. 626-629.

[4] Heermann KH, Goldmann U, Schwartz W, Seyffarth T, Baumgatten H, Gerlich WH. Large surface protein of Hepatitis B virus containing pre-S sequence. *J. virol.* 1984. 52: 396-402.

[5] Lu X, Block T. and Gerlich WH. Protease induced infectivity of Hepatitis B virus for human hepatoma cell line. *J. Virol.* 1996. 70: 2277-2285.

[6] Lu X, Hazbourne T. and Block T. Limited proteolysis induces woodchuck hepatitis virus for human Hep2G cells. *Virus Research*. 2001. 73 (1): 27-40.

[7] Tuttleman JS, Pourcel C. and Summers J. Formation of the pool of covalently closed circular DNA in hepadna virus infected cells. Cell. 1986. 47: 451-460.

[8] Ueda K, Tsurimoto K and Matsubara K. Three envelope proteins of hepatitis B virus: Large S, Middles S and major SHBs needed for the formation of Dane particles. *J. virol.* 1991. 65(7):3521-3529.

[9] Birnbaun F. and Nassal M. Hepatitis B nucleocapsid assembly: primary structure requirements in the core protein. *J. virol.* 1990. 64: 3319-3330.

[10] Huovila AJ, Eder AM, and Fuller SD. Hepatitis B surface assembler in a post-ER and pre-Golgi compartment. *J. Cell Biol.* 1992. 118: 1305-1320.

[11] Xuanyoang L and Block T. Study of the early steps of hepatitis B virus life cycle. *Int. J. Med. Sci.* 2004. 1(1): 21-33.

[12] Kidd-Ljungren K, Miyakawa Y, *et al.*, Genetic variability of hepatitis B virus. *J. Gen. virol.* 2002. 83: 1257-1280.

[13] Pan C. and Zhang JS. Natural history and clinical consequences of hepatitis B virus infection.2005. 2(1):36-40.

[14] Kao JH, Chen PJ, Lai MY, Chen DS. Genotypes and clinical phenotypes of hepatitis B virus in patients with chronic hepatitis B virus infection. *J. clin. microbiol.* 2002.83:2059-2093.

[15] McMahon BJ, Holck P, Bulkow L. *et al.* Serologic and clinical outcome of 1536 Alaska natives chronically infected with hepatitis B virus. *Annual Interna. Med.* 2001. 135:759-768.

[16] Sumi H, Yokosuka O, Seki N. *et al.* Influence of hepatitis B virus genotype on progression of chronic hepatitis B virus liver disease. *Hepatol.* 2003. 27:19-26.

[17] Chu CJ and Lok ASF. Clinical significance of hepatitis B virus genotype. *Hepatol.* 2002. 35:1274-1276.

[18] Chu CJ, Keeffe EB, Han SY. *et al.* Prevalence of HBV precore/core promoter among variants in USA. *Hepatol.* 2003. 38:619-928.

[19] Riordan SM, Williams R. Impact of hepatitis C virus ‘epidemics’ on clinical services. *AIDS and Hepatitis Digest.* 2004. 101: 1-5.

[20] Treifinger A, Van Dor Sandors S, Verde J. Hepatitis B and hepatitis C prevalence among blood donors and HIV 1 infected patients in Florianopolis, Brazil. *Braz.J.Infect. Dis.* 2000. 4: 192-6.

[21] Donahue JG, Mnnoz A, Ness PP, *et al.* The declining risk of post transfusion hepatitis C virus infection. *N. Eng. Med. J.* 1992. 372:369-73.

[22] Umolu PI. And Okoror LE. Sero-epidemiological survey of hepatitis B, hepatitis C and HIV infection in blood donors in Irrua and Ekpoma Nigeria. *AIDS and hepatitis digest* 2005.105

[23] Umolu PI, Okoror LE. and P Orhue. Human immune deficiency virus (HIV) seropositivity and hepatitis B surface antigenamea (HBSAG) among blood donors in Benin City. 2005. 5(1):55-58.

[24] Mast EE, Alter MJ. Prevention of Hepatitis B virus infection among health care worker. *In:* Ellis RW, Ed. Hepatitis B vaccines in clinical practice. Mercel Decker Inc. West point 1993. 295-307.

[25] Dienstag JL, Ryan DM. Occupational exposure of hepatitis B virus in hospital personnel: Infection or immunization? *Am. J. Epidemiol.* 1982. 115:26-29.

[26] Hadler SC, Doto IL, Maynard JD, Smith J, Clark B, Mosely J. *et al.* Occupational risk of hepatitis B virus infection in hospital workers. *Infect. Control.* 1985. 6:24-31.

[27] Mahony FJ, Stewart K, Hu H, Coleman P, Alter MJ. Progress toward the elimination of hepatitis B virus transmission among health workers in USA. *Arch. Of Intern. Med.* 1997. 157:2601-5.

[28] Agerton TB, Mahony FJ, Polish FB, Shapiro CN. Impact of bloodborne pathogens standard on vaccination of healthcare workers with hepatitis B vaccine. *Infect. Control Hosp. Epidemiol.* 1995. 16: 287-91.

[29] WHO. Global burden of disease. *In*: The World Health Report. 2002, Reducing Risk, Promoting Healthy Life. Geneva.2002.

[30] Chang MH, Chen CJ, Lai MS, Hsu HM, Wu TC, Kong MS, *et al.* Universal hepatitis B vaccination in Taiwan and incidence of hepatocellular carcinoma in children. Taiwan childhood hepato study group. *N. Engl. Med.* 1997. 336: 1855-9.

[31] Alter HJ, Purcell RH, Shih JW. *et al.* Detection of antibody to hepatitic C virus prospectively followed transfused recipients with acute and chronic non-A, non-B hepatitis. *N. Engl. J. Med.* 1989. 321:1494-1500.

[32] WHO. 45th World Health Assembly. Resolution No. WHA 45. 17. 1992.

[33] MacClennan S, Barbara JA, Hewitt P, Moore C, Contreras M. Screening blood donations for HCV. *Lancet* 1992. 339: 131-2.

[34] Neal KR, Jones DA, Killey D. and James V. Risk factors for hepatitis C virus infection. A case –control study of blood donors in the Trent Region (UK). *Epidemiol. And Infect.* 1994. 112. 595-601.

In: Hepatitis B Research Advances
Editor: Alicia P. Willis, pp. 113-140

ISBN: 978-1-60021-666-4

Chapter VIII

ROLES OF HEPATITIS B VIRUS IN HEPATOCARCINOGENESIS

***Xiong-Zhi Wu*[1] *and Dan Chen*[2]**

[1]Tianjin Medical University Cancer Institute and Hospital, Tianjin 300060, China
[2]Department of Biophysics, School of Basic Medical Sciences, Peking University, BeiJing 100083, China.

ABSTRACT

Although hepatitis B virus (HBV) has been documented to cause hepatocellular carcinoma (HCC), the exact role of HBV in the development of HCC remains enigmatic. Several hypotheses have been proposed to explain the potential mechanism, including insertional mutagenesis of HBV genomes, transcriptional activators of HBV gene products such as HBx and truncated middle S mutants and chromosomal alterations. HBx and integrated preS2/S sequences increased the expression levels of C-myc. C-myc inactivation resulted in HCC cells differentiating into hepatocytes and biliary cells forming bile duct structures. Malignant transformation of hepatocytes may occur in the context of chronic liver injury, regeneration and cirrhosis. Chronic liver inflammation and hepatic regeneration induced by cellular immune responses may favor the accumulation of genetic alterations and the proliferation of oval cells. Chronic liver inflammation is the setting for the accumulation of ECM, resulting in cirrhosis. ECM remodeling plays an important role in hepatocarcinogenesis through providing the survival signals, promoting the proliferation, invasion and metastasis and blocking the differentiation and apoptosis. Both mature cells and stem cells (oval cells and bone marrow stem cells) may be the targets of hepatocarcinogenesis. Two topics about the correlation between HBV and hepatocarcinogensis are very interesting and must be identified: whether the virus or viral protein directly induces HCC, or the long-term inflammatory changes caused by chronic HBV infection play more important roles in accelerating hepatocarcinogenesis; whether HCC originates from the de-differentiation of mature cells or differentiation block of stem cells.

INTRODUCTION

Hepatocellular carcinoma (HCC) is the most common primary cancer of the liver. The prevalence of HCC varies widely among different geographical areas, with the highest prevalence being in Africa and Asia. HCC in Asia is almost always associated with liver cirrhosis induced by chronic viral hepatitis, especially hepatitis B virus (HBV). Hence, there is a pressing need to understand the mechanism of HBV- associated hepatocarcinogenesis. Two topics about the correlation between HBV and hepatocarcinogensis are very interesting and must be identified: whether the virus or viral protein directly induces HCC, or the long-term inflammatory changes caused by chronic HBV infection play more important roles in accelerating hepatocarcinogenesis; whether HCC originates from the de-differentiation of mature cells or differentiation block of stem cells [1,2].

1. Does HBV Induce HCC Directly?

The HBV genome is a partial duplex circular genome whose circularity is maintained by 5' cohesive ends (Figure 1). Four open-reading frames (ORF) are present in the genome. The viral DNA polymerase that is encoded by the P ORF has reverse transcriptase activity. The C ORF encodes the structural protein of the nucleocapsid, while S ORF encodes the viral surface glycoproteins. Lastly, ORF X encodes a viral regulatory protein, HBx, which is best characterized as a transcriptional transactivator [3]. HBV can be classified into seven genotypes-A through H-based on an intergroup divergence of 8% or more in the nucleotide sequence. Genotype A is most common in the United States and northwest Europe, that genotypes B and C predominate in Asia, that genotype D is most frequently found in the Mediterranean countries, and that genotype F prevails in Central and South America. The geographic distribution of genotypes E, G, and H is less clear [4]. Viral DNA could integrate in hepatocyte. The HBV integrants are usually highly rearranged with deletions, inversions, and sequence reiterations. Elevated serum HBV DNA level (> or =10,000 copies/mL) is a strong risk predictor of HCC independent of HBeAg, serum alanine aminotransferase level, and liver cirrhosis [5,6]. Genotype C HBV was associated with an increased risk of HCC compared with other HBV genotypes [6].

Although HBV has been documented to cause HCC, the exact role of HBV in the development of HCC remains enigmatic. There are two general concepts about the mechanism of HBV-associated hepatocarcinogenesis. One is insertional (in-) activation of cellular genes, and the other is transactivation of cellular gene expression by HBx and truncated HBs proteins.

The first clue came from the discovery of integrated viral DNA in HCC and HCC-derived cell lines. The HBV integrants are usually highly rearranged with deletions, inversions, and sequence reiterations that are all commonly observed. The integrated viral DNA might therefore act as a mutagenic agent, causing secondary chromosomal rearrangement (duplications, translocations and deletions) and increasing genomic instability. Although the integration of WHV results in the activation of the transcription of the N-myc locus [7,8], common cellular target for HBV integration are not observed in HBV-infected patients with HCC. Moreover, integration at cellular sites that are important for regulation of hepatocyte proliferation appears to be a rare event [9].

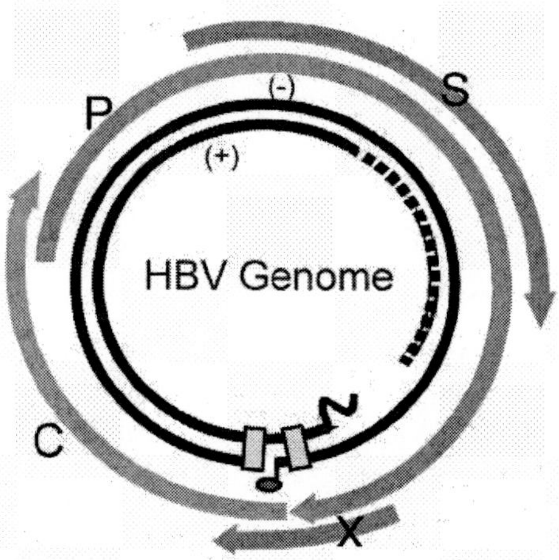

Figure 1. Genetic organization of hepatitis B virus genome. Four open-reading frames are indicated by open arrows: C (core), P (viral polymerase), S (surface glycoprotein), and X (HBx). DR1 and DR2 are two directly-repeated sequences of 11 bp at the 5' extremities of the minus- and plus-strand DNA.

1.1. HBx and Hepatocarcinogenesis

HBx, a 154 amino acid gene product of the X gene, is known as a promiscuous transcriptional transactivator, since it is capable of transactivating the gene expression by acting on a wide range of viral and cellular regulatory elements [10]. It is, therefore, suggested that HBx might play a role in hepatocarcinogenesis.

HBx does not directly bind to DNA, but HBx may stimulate transcription by interacting with transcription factors or with the basal transcription machinery of host RNA polymerase II and III [3]. For instance, HBx enhances AP-1 activation through interaction with Jab1 [11]. HBx binds to such protein targets as p53, proteasome subunits, and damaged DNA binding protein (DDB) [12-15]. Interestingly, HBx inactivates tumor suppressors, such as p53 (by direct binding) and Rb (by stimulating its phosphorylation), early in carcinogenesis that are mutated later during tumor progression [16,17].

P53-induced apoptosis has been implicated as its major tumor suppressor function. Dramatically, although HBx could induce apoptosis too, HBx binds to p53 to block p53-mediated apoptosis. The abrogation of p53-mediated apoptosis by integrated HBx mutants may provide a selective clonal advantage for preneoplastic or neoplastic hepatocytes and contribute to HCC [18]. HBX interacts with p53 to up-regulate AFP gene transcription by restoration of the p53-mediated repression of the AFP promotor activity [19,20].

HBx represses the transcription of p21 (waf1) by down-regulating the activity of Sp1. Because the tumor repressor p21 (waf1) protein is a universal inhibitor of cyclin-CDK complexes and DNA replication that induces cell cycle arrest at the G1-S checkpoint, the repression of p21 (waf1) by HBx might play an important role in a HBV-mediated pathogenesis [21].Transcription of p21 (waf1/cip1) was activated by HBx in the presence of functional p53, while it was repressed by HBx when p53 was absent or present at a low level. Thus, the opposite effects of HBx on the regulation of the cell cycle depend on the status of p53 [22]. HBx could inhibit the pRb tumor suppressor and increase the activity of E2F1, a positive regulator of the cell cycle [23]. E2F1 overcame the repressive effect of HBx on the p53 promoter through the E2F1 site. The pRb-binding domain of E2F1 was necessary for the functional interaction of these two proteins [24]. It also interacts with the cyclic AMP-responsive element binding protein, ATF-2, NFkappaB, and basal transcription factors [11,25-27].

Further implication of HBx in hepatocyte transformation has been demonstrated that it inhibits the repair of damaged hepatocyte DNA [28]. This effect may be mediated by interaction with p53 or through binding to DDB, which plays an accessory role in nucleotide excision repair [29,30]. Furthermore, HBX up-regulates the expression and activity of human telomerase reverse transcriptase (hTERT) in hepatoma cells [31].

Several studies indicated that HBx influences cellular signaling pathways [32]. HBx activates src [33] and the ras/raf/ ERK pathway, which leads to transcriptional transactivation and the stimulation of proliferation in quiescent cells [34,35]. HBx is primarily localized to the cytoplasm, where it interacts with and stimulates protein kinases, including protein kinase C, Janus kinase/STAT, IKK, PI-3-K, stress-activated protein kinase/Jun N-terminal kinase and protein kinase B/Akt [12,16,36]. HBx is likely to have wide-ranging effects on hepatocyte proliferation, apoptosis, cell cycle, signaling pathways, hTERT, DNA repair, oncogenes, tumor suppressors and transcription factors.

Numerous attempts have been made to examine the oncogenic potential of HBx in cell cultures [37-39]. However, most of the transgenic mice that harbored the HBx gene had no serious liver diseases or tumors [40,41]. Only in certain transgenic lineages of the CD-1 and FMH202 cells, HBx weakly promotes tumorigenesis [42,43]. Data obtained from these studies suggested that HBx had no or low acute transforming activity [32].

HBx may promote the apoptosis of hepatocytes by regulating the expressions of Fas/FasL and Bax/Bcl-2 gene in a dose-dependent manner [44].The effect of HBx on apoptosis may be important for the establishment of HBV infection. However, H-ras collaborates with HBx to transform cells by suppressing the HBx-mediated apoptosis [45]. Thus, HBx contributes to the neoplastic transformation in collaboration with H-ras that renders cells to counteract the HBx-mediated apoptosis. In addition, HBx was shown to potentate other oncogenes, such as c-myc and SV40 T-antigen, induced liver oncogenesis in transgenic mice [46,47]. Expression of HBx in a certain genetic background might induce tumor formation, possibly in collaboration with activated cellular oncogenes in the multistage transformation [32].

Most of the COOH-terminally truncated HBx sequences obtained from tumor tissues, in contrast to the full-length HBx isolated from the sera and nontumor tissue, enhance the transforming ability of ras and myc. The hypothesis is that natural HBx mutants might be selected in tumor tissues and plays a role in hepatocarcinogenesis by modifying the biological functions of HBx [48]. Rearrangements of HBV sequence, most frequently 3'-deleted X gene and consequent C-terminal truncated X protein, were observed in the HBV integration. These deletions cause the losses of p53-dependent transcriptional repression binding site, transcription factor Sp1 binding site and growth-suppressive effect domain, leading to cell proliferation and transformation. Thus, 3'-deleted X gene caused by the HBV integration may play an important role in the HCC development [9].

1.2. HBV Pre-S Mutants and Hepatocarcinogenesis

A second type of transactivator is encoded in the preS/S region of HBV. In contrast to HBx, HBs transactivators require carboxyterminal truncation to gain their transactivating function. The intracellular retention and accumulation of the normally secreted middle HBs (MHBs) leads to oxidative stress and activation of transcription factors NFkappaB and AP-1 [49]. Unlike full-length MHBs, the truncated MHBst is retained in the endoplasmic reticulum and not secreted into the surrounding medium [50]. The truncated MHBst is the authentic transactivating factor for many cellular genes [51-55].

Large HBs (LHBs), like MHBst, is indeed able to activate a variety of promoter elements. There is evidence for a PKC-dependent activation of AP-1 and NF-kappa B by LHBs. Downstream of the PKC, the functionality of c-Raf-1 kinase is a prerequisite for LHBs-dependent activation of AP-1 and NF-kappa B, since inhibition of c-Raf-1 kinase abolishes LHBs-dependent transcriptional activation of AP-1 and NF-kappa B [56].Two types of LHBs with deletions at the pre-S1 (DeltaS1-LHBs) and pre-S2 (DeltaS2-LHBs) regions have been identified. Pre-S mutant LHBs can initiate endoplasmic reticulum stress to induce oxidative DNA damage and genomic instability. Furthermore, pre-S mutant LHBs can up-regulate cyclooxygenase-2 and cyclin A to induce cell cycle progression and the proliferation of hepatocytes. In transgenic mice, the pre-S mutants can induce dysplasia of hepatocytes and the development of HCC [50]. The PreS2 domain binds of PKC alpha/beta and triggers a PKC-dependent activation of the c-Raf-1/MAP2-kinase signal transduction cascade, resulting in an activation of AP-1 and NF-kappa B. By activation of this signaling cascade, the PreS2 activators cause an increased proliferation rate of hepatocytes [57].

2. C-myc: A Molecular Target of HBV-Induced Hepatocarcinogenesis?

C-myc plays a pivotal role in hepatocarcingenesis. C-myc transgenic mice are prone to liver cancer [58-60]. Overexpression of c-myc has been frequently observed in HCC. C-myc amplification occurs more frequently in young patients with HBV infection, and is related to poorly differentiated, intrahepatic portal vein spread and worse survival rate in patients [61,62]. Hence, there is a critical need to understand the role of C-myc in HBV-associated hepatocarcinogenesis.

2.1. C-Myc and HBV-induced Hepatocarcinogenesis

C-myc is acted by two potential mechanisms: insertional mutagen and amplification. HCC has been observed in animals chronically infected with two hepadnaviruses: ground squirrel hepatitis virus (GSHV) and woodchuck hepatitis virus (WHV). A distinctive feature of WHV is the early onset of woodchuck tumors, which may be correlated with a direct role of the virus as an insertional mutagen of c-myc gene. However, the high frequency of c-myc amplification observed in ground squirrel HCC [63,64].

Many c-myc-regulated genes are involved in HBV-related HCC. 237 genes whose expression differed between HCC and non-tumorous livers, all of which were associated with genotype-C HBV infection, were identified by DNA microarray. Among the 237 genes, the top 35 up-regulated and top 35 down-regulated genes in tumor were highlighted. When overlapping genes were excluded, 12 of the top 34 up-regulated genes and 5 of the top 33 down-regulated genes were c-myc-regulated genes. That many c-myc-regulated genes are involved in genotype-C-HBV-related HCC suggest that c-myc is related to the hepatocarcinogenic activity of genotype-C HBV [65].

2.2. HBx and C-Myc Amplification

A consistent alteration of many cellular genes including a subset of oncogenes, such as c-myc, and tumor suppressor genes, such as APC, are regulated by HBx [66]. In transgenic mouse model, HBx alone has no direct pathological effect but it is shown to accelerate tumor development induced by c-myc [47]. Transgene incorporates HBx and c-myc gene, changes in the liver from birth with foci of multicentric dysplasia evolved into nodules and overt HCC. The hepatocytes are mitotically active and show increased proliferative capacity. This is accompanied by a high rate of apoptosis, which later declined as the tumors developed. The disturbances of cell growth and death because of the collaborative influence of HBx and c-myc genes result in the development of HCC after a prolonged latent period [67].

C-myc-induced apoptosis of hepatocyte is dependent on the expression of c-Fos [68]. Dramatically, although HBx could induce apoptosis too, co-expression of HBx along with myc abrogate the apoptotic signals. The HBx expression is associated with an increase in the levels of phosphorylated AKT and down-regulation of c-Fos by myc [30].

Co-expression of HBx and c-myc resulted in increasing stability of intracellular c-myc. HBx block the ubiquitination of myc through a direct interaction with the F box region of Skp2 and destabilization of the SCF (Skp2) complex. Sustained presence of c-myc combined with mitogenic activity inherent to HBx may be associated with cell cycle deregulation and transformation [69].

Most of the COOH-terminally truncated HBx sequences obtained from tumor tissues, in contrast to the full-length HBx isolated from the sera and nontumor tissue, enhance the transforming ability of myc. The hypothesis is that natural HBx mutants might be selected in tumor tissues and plays a role in hepatocarcinogenesis by modifying the biological functions of HBx [31].

2.3. Wnt Signaling Pathway and C-Myc

The Wnt signaling pathway is a major route by which the cell conveys information from its exterior to the nucleus [70]. The Wnt signaling pathway is activated by binding of Wnt to their receptors, leading to the release of beta-catenin from the degradation complex, and facilitating its entry into the nucleus, where it regulates target gene transcription (Figure 2). A genetic program regulated by beta-catenin control the transcription of a suite of genes promoting cellular proliferation and repressing differentiation during embryogenesis and carcinogenesis [71-73]. C-myc gene is a target of Wnt/beta-catenin pathway, and activation of the Wnt/ beta-catenin pathway is a dominant event during c-myc/E2F1 hepatocarcinogenesis [74,75]. Wnt/beta-catenin pathway has been implicated in the development of HCC [76-79].

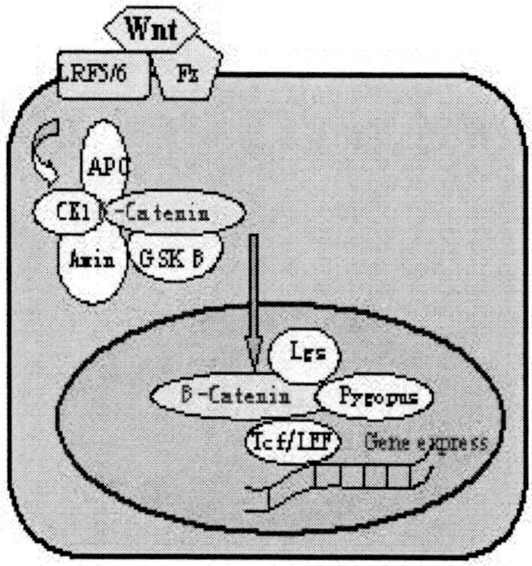

Figure 2. Wnt signaling pathway. The Wnt signaling pathway is activated by binding of Wnt to their receptors Fz and LRP5/6, leading to the release of beta-catenin from the degradation complex, which is composed by beta-catenin, APC, Axin, GSK3-beta and CK1α, and facilitating its entry into the nucleus, where it regulates target gene transcription through association with TcF/LEF, Lgs and Pygopus.

Abbreviations: Fz, Frizzled; LRP5/6, LDL-receptor related proteins 5 and 6; APC, adenomatous polyposis coli; GSK3-β, glycogen synthase kinase 3-β; CK1α, casein kinase 1a; Lgs, Legless; TcF/LEF, T-Cell Factor/Lymphoid Enhancer Factor.

Wnt-1 is necessary but insufficient to activate Wnt/beta-catenin signaling in hepatoma cells and the enhanced stabilization of beta-catenin by HBx, in addition to Wnt-1, is essential for the activation of Wnt/beta-catenin signaling in hepatoma cells [80]. HBx stabilizates beta-catenin by suppressing glycogen synthase kinase 3 activity via the activation of Src kinase [80,81]. HBx down-regulate APC gene and up-regulate c-myc gene [65]. Thus HBx up-regulate c-myc gene and promote hepatocarcinogenesis by activating Wnt signal pathway.

2.4. Integrated preS2/S Sequences and C-Myc Amplification

The integration of HBV Pre-S gene with cellular chromosome can activate myc, ras oncogenes and inactivate the p53 tumor suppressor gene [82]. 3'-truncated preS2/S sequences in integrated HBV DNA of liver cell carcinomas encode an unidentified transcriptional trans-activation activity of c-myc oncogene. This activity is also produced by an artificially 3'-truncated preS2/S gene of the wild-type HBV genome [83].

2.5. Myc Inactivation: Induce Differentiation of HCC

Despite the high mortality and frequency of HCC, surgical resection is an available option for only a small proportion of patients because metastases are often present when the cancer is discovered. Malignant transformation of hepatocytes may occur in the context of chronic liver injury, regeneration and cirrhosis. As it is difficulty to give sufficient dose due to the poor liver function and low sensitivity for the anti-cancer agents, chemotherapy adds little to the overall survival of HCC patients. Since prognosis and survival of patients with HCC is still very poor, novel strategies, which have greater targeting on HCC but lower toxicity for normal liver cells, are seen as a direction of enormous potential. The development of malignancies can be considered as the result of change of the normal process of cell differentiation. The induction of terminal differentiation in tumor cells represents a possible therapeutic strategy with less toxicity.

Myc inactivation result in HCC cells differentiating into hepatocytes and biliary cells forming bile duct structures. This is associated with rapid loss of expression of AFP, the increase in expression of liver cell markers cytokeratin 8 [84].

The human liver-specific antigen expression is enhanced and c-myc levels is reduced during sodium butyrate-induced differentiation of HCC [85,86]. Dramatically, the reduction of c-myc transcription and increase of liver-specific antigen expression during antisense oligodeoxynucleotide against c-myc mRNA-induced differentiation of HCC is similar to those induced by butyrate [87]. Tachyplesin, which is isolated from Chinese horseshoe crab (Tachypleus tridentatus) hemocytes, could effectively inhibit the proliferation and induce the differentiation of HCC. After tachyplesin treatment, the cell cycle arrested at G_0 / G_1 phase, and the protein and mRNA level of c-myc gene are decreased [88,89]. Thus, reduction of c-myc transcription is a key event of differentiation of HCC, and c-myc is a potential target of HCC therapy.

Mono- and bicistronic antisense recombinants against HBx and c-myc genes could inhibit in the expression levels of HBx and c-Myc [90]. The inhibitory effects with two different small hairpin RNAs (shRNAs) against two different regions each of the HBx and c-myc open reading frames were cumulative [91]. RNAi targeting HBx in PLC/PRF/5 cells demonstrated significant reduction in cell proliferation and tumor development in nude mice. In addition, depletion of HBx expression increase cell sensitivity to TNFalpha-mediated and serum-free-induced apoptosis, and reduce the expression levels of C-myc and Bcl-X (L) [92].

Although myc inactivation result in HCC cells differentiating into hepatocytes and biliary cells, and many of these tumor cells remained dormant as long as myc inactivated; however, myc reactivation immediately restored their neoplastic features [84]. Thus inducing differentiation through myc inactivation may have the high potential of recrudescence.

3. Inflammation and Hepatocarcinogenesis

The question about whether HBV themselves act as carcinogenic factors, independent of any hepatitis-related proliferative change, however, is still debated. The evidence that supports the former concept is mainly derived from the study of the HBx. The HBx is reported to transactivate many cellular genes associated with cell proliferation to cause HCC in the transgenic mouse. However, many clinical observations do not support this concept.

First, asymptomatic HBV carriers with extensive viral replication rarely develop HCC. Second, there has been no report to show the ability of HBx to transform or immortalize primary cells. Data obtained from transgenic studies suggested that HBx had no acute transforming activity, but its over-expression in a certain genetic background might induce tumor formation, possibly in collaboration with activated cellular oncogenes in the multistage transformation. Finally, among HBV carriers, HCC usually develops inpatients with chronic liver disease, such as chronic active hepatitis or cirrhosis. In a word, the continuous inflammatory changes play positive roles in hepatocarcinogenesis (Figure 3). Overproduction of HBV in transgenic mice initiates a process characterized by liver cell injury, inflammation and regenerative hyperplasia, which places large numbers of hepatocytes at risk for the development of transforming mutations, and inexorably progresses to HCC [93]. However, the distinct molecular pathway or molecules that could explain this concept are not yet known.

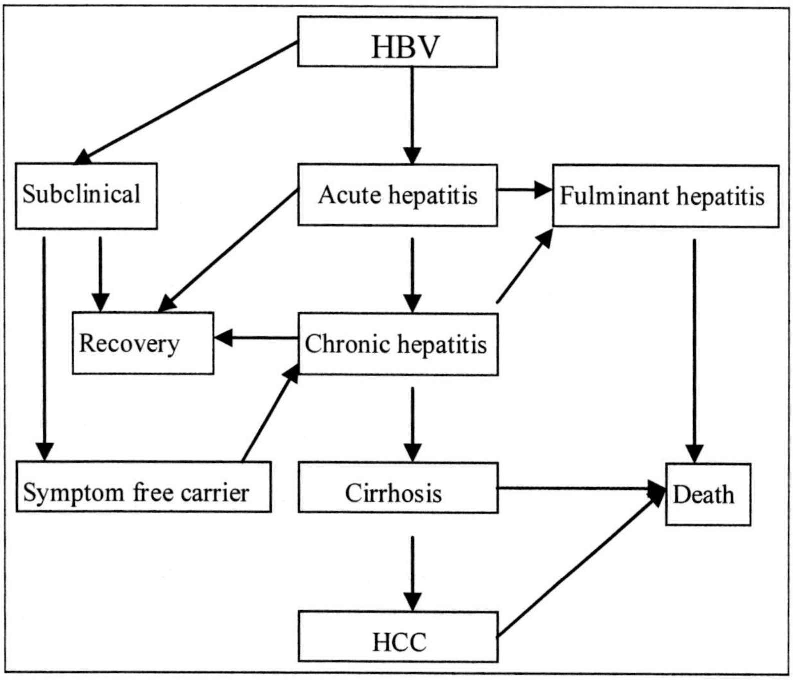

Figure 3. Chronic liver inflammation and HCC. HCC usually is developed in patients with chronic liver disease, such as chronic active hepatitis or cirrhosis. Chronic inflammation places large numbers of hepatocytes at risk for the development of transforming mutations, and inexorably progresses to HCC.

Moreover, persistent regeneration increases the rate of transforming mutations or epigenetic events that make transformed cells proliferate independently [94-96]. HBV transgenic mice with chronic active hepatitis display greatly increased hepatic oxidative DNA damage. Moreover, the DNA damage occurs in the presence of heightened hepatocellular proliferation, increasing the probability of fixation of the attendant genetic and chromosomal abnormalities and the development of HCC [97]. HBx might trigger an apoptotic process in HBV-infected hepatocytes, in turn possibly favoring liver regeneration and accumulation of genetic alterations, ultimately leading to liver cell transformation in chronically infected patients [98].

Recently, cancer is increasingly being viewed as a stem cell disease. But stem cell activity is tightly controlled, raising the question of how normal regulation might be subverted in carcinogenesis. The long-known association between cancer and chronic tissue injury, and the more recently appreciated roles of Hedgehog and Wnt signalling pathways in tissue regeneration, stem cell renewal and cancer growth together indicate that carcinogenesis is the response of chronic tissue injury [94]. Dramatically, HCC usually is developed in patients with chronic liver disease and activation of Hedgehog and Wnt signalling pathways [80,99-103].

Growth genes in stem cells are activated by tissue injury and many growth factors are secreted to stimulate the proliferation and differentiation of stem cells. However, if the wound is persistent, amplification of growth genes and the persistent stimulation of growth factors may lead to a clinical cancer [104]. Unfortunately, termination of injury could not induce the regression of most cancer. It suggests that cancer is not the normal response for persistent injury, because it could grow independently without the stimulation of growth factors which is secreted with tissue repair [105]. In fact, HCC cells could secret growth factor to stimulate the growth of self and neighboring cells. Dysregulation of pleiotropic growth factors, receptors and their downstream signaling pathway components, especially the insulin-like growth factor/insulin-like growth factor-1 receptor, hepatocyte growth factor, transforming growth factor alpha/epidermal growth factor receptor and transforming growth factor beta pathways, represent a central protumorigenic principle in human hepatocarcinogenesis [106,107]. Thus HCC may be the "abnormal repair tissue" with genetic or epigenetic change, which could escape the control of host [105].

4. Extracellular Matrix and Hepatocarcinogenesis: The Effect of Soil on Feed?

Extracellular matrix (ECM) surrounds hepatocyte as a capsule, and creates a permissive soil on hepatocyte. As the important component of niche, ECM is important in cell identify, differentiation, proliferation and gene expression, both in physiological and in pathological conditions [108,109]. Malignant transformation of hepatocytes may occur in the context of chronic liver injury, regeneration and cirrhosis. Proliferation of hepatocyte and production of ECM are response for the injury and closing the wound. When the injury is limited in time, the result of the repair is restoration of normal tissue structure. When the injury is persistent, however, there is net accumulation of ECM, result in cirrhosis [110]. Cirrhosis can be regarded as a continuous wound-healing process and which results in scar formation, which is characterized by accumulation of ECM proteins in response to liver injury [111,112]. The interaction between ECM and liver cells plays an important role in hepatocarcinogenesis [113].

4.1. Collagens and Hepatocarcinogenesis

Different event is a process that is dependent on stimulation of extracellular signals, signal transduction and gene express. Extracellular signals, involve either soluble factors (hormones and growth factors) or ECM, are transduced to the nucleus and modulate the expression of groups of genes. To be functionally stable along the adult stage, the liver has to maintain an ordered activity of cell renewal. This balance between proliferation and differentiation is, at least in part, controlled by ECM. ECM, which located in and around HCC, is different from normal organ stroma. Changes of collagens, especially type I and IV collagens, result in modifying the differentiation/proliferation balance [114-117]. Moreover, dipeptidyl peptidase IV, a protein of ECM that could binds to collagens, preferentially to the collagens I and III, is markedly reduced in rat hepatoma cells [118,119].

4.2. Integrins and Hepatocarcinogenesis

Integrins, the receptor for the laminin (Ln) family enable cells to recognize adhesive substrates in the ECM. The integrin alpha6 beta1 has been found to be over-expressed in HCC [120,121]. Poorer differentiation of HCC was characterized by down-regulation of Ln and integrins alpha 5 and beta 4 [122-126]. The interaction between integrin and Ln may be an import extracellular signal to induce differentiation of HCC [113].

Beta 1-integrin provides a strong anti-apoptotic signal via a mitogen-activated protein (MAP) kinase dependent pathway during TGF-beta 1-induced apoptosis in HCC [127]. Over-expression of Beta 1-integrin protects HCC from chemotherapy induced apoptosis via a MAP kinase dependent pathway [128]. Thus the interaction between integrin and Ln is closely linked to transduce survival signals.

In HCC, Ln and fibronectin could stimulate the secretion of matrix metalloproteinases (MMPs), especially MMP-9 and its activated type [129]. HBx-bearing cells showed decreased adhesion to fibronectin, which correlated with a decreased expression of the alpha5 integrin subunit [130]. The interaction between integrin and Ln could provide survival signals, induce differentiation and promote the metastasis of HCC.

4.3. Polysaccharides and Hepatocarcinogenesis

Sulfated oligosaccharides, which often bind to protein, are important intigrents of ECM. Members of this family include heparan, heparan sulfate, chondroitin sulfate, keratan sulfate and dermatan sulfate. The changes of sulfated glycosaminoglycans were detected in HCC. The major component of glycosaminoglycans in healthy adult rat liver is heparan sulfate, while chondroitin sulfate is more prevalent in the tumors [131]. Hepatoma cell could synthesize heparan sulfate and chondroitin sulfate proteoglycans, but the hepatoma heparan sulfate proteoglycans had a lower average charge density than the rat liver heparan sulfate proteoglycans. Furthermore, the hepatoma proteoglycan do not bind to the neoplastic cells, whereas heparan sulfate from normal rat liver bind to the hepatoma cells in a time-dependent reaction [132]. The increasing of chondroitin sulfate and the modification of chondroitin sulfate and heparan sulfate play an important role in hepatocarcinogenesis [133]. Recently, we separated sulfated polysaccharide from Gekko swinhonis Gūenther. Gekko sulfated polysaccharide (Gepsin) suppresses the proliferation and induces differentiation of hepatocarcinoma, but the toxicity to normal liver cells is negligible (Figure 4) [134].

4.5. The Role of ECM in Tumor Invasion and Metastasis

The degradation of ECM plays an important role in tumor invasion and metastasis [136]. Proteolytic enzymes, such as plasmin, collagenase and MMPs are thought to play a pivotal role in degradation of ECM. Enzymatic activity depends on balance between enzymes and their inhibitors. MMPs play a major role in the turnover of ECM during cancer invasion and metastasis, and tissue inhibitors of metalloproteinases (TIMPs) control MMPs, thus maintaining a balanced ECM catabolism under physiological conditions. HBV transfection affects the malignance of HCC by elevating MMP-9 activity, and suppressing TIMP-1 and

TIMP-3 [137]. HBx up-regulated the transcription, translation and secretion of MMP-3, manifest as a cell migratory phenotype [138]. HBx-bearing cells show decreased adhesion to fibronectin, which correlated with a decreased expression of the alpha5 integrin subunit [130].

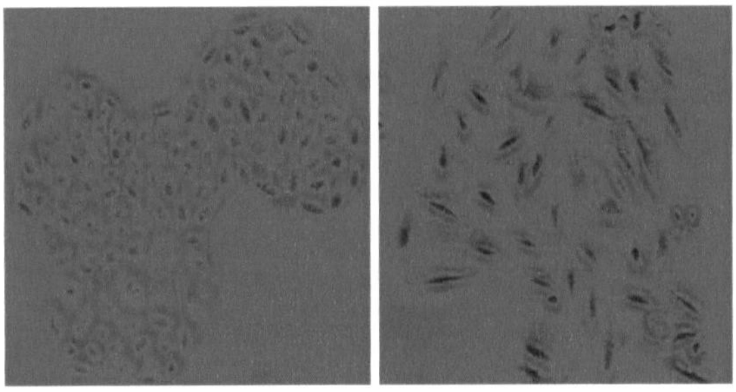

A B

Figure 4. Effect of Gepsin on morphologic variation of Bel-7402 cells. A: Cells cultured without Gepsin; B: Cells cultured with Gepsin. Chedid et al reported that hepatocellular carcinoma cells show two shapes: polygonal and spindle and spindle cells were associated with a better prognosis [135]. Bel-7402 cells showed abnormal features with a round shape, but cells changed to spindle shape after exposure to Gepsin.

In conclusion, ECM remodeling plays an important role in hepatocarcinogenesis. ECM provides the survival signals and controls the proliferation, differentiation and metastasis of HCC. Thus normalization of the soil, ECM, is a hopeful strategy to control the seed – HCC cells [113]. However, the activities of the ingredients of ECM are complicated. More experimental and clinical studies must be performed to evaluate the exact activity of each ingredient of ECM in the hepatocarcinogenesis.

5. Stem Cells and Hepatocarcinogenesis: The Trouble Maker?

A role for cancer stem cells has been demonstrated for some cancers, such as the hematopoietic system, breast and brain [139-146]. The clear similarities between stem cell and cancer stem cell genetic programs are the basis of a proposal that some cancer stem cells could derive from human adult stem cells. Adult mesenchymal stem cells (MSCs) may be targets for malignant transformation and undergo spontaneous transformation following long-term *in vitro* culture, supporting the hypothesis of cancer stem cell origin [147-149]. Stem cells are not only units of biological organization, responsible for the development and the regeneration of tissue and organ systems, but also are target of carcinogenesis. However, the origin of the cancer stem cell remains elusive.

Three levels of cells that can respond to liver tissue renewal or damage have been proved: (1) Mature liver cells, which proliferate after normal liver tissue renewal and respond rapidly to liver injury [150], (2) Oval cells, as bi-potential stem cells, which are activated to proliferate when the liver damage is extensive and chronic, or if proliferation of hepatocytes is inhibited, (3) Bone marrow stem cells, as multi-potential stem cells, which could differentiate into oval cell and hepatocyte and have a very long proliferation potential (Figure

5) [151]. There are two major nonexclusive hypotheses of the cellular origin of cancer: from stem cells due to maturation arrest or from dedifferentiation of mature cells [152]. Research on hepatic stem cells in hepatocarcinogenesis has entered a new era of controversy, excitement, and great expectations.

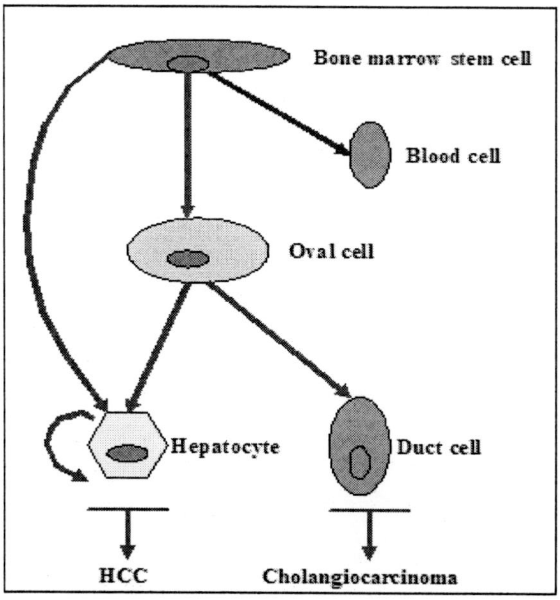

Figure 5. Hepatic stem cell and HCC. Bone marrow stem cells, as multipotent stem cells, could differentiate into oval cell. Oval cells, as bipotential stem cells, could differentiate into hepatocyte and duct cell. All of the three levels of cells may be the targets of hepatocarcinogenesis.

5.1. Oval Cell and HCC

The distribution of oval cells inside and outside the HCC nodes supports the concepts that hepatocarcinogenesis can be based on transformation of oval cells [153,154]. Two evidences support that oval cells is the troublemaker of HCC: (1) Oval cells transfected with activated oncogene or drop of tumor suppressor gene can give rise to HCC [155-159]. (2) C-myc over-express in oval cells during hepatocarcinogenesis [160,161]. Myc inactivation resulted in HCC cells differentiating into hepatocytes and biliary cells forming bile duct structures [84]. It support strongly that some HCC originate from the differentiation arrest of oval cells. (3) As bipotential stem cells, oval cells have the bipotent for differentiating into hepatocyte and bile cells. Dramatically, some liver tumor cells present intermediate (hepatocyte-bile duct cell) phenotype [162-164]. Moreover, some hepatocarcinomas combined with hepatocellular / cholangiocarcinomas contained oval cells [165-166]. These intermediate and combined types can be more easily explained as deriving from bipotential stem cells.

HBs protein could be detected in oval cells and mature hepatocytes, but not in bile duct or ductule cells in patients with HCC. Transforming growth factor-alpha (TGF-alpha) is expressed in oval cells, mature hepatocytes and bile duct cells in patients with HCC. Co-expression of HBs protein and TGF-alpha is identified in the same cells in populations of oval cells of selected patients [167,168]. Thus HBV infection of oval cells could be a mechanism of human hepatocarcinogenesis.

The long-known association between cancer and chronic tissue injury, and the more recently appreciated roles of Hedgehog and Wnt signalling pathways in tissue regeneration, stem cell renewal and cancer growth together indicate that carcinogenesis is the response of chronic tissue injury [94]. Dramatically, HCC usually develops inpatients with chronic liver disease and activation of Hedgehog and Wnt signalling pathways [80,99-103]. The hypothesis is that the activation of Hedgehog and Wnt signalling pathways by chronic liver inflammation and repeat regeneration may contribute for transformation of oval cells.

5.2. Bone Marrow Cell and HCC

Hematopoiesis and the hepatic environment are known to have a close relationship at the time of hepatic development and systemic diseases. During development, blood cell formation moves from extraembryonic regions to the aorto-gonadalmesonephros in the embryo and then to the liver in the first trimester. Liver provides a more conducive microenvironment to support hematopoietic stem cells (HSCs) [169]. HSCs could be detected in the fetal and adult liver [170,171]. Oval cells express many markers, such as C-kit, CD_{34} and Thy-1, also found on HSCs [172-177]. Recently, some research reported that bone marrow stem cells could differentiate into oval cells, hepatocytes and cholangiocytes, especially when proliferation of hepatocyte was suppressed (Figure 6) [178-186].

HBs antigen was detected in nuclei of immature hematopoietic cells including myeloblasts, normoblasts, and lymphoblasts; granulocytes had mostly cytoplasmic HBs antigen. Hepatitis B virus core antigen was also detected in HBV infected bone marrow cells. [187] Exposure to HBV suppressed the ability of hematopoietic cell lines HL-60 cells to differentiate into granulocytes after treatment with retinoic acid (RA) or dimethyl sulfoxide, and RA-induced activation of the monocytic cell line THP-1 was also suppressed. Terminal differentiation of both cell lines by phorbol 12-myristate 13-acetate (PMA) was not affected by HBV. At 5 days postinfection, extracellular viral DNA was detected in immature but not in differentiated cultures and higher levels of core antigen and surface antigen were seen in undifferentiated cells than in RA- or PMA-treated cells. In addition, release of HBs antigen into the medium was 2 to 12 times greater in untreated cultures than for RA- or PMA-treated cells. Thus, HBV block the maturational development of progenitors and selectively infects immature myeloid cells compared with mature end-stage cells [188]. The infection of HBV may contribute to the pathogenesis of hematopoietic tumors [189,190].

Adult MSCs may be targets for malignant transformation and undergo spontaneous transformation following long-term *in vitro* culture [147-149]. Chronic gastric inflammation, which develops as a consequence of *H. pylori*, leads over time to repetitive injury and repair resulting in hyperproliferation, an increased rate of mitotic error, and progression to adenocarcinoma. Wang *et al.* reported that chronic infection of C57BL/6 mice with *H. pylori*, induced repopulation of the stomach with bone mesenchymal stem cells. Subsequently, these cells progressed through metaplasia and dysplasia to intraepithelial cancer [191]. Ishikawa *et a.l* reported that bone marrow cells could not progress to HCC in transgenic mouse induced HCC by treatment with diethylnitrosamine and phenobarbital [192]. The hypothesis is that chronic liver inflammation, which may develop as a consequence of HBV, plays a possible role of leading over time to repetitive injury and repair resulting in hyper-proliferation of bone marrow stem cells, an increased rate of mitotic error, and progression to HCC [193].

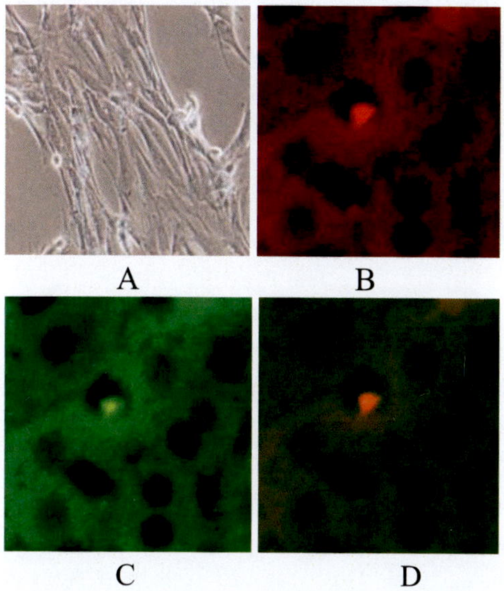

Figure 6. Bone mesenchymal stem cells differentiate into hepatocytes. A: Bone mesenchymal stem cells; B: cytokeratin 18 (Cy3); C: Y-chromosome (FITC); D: photo superposition. Bone mesenchymal stem cells (BMSCs) were isolated from the bone marrow of BALB/C male donor mouse by adherence selecting. Mice were hepatectomined, and transplant group immediately accepted BMSCs transplant. Simultaneous detection were performed on regenerated liver for both the Y-chromosome by fluorescence in situ hybridization and the albumin or cytokeratin 18 (CK18) by fluorescence immunoassays. The cells which showed both Y chromosome and albumin (or CK18) positive can be detected in both rejected liver lobe and other lobe. These cells located in hepatic plate. Most of these cells exist separate, but some cells are close or form a node. Some of these cells have two Y chromosome in karyon.

Whether there are common stem cells for the hematopoietic and hepatic systems in bone is uncertain [194]. Some researches suggest that there are multi-potent adult progenitor cells in bone, which could differentiate into hepatocyte [195-197]. Moreover, some research indicates that bone marrow is a "home" of liver stem cells [198,199]. Both HSCs and MSCs could differentiate into hepatocyte in vitro and in vivo. If bone marrow stem cells could differentiate to HCC cells, who is the real troublemaker?

Two major hypotheses about the cellular origination of HCC have been discussed for almost 20 years. Debate has centered on whether HCC originates from the differentiation block of stem cells or dedifferentiation of mature cells. In fact, there might be more than one type of carcinogen target cell [200-202]. Both mature cells and stem cells may be the targets of hepatocarcinogenesis. However, the role of HBV infection in stem cells-originated hepatocarcinogensis remains enigmatic.

CONCLUSION

Although HBV has been documented to cause HCC, the exact role of HBV in the development of HCC remains enigmatic. Several hypotheses have been proposed to explain the potential mechanism, including insertional mutagenesis of HBV genomes, transcriptional activators of HBV gene products such as HBx and truncated middle S mutants and chromosomal alterations. The collaborative influence of HBx and c-myc genes result in the development of HCC, and C-myc inactivation resulted in HCC cells differentiating into hepatocytes and biliary cells forming bile duct structures. Reduction of c-myc transcription is a key event of differentiation of HCC, and c-myc is a potential target of HCC therapy. Malignant transformation of hepatocytes may occur in the context of chronic liver injury, regeneration and cirrhosis. Chronic liver inflammation and hepatic regeneration induced by cellular immune responses may favor the accumulation of genetic alterations and proliferation of oval cells. Chronic liver inflammation is the setting for the accumulation of ECM, resulting in cirrhosis. ECM remodeling plays an important role in hepatocarcinogenesis through providing the survival signals, promoting the proliferation, invasion and metastasis and blocking the differentiation and apoptosis. There is more than one type of carcinogen target cell. Both mature cells and stem cells (oval cells and bone marrow stem cells) may be the targets of hepatocarcinogenesis.

REFERENCES

[1] Hino O, Kajino K, Umeda T, Arakawa Y. Understanding the hypercarcinogenic state in chronic hepatitis: a clue to the prevention of human hepatocellular carcinoma. *J Gastroenterol.* 2002;37:883-887.

[2] Wu XZ, Chen D. Origin of hepatocellular carcinoma: role of stem cells. *J Gastroenterol Hepatol.* 2006;21:1093-1098.

[3] Murakami, S. Hepatitis B virus X protein: a multifunctional viral regulator. *J Gastroenterol.* 2001,36: 651-660.

[4] Enomoto M, Tamori A, Nishiguchi S. Hepatitis B virus genotypes and response to antiviral therapy. *Clin Lab.* 2006;52:43-47.

[5] Chen CJ, Yang HI, Su J, Jen CL, You SL, Lu SN, *et al.* Risk of hepatocellular carcinoma across a biological gradient of serum hepatitis B virus DNA level. *JAMA.* 2006;295:65-73.

[6] Yu MW, Yeh SH, Chen PJ, Liaw YF, Lin CL, Liu CJ, *et al.* Hepatitis B virus genotype and DNA level and hepatocellular carcinoma: a prospective study in men. *J Natl Cancer Inst.* 2005;97:265-272.

[7] Fourel G, Couturier J, Wei Y, Apiou F, Tiollais P, Buendia MA. Evidence for long-range oncogene activation by hepadnavirus insertion. *EMBO J.* 1994;13: 2526-2534.

[8] Fourel G, Trepo C, Bougueleret L, Henglein B, Ponzetto A, Tiollais P *et al.* Frequent activation of N-myc genes by hepadnavirus insertion in woodchuck liver tumors. Nature 1990;347:294-298.

[9] Wang Y, Sze HL, Jonathan STS, Wu MC, Wang T, Guan XY. Characterization of HBV integrants in 14 hepatocellular carcinomas: association of truncated X gene and hepatocellular carcinogenesis. *Oncogene.* 2004;23: 142-148.

[10] Yen TSB. Hepadnaviral X protein: review of recent progress. *J Biomed Sci.* 1996; 3:20-30.

[11] Tanaka Y, Kanai F, Ichimura T, Tateishi K, Asaoka Y, Guleng B, *et al.* The hepatitis B virus X protein enhances AP-1 activation through interaction with Jab1. *Oncogene.* 2006 Jan 26;25:633-642.

[12] Zhang X, Zhang H, Ye L. Effects of hepatitis B virus X protein on the development of liver cancer. *J Lab Clin Med.* 2006 ;147:58-66.

[13] Lee SG, Rho HM. Transcriptional repression of the human p53 gene by hepatitis B viral X protein. *Oncogene.* 2000;19:468-471.

[14] Wang XW, Forrester K, Yeh H, Feitelson MA, Gu JR, Harris CC. Hepatitis B virus X protein inhibits p53 sequence-specific DNA binding, transcriptional activity, and association with transcription factor ERCC3. *Proc Natl Acad Sci U S A.* 1994;91:2230-2234.

[15] Dewantoro O, Gani RA, Akbar N. Hepatocarsinogenesis in Viral Hepatitis B Infection: The Role of HBx and p53. *Acta Med Indones.* 2006;38:154-9.

[16] Arbuthnot P, Capovilla A, Kew M. Putative role of hepatitis B virus X protein in hepatocarcinogenesis: effects on apoptosis, DNA repair, mitogen-activated protein kinase and JAK/STAT pathways. *J Gastroenterol Hepatol.* 2000;15:357-68.

[17] Feitelson MA, Pan J, Lian Z. Early molecular and genetic determinants of primary liver malignancy. *Surg Clin North Am.* 2004;84:339-354.

[18] Huo TI, Wang XW, Forgues M, Wu CG, Spillare EA, Giannini C, *et al.* Hepatitis B virus X mutants derived from human hepatocellular carcinoma retain the ability to abrogate p53-induced apoptosis. *Oncogene.* 2001;20:3620-3628.

[19] Ogden SK, Lee KC, Barton MC. Hepatitis B viral transactivator HBx alleviates p53-mediated repression of alpha-fetoprotein gene expression. *J Biol Chem.* 2000;275:27806-27814.

[20] Arima T, Nakao K, Nakata K, Ishikawa H, Ichikawa T, Hamasaki K, *et al.* Transactivation of human alpha-fetoprotein gene by X-gene product of hepatitis B virus in human hepatoma cells. *Int J Mol Med.* 2002;9:397-400.

[21] Ahn JY, Chung EY, Kwun HJ, Jang KL. Transcriptional repression of p21(waf1) promoter by hepatitis B virus X protein via a p53-independent pathway. *Gene.* 2001;275:163-168.

[22] Ahn JY, Jung EY, Kwun HJ, Lee CW, Sung YC, Jang KL. Dual effects of hepatitis B virus X protein on the regulation of cell-cycle control depending on the status of cellular p53. *J Gen Virol.* 2002;83:2765-2772.

[23] Choi BH, Choi M, Jeon HY, Rho HM. Hepatitis B viral X protein overcomes inhibition of E2F1 activity by pRb on the human Rb gene promoter. *DNA Cell Biol.* 2001;20:75-80.

[24] Choi M, Lee H, Rho HM. E2F1 activates the human p53 promoter and overcomes the repressive effect of hepatitis B viral X protein (Hbx) on the p53 promoter. *IUBMB Life.* 2002;53:309-317.

[25] Lucito R, and Schneider R J. Hepatitis B virus X protein activates transcription factor NF-kappa B without a requirement for protein kinase C. *J Virol.* 1992;66: 983-991.

[26] Chirillo P, Falco M, Puri PL, Artini M, Balsano C, Levrero M, *et al.* Hepatitis B virus pX activates NF-kappa B-dependent transcription through a Rafindependent pathway. *J Virol.* 1996;70:641-646.

[27] Su F, Schneider RJ. Hepatitis B virus HBx protein activates transcription factor NF-kappaB by acting on multiple cytoplasmic inhibitors of rel-related proteins. *J Virol.* 1996; 70: 4558- 4566.

[28] Arbuthnot P, Kew M. Hepatitis B virus and hepatocellular carcinoma. *Int J Exp Pathol.* 2001;82:77-100.

[29] Groisman IJ, Koshy R, Henkler F, Groopman JD, Alaoui-Jamali MA. Downregulation of DNA excision repair by the hepatitis B virus-x protein occurs in p53-proficient and p53-deficient cells. *Carcinogenesis.* 1999;20:479-483.

[30] Jia L, Wang XW, Harris CC. Hepatitis B virus X protein inhibits nucleotide excision repair. *Int J Cancer.* 1999;80:875-879.

[31] Zhang X, Dong N, Zhang H, You J, Wang H, Ye L. Effects of hepatitis B virus X protein on human telomerase reverse transcriptase expression and activity in hepatoma cells. *J Lab Clin Med.* 2005;145:98-104.

[32] Wang-Shick Ryu. Molecular Aspects of Hepatitis B Viral Infection and the Viral Carcinogenesis. *J Biochem Mol Biol.*2003;36: 138-143.

[33] Klein NP, Schneider RJ. Activation of Src family kinases by hepatitis B virus HBx protein and coupled signaling to Ras. *Mo. Cell Biol.* 1997;17: 6427-6436.

[34] Natoli G, Avantaggiati M L, Chirillo P, Puri P L, Ianni A, Balsano C, *et al.* (1994) Ras- and Raf-dependent activation of c-jun transcriptional activity by the hepatitis B virus transactivator pX. *Oncogene* 1994;9: 2837-2843.

[35] Benn J, Su F, Doria M, Schneider RJ. Hepatitis B virus HBx protein induces transcription factor AP-1 by activation of extracellular signal-regulated and c-Jun N-terminal mitogen-activated protein kinases. *J Virol.* 1996;70:4978-4985.

[36] Lee YH, Yun Y. HBx protein of hepatitis B virus activates Jak1-STAT signaling. *J Biol Chem.* 1998;273:25510-25515.

[37] Shirakata Y, Kawada M, Fujiki Y, Sano H, Oda M, Yaginuma K, *et al.* (1989) The X gene of hepatitis B virus induced growth stimulation and tumorigenic transformation of mouse NIH3T3 cells. *Jpn J Cancer Res.* 1989;80: 617-621.

[38] Oguey D, Dumenco LL, Pierce RH, Fausto N. Analysis of the tumorigenicity of the X gene of hepatitis B virus in a non-transformed hepatocyte cell line and the effects of co-transfection with a murine p53 mutant equivalent to human codon 249. *Hepatology* 1996;24: 1024-1033.

[39] Tarn C, Bilodeau ML, Hullinger RL, Andrisani OM. () Differential immediate early gene expression in conditional hepatitis B virus pX-transforming versus nontransforming hepatocyte cell lines. *J Biol Chem.* 1999;274:2327-2336.

[40] Koike K, Moriya K, Iino S, Yotsuyanagi H, Endo Y, Miyamura T , *et al.* (1994a) High-level expression of hepatitis B virus HBx gene and hepatocarcinogenesis in transgenic mice. *Hepatology* 1994;19: 810-819.

[41] Guidotti LG, Matzke B, Schaller H, Chisari FV. (1995) High-level hepatitis B virus replication in transgenic mice. *J Virol.* 1995;69: 6158-6169.

[42] Kim CM, Koike K, Saito I, Miyamura T, Jay G. HBx gene of hepatitis B virus induces liver cancer in transgenic mice. *Nature* 1991;351: 317-320.

[43] Seifer M, Hohne M, Schaefer S, Gerlich WH. In vitro tumorigenicity of hepatitis B virus DNA and HBx protein. *J Hepatol.* 1991;13:S61-S65.

[44] Zhang SJ, Chen HY, Chen ZX, Wang XZ. Possible mechanism for hepatitis B virus X gene to induce apoptosis of hepatocytes. *World J Gastroenterol.* 2005;11:4351-4356.

[45] Kim YC, Song KS, Yoon G, Nam MJ, Ryu WS. Activated ras oncogene collaborates with HBx gene of hepatitis B virus to transform cells by suppressing HBxmediated apoptosis. *Oncogene* 2001;20:16-23.

[46] Hohne M, Schaefer S, Seifer M, Feitelson MA, Paul D, Gerlich WH. Malignant transformation of immortalized transgenic hepatocytes after transfection with hepatitis B virus DNA. 1990;9:1137-1145.

[47] Terradillos O, Billet O, Renard CA, Levy R, Molina T, Briand P, *et al.* The hepatitis B virus X gene potentates c-myc-induced liver oncogenesis in transgenic mice. *Oncogene* 1997;14: 395-404.

[48] Tu H, Bonura C, Giannini C, Mouly H, Soussan P, Kew M, *et al.* Biological impact of natural COOH-terminal deletions of hepatitis B virus X protein in hepatocellular carcinoma tissues. *Cancer Res.* 2001;61:7803-7810.

[49] Schluter V, Rabe C, Meyer M, Koshy R, Caselmann WH. Intracellular accumulation of middle hepatitis B surface protein activates gene transcription. *Dig Dis.* 2001;19:352-363.

[50] Wang HC, Huang W, Lai MD, Su IJ. Hepatitis B virus pre-S mutants, endoplasmic reticulum stress and hepatocarcinogenesis. *Cancer Sci.* 2006;97:683-688.

[51] Caselmann WH. Transactivation of cellular gene expression by hepatitis B viral proteins: a possible molecular mechanism of hepatocarcinogenesis. *J Hepatol.* 1995;22:S34-S37.

[52] Hildt E, Urban S, Lauer U, Hofschneider PH, Kekule AS. ER-localization and functional expression of the HBV transactivator MHBst. *Oncogene.* 1993;8:3359-3367.

[53] Lauer U, Weiss L, Hofschneider PH, Kekule AS. The hepatitis B virus pre-S/S(t) transactivator is generated by 3' truncations within a defined region of the S gene. *J Virol.* 1992;66:5284-5289.

[54] Hildt E, Urban S, Hofschneider PH. Characterization of essential domains for the functionality of the MHBst transcriptional activator and identification of a minimal MHBst activator. *Oncogene.* 1995;11:2055-2066.

[55] Kim DG. Differentially expressed genes associated with hepatitis B virus HBx and MHBs protein function in hepatocellular carcinoma. *Methods Mol Biol.* 2006;317:141-155.

[56] Hildt E, Saher G, Bruss V, Hofschneider PH. The hepatitis B virus large surface protein (LHBs) is a transcriptional activator. *Virology.* 1996;225:235-9.

[57] Hildt E, Hofschneider PH. The PreS2 activators of the hepatitis B virus: activators of tumour promoter pathways. *Recent Results Cancer Res.* 1998;154:315-329.

[58] Calvisi DF, Thorgeirsson SS. Molecular mechanisms of hepatocarcinogenesis in transgenic mouse models of liver cancer. *Toxicol Pathol.* 2005;33:181-184.

[59] Cavin LG, Wang F, Factor VM, Kaur S, Venkatraman M, Thorgeirsson SS, *et al.* Transforming growth factor-alpha inhibits the intrinsic pathway of c-Myc-induced apoptosis through activation of nuclear factor-kappaB in murine hepatocellular carcinomas. *Mol Cancer Res.* 2005;3: 403-412.

[60] Cadoret A, Desbois-Mouthon C, Wendum D, Leneuve P, Perret C, Tronche F, *et al.* c-myc-induced hepatocarcinogenesis in the absence of IGF-I receptor. *Int J Cancer.* 2005;114: 668-672.

[61] Peng SY, Lai PL, Hsu HC. Amplification of the c-myc gene in human hepatocellular carcinoma: biologic significance. *J Formos Med Assoc.* 1993;92:866-870.

[62] Kawate S, Fukusato T, Ohwada S, Watanuki A, Morishita Y. Amplification of c-myc in hepatocellular carcinoma: correlation with clinicopathologic features, proliferative activity and p53 overexpression. *Oncology.* 1999;57:157-163.

[63] Transy C, Fourel G, Robinson WS, Tiollais P, Marion PL, Buendia MA. Frequent amplification of c-myc in ground squirrel liver tumors associated with past or ongoing infection with a hepadnavirus. *Proc Natl Acad Sci U S A.* 1992;89:3874-3878.

[64] Hansen LJ, Tennant BC, Seeger C, Ganem D. Differential activation of myc gene family members in hepatic carcinogenesis by closely related hepatitis B viruses. *Mol Cell Biol.* 1993 ;13:659-667.

[65] Iizuka N, Tsunedomi R, Tamesa T, Okada T, Sakamoto K, Hamaguchi T, *et al.* Involvement of c-myc-regulated genes in hepatocellular carcinoma related to genotype-C hepatitis B virus. *J Cancer Res Clin Oncol.* 2006;132:473-481.

[66] Wu CG, Salvay DM, Forgues M, Valerie K, Farnsworth J, Markin RS, *et al.* Distinctive gene expression profiles associated with Hepatitis B virus x protein. *Oncogene.* 2001;20:3674-3682.

[67] Lakhtakia R, Kumar V, Reddi H, Mathur M, Dattagupta S, Panda SK. Hepatocellular carcinoma in a hepatitis B 'x' transgenic mouse model: A sequential pathological evaluation. *J Gastroenterol Hepatol.* 2003;18:80-91.

[68] Kalra N, Kumar V. c-Fos is a mediator of the c-myc-induced apoptotic signaling in serum-deprived hepatoma cells via the p38 mitogen-activated protein kinase pathway. *J Biol Chem.* 2004;279:25313-25319.

[69] Kalra N, Kumar V. The X protein of hepatitis B virus binds to the F box protein Skp2 and inhibits the ubiquitination and proteasomal degradation of c-Myc. *FEBS Lett.* 2006;580:431-436.

[70] Nusse R. Relay at the membrane. *Nature.*2005,438:747-749.

[71] Cadigan KM, Nasse R. Wint signaling: a common theme in animal development. *Genes Dev* 1997,11:3286-3305

[72] Giles RH, van Es JH, Clevers H. Caught up in a Wnt storm: Wnt signaling in cancer. *Biochim Biophys Acta* 2003;1653:1-24.

[73] Wu XZ, Chen D. Cell-matrix talks: Effects on differentiation of hepatocellular carcinoma. *Minerva INERVA Gastroenterol. E Dietologica.* 2007, In press.

[74] Calvisi DF, Conner EA, Ladu S, Lemmer ER, Factor VM, Thorgeirsson SS. Activation of the canonical Wnt/beta-catenin pathway confers growth advantages in c-Myc/E2F1 transgenic mouse model of liver cancer. *J Hepatol* 2005;42:842-849.

[75] Jung HC, Kim K. Identification of MYCBP as a beta-catenin/LEF-1 target using DNA microarray analysis. *Life Sci* 2005;77:1249-1262.

[76] Colnot S, Decaens T, Niwa-Kawakita M, Godard C, Hamard G, Kahn A, *et al.* Liver-targeted disruption of Apc in mice activates beta-catenin signaling and leads to hepatocellular carcinomas. *Proc Natl Acad Sci U S A* 2004;101:17216-17221.

[77] Ishizaki Y, Ikeda S, Fujimori M, Shimizu Y, Kurihara T, Itamoto T, *et al.* Immunohistochemical analysis and mutational analyses of beta-catenin, Axin family and APC genes in hepatocellular carcinomas. *Int J Oncol* 2004;24:1077-1083.

[78] Ikenoue T, Ijichi H, Kato N, Kanai F, Masaki T, Rengifo W, *et al.* Analysis of the beta-catenin/T cell factor signaling pathway in 36 gastrointestinal and liver cancer cells. *Jpn J Cancer Res* 2002;93:1213-1220.

[79] Han Chu Lee, Miran Kim, and Jack R. Wands. Wnt/frizzled signaling in hepatocellular carcinoma. *Front Biosci* 2006;11: 1901-1915.

[80] Cha MY, Kim CM, Park YM, Ryu WS. Hepatitis B virus X protein is essential for the activation of Wnt/beta-catenin signaling in hepatoma cells. *Hepatology*. 2004; 39: 1683-1693.

[81] Ding Q, Xia W, Liu JC, Yang JY, Lee DF, Xia J, *et al.* Erk associates with and primes GSK-3beta for its inactivation resulting in upregulation of beta-catenin. *Mol Cell.* 2005;19:159-170.

[82] Zhang L, Cao Y, Song J. The correlation between integration of HBV X, S, Pre-S, C gene and the expression of oncogenes/tumor suppressor genes in primary hepatocellular carcinoma. *Zhonghua Gan Zang Bing Za Zhi.* 1999;7:138-139.

[83] Kekule AS, Lauer U, Meyer M, Caselmann WH, Hofschneider PH, Koshy R. The preS2/S region of integrated hepatitis B virus DNA encodes a transcriptional transactivator. *Nature*. 1990;343:457- 461.

[84] Shachaf CM, Kopelman AM, Arvanitis C, Karlsson A, Beer S, Mandl S, *et al.* MYC inactivation uncovers pluripotent differentiation and tumour dormancy in hepatocellular cancer. *Nature*. 2004;431:1112-1117.

[85] Saito H, Morizane T, Watanabe T, Kagawa T, Miyaguchi S, Kumagai N, *et al.* Differentiating effect of sodium butyrate on human hepatoma cell lines PLC/PRF/5, HCC-M and HCC-T. *Int J Cancer*. 1991;48:291-296.

[86] Tada S, Saito H, Ebinuma H, Atsukawa K, Masuda T, Tsunematsu S, *et al.* Reduction of LAK-sensitivity and changes in antigen expression on hepatoma cells by sodium butyrate. *Cancer Biochem Biophys*. 1996;15:177-186.

[87] Ebinuma H, Saito H, Saito Y, Wakabayashi K, Nakamura M, Kurose I, *et al.* Antisense oligodeoxynucleotide against c-myc mRNA induces differentiation of human hepatocellular carcinoma cells. *Int J Oncol*. 1999;15:991-999.

[88] Ouyang GL, Li QF, Peng XX, Liu QR, Hong SG.. Effects of tachyplesin on proliferation and differentiation of human hepatocellular carcinoma SMMC-7721 cells. *World J Gastroenterol.* 2002;8:1053-1058.

[89] Li QF, Ou-Yang GL, Peng XX, Hong SG. Effects of tachyplesin on the regulation of cell cycle in human hepatocarcinoma SMMC-7721 cells. *World J Gastroenterol.* 2003;9:454-458.

[90] Hung L, Kumar V. Antisense regulation of expression and transactivation functions of the tumorigenic HBx and c-myc genes. *Biochem Biophys Res Commun.* 2006;344:293-299.

[91] Hung L, Kumar V. Specific inhibition of gene expression and transactivation functions of hepatitis B virus X protein and c-myc by small interfering RNAs. *FEBS Lett.* 2004;560:210-214.

[92] Chan DW, Ng IO. Knock-down of hepatitis B virus X protein reduces the tumorigenicity of hepatocellular carcinoma cells. *J Pathol.* 2006;208:372-380.

[93] Dunsford HA, Sell S, Chisari FV. Hepatocarcinogenesis due to chronic liver cell injury in hepatitis B virus transgenic mice. *Cancer Res.* 1990;50:3400-3407.

[94] Beachy PA, Karhadkar SS, Berman DM. Tissue repair and stem cell renewal in carcinogenesis. *Nature.* 2004;432:324-331.

[95] Bissell DM. Chronic liver injury, TGF-beta, and cancer. *Exp Mol Med.* 2001; 33: 179-190.

[96] Hino O, Kajino K, Umeda T, Arakawa Y. Understanding the hypercarcinogenic state in chronic hepatitis: a clue to the prevention of human hepatocellular carcinoma. *J Gastroenterol.* 2002;37:883-887.

[97] Hagen TM, Huang S, Curnutte J, Fowler P, Martinez V, Wehr CM, *et al.* Extensive oxidative DNA damage in hepatocytes of transgenic mice with chronic active hepatitis destined to develop hepatocellular carcinoma. *Proc Natl Acad Sci U S A.* 1994;91: 12808-12812.

[98] Pollicino T, Terradillos O, Lecoeur H, Gougeon ML, Buendia MA. Pro-apoptotic effect of the hepatitis B virus X gene. *Biomed Pharmacother.* 1998;52:363-368.

[99] Huang S, He J, Zhang X, Bian Y, Yang L, Xie G, *et al.* Activation of the hedgehog pathway in human hepatocellular carcinomas. *Carcinogenesis.* 2006;27:1334-1340.

[100] Patil MA, Zhang J, Ho C, Cheung ST, Fan ST, Chen X. Hedgehog signaling in human hepatocellular carcinoma. *Cancer Biol Ther.* 2006;5:111-117.

[101] Sicklick JK, Li YX, Jayaraman A, Kannangai R, Qi Y, Vivekanandan P, *et al.* Dysregulation of the Hedgehog pathway in human hepatocarcinogenesis. *Carcinogenesis.* 2006;27:748-757.

[102] Osipo C, Miele L. Hedgehog signaling in hepatocellular carcinoma: novel therapeutic strategy targeting hedgehog signaling in HCC. *Cancer Biol Ther.* 2006;5:238-239.

[103] Lee HC, Kim M, Wands JR. Wnt/Frizzled signaling in hepatocellular carcinoma. *Front Biosci.* 2006;11:1901-1915.

[104] Meng X, Riordan NH. Cancer is a functional repair tissue. *Medical Hypotheses.* 2006;66: 486-490.

[105] Wu XZ. Cancer and chronic tissue injury: abnormal repair tissue or functional repair tissue? *Med Hypotheses.* 2006;67:676-677.

[106] Breuhahn K, Longerich T, Schirmacher P. Dysregulation of growth factor signaling in human hepatocellular carcinoma. *Oncogene.* 2006;25:3787-3800.

[107] Yang EB, Qin LL, Zhao YN, Zhang K, Chow P. Genetic changes and expression of the mannose 6-phosphate/insulin-like growth factor II receptor gene in human hepatitis B virus-associated hepatocellular carcinoma. *Int J Mol Med.* 2003;11:773-778.

[108] Boudreau N, Bissell MJ. Extracellular matrix signaling: integration of form and function in normal and malignant cells. *Curr Opin Cell Biol.* 1998; 10: 640-646.

[109] Tennenbaum T, Belanger AJ, Quaranta V, Yuspa SH. Differential regulation of integrins and extracellular matrix binding in epidermal differentiation and squamous tumor progression. *J Investig Dermatol Symp Proc.* 1996; 1: 157-161.

[110] Bissell DM. Chronic liver injury, TGF-beta, and cancer. *Exp Mol Med.* 2001; 33: 179-190.

[111] Kershenobich Stalnikowitz D, Weissbrod AB. Liver fibrosis and inflammation. A review. *Ann Hepatol.* 2003;2:159-163.

[112] Schuppan D, Ruehl M, Somasundaram R, Hahn EG. Matrix as a modulator of hepatic fibrogenesis. *Semin Liver Dis.* 2001;21:351-372.

[113] Wu XZ. Extracellular matrix and hepatocarcinogenesis: The effect of soil on feed? *Med Hypotheses.* 2006;66:1115-1120.

[114] Zhao M, Laissue JA, Zimmermann A. Tenascin and type IV collagen expression in liver cell dysplasia and in hepatocellular carcinoma. *Histol Histopathol.* 1996; 11: 323-333.

[115] Fujii M, Yamashita Y, Shirabe K, Ijima H, Nakazawa K, Funatsu K, *et al.* Basic study about the development of the hybrid-artificial liver support system using human hepatoma cell lines (Hep G2, Huh 7): effects on liver functions by extracellular matrix (type I collagen) in monolayer culture. *Fukuoka Igaku Zasshi.* 2001; 92: 299-305.

[116] Kudriavtseva EI, Morozova OV, Rudinskaia TD, Engel'gard NV. Disruption of intercellular contacts and cell-extracellular matrix interaction in rapidly growing murine hepatocarcinoma. *Arkh Patol.* 2001; 63: 33-37.

[117] Kudriavtseva EI, Morozova OV, Rudinskaia TD, Engel'gard NV. Disruption of intercellular contacts and cell-extracellular matrix interaction in rapidly growing murine hepatocarcinoma. *Arkh Patol.* 2001; 63: 33-37.

[118] McCaughan GW, Siah CL, Abbott C, Wickson J, Ballesteros M, Bishop GA. Dipeptidyl peptidase IV is down-regulated in rat hepatoma cells at the mRNA level. *J Gastroenterol Hepatol.* 1993; 8: 142-145.

[119] Loster K, Zeilinger K, Schuppan D, Reutter W. The cysteine-rich region of dipeptidyl peptidase IV (CD 26) is the collagen-binding site. *Biochem Biophys Res Commun.* 1995; 217: 341-348.

[120] Le Bail B, Faouzi S, Boussarie L, Balabaud C, Bioulac-Sage P, Rosenbaum J. Extracellular matrix composition and integrin expression in early hepatocarcinogenesis in human cirrhotic liver. *J Pathol.* 1997; 181: 330-337.

[121] Carloni V, Romanelli RG, Mercurio AM, Pinzani M, Laffi G, Cotrozzi G, *et al.* Knockout of alpha6 beta1-integrin expression reverses the transformed phenotype of hepatocarcinoma cells. *Gastroenterology.* 1998; 115: 433-442.

[122] Jaskiewicz K, Chasen MR, Robson SC. Differential expression of extracellular matrix proteins and integrins in hepatocellular carcinoma and chronic liver disease. *Anticancer Res.* 1993; 13: 2229-2237.

[123] Seebacher T, Medina JL, Bade EG. Laminin alpha 5, a major transcript of normal and malignant rat liver epithelial cells, is differentially expressed in developing and adult liver. *Exp Cell Res*. 1997; 237: 70-76.

[124] Szendroi M, Lapis K. Distribution of fibronectin and laminin in human liver tumors. *J Cancer Res Clin Oncol.* 1985; 109: 60-64.

[125] Torimura T, Ueno T, Inuzuka S, Kin M, Ohira H, Kimura Y, *et al.* The extracellular matrix in hepatocellular carcinoma shows different localization patterns depending on the differentiation and the histological pattern of tumors: immunohistochemical analysis. *J Hepatol.* 1994; 21: 37-46.

[126] Yao M, Zhou XD, Zha XL, Shi DR, Fu J, He JY, *et al.* Expression of the integrin alpha5 subunit and its mediated cell adhesion in hepatocellular carcinoma. *J Cancer Res Clin Oncol*. 1997; 123: 435-440.

[127] Zhang H, Ozaki I, Mizuta T, Yoshimura T, Matsuhashi S, Eguchi Y, *et al.* Transforming growth factor-beta 1-induced apoptosis is blocked by beta 1-integrin-mediated mitogen-activated protein kinase activation in human hepatoma cells. *Cancer Sci*. 2004; 95: 878-886.

[128] Zhang H, Ozaki I, Mizuta T, Matsuhashi S, Yoshimura T, Hisatomi A, *et al.* Beta 1-integrin protects hepatoma cells from chemotherapy induced apoptosis via a mitogen-activated protein kinase dependent pathway. *Cancer.* 2002; 95: 896-906.

[129] Tian B, Li Y, Ji XN, Chen J, Xue Q, Ye SL, *et al.* Basement membrane proteins play an active role in the invasive process of human hepatocellular carcinoma cells with high metastasis potential. *J Cancer Res Clin Oncol*. 2005; 131: 80-86.

[130] Lara-Pezzi E, Majano PL, Yanez-Mo M, Gomez-Gonzalo M, Carretero M, Moreno-Otero R, *et al.* Effect of the hepatitis B virus HBx protein on integrin-mediated adhesion to and migration on extracellular matrix. *J Hepatol*. 2001;34:409- 415.

[131] Kojima J, Nakamura N, Kanatani M, Akiyama M. Glycosaminoglycans in 3'-methyl-4-dimethylaminoazobenzene- induced rat hepatic cancer. *Cancer Res*. 1982; 42: 2857-2860.

[132] Robinson J, Viti M, Hook M. Structure and properties of an under-sulfated heparan sulfate proteoglycan synthesized by a rat hepatoma cell line. *J Cell Biol.* 1984; 98: 946-953.

[133] Wu XZ. Sulfated oligosaccharides and tumor: promoter or inhibitor? *Panminerva Med.* 2006;48:27-31.

[134] Wu XZ, Chen D, Xie GR. Effects of Gekko sulfated polysaccharide on the proliferation and differentiation of hepatic cancer cell line. *Cell Biol Int*. 2006;30:659-664.

[135] Chedid A, Ryan LM, Dayal Y, Wolf BC, Falkson G. Morphology and other prognostic factors of hepatocellular carcinoma. *Arch Patholo Lab Med* 1999; 123:524-528.

[136] Wu XZ. The role of extracellular matrix remodeling in carcinogenesis and metastasis. *Med Hypotheses*. 2006;67:425.

[137] Kim JR, Kim CH. Association of a high activity of matrix metalloproteinase-9 to low levels of tissue inhibitors of metalloproteinase-1 and -3 in human hepatitis B-viral hepatoma cells. *Int J Biochem Cell Biol*. 2004;36:2293-2306.

[138] Yu FL, Liu HJ, Lee JW, Liao MH, Shih WL. Hepatitis B virus X protein promotes cell migration by inducing matrix metalloproteinase-3. *J Hepatol*. 2005;42:520-527.

[139] Lapidot T, Sirard C, Vormoor J, Murdoch B, Hoang T, Caceres-Cortes J, *et al.* A cell initiating human acute myeloid leukaemia after transplantation into SCID mice. *Nature.* 1994;367:645–648.

[140] George AA, Franklin J, Kerkof K, Shah AJ, Price M, Tsark E, *et al.* Detection of leukemic cells in the CD34(-)CD38(-) bone marrow progenitor population in children with acute lymphoblastic leukemia. *Blood.* 2001;97:3925–3930.

[141] Nilsson L, Astrand-Grundstrom I, Anderson K, Arvidsson I, Hokland P, Bryder D, *et al.* Involvement and functional impairment of the CD34(-)CD38(-)Thy-1(-) hematopoietic stem cell pool in myelodysplastic syndromes with trisomy 8. *Blood.* 2002;100:259–267.

[142] Al Hajj M, Wicha MS, Benito-Hernandez A, Morrison SJ, Clarke MF. Prospective identification of tumorigenic breast cancer cells. *Proc Natl Acad Sci USA.* 2003;100: 3983–3988.

[143] Matsui W, Huff CA, Wang Q, Malehorn MT, Barber J, Tanhehco Y, *et al.* Characterization of clonogenic multiple myeloma cells. *Blood. 2004*; 103:2332–2336.

[144] Fomchenko EI, Holland EC. Stem cells and brain cancer. *Exp Cell Res.* 2005;306:323-329.

[145] Reya T, Morrison SJ, Clarke MF, Weissman IL. Stem cells, cancer, and cancer stem cells. *Nature.* 2001; 414:105-111.

[146] Pardal R, Clarke MF, Morrison SJ. Applying the principles of stem-cell biology to cancer. *Nat Rev Cancer.* 2003; 3:895-902.

[147] Rubio D, Garcia-Castro J, Martín MC, de la Fuente R, Cigudosa JC, Lloyd AC, *et al.* Spontaneous human adult stem cell transformation. *Cancer Res.* 2005; 65: 3035-3039.

[148] Burns JS, Abdallah BM, Guldberg P, Rygaard J, Schrøder HD, Kassem M. Tumorigenic heterogeneity in cancer stem cells evolved from long-term cultures of telomerase-immortalized human mesenchymal stem cells. *Cancer Res.* 2005; 65: 3126-3135.

[149] Serakinci N, Guldberg P, Burns JS, Abdallah B, Schrodder H, Jensen T, *et al.* Adult human mesenchymal stem cell as a target for neoplastic transformation. *Oncogene.* 2004;23:5095-5098.

[150] Grompe M, Finegold MJ. Liver stem cells; in Marshak DR, Gardner RL, Gottlieb D(ed): *Stem cell Biology.* Cold Spring Harbor Laboratory Press. 2001, PP 455-497.

[151] Sell S. Heterogeneity and plasticity of hepatocyte lineage cells. *Hepatology.* 2001;33:738-50.

[152] Sell S. Cellular origin of cancer: dedifferentiation or stem cell maturation arrest? *Environ Health Perspect.* 1993;101:15-26.

[153] Lee ES, Han EM, Kim YS, Shin BK, Kim CH, Kim HK, *et al.* Occurrence of c-kit+ tumor cells in hepatitis B virus-associated hepatocellular carcinoma. *Am J Clin Pathol.* 2005;124:31-36.

[154] Fang CH, Gong JQ, Zhang W. Function of oval cells in hepatocellular carcinoma in rats. *World J Gastroenterol.* 2004;10:2482-2487.

[155] Braun L, Goyette M, Yaswen P, Thompson NL, Fausto N. Growth in culture and tumorigenicity after transfection with the ras oncogene of liver epithelial cells from carcinogen- treated rats. *Cancer Res.* 1987;47:4116-4124.

[156] Richards WG, Yoder BK, Isfort RJ, Detilleux PG, Foster C, Neilsen N, *et al.* Oval cell proliferation associated with the murine insertional mutation TgN737Rpw. *Am J Pathol.* 1996;149:1919- 1930.

[157] Dumble ML, Croager EJ, Yeoh GC, Quail EA. Generation and characterization of p53 null transformed hepatic progenitor cells: oval cells give rise to hepatocellular carcinoma. *Carcinogenesis*. 2002; 23: 435-445.

[158] Iidaka T, Tsukamoto T, Totsuka Y, Hirata A, Sakai H, Shirai N, *et al.* Lack of elevated liver carcinogenicity of aminophenylnorharman in p53-deficient mice. *Cancer Lett.* 2005; 217: 149-159.

[159] Becker R, Luthgens B, Oesch F, Dienes HP, Steinberg P. Ha-rasVal12 but not p53Ser247 leads to a significant neoplastic transformation rate of the putative rat liver stem cells (oval cell). *Carcinogenesis*. 1996;17: 2635-2640.

[160] Yaswen P, Goyette M, Shank PR, Fausto N. Expression of c-Ki-ras, c-Ha-ras, and c-myc in specific cell types during hepatocarcinogenesis. *Mol Cell Biol.* 1985; 5:780-786.

[161] Lemmer ER, de la Motte Hall P, Omori N, Omori M, Shephard EG, Gelderblom WC, *et al.* Histopathology and gene expression changes in rat liver during feeding of fumonisin B1, a carcinogenic mycotoxin produced by Fusarium moniliforme. *Carcinogenesis*. 1999; 20:817-824.

[162] Libbrecht L, De Vos R, Cassiman D, Desmet V, Aerts R, Roskams T. Hepatic progenitor cells in hepatocellular adenomas. *Am J Surg Pathol.* 2001; 25:1388-1396.

[163] Robrechts C, De Vos R, Van den Heuvel M, Van Cutsem E, Van Damme B, Desmet V, *et al.* Primary liver tumour of intermediate (hepatocyte- bile duct cell) phenotype: a progenitor cell tumour. *Liver* 1998; 18: 288-293.

[164] Kim H, Park C, Han KH, Choi J, Kim YB, Kim JK, *et al.* Primary liver carcinoma of intermediate (hepatocyte-cholangiocyte) phenotype. *J Hepatol*. 2004; 40:298-304.

[165] Kim H, Park C, Han KH, Choi J, Kim YB, Kim JK, *et al.* Primary liver carcinoma of intermediate (hepatocyte-cholangiocyte) phenotype. *J Hepatol*. 2004; 40:298-304.

[166] Robrechts C, De Vos R, Van den Heuvel M, Van Cutsem E, Van Damme B, Desmet V, *et al.* Primary liver tumour of intermediate (hepatocyte- bile duct cell) phenotype: a progenitor cell tumour. *Liver.* 1998; 18: 288-293.

[167] Hsia CC, Thorgeirsson SS, Tabor E. Expression of hepatitis B surface and core antigens and transforming growth factor-alpha in "oval cells" of the liver in patients with hepatocellular carcinoma. *J Med Virol*. 1994;43:216-221.

[168] Thorgeirsson SS. Target cell populations in virus-associated hepatocarcinogenesis. *Princess Takamatsu Symp*. 1995;25:163-70.

[169] Heissig B, Ohki Y, Sato Y, Rafii S, Werb Z, Hattori K. A role for niches in hematopoietic cell development. *Hematology*. 2005;10:247-253.

[170] Martin MA, Bhatia M. Analysis of the human fetal liver hematopoietic microenvironment. *Stem Cells Dev.* 2005;14:493- 504.

[171] Kotton DN, Fabian AJ, Mulligan RC. A novel stem-cell population in adult liver with potent hematopoietic-reconstitution activity. *Blood*. 2005;106:1574-1580.

[172] Theise ND, Badve S, Saxena R, Henegariu O, Sell S, Crawford JM, *et al.* Derivation of hepatocytes from bone marrow cells in mice after radiation-induced myeloablation. *Hepatology*. 2000; 31: 235-240.

[173] Krause DS, Theise ND, Collector MI, Henegariu O, Hwang S, Gardner R, *et al.* Multi-organ, multi-lineage engraftment by a single bone marrow-derived stem cell. *Cell.* 2001; 105: 369-377.

[174] Petersen BE, Goff JP, Greenberger JS, Michalopoulos GK. Hepatic oval cells express the hematopoietic stem cell marker Thy-1 in the rat. *Hepatology.* 1998; 27: 433-445.

[175] Baumann U, Crosby HA, Ramani P, Kelly DA, Strain AJ. Expression of the stem cell factor receptor c-kit in normal and diseased pediatric liver: identification of a human hepatic progenitor cell. *Hepatology.* 1999; 30: 112-117.

[176] Lemmer ER, Shepard EG, Blakolmer K, Kirsch RE, Robson SC. Isolation from human fetal liver of cells co-expressing CD34 haematopoietic stem cell and CAM 5.2 pancytokeratin markers. *J Hepatol.* 1998; 29: 450- 454.

[177] Petersen BE, Grossbard B, Hatch H, Pi L, Deng J, Scott EW. Mouse A6-positive hepatic oval cells also express several hematopoietic stem cell markers. *Hepatology.* 2003;37:632-640.

[178] Petersen BE, Bowen WC, Patrene KD, Mars WM, Sullivan AK, Murase N, *et al.* Bone marrow as a potential source of hepatic oval cells. *Science.* 1999; 284: 1168-1170.

[179] Fukuda K, Sugihara A, Nakasho K, Tsujimura T, Yamada N, Okaya A, *et al.* The origin of biliary ductular cells that appear in the spleen after transplantation of hepatocytes. *Cell Transplant.* 2004; 13: 27-33.

[180] Minguet S, Cortegano I, Gonzalo P, Martinez-Marin JA, de Andres B, Salas C, *et al.* A population of c-Kit (low) (CD45/ TER119) hepatic cell progenitors of 11-day postcoitus mouse embryo liver reconstitutes cell- depleted liver organoids. *J Clin Invest.* 2003; 112: 1152-1163.

[181] Taniguchi H, Kondo R, Suzuki A, Zheng YW, Takada Y, Fukunaga K, *et al.* Clonogenic colony-forming ability of flow cytometrically isolated hepatic progenitor cells in the murine fetal liver. *Cell Transplant.* 2000; 9: 697-700.

[182] Wu XZ, Zhao LS, Xu Q, Zhang Y, Tang H. Differentiation of Bone Marrow Mesenchymal Stem Cells into Hepatocytes in Hepatectomized Mouse. *J Biomed Eng.* 2005; 22: 1234-1237.

[183] Collector MI, Baylin S B, Diehl A M, Sharkis S J. Hematopoietic stem cells convert into liver cells within days without fusion. *Nat Cell Biol.* 2004;6: 532-539.

[184] Jiang Y, Jahagirdar BN, Reinhardt RL, Schwartz RE, Keene CD, Ortiz-Gonzalez XR, *et al.* Pluripotency of mesenchymal stem cells derived from adult marrow. *Nature.* 2002; 418:41-49.

[185] Fiegel HC, Lioznov MV, Cortes-Dericks L, Lange C, Kluth D, Fehse B, *et al.* Liver-specific gene expression in cultured human hematopoietic stem cells. *Stem Cells.* 2003;21:98-104.

[186] Yamazaki S, Miki K, Takayama T, Hasegawa K, Sata M, Midorikawa Y, *et al.* Hepatic gene induction in murine bone marrow after hepatectomy. *J Hepatol.* 2006;44:325-333.

[187] Zeldis JB, Mugishima H, Steinberg HN, Nir E, Gale RP. In vitro hepatitis B virus infection of human bone marrow cells. *J Clin Invest.* 1986;78:411-417.

[188] Sing GK, Prior S, Fernan A, Cooksley G. Hepatitis B virus differentially suppresses myelopoiesis and displays tropism for immature hematopoietic cells. *J Virol.* 1993;67:3454-3460.

[189] Galun E, Ilan Y, Livni N, Ketzinel M, Nahor O, Pizov G, *et al.* Hepatitis B virus infection associated with hematopoietic tumors. *Am J Pathol* 1994;145:1001-1007.

[190] Pontisso P, Locasciulli A, Schiavon E, Cattoretti G, Schiro R, Stenico D, *et al.* Detection of hepatitis B virus DNA sequences in bone marrow of children with leukemia. *Cancer* 1987;59:292-296.

[191] Houghton J, Stoicov C, Nomura S, Rogers AB, Carlson J, Li H, *et al.* Gastric cancer originating from bone marrow– derived cells. *Science*. 2004,306:1568-1571.

[192] Ishikawa H, Nakao K, Matsumoto K, Nishimura D, Ichikawa T, Hamasaki K, *et al.* Bone marrow engraftment in a rodent model of chemical carcinogenesis but no role in the histogenesis of hepatocellular carcinoma. *Gut*. 2004; 53: 884-889.

[193] Wu XZ, Yu XH. Bone Marrow Cells: The Source of Hepatocellular Carcinoma? *Medical Hypotheses*. 2007 2007 Feb 12; [Epub ahead of print].

[194] Suskind DL, Muench MO. Searching for common stem cells of the hepatic and hematopoietic systems in the human fetal liver: CD34+ cytokeratin 7/8+ cells express markers for stellate cells. *J Hepatol*. 2004;40:261-268.

[195] Coussens LM, Werb Z. Inflammation and cancer. *Nature*. 2002,420, 860–867.

[196] Ratajczak MZ, Kucia M, Reca R, Majka M, Janowska-Wieczorek A, Ratajczak J. Stem cell plasticity revisited: CXCR4-positive cells expressing mRNA for early muscle, liver and neural cells 'hide out' in the bone marrow. *Leukemia*. 2004; 18: 29-40.

[197] Kucia M, Ratajczak J, Ratajczak MZ. Bone marrow as a source of circulating CXCR4 (+) tissue-committed stem cells. *Biol Cell*. 2005; 97: 133-146.

[198] Avital I, Feraresso C, Aoki T, Hui T, Rozga J, Demetriou A, *et al.* Bone marrow-derived liver stem cell and mature hepatocyte engraftment in livers undergoing rejection. *Surgery*. 2002;132: 384-390.

[199] Avital I, Inderbitzin D, Aoki T, Tyan DB, Cohen AH, Ferraresso C, *et al.* Isolation, characterization, and transplantation of bone marrow-derived hepatocyte stem cells. *Biochem Biophys Res Commun*. 2001;288:156-164.

[200] Sell S. Cellular origin of hepatocellular carcinomas. *Semin Cell Dev Biol*. 2002; 13:419-424.

[201] Guettier C. Which stem cells for adult liver? *Ann Pathol*. 2005;25:33-44.

[202] Alison MR, Lovell MJ. Liver cancer: the role of stem cells. *Cell Prolif*. 2005;38:407-421.

In: Hepatitis B Research Advances
Editor: Alicia P. Willis, pp. 141-169

ISBN: 978-1-60021-666-4

Chapter IX

HEPATITIS B VIRAL FACTORS AFFECTING LONG-TERM OUTCOMES OF CHRONIC HEPATITIS B

***Chih-Lin Lin*[1] *and Jia-Horng Kao*[2,3,4,5,*]**

[1]Department of Gastroenterology, Ren-Ai branch, Taipei City Hospital, Taiwan
[2]Department of Internal Medicine, National Taiwan University Hospital, Taiwan
[3]Graduate Institute of Clinical Medicine, [4]Hepatitis Research Center, and
[5]Department of Medical Research, National Taiwan University College of Medicine and National Taiwan University Hospital, Taipei, Taiwan.

ABSTRACT

Hepatitis B virus (HBV) infection is a global health problem and causes a wide spectrum of clinical manifestations, ranging from acute or fulminant hepatitis to various forms of chronic liver disease, including inactive carrier state, chronic hepatitis, cirrhosis and hepatocellular carcinoma (HCC). Most HBV carriers in the endemic regions acquire the virus during birth or early childhood. Liver injury associated with HBV infection is predominantly mediated through immune mediated mechanisms. The natural history of HBV carriers who are infected early in life can thus be divided into 4 dynamic phases based on the virus-host interaction. During the immune tolerance phase, serum HBV DNA levels are high and hepatitis B e antigen (HBeAg) is present. In the immune clearance phase, the majority of carriers seroconvert from HBeAg to anti-HBe. After HBeAg seroconversion, patients are usually in the integration or low replication phase, with low HBV DNA level and normal serum alanine aminotransferase activity. However, a small proportion of patients continue to have moderate level of HBV replication and

* Correspondence concerning this article should be addressed to Prof. Jia-Horng Kao, Director and Professor, Hepatitis Research Center, National Taiwan University Hospital, 1 Chang-Te St., Taipei 100, Taiwan. Tel.: 886-2-23123456 ext 7307; Fax: 886-2-23825962; E-mail: kaojh@ntu.edu.tw.

active liver disease designated reactivation phase. The frequency and severity of hepatitis flares during the immune clearance and/or reactivation phase predicts progression of liver disease. In general, early HBeAg seroconversion typically confers a favorable outcome, whereas late or absent HBeAg seroconversion after multiple hepatitis flares may accelerate the progression of chronic hepatitis to cirrhosis, and therefore, has a poor clinical outcome. Other factors identified as risk factors of cirrhosis and HCC development include male gender, older age, presence of cirrhosis, family history of HCC, persistence of ALT elevations, co-infection with HCV or HDV, cigarette smoking, alcohol drinking, aflatoxin exposure, and co-morbidities of diabetes and obesity. Recently, new hepatitis B viral factors predictive of clinical outcomes have been identified. Three large-scale, population-based prospective cohort studies (7 townships in Taiwan, Haimen city in China, and Philadelphia in the US) of Asian HBV carriers aged between 25-65 years all indicated that the best predictor of adverse outcomes (cirrhosis, HCC and death from liver disease) in chronic HBV infection is the serum HBV DNA level at enrollment, independent of HBeAg status, baseline serum ALT level and other risk factors. The higher the serum HBV DNA level in the immune clearance phase, the higher the incidence of adverse outcomes over time. In addition, several hospital-based cohort or case control studies from Taiwan and Hong Kong indicated that high HBV DNA level, HBV genotype C, basal core promoter mutation and pre-S deletion are associated with increased risk of liver disease progression as well as HCC development. In conclusion, the lessons learned from the natural history of chronic HBV infection in adult HBV carriers from endemic areas can help us better define the clinical threshold as well as therapeutic endpoint of "safe" HBV DNA level (e.g. 10,000 copies or 2,000 IU/ml) for the prevention of long-term liver related complications in patients during later phases of chronic HBV infection.

INTRODUCTION

Hepatitis B virus (HBV) is an important public health problem and the major cause of chronic hepatitis, cirrhosis, and hepatocellular carcinoma (HCC) worldwide. HBV is the smallest human DNA virus with a genome of 3,200 base pairs [1,2], which belongs to the family *Hepadnaviridae.* The partially double-stranded circular DNA encodes four overlapping open reading frames (Figure 1): S for the surface or envelope gene, C for the core gene, P for the polymerase gene and X for the X gene [3,4]. The S and C genes also have up-stream regions designated pre-S and pre-C. The infectious virion, or Dane particle, is a 42-nm sphere that contains the nucleocapsid. The HBsAg is presumably responsible for receptor binding and composed large, middle and major (or small) proteins that are synthesized by beginning transcription with pre-S1, pre-S2 or S gene alone, respectively. The major protein serves as a membrane anchor and plays an important role in virus assembly and, possibly, membrane fusion. The middle protein contains the pre-S2 and the S regions. The large protein contains all three regions; it is preferentially present on the infectious virus particle and is essential for both viral assembly and infectivity [5]. The pre-S1 and pre-S2 proteins are highly immunogenic components of HBsAg [6]. Hepatitis B core antigen (HBcAg) is an inner nucleocapsid surrounding the viral DNA. HBcAg is the major target of cytotoxic T-cell. Expressed HBcAg on the surface of liver cells can induce a cellular immune response to kill infected cells and clear the virus. Hepatitis B e antigen (HBeAg) is a circulating peptide derived from the core gene, then modified and secreted from liver cells [7]. It usually serves as a marker of active viral replication. HBeAg can act as a tolerogen to diminish host immune response against HBV because of its close resemblance to HBcAg, the putative target of the immune response [8]. The long P gene encodes the DNA polymerase. It also provides reverse transcription function to HBV. Because of the spontaneous error rate of viral reverse transcriptase, HBV genome evolves with an estimated rate of nucleotide substitution at 1.4–3.2 x 10^{-5}/sites/year [9]. This unique replication strategy accounts for the majority of point mutations and deletions or insertions observed in HBV genome. The long time evolution of HBV therefore leads to the occurrence of various genotypes, subgenotypes, mutants, recombinants, and even quasispecies [4,10]. The X gene encodes two proteins that have transactivation activities on HBV enhancer in aiding viral replication [11]. These proteins can also transactivate other cellular genes that may play a role in hepatocarcinogenesis [12].

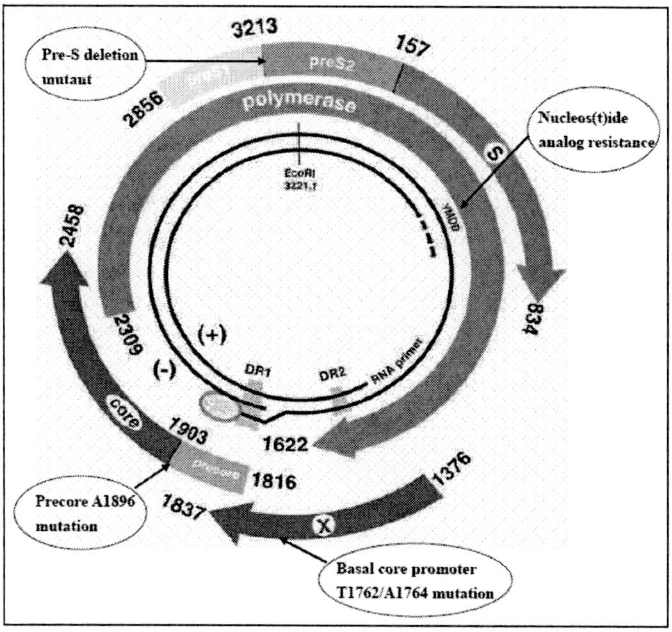

Figure 1. The partially double-stranded circular DNA of hepatitis B virus encodes four overlapping open reading frames: S for the surface or envelope gene, C for the core gene, P for the polymerase gene and X for the X gene. Naturally occurring mutant strains including mutations in precore, core promoter and deletion mutation in pre-S genes have been reported to be associated with the pathogenesis of progressive liver disease. Modified from Hunt et al. with permission [4].

NATURAL HISTORY OF HBV INFECTION

HBV infection is one of the most common viral infections in humans [13]. It is prevalent in Asia, Africa, Southern Europe and Latin America, where the prevalence of HBsAg in general population ranges from 2% to 20%. HBV can cause acute and chronic infection in humans. The acute infection may result in classical acute hepatitis or fulminant hepatitis. In chronic infection, HBV replication persists throughout the course of chronic HBV infection, and host immune response plays a pivotal role in HBV-related liver injury. In addition, HBV carriers are usually highly infectious. They can spread HBV through horizontal or perinatal transmission [14,15].

In Asian countries, HBV carriers mostly acquire the virus in perinatal period or early childhood. Based on the virus and host interactions, the natural history of perinatally acquired HBV infection can be divided into four dynamic phases (Figure 2) [13,16]:

1. Immune tolerance phase
2. Immune clearance phase
3. Integration or low replication phase
4. Reactivation phase

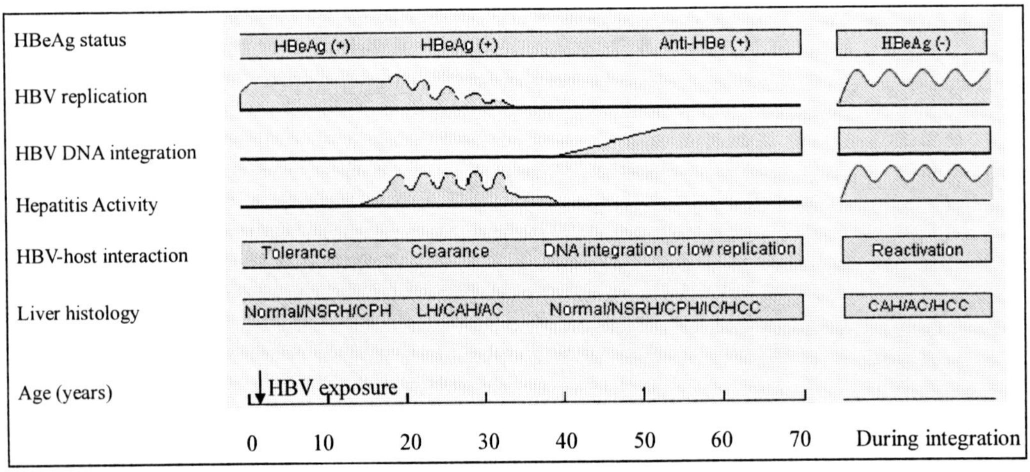

Figure 2. The natural history can be divided into four dynamic phases based on virus-host interactions: immune tolerance phase, immune clearance phase, HBV DNA integration or low replication phase, reactivation phase. Modified from The Lancet Infectious Diseases, Vol 2, Kao JH, Chen DS, Global control of hepatitis B virus infection, Pages 395-403, Copyright 2002, with permission from Elsevier [13]. (AC=active cirrhosis; CAH=chronic active hepatitis; CPH=chronic persistent hepatitis; HBeAg=hepatitis B e antigen; HCC=hepatocellular carcinoma; IC=inactive cirrhosis; LH=lobular hepatitis; NSRH=non-specific reactive hepatitis).

Immune Tolerance Phase

This phase, typically represented in the chronically infected children or young adults, is associated with high serum levels of HBV DNA (> 10^8 copies/ml), limited immunological reactivity to HBV, extensive liver replication of HBV, and expression of HBeAg. Despite lack of symptoms, the liver in young HBV carriers shows some abnormalities, albeit mild and non-specific. This is supported by the frequent findings of mildly elevated serum ALT levels. The disease activities are low in this phase despite active HBV replication as reflected by high serum HBV DNA and HBeAg levels, as well as intrahepatic HBcAg expression, which is abundant in the nucleus of hepatocyte at this phase [17].

Immune Clearance Phase

After 2 to 3 decades of persistent infection, the disease activities begin to increase. Clinically, the previously symptomless carriers may start to have bouts of symptoms and signs suggestive of acute hepatitis flare, so-called "acute exacerbations" of chronic HBV infection [18,19]. The infection now enters the clearance phase when previous immune tolerance no longer exists, probably because the levels of HBV replication decline with time. The decrease of tolerogen (HBeAg) possibly contributed to the emergence of HBV antigen-specific thymocyte from the thymus. The T cells then have specific responses to viral antigens [8]. As a result, the liver suffers continuous and repeated bouts of damage, documented by elevated serum ALT levels during acute exacerbation. The bouts of acute exacerbation are usually self-limited, although a small proportion of patients may have liver failure during the acute exacerbation [20]. Histologic changes vary from chronic persistent hepatitis (CPH), chronic lobular hepatitis (CLH), chronic active hepatitis (CAH) and active cirrhosis [21]. After a series of acute exacerbations the liver starts to have cirrhotic changes in about 40% of those with severe CAH. The incidence of cirrhosis has been shown to be 2% per year [22]. Those with persistent HBcAg in the liver and higher serum HBV DNA levels are more likely to have aggressive forms of liver disease and even cirrhosis [23].

Integration or Low Replication Phase

After destruction of the liver cells producing HBV, active replication of HBV ceases and anti-HBe is detected in the serum. However, HBsAg is continuously expressed from liver cells that contain integrated HBV genome. Although we do not know exactly when the HBV DNA integrates into the host chromosomal DNA, it is certain that the integration can be demonstrated readily at this phase. Because of the absence or presence of minimally active HBV replication in the liver, the liver cells are spared from attacks by the immune cells, thus the patients were under inactive HBV carrier status. The third phase is characterized by absence of HBeAg, presence of anti-HBe, persistently normal ALT levels, low or undetectable serum HBV DNA ($< 10^4$ copies/ml), and even HBsAg seroclearance. In this phase, liver biopsy usually shows mild hepatitis and minimal fibrosis. HBV carriers in this phase usually confer a favorable prognosis [24]; however, a significant proportion of Asian carriers still develop HCC from a background of cirrhosis [25].

Reactivation Phase

HBV carriers negative for HBeAg were considered to have nonreplicative HBV infection, and their serum ALT levels were normal or nearly normal. In the early 1980s it became apparent that HBV could replicate in the absence of HBeAg, HBV reactivation phase was thus designated. Reactivation may occur spontaneously or as a result of immunosuppression [26,27]. In this phase, detectable HBV DNA ($> 10^4$ copies/ml), elevated ALT, and progressive liver disease develop. The long-term outcome is heterogeneous. In one study of 283 Taiwanese patients followed for a median of 8.6 years after spontaneous HBeAg seroconversion, 67% had sustained remission, 4% had HBeAg reversion, and 24% had HBeAg-negative chronic hepatitis B. Cirrhosis developed in 8% and HCC in 2%. The annual incidence of cirrhosis and HCC development in HBeAg-negative patients has been estimated to be 3.7% and 0.5%, respectively [28]. Thus the clinical spectrum of HBeAg-negative chronic HBV infection may range from inactive carrier to aggressive chronic hepatitis with or without cirrhosis [29,30].

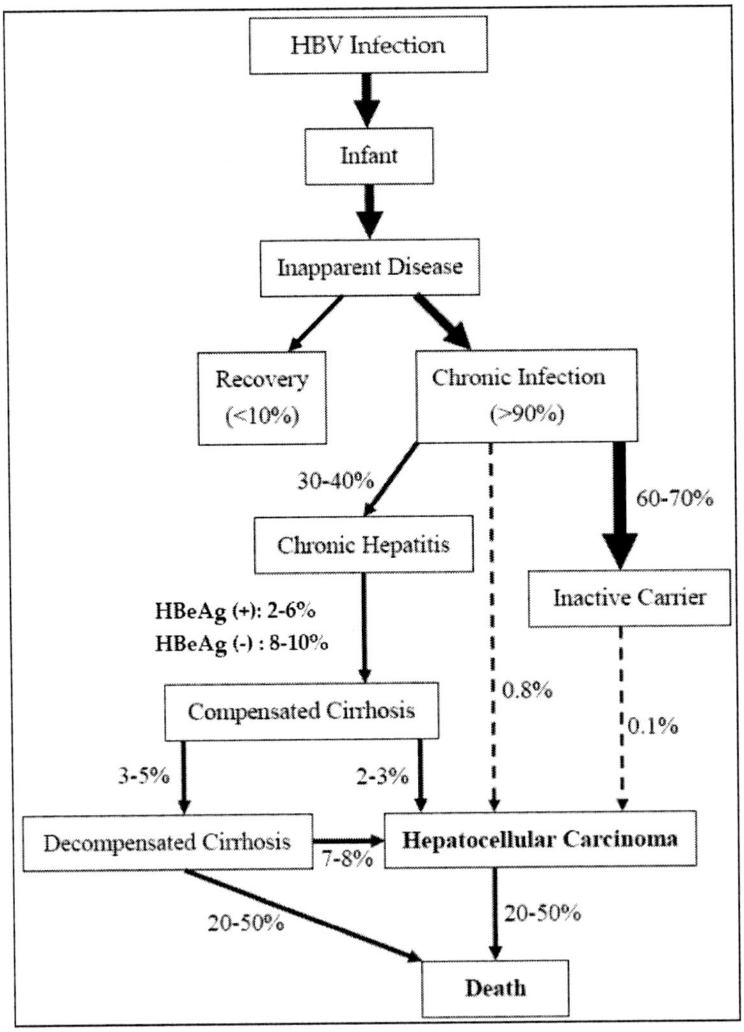

Figure 3. Annual rates of liver disease progression during the course of chronic hepatitis B virus infection. Modified from Kao et al. [34].

Hepatitis B Viral Factors and Long-Term Outcomes

In a population study, the relative risk of HCC in Taiwanese patients with persistent HBV infection was estimated to be 200 times higher than in non-infected individuals [31].

The lifetime risk of HBV carriers to develop cirrhosis, liver failure, or HCC may be as high as 15-40% [32]. The annual incidence of cirrhosis has been estimated to be 2% to 6% for HBeAg-positive and 8% to 10% for HBeAg-negative patients. The annual incidence of HCC has been estimated to be less than 1% for non-cirrhotic carriers and 2% to 3% for patients with cirrhosis (Figure 3) [33,34].

The identification of risk factors for the development of advanced liver disease, including cirrhosis and HCC, in HBV carriers is important for developing appropriate treatment. The risk factors associated with the development of HCC include chronic infection with either HBV or HCV, the presence of cirrhosis, carcinogen exposure especially aflatoxin, alcohol abuse, genetic factors, male gender, cigarette smoking and advanced age [35,36]. These factors have been found to act synergistically to induce liver cirrhosis and HCC. Among these risk factors, chronic hepatitis viral infections, particularly those with cirrhosis and HBsAg-positive family members of patients with HBV-related HCC, show the strongest association with the development of HCC in Asian countries (Table 1) [37- 40].

Table 1. Risk factors associated with the development of advanced liver disease, including cirrhosis and hepatocellular carcinoma in chronic hepatitis B

Host factors	Viral factors	External factors
Advanced age	High viral load	Alcohol consumption
Male gender	Genotype (C>B, D>A)	Aflatoxin exposure
Genetic alteration Family history of HCC Ethnicity (Asian > Caucasian)	Specific HBV mutants	Cigarette smoking Concurrent HCV, HDV or HIV infection Diabetes mellitus Obesity

HBV Serotype and Genotype

After a long-time evolution, HBsAg derived from different strains carries serologically group-specific antigenic determinants, including the '*a*' determinant are common to all HBsAg, whereas the *d, y, w*, and *r* determinants are mainly of epidemiological interest. Based on different serological reactivities of HBsAg, HBV has been classified into 4 serotypes, adw, adr, ayw and ayr. Each serotype comprises the '*a*' determinant together with two allelic determinants '*d/y*' and '*w/r*' [41]. Serotypes of HBV have specific geographic distributions [42,43]. Recently, according to the homogeneity of the virus sequence, at least 8 HBV genotypes (A to H) are defined by divergence in the entire HBV genomic sequence > 8% [44]. Currently, there were many methods available for HBV genotyping, including direct sequencing and subsequent homology comparison or phylogenetic tree analysis, polymerase chain reaction-restriction fragment length polymorphism (PCR-RFLP), PCR with type specific primers, enzyme-linked immunosorbant assay, real-time PCR with melting curve analysis [45] and line probe assay using reverse hybridization technology [46].

Epidemiologic studies have shown that each genotype has its distinct geographic and ethnic distribution [10,44]. Genotypes A and D occur frequently in Africa, Europe and India, while genotypes B and C are prevalent in Asia. Genotype E is restricted to West Africa, and F is found in Central and South America. Genotype G has been reported in France, Germany and the United States. Recently, the eighth genotype H was described in Central America (Figure 4). Interestingly, it is noted that genotypes B and C are prevalent in highly endemic areas, such as Asian countries, where perinatal or vertical transmission plays an important role in spreading the virus and the same genotype may be conserved in the same population, whereas genotypes A, D, E, F and G are frequently found in areas where horizontal transmission is the main mode of transmission. The correlation between serologic subtypes and genotypes has been clarified [47,48]. A recent study from Taiwan consistently showed that *adw* and *adr* account for 70 and 30% of HBV strains, respectively. In contrast, all *adr* strains are genotype C, whereas 81 and 12% of the *adw* strains are genotype B and genotype C, respectively [47].

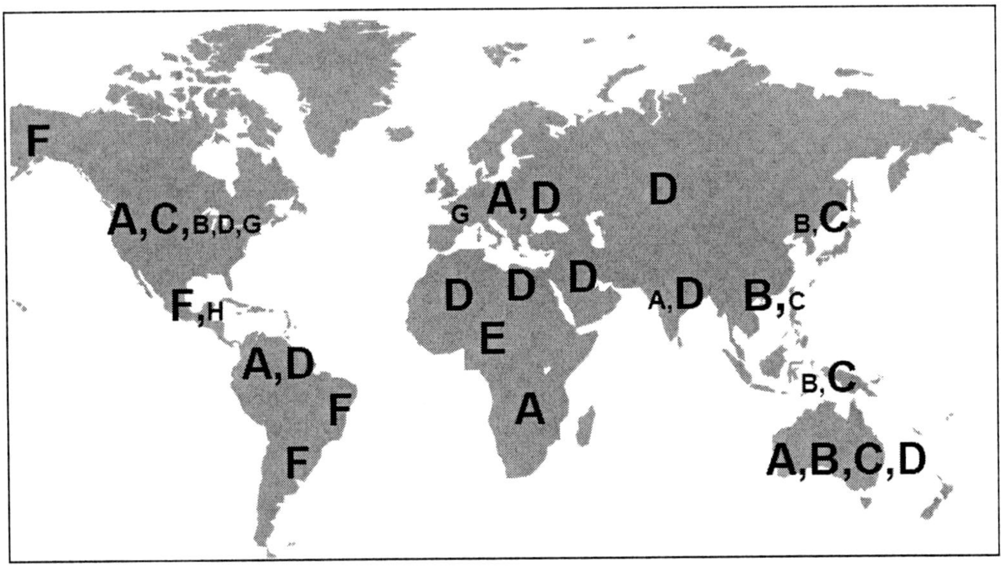

Figure 4. Worldwide distribution of HBV genotypes. The size of capitals indicates the relative prevalence of each genotype in a given area [10].

Previous studies have demonstrated that both serotype and genotype of HBV can serve as useful epidemiologic tools for the investigation of maternal transmission, familial clustering and geographic distribution of HBV strains [42,49,50]. In our previous study, we performed HBV genotyping and phylogenetic analysis to elucidate the modes of intrafamilial HBV transmission in a cohort of 103 individuals from 20 families. Three patterns of intrafamilial clustering of HBV infection, including family with HBsAg-positive mother, family with HBsAg-positive father and both parents positive for HBsAg, were identified. The identical genotyping results between index parent and carrier children indicated that HBV clustering was caused by index parental transmission. The modes of transmission were confirmed by phylogenetic analysis of the hypervariable pre-S gene of HBV genome. Accordingly, these lines of evidence highlight that genotyping of HBV can serve as a screening tool for possible sources of intrafamilial transmission [50].

The Impact of HBV Genotype on Natural History of Chronic Hepatitis B

Contrary to HCV genotyping, HBV genotyping remained an investigational tool with limited application to the study of the natural history and treatment of HBV infection few years ago. In addition, due to the unique distribution of HBV genotypes in Asian and Western countries, the clinical significance of HBV genotype could only be reliably compared between genotype B and C (Table 2) or genotype A and D (Table 3).

Table 2. Comparison of clinical and virologic differences between hepatitis B virus genotype B and C

Characteristics	Genotype B	Genotype C
Clinical		
Positivity of HBeAg	Lower	Higher
Seroconversion of HBeAg	Earlier	Later
Immunoclearance phase	Shorter	Longer
Seroclearance of HBsAg	More	Less
Reactivation after HBeAg seroconversion	Less	More
Histologic activity	Lower	Higher
Clinical outcome (cirrhosis and hepatocellular carcinoma)	Better	Worse
Recurrence after liver transplantation	Lower	Higher
Virologic		
Serum HBV DNA level	Lower	Higher
Frequency of precore A1896 mutation	Higher	Lower
Frequency of basal core promoter T1762/A1764 mutation	Lower	Higher

Table 3. Comparison of clinical and virologic differences between hepatitis B virus genotype A and D

Characteristics	Genotype A	Genotype D
Clinical		
Acute hepatitis	Less	More
Chronic hepatitis	More	Less
Reactivation after HBeAg seroconversion	Less	More
Histologic activity	Lower	Higher
Clinical outcome (cirrhosis and hepatocellular carcinoma)	Better	Worse
Recurrence after liver transplantation	Lower	Higher
Virologic		
Frequency of precore A1896 mutation	Lower	Higher
Frequency of basal core promoter T1762/A1764 mutation	Higher	Lower

HBV Genotypes and the Tendency of Chronic Infection

The relationship of HBV genotypes and the tendency of chronic infection has been elucidated. Suzuki et al. reported 97 adult patients with acute hepatitis B recruited from 1976 to 2003 in Japan [51]. The persistence of HBV infection was higher in patients with genotype A infection (23%) than those with genotype B (11%) or C (7%) infection. These data suggest that infection with genotype A prevails in patients with acute hepatitis B in Japan where genotypes B and C are common, and tends to persist. In a European study of 65 patients, genotype D was more prevalent in patients with acute, self-limited hepatitis B as compared with genotype A (80% vs. 10%, $P < 0.01$). In contrast, genotype A predominated over genotype D in patients with chronic HBV infection (80% vs. 11%, $P < 0.01$) [52]. In general, the rate of chronicity of acute genotype A and D infection were reported to be high compared with genotype B and C [53-55].Taken together, the persistence of HBV infection after acute infection may be attributed to the variable strength of host-viral interactions, the modes of transmission as well as the varying distribution of genotypes.

HBV Genotypes and HBeAg Seroconversion

Seroconversion of HBeAg has been recognized as an important event in the natural history of Asian HBV carriers. Early HBeAg seroconversion typically confers a favorable outcome, whereas late or absent HBeAg seroconversion after multiple hepatitis flares may accelerate the progression of chronic hepatitis to cirrhosis, and therefore, has a poor clinical outcome [28,56]. Patients with genotype C infection are shown to more often HBeAg positive than those with genotype B infection [44], it is therefore reasonable to examine whether genotype C may have lower rates of spontaneous HBeAg seroconversion and therefore stay longer in the replicative phase of chronic HBV infection than genotype B. Chu et al. first reported that genotype B is associated with earlier and frequent HBeAg seroconversion than genotype C in Chinese patients [56]. In Taiwan, we examined 146 HBeAg-positive HBV carriers followed-up for a mean of 52 months (range, 12-120 months) and found that genotype C infection has lower rates of spontaneous HBeAg seroconversion than those with genotype B infection at the end of follow-up (27% vs. 47%, $P < 0.025$). The estimated rate of HBeAg seroconversion in all HBV carriers is 12.6% per year, and the rates in genotype B and C patients are 15.5% and 7.9% per year, respectively. In addition, the mean age at HBeAg seroconversion of genotype C patients was one decade older than that of genotype B patients (41 ± 10 vs. 30 ± 8 years, $P < 0.001$), suggesting a delayed HBeAg seroconversion and a longer duration of high HBV replication in genotype C patients [57]. These results have also been found in Hong Kong and Japan [58,59]. We further studied the clinical relevance of HBV genotype in 460 Taiwanese HBV carrier children [60], and the data indicated that the seropositive rates of HBeAg after 20 years of follow-up was 70% in genotype C and 40% in genotype B carriers. The frequency and severity of hepatitis flare of chronic hepatitis B are closely associated with the development of liver cirrhosis in HBV carriers [20,61]. To explore the clinical phenotypes, with special reference to the seroconversion of HBeAg and frequency of acute exacerbation between patients infected with HBV genotypes B and C, a cohort of 272 Taiwanese with chronic HBV infection were analyzed. Genotype C patients are more likely associated with persistently HBeAg positive chronic HBV infection despite multiple episodes of hepatitis flare [62]. In a prospective study of 146 HBeAg-positive chronic hepatitis B patients with a mean follow-up of 32 months, Chan et al. consistently found that the disease activity in the HBeAg-positive phase was higher in genotype C patients than in genotype B patients (78% vs. 50%, $P = 0.032$) [63]. Regarding the fibrosis progression in chronic hepatitis, a Japanese study including 258 patients with histologically verified chronic hepatitis B showed that the ratio of patients with advanced fibrosis in genotype B was significantly lower than in genotype C (13% vs. 33%, $P = 0.034$), and the difference was more evident in younger patients (< 45 years; 4% vs. 26%, $P = 0.02$) [64].

Regarding genotypes A and D, one prospective study evaluated the clinical outcomes of 258 Spanish patients with chronic HBV infection with a mean follow-up of 94 months (range, 24-180). The baseline HBeAg positivity was significantly lower in patients with genotype D than those with genotype A (36% vs. 80%, $P < 0.0001$). In addition, the rate of sustained remission after seroconversion was higher in genotype A than in genotype D patients (55% vs. 32%, $P < 0.01$) [65]. Taken together, these facts suggest the phenotype of HBeAg seroconversion between genotype B and C as well as genotype A and D differs in the early phase of chronic HBV infection, and genotype C and D patients, compared to genotype B and A patients, have late or absent HBeAg seroconversion after multiple hepatitis flares may accelerate the progression of chronic hepatitis and therefore, have a poor clinical outcome.

HBV Genotypes and Disease Progression

Most retrospective or case control studies indicated that the patients with genotype C have more severe liver disease including cirrhosis and HCC than those with genotype B [66-69]. In a cross-sectional study, the prevalence of HBV genotypes and the association between distinct genotypes and severity of liver disease has been studied in 270 Taiwanese HBV carriers with various forms of liver disease [67]. The results suggested that genotypes B and C are the predominant strains in Taiwan and genotype C is more prevalent in patients with cirrhosis and in patients with HCC aged above 50 years compared with age-matched asymptomatic carriers (60% vs. 23%, $P < 0.001$ and 41% vs. 15%, $P = 0.005$). A further survey of 200 surgical cases also showed the same tendency: the prevalence of genotype C was higher in old HCC patients (Figure 5) [44]. Our recent 14-year prospective study on 4841 Taiwanese men who were HBV carriers also demonstrated that HBV genotype C was associated with an increased risk of HCC compared with other HBV genotypes (adjusted OR = 5.11, 95% CI = 3.20 to 8.18) [70]. These findings indicate that genotype C is indeed correlated with a higher risk of developing HCC. Of particular note, we also found genotype B was significantly more common in patients with HCC aged less than 50 years compared with age-matched asymptomatic carriers in Taiwan (80% vs. 52%; $P = 0.03$). This predominance was more remarkable in younger patients with HCC, being 90% in those aged less than 35 years, and most were non-cirrhotic. These data thus suggested that certain genotype B strains may be associated with the development of HCC in young non-cirrhotic HBV carriers [67]. Similar findings also documented in Taiwanese pediatric patients with chronic HBV infection [60]. The results revealed that among 26 children with HBV-related HCC, genotype B was the major genotype (74%). Studies from Japan and China have confirmed the findings that HBV genotype C is associated with the development of HCC [34,69]. In summary, the data indicated that genotype B is rarely associated with the development of HCC in Japan and China. In contrast, more than 50% of HBV-related HCC patients in Taiwan are infected with HBV genotype B [67]. Accordingly, the genotype B strains in Taiwan are somewhat different from those in Japan and China and may be provisionally divided into three phenotypic subtypes, slowly progressive subtype, intermediately progressive subtype, and rapidly progressive subtype, based on the rate of liver disease progression [34]. However, these speculations need further confirmation. In addition to clinical and pathogenic differences between HBV genotype B and C, HBV genotypes also influence the clinicopathological features of patients with resectable HCC. Recently, in our 193 patients with resectable HBV-related HCC, 107 (55%) and 86 (45%) were infected with genotype B and C, respectively. Compared with genotype C patients, genotype B patients were less associated with liver cirrhosis (33% vs. 51%, P=0.01). Pathologically, genotype B patients had a higher rate of solitary tumor (94% vs. 86%, P=0.048) and more satellite nodules (22% vs. 12%, P=0.05) than genotype C patients. These characteristics may contribute to the recurrence patterns and prognosis of HBV-related HCC patients with genotype B or C infection [71,72].

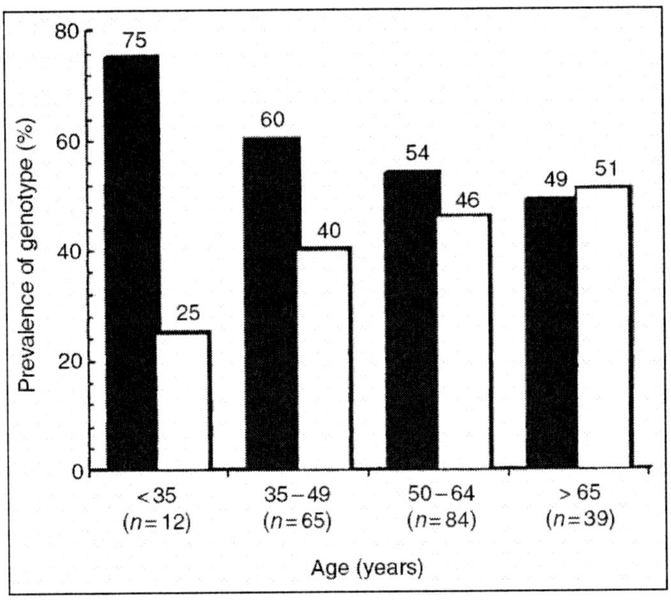

Figure 5. Genotypes of hepatitis B virus in 200 patients with resectable hepatocellular carcinoma (HCC) stratified by age. The prevalence of genotype B (■) in HCC patients showed a gradual decrease from 75% in HCC patients aged below 35 years to 49% in those aged above 65 years. The prevalence of genotype C (□) gradually increased from 25% in HCC patients aged below 35 years to 51% in those aged above 65 years [44].

As for other genotypes, Thakur et al. prospectively studied the prevalence and clinical significance of HBV genotypes A and D in 130 histologically proven chronic HBV infected Indian patients [73]. Their results showed the prevalence of genotype D tended to be higher in HCC patients younger than 40 years of age than in age-matched inactive carriers. Another report from Spain indicated that death related to liver disease was more frequent in genotype F than in genotype A (P = 0.02) or genotype D (P = 0.002) hepatitis [65].

Although the influence of HBV genotypes on disease progression and clinical outcome has been increasingly recognized; however, the molecular mechanisms remain largely unknown. Sugiyama et al. recently reported the intra- and extracellular expression of HBV DNA and antigen [74]. The intracellular expression of HBV DNA and HBcAg were higher for genotypes B and C than genotypes A and D. The extracellular expression of HBV DNA and HBeAg were also higher for genotypes B and C than genotypes A and D (Table 4). The intracellular accumulation of HBV DNA and antigens may play a role in inducing liver cell damage. In addition, the highest replication capacity of genotype C may explain why genotype C is associated with more severe histological liver damage than other genotypes. On the other hand, a strong extracellular virion secretion may endow a high infectious capacity to blood from individuals infected with this genotype. These data suggest that virologic differences indeed exist among HBV genotypes that may influence their clinical outcomes and epidemiological characteristics. Nevertheless, whether immunopathogenesis differs between various HBV genotypes need further studies.

Table 4. Influence of hepatitis B virus genotypes on the intra- and extra-cellular expression of viral DNA and antigens. Adapted from Sugiyama et al. [74]

Expression	Genotypes
Intracellular	
HBV DNA	C > B > D > A
HBcAg	B > C > D > A
Extracellular	
HBV DNA	B > C = D > A
HBeAg	B > C > D > A
HBsAg	A > B > C > D

HBV Genotypes and Response to Anti-Viral Therapy

Currently, six drugs have been approved for the treatment of chronic hepatitis B: conventional interferon (IFN) alfa, lamivudine, adefovir dipivoxil, entecavir, pegylated interferon alfa-2a and telbivudine [75-78]. HBV genotype has been partly clarified to influence response to both nucleoside analogue and interferon-based treatment [79]. In patients treated with conventional IFN, The response rate, defined as normalization of serum ALT level and HBeAg seroconversion, was better in patients with genotype A and B than in those with genotype C and D [80-83]. As to pegylated IFN alfa-2a, Cooksley et al. showed that the response rate of using pegylated IFN alfa-2a or conventional IFN alfa-2a was higher in genotype B than genotype C (33% vs. 21%; 25% vs. 6%; respectively) [84]. In a multi-center study, the overall response rate also differed according to HBV genotype: genotype A, 47%; genotype B, 44%; genotype C, 28%; and genotype D, 25% [85]. Another study consistently demonstrated a higher rate of treatment response in genotype A compared to the other 3 genotypes in terms of HBsAg seroconversion, in both HBeAg-positive and HBeAg-negative chronic hepatitis B [86].

In lamivudine-treated patients, Chien et al. reported that the sustained response rate to lamivudine was much higher in patients with genotype B than those with genotype C (61% vs. 20%, P = 0.009) [87]. However, two studies from Hong Kong contradicted this finding [88,89]. In addition, our previous study showed that the development of lamivudine resistance was similar between genotype B and C [90]. In Spain, Buti et al. suggested that the outcome after lamivudine treatment as well as the emergence of lamivudine resistance were comparable between genotype A and D [91]. No statistical differences were found in response to adefovir dipivoxil, entecavir and telbivudine among patients with different genotypes [92-94]. In summary, these lines of evidence imply that HBV genotype appears to have no substantial impact on the response to nucleoside analogue treatment.

Based on these data, it is recommended that HBV carriers should be routinely genotyped to help identify those who may be at higher risk of liver disease progression, and who are most appropriate for interferon treatment [95].

Naturally Occurring HBV Mutants and Disease Progression

Due to the spontaneous error rate of viral reverse transcription, naturally occurring variations between HBV strains as well as mutations arising during the course of a patient's infection have implications at both the clinical and epidemiological levels. Several HBV mutant strains including mutations in precore, core promoter and deletion mutation in pre-S/S genes have been reported to be associated with the pathogenesis of progressive liver disease, including cirrhosis and HCC (Figure 1). HBV precore nucleotide 1896 mutation from guanine (G) to adenine (A) as well as changes of 2 nucleotides, an adenine (A) to thymine (T) transversion at nucleotide 1762 together with a guanine (G) to adenine (A) transition at nucleotide 1764 within the basal core promoter (BCP) lead to a proportion of HBeAg-negative patients continue to have moderate levels of HBV replication and active liver disease [4,96-98]. In addition, the dual mutation in BCP T1762/A1764 mutation may increase the risk of liver disease progression and HCC development for both genotypes B and C infection [66,67,99-103]. In a cohort study, we investigated the prevalence of BCP T1762/A1764 mutation in 250 genotype B- or C-infected HBV carriers with different stages of liver disease. The results showed genotype C has a higher prevalence of BCP T1762/A1764 mutation than genotype B (odds ratio, 5.18; 95% confidence interval [CI], 2.59-10.37; P < 0.001). The likelihood of T1762/A1764 mutation parallels the progression of liver disease, from 3% in inactive carriers to 64% in HCC patients (odds ratio, 20.04; 95% CI, 7.25-55.41; P < 0.001). Patients with BCP T1762/A1764 mutation were significantly associated with the development of HCC than those without (odds ratio, 10.60; 95% CI, 4.92-22.86; P < 0.001), and the risk was observed for both genotypes B and C [66]. Taking together, BCP T1762/A1764 mutation is the strongest viral factor associated with risk of HCC in HBV carriers. These findings were in accordance with a long-term follow-up study involving 400 HBV carriers that showed presence of BCP T1762/A1764 mutation (odds ratio, 2.93; 95% CI, 1.24-7.57; P = 0.02) were independent predictors for progression to HCC [104]. Therefore, BCP T1762/A1764 mutation may play an important role in the pathogenesis of liver disease progression.

Other naturally occurring mutations or deletions in the pre-S gene of HBV genome frequently occurred in chronic HBV infection [105,106]. The deletion over pre-S gene may affect the expression of middle and small surface proteins, resulting in intracellular accumulation of large surface protein [107], and contribute to more progressive liver cell damage and finally hepatocarcinogenesis [108,109]. In our case-control study, pre-S deletion mutant of HBV were determined in 202 asymptomatic carriers and 64 HCC patients with chronic HBV genotype B or C infection. The presence of pre-S deletion mutant was independently associated with the development of HCC (odds ratio, 3.72; 95% CI, 1.44-9.65, P=0.007) [110]. Our further mapping study of pre-S region revealed all the deletion regions encompassed T- and B-cell epitopes, and most of them lost one or more functional sites, including polymerized human serum albumin-binding site, nucleocapsid-binding site. These finding lend support to the biologic significance of emerging HBV pre-S deletion mutants, which may contribute to more progressive liver cell damage and finally hepatocarcinogenesis [102].

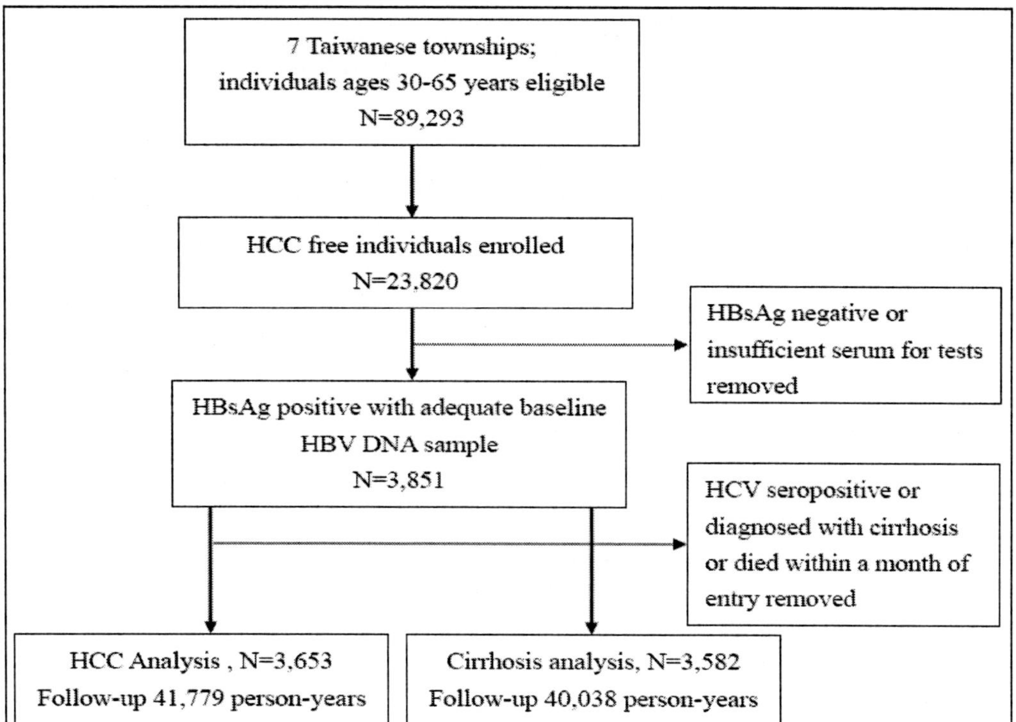

Figure 6. The flow of patients in a population-based prospective cohort study to assess the impact of viral load on the risk of cirrhosis and hepatocellular carcinoma (HCC). Adapted from Iloeje et al and Chen et al. [115,116].

Hepatitis B Viral Load and Disease Progression

Recently, new hepatitis B viral factors predictive of clinical outcomes have been identified. In a longitudinal follow-up study, Chan et al. reported that an HBV DNA level below 10^4 copies/ml was predictive of inactive liver disease among patients undergoing HBeAg seroconversion and in HBeAg-negative patients. On the other hand, an HBV DNA level above 10^5 copies/ml was predictive of HBeAg reversion and viral recurrence [111], in line with the findings of other Asian and European studies [112-114]. Therefore, measurement of HBV DNA after HBeAg seroconversion and in HBeAg-negative patients is useful to assess the risk of HBeAg reversion. More recently, the impact of viral load on the risk of cirrhosis was assessed in a population-based prospective cohort of 3,582 untreated Taiwanese with chronic hepatitis B infection, including 7 townships in Taiwan. Of them, 85% were HBeAg-negative and were followed for a mean duration of 11 years (Figure 6) [115,116]. The cumulative incidence of cirrhosis increased with the HBV-DNA level and ranged from 4.5% to 36.2% for patients with a hepatitis B viral load of less than 300 copies/ml and 10^6 copies/ml or more, respectively ($P < 0.001$). After adjusting for hepatitis B e-antigen status and serum ALT level among other variables, hepatitis B viral load was the strongest predictor of progression to cirrhosis. The relative risk started to increase at an entry HBV DNA level of 10^4 copies/ml (relative risk 2.5; 95% CI, 1.6-3.8). Those with HBV-DNA levels of 10^6 copies/ml or more had the greatest risk 6.5 (relative risk 6.5 ; 95% CI,4.1-10.2; $P<0.001$). Of particular note, in the HBeAg-negative patients with normal serum ALT levels at cohort entry, the risk of cirrhosis was also increased significantly as the HBV-DNA level increased (Figure 7) [115]. The relationship between serum HBV DNA level and risk of HCC has also been evaluated in several prospective clinical and population-based studies [70,116-118]. In the same prospective cohort in Taiwan, the risk factors associated with the development of HCC were assessed in 3,653 HBV carriers age between 30-65 years [116]. A significant biological gradient of hepatocellular carcinoma risk by serum HBV DNA level from 300 copies/ml (undetectable) to 1 million copies/ml or greater was observed in this study. The dose-response relationship was most prominent for participants who were seronegative for HBeAg with normal serum ALT levels and no liver cirrhosis at study entry (Figure 8). Participants with persistent elevation of serum HBV DNA level during follow-up had the highest hepatocellular carcinoma risk. These results were consistent with another prospective cohort study in 2,763 adult HBV carriers with 11 years of follow-up from Haimen city in China and Philadelphia in the US, that assessed the relationship between past hepatitis B virus (HBV) viral load and mortality [118]. Compared to the HBV undetected carriers, the relative risk for HCC mortality in carriers with low viral load ($< 10^5$ copies/ml) was 1.7 (95% CI, 0.5-5.7) and 11.2 (95% CI, 3.6-35.0) in those with high viral load ($\geq 10^5$ copies/ml). Overall, the ample evidence from these studies strongly indicate that the best predictor of adverse outcomes (cirrhosis, HCC and death from liver disease) in chronic HBV infection is the serum HBV DNA level at enrollment, independent of HBeAg status, baseline serum ALT level and other risk factors. However, because of the heterogeneity of HCC populations, risk factors may differ between old HCC patients and young HCC patients. In our case-control study, including 183 HBV-related HCC patients and 202 HBV carriers, showed that young ($\leq$ 40 years old) HCC patients had lower serum HBV DNA level than old

HCC patients (log_{10}HBV DNA: 4.2 vs. 4.8, P = 0.056). In addition, high serum HBV DNA level was associated with the development of HCC in old patients (odds ratio, 1.584, 95% CI, 1.075–2.333; P = 0.02) rather than in young patients (odds ratio, 0.848, 95% CI 0.645–1.116; P = 0.239) [119]. Thus, viral factors in association with the development of HCC in young and old patients await more investigation.

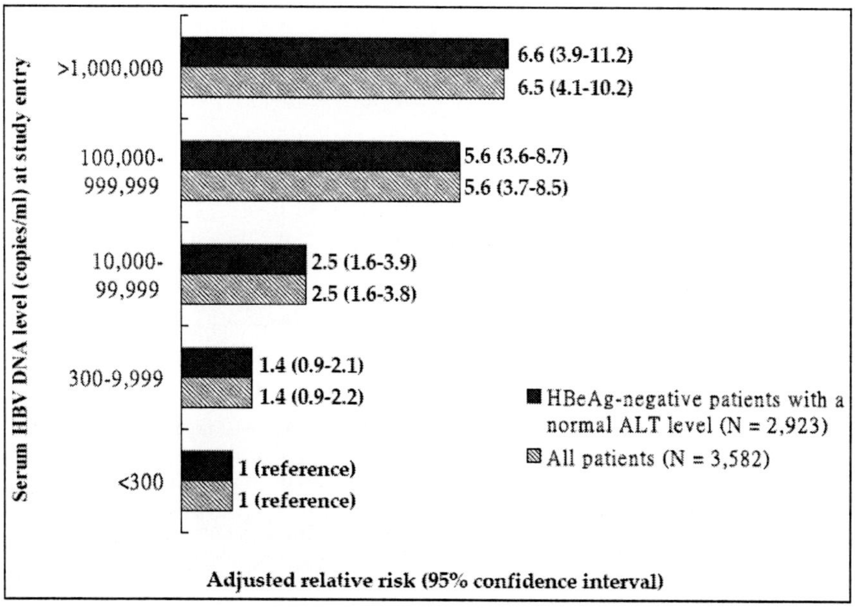

Figure 7. Adjusted relative risks of cirrhosis for HBV carriers by baseline serum HBV DNA level in a population-based prospective cohort study. Adapted from Iloeje et al. [115].

Hepatitis B Viral Factors and Serum Alanine Aminotransferase Levels

The differential diagnosis of HBeAg-negative chronic hepatitis from inactive carrier mainly depends on sequential determinations of serum ALT level [120]. However, slightly increased serum ALT level, although within the normal range, has been reported to be significantly associated with risk of liver-related mortality in the general population [121]. Furthermore, recent large-scale cohort studies showed that chronic hepatitis B patients with a normal serum ALT level, irrespective of HBeAg status, were also at a risk for the development of cirrhosis and HCC [116,122]. As the distribution of serum ALT level is continuous, it is difficult to arbitrarily define the cut-off concentration of ALT to separate the clinical significant HBV patients from inactive carriers. A recent study on Chinese chronic hepatitis B patients showed that patients with serum ALT levels of 0.5-1 x upper limit of normal (ULN) had a significantly increased risk of complications compared with patients with serum ALT levels < 0.5 x ULN [122]. Therefore, chronic hepatitis B patients with high-normal serum ALT levels (0.5-1 x ULN) may be at risk of progressive liver disease. Recently, we investigated the correlation between serum ALT level and hepatitis B viral factors in 414 HBeAg-negative carriers with persistently normal serum ALT level [123]. Compared to HBV carriers with low-normal ALT, those with high-normal ALT had a greater frequency of serum HBV DNA level > 10^4 copies/ml (63.4% vs. 47.5%, P < 0.001) as well as a higher prevalence of BCP T1762/A1764 mutant (36.5% vs. 24.2%, P = 0.01). Multivariate analysis showed that factors associated with a high-normal serum ALT level included male gender [relative risk (RR), 1.82; 95% CI, 1.10-3.01, P = 0.019], increasing age (RR, <30 years: 1, reference; 30-39 years: 2.43, 95% CI, 1.18-5.03, P = 0.016; 40-49 years: 4.22, 95% CI, 1.99-8.93, P < 0.001; ≥50 years: 4.06, 95% CI, 1.69-9.78, P = 0.002) and serum HBV DNA level > 10^4 copies/ml (RR, 1.83; 95% CI, 1.07-3.13, P = 0.027) (Table 5). Our findings convincingly indicate that persistent HBV viremia may cause subclinical yet continuous disease activity in HBeAg-negative carriers with persistently normal serum ALT level. In a retrospective cohort study from Japan, Ikeda et al. elucidate the incidence of hepatitis activation during long-term follow-up (median follow-up of 10.2 years) in 116 HBeAg-negative carriers with persistently normal serum ALT level. They found that hepatitis activation rates with twice as high as normal ALT level at the end of the third year follow-up were 12.1% in the low DNA group ($\leq 10^4$ copies/ml), 43.4% in the intermediate Group (10^4-10^6 copies/ml), and 66.7% in the high DNA group ($\geq 10^6$ copies/ml). Initial HBV DNA values were significantly associated with future increase in aminotransferase (P = 0.0001). Particularly, carcinogenesis rate in patients with and without high DNA of 10^6 copies/ml was 11.5% and 1.8%, respectively, at the 10th year follow-up, (P = 0.021) [124]. Taken together, these results were consistent with previous reports that a normal ALT level alone was not an accurate indicator of inactive disease [125,126], and the inactive range of serum ALT level should be redefined to 30 U/L for male and 19 U/L for female [127]. In addition, serum HBV DNA should be monitored even in HBeAg-negative carriers with persistently normal serum ALT level, and serum HBV DNA level of 10^4 copies/ml might serve as a critical cutoff level to predict disease progression.

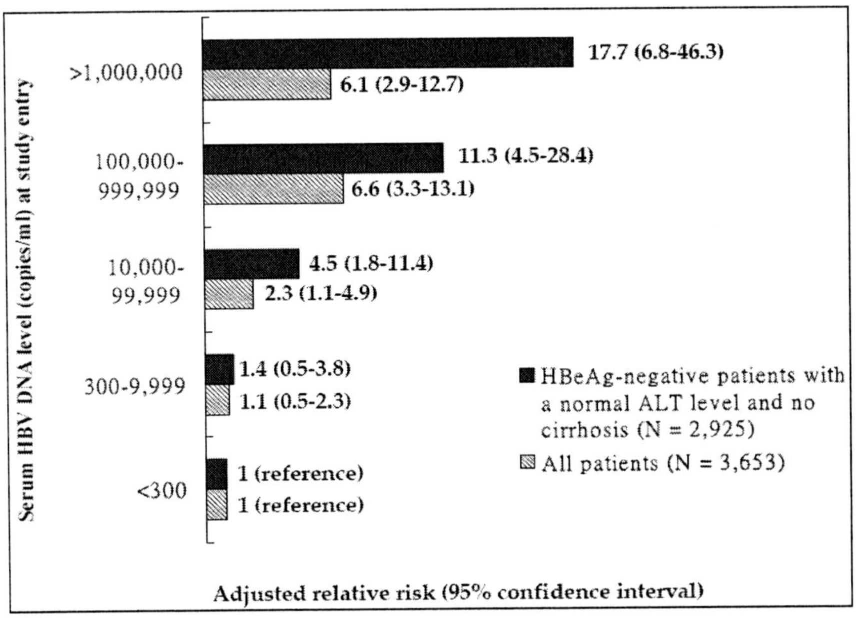

Figure 8. Adjusted relative risk for hepatocellular carcinoma for HBV carriers by baseline serum HBV DNA level in a population-based prospective cohort study. Adapted from Chen et al. [116].

Table 5. Factors associated with high-normal serum alanine aminotransferase level in 414 HBeAg-negative HBV carriers with persistently normal alanine aminotransferase. Adapted from Lin et al. [123]

	Relative risk	95% confidence interval	P value
Gender			0.019
Female	1		
Male	1.82	1.10-3.01	
Age			
< 30 years	1		
30-39 years	2.43	1.18-5.03	0.016
40-49 years	4.22	1.99-8.93	<0.001
≥50 years	4.06	1.69-9.78	0.002
HBV DNA level			0.027
< 4 Log_{10}	1		
≥ 4 Log_{10}	1.83	1.07-3.13	

Potential Interactions between Hepatitis B Viral Factors

In light of these emerging data, HBV genotypes, mutant stains and HBV DAN level are closely associated with the long-term outcomes of HBV-related chronic liver disease. In our earlier study, we already found that genotype C has a higher frequency of BCP T1762/A1764 mutation than genotype B that is 50% vs. 6% [80]. However, it is unclear whether a specific combination of these factors is associated with the development of severe liver disease. In a prospective study, Yu et al. provide strong evidence that the risk of HCC was increased approximately 5 folds among men infected with HBV genotype C compared with genotype B. They also found HBV viral load was higher with HBV genotype C than with HBV genotype B, and men who had both HBV genotype C and a very high HBV viral load had a 26-fold higher risk of HCC than those with other genotypes and low or undetectable viral loads (Figure 9) [70,79]. These observations suggest additive associations of viral load and HBV genotype C with HCC risk. We recently investigated the independent and interactive effects of each known viral factor on the development of HCC. Compared with patients with low HBV load and the BCP A1762/G1764 wild-type strain, the adjusted OR of developing HCC was more than 30 folds in patients with an HBV load $\geq 10^5$ copies/ml and the BCP T1762/A1764 mutant, irrespective of the presence of the precore A1896 mutation and viral genotype [100]. Similar to cirrhotic HCC, BCP T1762/A1764 mutation, and viral load $\geq 10^5$ copies/ml were independently associated with the risk of noncirrhotic HCC [101]. We therefore studied the relationship between viral load and HBV mutants in 414 HBeAg-negative carriers with persistently normal serum ALT level. Patients with BCP T1762/A1764 mutant alone had a significantly higher serum HBV DNA level than those with BCP A1762/G1764 wild-type strain, regardless of precore 1896 status [123]. These results confirmed in vitro data that BCP T1762/A1764 mutant may increase of HBV replication [128,129]. We also investigated the interactions among pre-S deletion, precore mutation, and

BCP T1762/A1764 mutation in various stages of chronic HBV infection [102]. The results revealed that the presence of pre-S deletion and BCP T1762/A1764 mutation were significantly associated with the development of progressive liver diseases. In addition, combination of mutations rather than single mutation was associated with the development of progressive liver diseases, especially in combination with pre-S deletion. These findings suggest that in addition to HBV DNA level, accumulation of complex viral mutants with precore mutation, BCP T1762/A1764 mutation and pre-S deletion mutation may all affect the long-term outcomes of chronic HBV infection.

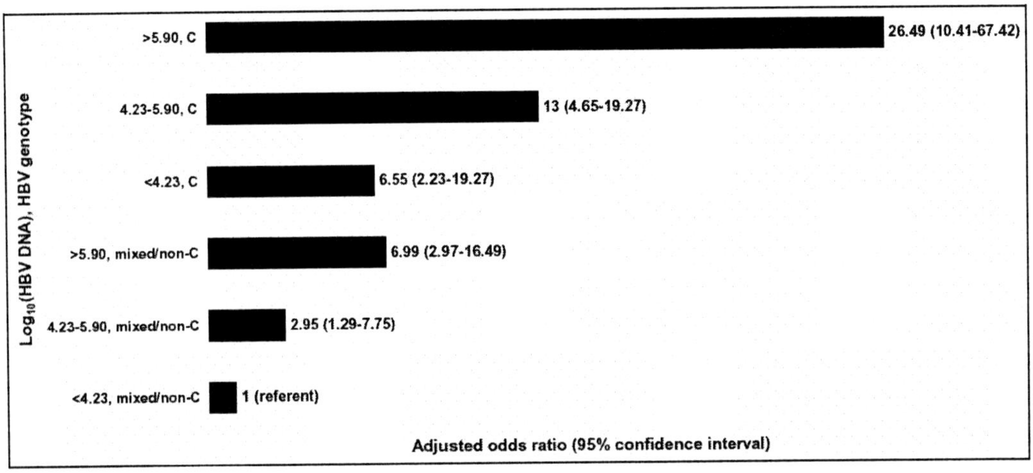

Figure 9. Combined risks of hepatocellular carcinoma associated with baseline serum HBV DNA level and genotype [79].

Summary and Prospective

HBV infection is a global public health problem and causes a wide spectrum of clinical manifestations, ranging from acute or fulminant hepatitis to various forms of chronic liver disease, including inactive carrier state, chronic hepatitis, cirrhosis and HCC. Most HBV carriers in the endemic regions acquire the virus during birth or early childhood. Liver injury associated with HBV infection is predominantly mediated through immune mediated mechanisms. The natural history of HBV carriers who are infected early in life can thus be divided into 4 dynamic phases based on the virus-host interaction. During the immune tolerance phase, serum HBV DNA levels are high and hepatitis B e antigen (HBeAg) is present. In the immune clearance phase, the majority of carriers seroconvert from HBeAg to anti-HBe. After HBeAg seroconversion, patients are usually in the integration or low replication phase, with low HBV DNA level and normal serum alanine aminotransferase activity. However, a small proportion of patients continue to have moderate level of HBV replication and active liver disease designated reactivation phase. The frequency and severity of hepatitis flares during the immune clearance and/or reactivation phase predicts progression of liver disease. In general, early HBeAg seroconversion typically confers a favorable outcome, whereas late or absent HBeAg seroconversion after multiple hepatitis flares may accelerate the progression of chronic hepatitis to cirrhosis, and therefore, has a poor clinical outcome. Other factors identified as risk factors of cirrhosis and HCC development include male gender, older age, presence of cirrhosis, family history of HCC, persistence of ALT elevations, co-infection with HCV or HDV, cigarette smoking, alcohol drinking, aflatoxin exposure, and co-morbidities of diabetes and obesity. Recently, new hepatitis B viral factors predictive of clinical outcomes have been identified. The higher the serum HBV DNA level in the immune clearance phase, the higher the incidence of adverse outcomes over time. In addition, several hospital-based cohort or case control studies from Taiwan and Hong Kong indicated that high HBV DNA level, HBV genotype C, basal core promoter mutation and pre-S deletion are associated with increased risk of liver disease progression as well as HCC development. These lines of evidence indicate additive associations of viral load, HBV genotype, and genome mutations with the progression of chronic hepatitis B. Further large-scale prospective studies are needed to confirm causal relationship

In summary, several viral factors has already been identified to influence liver disease progression of chronic hepatitis B, and the lessons learned from the natural history of chronic HBV infection in adult HBV carriers from endemic areas can help us better define the clinical threshold as well as therapeutic endpoint of "safe" HBV DNA level (e.g. 10,000 copies or 2,000 IU/ml) for the prevention of long-term liver-related complications in patients during later phases of chronic HBV infection worldwide.

REFERENCES

[1] Robinson WS. The genome of hepatitis B virus. *Ann Rev Microbiol* 1977;31:357-377.

[2] Ganem D, Varmus HE. The molecular biology of the hepatitis B viruses. *Annu Rev Biochem* 1987;56:651-693.

[3] Lau JY, Wright TL. Molecular virology and pathogenesis of hepatitis B. *Lancet* 1993;342:1335-1340.

[4] Hunt CM, McGill JM, Allen MI, Condreay LD. Clinical relevance of hepatitis B viral mutations. *Hepatology* 2000;31:1037-1044.

[5] Heermann KH, Goldmann U, Schwartz W, Seyffarth T, Baumgarten H, Gerlich WH. Large surface proteins of hepatitis B virus containing the pre-s sequence. *J Virol* 1984;52:396-402.

[6] Heermann KH, Kruse F, Seifer M, Gerlich WH. Immunogenicity of the gene S and Pre-S domains in hepatitis B virions and HBsAg filaments. *Intervirology* 1987;28:14-25.

[7] Ou JH, Laub O, Rutter WJ. Hepatitis B virus gene function: the precore region targets the core antigen to cellular membranes and causes the secretion of the e antigen. *Proc Natl Acad Sci* 1986;83:1578-1582.

[8] Milich DR, Jones JE, Hughes JL, Price J, Raney AK, McLachlan A. Is a function of the secreted hepatitis B e antigen to induce immunologic tolerance in utero? *Proc Natl Acad Sci U S A* 1990;87:6599-603.

[9] Okamoto H, Imai M, Kametani M, Nakamura T, Mayumi M. Genomic heterogeneity of hepatitis B virus in a 54-year-old woman who contracted the infection through materno-fetal transmission. *Jpn J Exp Med* 1987;57:231-236.

[10] Kao JH, Chen DS. HBV Genotypes: Epidemiology and Implications Regarding Natural History. *Current Hepatitis Reports* 2006; 5:5–13.

[11] Murakami S. Hepatitis B virus X protein: structure, function and biology. *Intervirology* 1999;42:81-99.

[12] Lin Y, Nomura T, Yamashita T, Dorjsuren D, Tang H, Murakami S. The transactivation and p53-interaction functions of HBx are mutually interfering but distinct. *Cancer Res* 1997;57:5137-5142.

[13] Kao JH, Chen DS. Global control of hepatitis B virus infection. *Lancet Infect Dis* 2002; 2: 395-403.

[14] Stevens CE, Beasley RP, Tsui J, Lee WC. Vertical transmission of hepatitis B antigen in Taiwan. *N Engl J Med* 1975;292:771-4.

[15] Hsu SC, Chang MH, Ni YH, Hsu HY, Lee CY. Horizontal transmission of hepatitis B virus in children. *J Pediatr Gastroenterol Nutr* 1993;16:66-69.

[16] Chen DS. Natural history of chronic hepatitis B virus infection: new light on an old story. *J Gastroenterol Hepatol* 1993;8:470-475.

[17] Chu CM, Liaw YF. Intrahepatic distribution of hepatitis B surface and core antigens in chronic hepatitis B virus infection. Hepatocyte with cytoplasmic/membranous hepatitis B core antigen as a possible target for immune hepatocytolysis. *Gastroenterology* 1987;92:220-225.

[18] Liaw YF, Chu CM, Su IJ, Huang MJ, Lin DY, Chang-Chien CS. Clinical and histological events preceding hepatitis B e antigen seroconversion in chronic type B hepatitis. *Gastroenterology* 1983;84:216-9.

[19] Liaw YF, Yang SS, Chen TJ, Chu CM. Acute exacerbation in hepatitis B e antigen positive chronic type B hepatitis. A clinicopathological study. *J Hepatol* 1985;1:227-33.

[20] Chu CM, Hung SJ, Lin J, Tai DI, Liaw YF. Natural history of hepatitis B e antigen to antibody seroconversion in patients with normal serum aminotransferase levels. *Am J Med* 2004;116:829-834.

[21] Ishak K, Baptista A, Bianchi L, Callea F, De Groote J, Gudat F, Denk H, Desmet V, Korb G, MacSween RN, et al. Histological grading and staging of chronic hepatitis. *J Hepatol* 1995;22:696-699.

[22] Chu CM. Natural history of chronic hepatitis B virus infection in adults with emphasis on the occurrence of cirrhosis and hepatocellular carcinoma. *J Gastroenterol Hepatol* 2000;15 Suppl:E25-30.

[23] Kao JH, Chen DS. The Natural History of Hepatitis B Virus Infection. In: Lai CL and Locarnini S ed. *Hepatitis B virus*. London: International Medical Press Ltd., 2002;161–172.

[24] Chen YC, Sheen IS, Chu CM, Liaw YF. Prognosis following spontaneous HBsAg seroclearance in chronic hepatitis B patients with or without concurrent infection. *Gastroenterology* 2002;123:1084-1089.

[25] Huo TI, Wu JC, Lee PC, Chau GY, Lui WY, Tsay SH, Ting LT, Chang FY, Lee SD. Sero-clearance of hepatitis B surface antigen in chronic carriers does not necessarily imply a good prognosis. *Hepatology* 1998;28:231-236.

[26] Lok AS, Lai CL, Wu PC, Leung EK, Lam TS. Spontaneous hepatitis B e antigen to antibody seroconversion and reversion in Chinese patients with chronic hepatitis B virus infection. *Gastroenterology* 1987;92:1839-1843.
[27] Lok AS, Liang RH, Chiu EK, Wong KL, Chan TK, Todd D. Reactivation of hepatitis B virus replication in patients receiving cytotoxic therapy: report of a prospective study. *Gastroenterology* 1991;100:182-188.
[28] Hsu YS, Chien RN, Yeh CT, Sheen IS, Chiou HY, Chu CM, Liaw YF. Long-term outcome after spontaneous HBeAg seroconversion in patients with chronic hepatitis B. *Hepatology* 2002;35:1522-1527.
[29] Hadziyannis SJ, Vassilopoulos D. Hepatitis B e antigen-negative chronic hepatitis B. *Hepatology* 2001;34:617-624.
[30] Bonino F, Brunetto MR. Chronic hepatitis B e antigen (HBeAg) negative, anti-HBe positive hepatitis B: an overview. *J Hepatol* 2003;39:S160-163.
[31] Beasley RP, Hwang LY, Lin CC, Chien CS. Hepatocellular carcinoma and hepatitis B virus: a prospective study of 22707 men in Taiwan. *Lancet* 1981;2:1129-1133.
[32] Lok AS. Chronic hepatitis B. *N Engl J Med* 2002;346:1682-1683.
[33] Fattovich G, Stroffolini T, Zagni I, Donato F. Hepatocellular carcinoma in cirrhosis: incidence and risk factors. *Gastroenterology* 2004;127 (Suppl 1):S35-S50.
[34] Kao JH: Hepatitis B virus genotypes and hepatocellular carcinoma in Taiwan. *Intervirology* 2003;46:400-407.
[35] Colombo M. Hepatocellular carcinoma. *J Hepatol* 1992;15: 225–36.
[36] Kao JH, Chen DS. Changing disease burden of hepatocellular carcinoma in the Far East and Southeast Asia. *Liver Int* 2005: 25: 696–703.
[37] Chen DS. From hepatitis to hepatoma: lessons from type B viral hepatitis. *Science* 1993; 262: 369–70.
[38] Kao JH, Chen DS. Overview of hepatitis B and C viruses. In: Goedert JJ, ed. *Infectious Causes of Cancer: Targets for Intervention.* Tottowa: Humana Press Inc., 2000;313–30.
[39] Kao JH, Chen DS. Hepatocellular carcinoma in Taiwan: progress in the past decade 1988–1997. In: Leong ASY, Liew CT, Lau JWY, Johnson PJ, eds. *Hepatocellular Carcinoma: Contemporary Diagnosis, Investigation and Management.* London: Arnold, 1999; 235–50.
[40] Wild CP, Hall AJ. Primary prevention of hepatocellular carcinoma in developing countries. *Mutat Res* 2000; 462:381–93.
[41] Tiollais P, Pourcel C, Dejean A. The hepatitis B virus. *Nature* 1985 16;317:489-95.
[42] Sung JL, Chen DS: Geographical distribution of the subtype of hepatitis B surface antigen in Chinese. *Gastroenterol Jpn* 1977;12:58–63.
[43] Nishioka K, Levin AG, Simons MJ. Hepatitis B antigen, antigen subtypes, and hepatitis B antibody in normal subjects and patients with liver disease. *Bull World Health Organ* 1975;52:293-300.
[44] Kao JH. Hepatitis B viral genotypes: clinical relevance and molecular characteristics. *J Gastroenterol Hepatol* 2002;17:643-650.

[45] Yeh SH, Tsai CY, Kao JH, Liu CJ, Kuo TJ, Lin MW, Huang WL, Lu SF, Jih J, Chen DS, Chen PJ. Quantification and genotyping of hepatitis B virus in a single reaction by real-time PCR and melting curve analysis. *J Hepatol* 2004;41:659-666.

[46] Chen BF, Chen PJ, Jow GM, Sablon E, Liu CJ, Chen DS, Kao JH. High prevalence of mixed genotype infections in hepatitis B virus infected intravenous drug users. *J Med Virol* 2004;74:536-542.

[47] Liu CJ, Kao JH, Chen PJ, Lai MY, Chen DS. Molecular epidemiology of hepatitis B viral serotypes and genotypes in Taiwan. *J Biomed Sci* 2002;9:166-170.

[48] Magnius LO, Norder H. Subtypes, genotypes and molecular epidemiology of the hepatitis B virus as reflected by sequence variability of the S-gene. *Intervirology* 1995; 38:24-34.

[49] Sung JL, Chen DS. Clustering of different subtypes of hepatitis B surface antigen in families of patients with chronic liver diseases. *Am. J. Gastroenterol.* 1978; 69: 559–564.

[50] Lin CL, Kao JH, Chen BF, Chen PJ, Lai MY, Chen DS. Application of hepatitis B virus genotyping and phylogenetic analysis in intrafamilial transmission of hepatitis B virus. *Clin Infect Dis* 2005;41:1576-1581.

[51] Suzuki Y, Kobayashi M, Ikeda K, Suzuki F, Arfase Y, Akuta N, Hosaka T, Saitoh S, Kobayashi M, Someya T, Matsuda M, Sato J, Watabiki S, Miyakawa Y, Kumada H. Persistence of acute infection with hepatitis B virus genotype A and treatment in Japan. *J Med Virol* 2005;76:33-39.

[52] Mayerat C, Mantegani A, Frei PC. Does hepatitis B virus (HBV) genotype influence the clinical outcome of HBV infection? *J Viral Hepat* 1999;6:299–304.

[53] Heijtink RA, Paulij W, van Roosmalen M, Hellings JA, Niesters HG, Schalm SW, Osterhaus AD. Characteristics of the early phase of chronicity in acute hepatitis B infection. *J Med Virol* 1999; 57: 331-336.

[54] Kobayashi M, Suzuki F, Arase Y, Akuta N, Suzuki Y, Hosaka T, Saitoh S, Kobayashi M, Tsubota A, Someya T, Ikeda K, Matsuda M, Sato J, Kumada H. Infection with hepatitis B virus genotype A in Tokyo, Japan during 1976 through 2001. *J Gastroenterol* 2004;39:844-850.

[55] Leblebicioglu H, Eroglu C; Members of the Hepatitis Study Group. Acute hepatitis B virus infection in Turkey: epidemiology and genotype distribution. *Clin Microbiol Infect* 2004;10:537-541.

[56] Chu CJ, Hussain M, Lok AS. Hepatitis B virus genotype B is associated with earlier HBeAg seroconversion compared with hepatitis B virus genotype C. *Gastroenterology* 2002;122:1756–1762.

[57] Kao JH, Chen PJ, Lai MY, Chen DS. Hepatitis B virus genotypes and spontaneous hepatitis B e antigen seroconversion in Taiwanese hepatitis B carriers. *J Med Virol* 2004;72:363-369.

[58] Yuen MF, Fung SK, Tanaka Y, Kato T, Mizokami M, Yuen JC, Wong DK, Yuan HJ, Sum SM, Chan AO, Wong BC, Lai CL. Longitudinal study of hepatitis activity and viral replication before and after HBeAg seroconversion in chronic hepatitis B patients infected with genotypes B and C. *J Clin Microbiol* 2004;42:5036-5040.

[59] Watanabe K, Takahashi T, Takahashi S, Okoshi S, Ichida T, Aoyagi Y. Comparative study of genotype B and C hepatitis B virus-induced chronic hepatitis in relation to the basic core promoter and precore mutations. *J Gastroenterol Hepatol* 2005;20:441-449.
[60] Ni YH, Chang MH, Wang KJ, Hsu HY, Chen HL, Kao JH, Yeh SH, Jeng YM, Tsai KS, Chen DS. Clinical relevance of hepatitis B virus genotype in children with chronic infection and hepatocellular carcinoma. *Gastroenterology* 2004;127:1733-1738.
[61] Chu CM, Liaw YF. Genotype C hepatitis B virus infection is associated with a higher risk of reactivation of hepatitis B and progression to cirrhosis than genotype B: a longitudinal study of hepatitis B e antigen-positive patients with normal aminotransferase levels at baseline. *J Hepatol* 2005;43:411-417.
[62] Kao JH, Chen PJ, Lai MY, Chen DS. Genotypes and clinical phenotypes of hepatitis B virus in patients with chronic hepatitis B virus infection. *J Clin Microbiol* 2002;40:1207-1209.
[63] Chan HL, Wong ML, Hui AY, Hung LC, Chan FK, Sung JJ. Hepatitis B virus genotype C takes a more aggressive disease course than hepatitis B virus genotype B in hepatitis B e antigen-positive patients. *J Clin Microbiol* 2003;41:1277-1279.
[64] Sumi H, Yokosuka O, Seki N, Arai M, Imazeki F, Kurihara T, Kanda T, Fukai K, Kato M, Saisho H. Influence of hepatitis B virus genotypes on the progression of chronic type B liver disease. *Hepatology* 2003;37:19–26.
[65] Sanchez-Tapias JM, Costa J, Mas A, Bruguera M, Rodes J. Influence of hepatitis B virus genotype on the long-term outcome of chronic hepatitis B in western patients. *Gastroenterology* 2002;123:1848–1856.
[66] Kao JH, Chen PJ, Lai MY, Chen DS. Basal core promoter mutations of hepatitis B virus increase the risk of hepatocellular carcinoma in hepatitis B carriers. *Gastroenterology* 2003;124:327-334.
[67] Kao JH, Chen PJ, Lai MY, Chen DS. Hepatitis B genotypes correlate with clinical outcomes in patients with chronic hepatitis B. *Gastroenterology* 2000;118:554-559.
[68] Yuen MF, Tanaka Y, Mizokami M, Yuen JC, Wong DK, Yuan HJ, Sum SM, Chan AO, Wong BC, Lai CL. Role of hepatitis B virus genotypes Ba and C, core promoter and precore mutations on hepatocellular carcinoma: a case control study. *Carcinogenesis* 2004;25:1593-1598.
[69] Chan HL, Hui AY, Wong ML, Tse AM, Hung LC, Wong VW, Sung JJ. Genotype C hepatitis B virus infection is associated with an increased risk of hepatocellular carcinoma. *Gut* 2004;53:1494-1498.
[70] Yu MW, Yeh SH, Chen PJ, Liaw YF, Lin CL, Liu CJ, Shih WL, Kao JH, Chen DS, Chen CJ. Hepatitis B virus genotype and DNA level and hepatocellular carcinoma: a prospective study in men. *J Natl Cancer Inst* 2005; 97: 265–272.
[71] Chen JD, Liu CJ, Lee PH, Chen PJ, Lai MY, Kao JH, Chen DS. Hepatitis B genotypes correlate with tumor recurrence after curative resection of hepatocellular carcinoma. *Clin Gastroenterol Hepatol* 2004;2:64-71.
[72] Lin CL, Chen JD, Liu CJ, Lee PH, Chen PJ, Lai MY, Kao JH, Chen DS. Clinicopathological differences between hepatitis B viral genotype B- and C-related resectable hepatocellular carcinoma. *J Viral Hepat* 2007;14:64-69.

[73] Thakur V, Guptan RC, Kazim SN, Malhotra V, Sarin SK. Profile, spectrum and significance of HBV genotypes in chronic liver disease patients in the Indian subcontinent. *J Gastroenterol Hepatol* 2002;17:165–170.

[74] Sugiyama M, Tanaka Y, Kato T, Orito E, Ito K, Acharya SK, Gish RG, Kramvis A, Shimada T, Izumi N, Kaito M, Miyakawa Y, Mizokami M. Influence of hepatitis B virus genotypes on the intra- and extracellular expression of viral DNA and antigens. *Hepatology* 2006;44:915-924.

[75] Liaw YF, Leung N, Guan R, Lau GK, Merican I; Asian-Pacific Consensus Working Parties on Hepatitis B. Asian-Pacific consensus statement on the management of chronic hepatitis B: an update. *J Gastroenterol Hepatol* 2003;18:239–245.

[76] Lok AS, McMahon BJ. Chronic hepatitis B: update of recommendations. *Hepatology* 2004;39:857-61.

[77] EASL International Consensus Conference on Hepatitis B: 13-14 September, 2002 Geneva, Switzerland: consensus statement (long version). *J Hepatol* 2003;39(Suppl1):S3-S25.

[78] Idenix Pharmaceuticals. Tyzeka (telbivudine) Approved by U.S. Food and Drug Administration (FDA) as a New Treatment for Patients with Chronic hepatitis B. *Press Release*. October 26, 2006.

[79] Liu CJ, Kao JH, Chen DS. Therapeutic implications of hepatitis B virus genotypes. *Liver Int* 2005;25:1097-1107.

[80] Kao JH, Wu NH, Chen PJ, Lai MY, Chen DS. Hepatitis B genotypes and the response to interferon therapy. *J Hepatol* 2000;33:998–1002.

[81] Wai CT, Chu CJ, Hussain M, Lok AS. HBV genotype B is associated with better response to interferon therapy in HBeAg(+) chronic hepatitis than genotype C. *Hepatology* 2002;36:1425–1430.

[82] Hou J, Schilling R, Janssen HLA. Molecular characteristics of hepatitis B virus genotype A confer a higher response to interferon treatment. *J Hepatol* 2001;34(Suppl 1):15.

[83] Erhardt A, Blondin D, Hauck K, Sagir A, Kohnle T, Heintges T, Haussinger D. Response to interferon alfa is hepatitis B virus genotype dependent: genotype A is more sensitive to interferon than genotype D. *Gut* 2005;54:1009-1013.

[84] Cooksley WG, Piratvisuth T, Lee SD, Mahachai V, Chao YC, Tanwandee T, Chutaputti A, Chang WY, Zahm FE, Pluck N. Peginterferon alpha-2a (40 kDa): an advance in the treatment of hepatitis B e antigen-positive chronic hepatitis B. *J Viral Hepat* 2003;10:298-305.

[85] Janssen HL, van Zonneveld M, Senturk H, Zeuzem S, Akarca US, Cakaloglu Y, Simon C, So TM, Gerken G, de Man RA, Niesters HG, Zondervan P, Hansen B, Schalm SW; HBV 99-01 Study Group; Rotterdam Foundation for Liver Research. Pegylated interferon alfa-2b alone or in combination with lamivudine for HBeAg-positive chronic hepatitis B: a randomised trial. *Lancet* 2005;365:123-129.

[86] Hadziyannis S, Lau GKK, Marcellin P, Piratvisuth T, Cooksley G, Bonino F, et al. Sustained HBsAg seroconversion in patients with chronic hepatitis B treated with peginterferon alfa-2a (40KD) (Pegasys). *J Hepatol* 2005;42(suppl 2):17

[87] Chien RN, Yeh CT, Tsai SL, Chu CM, Liaw YF. Determinants for sustained HBeAg response to lamivudine therapy. *Hepatology* 2003;38:1267–1273.

[88] Yuen MF, Wong DK, Sablon E, Yuan HJ, Sum SM, Hui CK, Chan AO, Wang BC, Lai CL. Hepatitis B virus genotypes B and C do not affect the antiviral response to lamivudine. *Antiviral Therapy* 2003;8:531–534.

[89] Chan HL, Wong ML, Hui AY, Chim AM, Tse AM, Hung LC, Chan FK, Sung JJ. Hepatitis B virus genotype has no impact on hepatitis B e antigen seroconversion after lamivudine treatment. *World J Gastroenterol* 2003;9:2695-2697.

[90] Kao JH, Liu CJ, Chen DS. Hepatitis B viral genotypes and lamivudine resistance. *J Hepatol* 2002;36:303–304.

[91] Buti M, Cotrina M, Valdes A, Jardi R, Rodriguez-Frias F, Esteban R. Is hepatitis B virus subtype testing useful in predicting virological response and resistance to lamivudine? *J Hepatol* 2002;36:445-446.

[92] Westland C, Delaney W 4th, Yang H, Chen SS, Marcellin P, Hadziyannis S, Gish R, Fry J, Brosgart C, Gibbs C, Miller M, Xiong S. Hepatitis B virus genotypes and virologic response in 694 patients in phase III studies of adefovir dipivoxil. *Gastroenterology* 2003;125:107–116.

[93] Lurie Y, Manns MP, Gish RG, Chang TT, Yurdaydin C, Lai CL, et al. The efficacy of entecavir is similar regardless of disease-related baseline subgroups in treatment of nucleoside-naive, HBeAg(+) and HBeAg(-) patients wth chronic hepatitis B. *J Hepatol* 2005;42(suppl 2):184.

[94] Rajendra A, Shah BB, Wong J. Impact of Hepatitis B Genotype on Treatment Response: A Meta-Analysis of Controlled and Uncontrolled Trials. *57th AASLD*. 2006. Abstract 987.

[95] Keeffe EB, Dieterich DT, Han SH, Jacobson IM, Martin P, Schiff ER, Tobias H, Wright TL. A treatment algorithm for the management of chronic hepatitis B virus infection in the United States: an update. *Clin Gastroenterol Hepatol.* 2006;4:936-962.

[96] Carman WF, Jacyna MR, Hadziyannis S, Karayiannis P, McGarvey MJ, Makris A, Thomas HC. Mutation preventing formation of hepatitis B e antigen in patients with chronic hepatitis B infection. *Lancet* 1989; 2: 588-591.

[97] Okamoto H, Yotsumoto S, Akahane Y, Yamanaka T, Miyazaki Y, Sugai Y, Tsuda F, Tanaka T, Miyakawa Y, Mayumi M. Hepatitis B viruses with precore region defects prevail in persistently infected hosts along with seroconversion to the antibody against e antigen. *J Virol* 1990; 64: 1298-1303.

[98] Okamoto H, Tsuda F, Akahane Y, Sugai Y, Yoshiba M, Moriyama K, Tanaka T, Miyakawa Y, Mayumi M. Hepatitis B virus with mutations in the core promoter for an e antigen-negative phenotype in carriers with antibody to e antigen. *J Virol* 1994; 68: 8102-8110.

[99] Lin CL, Liao LY, Wang CS, Chen PJ, Lai MY, Chen DS, Kao JH. Basal core-promoter mutant of hepatitis B virus and progression of liver disease in hepatitis B e antigen-negative chronic hepatitis B. *Liver Int* 2005;25:564-570.

[100] Liu CJ, Chen BF, Chen PJ, Lai MY, Huang WL, Kao JH, Chen DS. Role of hepatitis B viral load and basal core promoter mutation in hepatocellular carcinoma in hepatitis B carriers. *J Infect Dis* 2006;193:1258-1265.

[101] Liu CJ, Chen BF, Chen PJ, Lai MY, Huang WL, Kao JH, Chen DS. Role of hepatitis B virus precore/core promoter mutations and serum viral load on noncirrhotic hepatocellular carcinoma: a case-control study. *J Infect Dis* 2006;194:594-599.

[102] Chen BF, Liu CJ, Jow GM, Chen PJ, Kao JH, Chen DS. High prevalence and mapping of pre-S deletion in hepatitis B virus carriers with progressive liver diseases. *Gastroenterology* 2006;130:1153-1168.

[103] Kuang SY, Jackson PE, Wang JB, Lu PX, Munoz A, Qian GS, Kensler TW, Groopman JD. Specific mutations of hepatitis B virus in plasma predict liver cancer development. *Proc Natl Acad Sci U S A* 2004 9;101:3575-80.

[104] Tong MJ, Blatt LM, Kao JH, Cheng JT, Corey WG. Precore/basal core promoter mutants and hepatitis B viral DNA levels as predictors for liver deaths and hepatocellular carcinoma. *World J Gastroenterol* 2006;12:6620-6626.

[105] Gerken G, Kremsdorf D, Capel F, Petit MA, Dauguet C, Manns MP, Meyer zum Buschenfelde KH, Brechot C. Hepatitis B defective virus with rearrangements in the preS gene during chronic HBV infection. *Virology* 1991;183:555-565.

[106] Fernholz D, Stemler M, Brunetto M, Bonino F, Will H. Replicating and virion secreting hepatitis B mutant virus unable to produce preS2 protein. *J Hepatol* 1991;13:S102-S104.

[107] Xu Z, Yen TSB. Intracellular retension of surface protein by a hepatitis B virus mutant that releases virion particles. *J. Virol.* 1996;70:133-140.

[108] Fan YF, Lu CC, Chen WC, Yao WJ, Wang HC, Chang TT, Lei HY, Shiau AL, Su IJ. Prevalence and significance of hepatitis B virus (HBV) pre-S mutants in serum and liver at different replicative stages of chronic HBV infection. *Hepatology* 2001;33:277-286.

[109] Sugauchi F, Ohno T, Orito E, Sakugawa H, Ichida T, Komatsu M, Kuramitsu T, Ueda R, Miyakawa Y, Mizokami M. Influence of hepatitis B virus genotypes on the development of preS deletions and advanced liver disease. *J Med Virol* 2003;70:537-544.

[110] Lin CL, Liu CH, Chen Wendy, Huang WL, Chen PJ, Lai MY, Chen DS, Kao JH. Association of pre-S deletion mutant of hepatitis B virus with risk of hepatocellular carcinoma. *J Gastroenterol Hepatol* Published article online: 18-Jul-2006.

[111] Chan HL, Wong ML, Hui AY, Hung LC, Chan FK, Sung JJ. Use of hepatitis B virus DNA quantitation to predict hepatitis B e antigen reversion in cases of chronic hepatitis B. *J Clin Microbiol* 2003;41:4793-4795.

[112] Chu, CJ, Hussain M, Lok ASF. Quantitative serum HBV DNA levels during different stages of chronic hepatitis B infection. *Hepatology* 2002;36:1408–1415.

[113] Manesis EL, G. V. Papatheodoridis, and S. J. Hadziyannis. Serum HBV-DNA levels in inactive hepatitis B virus carriers. *Gastroenterology* 2002;122:2092–2093.

[114] Martinot-Peignoux, M., N. Boyer, M. Colombat, R. Akremi, B. N. Pham, S. Ollivier, C. Castelnau, D. Valla, C. Degott, and P. Marcellin. Serum hepatitis B virus DNA levels and liver histology in inactive HBsAg carriers. *J Hepatol* 2002;36:543–546.

[115] Iloeje UH, Yang HI, Su J, Jen CL, You SL, Chen CJ. Predicting liver cirrhosis risk based on the level of circulating hepatitis B viral load. *Gastroenterology* 2006; 130: 678–686.

[116] Chen CJ, Yang HI, Su J, Jen CL, You SL, Lu SN, Huang GT, et al. Risk of hepatocellular carcinoma across a biological gradient of serum hepatitis B virus DNA level. *JAMA* 2006;295:65-73.

[117] Tang B, Kruger WD, Chen G, Shen F, Lin WY, Mboup S, London WT, Evans AA. Hepatitis B viremia is associated with increased risk of hepatocellular carcinoma in chronic carriers. *J Med Virol* 2004; 72: 35-40.

[118] Chen G, Lin W, Shen F, Iloeje UH, London WT, Evans AA. Past HBV viral load as predictor of mortality and morbidity from HCC and chronic liver disease in a prospective study. *Am J Gastroenterol* 2006;101:1797-803.

[119] Tsai FC, Liu CJ, Chen CL, Chen PJ, Lai MY, Kao JH, Chen DS. Lower serum viral loads in young patients with hepatitis-B-virus-related hepatocellular carcinoma. *J Viral Hepat* 2007;14:153-160.

[120] Papatheodoridis GV, Hadziyannis SJ. Diagnosis and management of precore mutant chronic hepatitis B. *J Viral Hep* 2001;8:311-321.

[121] Kim HC, Nam CM, Jee SH, Han KH, Oh DK, Suh I. Normal serum aminotransferase concentration and risk of mortality from liver diseases: prospective cohort study. *BMJ* 2004;328:983-988.

[122] Yuen MF, Yuan HJ, Wong DK, Yuen JC, Wong WM, Chan AO, Wong BC, Lai KC, Lai CL. Prognostic determinants for chronic hepatitis B in Asians: therapeutic implications. *Gut* 2005;54:1610-1614.

[123] Lin CL, Liao LY, Liu CJ, Yu MW, Chen PJ, Lai MY, Chen DS, Kao JH. Hepatitis B viral factors in HBeAg-negative carriers with persistently normal serum alanine aminotransferase levels. *Hepatology* 2007;45:1193-1198.

[124] Ikeda K, Arase Y, Saitoh S, Kobayashi M, Someya T, Hosaka T, Sezaki H, Akuta N, Suzuki Y, Suzuki F, Kumada H. Long-term outcome of HBV carriers with negative HBe antigen and normal aminotransferase. *Am J Med* 2006;119:977-985.

[125] Chan HL, Tsang SW, Liew CT, Tse CH, Wong ML, Ching JY, Leung NW, Tam JS, Sung JJ. Viral genotype and hepatitis B virus DNA levels are correlated with histologic liver damage in HBeAg-negative chronic hepatitis B virus infection. *Am J Gastroenterol* 2002;97:406-412.

[126] Sung JJ, Chan HL, Wong ML, Tse CH, Yuen SC, Tam JS, Leung NW. Relationship of clinical and virological factors with hepatitis activity in hepatitis B e antigen-negative chronic hepatitis B virus-infected patients. *J Viral Hepat* 2002;9:229-234.

[127] Prati D, Taioli E, Zanella A, Della Torre E, Butelli S, Del Vecchio E, Vianello L, Zanuso F, Mozzi F, Milani S, Conte D, Colombo M, Sirchia G. Updated definitions of healthy ranges for serum alanine aminotransferase levels. *Ann Intern Med* 2002;137:1-10.

[128] Kidd AH, Kidd-Ljunggren K. A revised secondary structure model for the 3-end of hepatitis B virus pregenomic RNA. *Nucleic Acids Res* 1996; 24:3295–3301.

[129] Li J, Buckwold VE, Hon MW, Ou JH. Mechanism of suppression of hepatitis B virus precore RNA transcription by a frequent double mutation. *J Virol* 1999;73:1239-1244.

In: Hepatitis B Research Advances
Editor: Alicia P. Willis, pp. 171-184

ISBN: 978-1-60021-666-4

Chapter X

SURVEILLANCE AND PREVENTION OF HEPATOCELLULAR CARCINOMA IN CHRONIC HEPATITIS B

Vincent Wai-Sun Wong and Henry Lik-Yuen Chan *
Department of Medicine and Therapeutics and Institute of Digestive Disease,
The Chinese University of Hong Kong, Hong Kong SAR, China

ABSTRACT

Chronic hepatitis B virus infection is the most important cause of hepatocellular carcinoma (HCC) in Asia. Regular surveillance of HCC by ultrasound and alfa-fetoprotein can detect early HCC that may be amendable to surgical resection. However, there is still much controversy on the survival benefit and cost-effectiveness of HCC surveillance programs. Lead-time bias and length-time bias impose major difficulties in the interpretation of clinical studies. The high false positive rate of alfa-fetoprotein and large demand for ultrasound examination limit the cost-effectiveness of surveillance programs. Risk stratification of patients may direct the resource allocation in the public health perspective. On top of the clinical factors of HCC, viral factors including HBV genotypes, basal core promoter mutations and viral load are emerging as hot research areas. Chemoprevention of HCC by treatment of HBV has shown preliminary success. Incidence of HCC is reduced among responders to conventional interferon-alfa treatment on long-term follow-up. Peginterferon can potentially improve the virological response and may offer a better hope for HCC prevention. Virological suppression by nucleotide analogues particularly among cirrhotic patients can also reduce of risk of HCC.

* Correspondence concerning this article should be addressed to Henry L.Y. Chan, M.D., Department of Medicine and Therapeutics, 9/F Prince of Wales Hospital, 30-32 Ngan Shing Street, Shatin, Hong Kong SAR, China. Phone: 852-26323140; Fax: 852-26373852; E-mail: hlychan@cuhk.edu.hk.

INTRODUCTION

Hepatocellular carcinoma (HCC) is the fifth most common cancer in the world. Since most patients present late and have poor liver function, the incidence of HCC is almost equal to the rate of HCC-related mortality. Worldwide, it is the third most common cause of cancer-related death (Parkin et al., 2001). The incidence of HCC is also rising rapidly in Western countries. From 1970s to 1990s, the mortality rate due to HCC rose by 41% in the United States (El Serag et al., 1999). Chronic hepatitis B is the most important cause of HCC worldwide, especially in Asian countries. An estimated 400 million people are chronically infected by hepatitis B virus (HBV) (Lee WM, 1997). More than a quarter of these chronic hepatitis B patients will die from liver-related diseases (Beasley, 1988). Unlike other chronic liver diseases such as chronic hepatitis C and alcoholic liver disease, in which HCC almost never develops before cirrhosis occurs, HBV itself is carcinogenic and may induce HCC in a non-cirrhotic liver. In this chapter, the epidemiology, the rationale and controversies of surveillance, the risk factors and the prevention of HBV-related HCC will be discussed.

EPIDEMIOLOGY OF HCC IN CHRONIC HEPATITIS B

In countries endemic with HBV, the incidence of HCC exceeds 30 per 100,000 population per year. Overall, the adjusted relative risk of HCC in patients with chronic hepatitis B is 60 in hepatitis B e-antigen (HBeAg)-positive cases and 10 in HBeAg-negative cases, as compared to people without HBV infection (Yang et al., 2002). When only people with chronic hepatitis B are considered, the incidence of HCC is even higher. In a recent cohort of 1018 chronic hepatitis B patients followed up for a median of 4.1 years in Hong Kong, 56 developed HCC. In patients who underwent intensive 3-monthly surveillance after a single abnormal screening results, the annual incidence of HCC was as high as 760 per 100,000 (Mok et al., 2005). The incidence rate was similar to a Taiwan study conducted around 20 years ago. In 432 Taiwan patients with chronic hepatitis B, HCC developed in 8 during a median follow-up of 23 months. The annual incidence of HCC in this study was 826 per 100,000, or 2768 per 100,000 for those over age 35 years (Liaw et al, 1986).

In Asia, most cases of HBV infection are due to maternal transmission or infection during early childhood. Since neonates and children below 1 year of age have immature immune system and tend to be immunotolerant to foreign antigens already present at birth, the risk of HBV infection becoming chronic is as high as 90% (Hyams, 1995). By contrast, the risk of acute HBV infection becoming chronic is less than 5% in adolescents and adults. This accounts for the high burden of chronic hepatitis B patients in Asia. In patients with chronic hepatitis B, the annual incidence of cirrhosis is 2.4% in HBeAg-positive cases and 1.3% in HBeAg-negative cases (Liaw et al., 1988).

Because of the differences between Asian and Western countries regarding the age of HBV infection, the epidemiology of HCC also differs. This has important bearing on the decision on HCC surveillance. In Montreal, no HCC was detected in 317 asymptomatic chronic hepatitis B patients after 16 years of follow-up (Villeneuve et al., 1994). By contrast, the annual incidence of HCC was 387 per 100,000 in men and 63 per 100,000 in women in

Alaska, an American state that was also affected by HBV endemic and maternal transmission (McMahon et al., 1990). The similar incidence of HCC in Alaska and Asia argues strongly that the age of infection is much more important than the genetic background in determining the risk of HCC.

CONTROVERSY IN SURVEILLANCE OF HCC

Strategy: Ultrasonography and Alpha-Fetoprotein

Screening is defined as a one-time application of a test to detect a disease at a stage when intervention may improve the outcome. Surveillance is the repeated application of such a test over time. Since HCC is such a deadly disease, it has been a routine practice to survey for HCC in patients with chronic liver disease in many parts of the world despite the lack of supportive evidence for this practice. It is important to note that the performance of an investigation as a diagnostic test differs from its performance as a surveillance test, and one should take this into consideration when reading literature on various surveillance tools.

Currently, ultrasonography and serum alpha-fetoprotein measurement are the most frequently used surveillance tools for HCC. Although computed tomography and magnetic resonant imaging are more sensitive in diagnosing HCC, their greater cost, repeated exposure to radiation and the use of contrast material make it impractical to use them as first-line surveillance tests at present.

Ultrasonography was evaluated both in cirrhotic and non-cirrhotic patients with chronic hepatitis B (Paterson et al., 1994; Sherman et al., 1995). Overall, the sensitivity is around 75% and specificity is 90%. The positive predictive value is 73% in cirrhotic patients and 14% in non-cirrhotic patients because of the difference in subgroup disease prevalence. Ultrasonography is non-invasive and carries no adverse effect. However, it is operator dependent and may be hampered by difficult anatomy such as high-riding liver. It is often difficult to differentiate HCC from regenerative nodules in a cirrhotic background.

The performance of alpha-fetoprotein is inferior. At a cutoff of 20 mg/l, alpha-fetoprotein has a sensitivity of only 39% in detecting HCC (Oka et al., 1994). This cutoff value is also associated with many false positives. Alpha-fetoprotein frequently increases above the normal range during flare of hepatitis (Bisceglie and Hoofnagle, 1989). However, if the cutoff is set higher at 100 mg/l, the sensitivity would drop markedly to 13%. Moreover, in a study involving 9373 Chinese patients with chronic hepatitis B, most (84%) of the HCC were detected by ultrasonography alone (Zhang and Yang, 1999). The addition of alpha-fetoprotein to the surveillance program only marginally increased the detection rate of HCC, but increased the false positivity rate from 2.9% to 7.5%. These data cast doubt on the role of alpha-fetoprotein.

In most surveillance programs, ultrasonography and/or alpha-fetoprotein are performed at 3 to 12 month intervals. The screening intervals are somewhat arbitrary, and there is no study showing that a shorter surveillance interval improves cancer-related mortality. According to studies in China, the doubling time of HCC was estimated to be 117 days, and the fastest growing tumor expanded from 1 cm to 3 cm in 5 months (Sheu et al., 1985). Therefore, 6-monthly surveillance seems to be reasonable.

Survival Benefit

Since the currently available surveillance tools are far from perfect and many detected HCC cannot be cured, surveillance programs can only be justified if they improve the prognosis of patients. Currently, there have been two big randomized controlled studies on HCC surveillance (Chen et al., 2003; Zhang et al., 2004). Both were conducted in China and used 6-monthly ultrasonography plus alpha-fetoprotein as surveillance tests. The first study was conducted in Jiangsu province and included 5581 HBsAg positive individuals (Chen et al., 2003). After a mean follow-up of 62 months, 374 HCC were found. Patients in the surveillance group were more likely to have early stage cancer. Thirty percent of patients in the surveillance group, compared to 6% of those in the control group, had stage I HCC. Nevertheless, over 85% of HCC patients in either group died during follow-up, and the study failed to show a survival benefit. In the second study conducted in urban Shanghai, 18,816 people were randomized to have surveillance or no surveillance for around 5 years (Zhang et al., 2004). The inclusion criteria were less stringent. The authors allowed inclusion of patients with a history of 'chronic hepatitis' only. Similar to the Jiangsu study, 61% of patients in the surveillance group and no patient in the control group had stage I HCC. Forty-seven percent of the HCC cases in the surveillance group and 8% of those in the control group could undergo liver resection. More importantly, the HCC patients in the surveillance group enjoyed a 5-year survival rate of 46%, compared to 0% in the control group. The reason why the findings of these two studies differ is not clear. However, both studies have been criticized for non-adherence to group assignment and high dropout rate. The high mortality rate even for stage I cancer in the Jiangsu study probably reflects the lack of effective treatment for early HCC in the province.

Observational studies also consistently show that people under surveillance programs have HCC detected at an earlier stage. Among 1018 HBV carriers in Hong Kong, an intensive surveillance program allowed the detection of early HCC with a mean diameter of 3 cm (Mok et al., 2005). In this intensive surveillance program, patients underwent 6-monthly ultrasonography and alpha-fetoprotein testing. Whenever an abnormal result was found, a lipiodol computed tomography was performed. After the exclusion of HCC, patients continued 3-monthly ultrasonography and alpha-fetoprotein surveillance. Thirty-six percent of the HCC patients in this study had liver resection and another 30% underwent local ablative therapy.

Observational studies are limited by lead time bias and length bias. Lead time bias is the detection of cancer at an earlier time without altering the natural history. Just because the cancer is detected earlier, the time from diagnosis to death would seem to be longer even if no effective treatment exists. Length bias is the preferential detection of slow-growing tumors by the surveillance program. Fast-growing tumors, on the other hand, tend to produce symptoms in between surveillance sessions, and may not be considered as tumors identified by surveillance. Both types of bias increase the apparent survival benefit of surveillance programs. These biases can only be eliminated by conducting properly-designed randomized controlled trial with sufficient length of follow-up. Few observational studies tried to adjust for these biases.

To Improve Cost-Effectiveness: Risk Stratification and Prevention

Taking chronic hepatitis B population as a whole, HCC surveillance is not cost-effective. Based on a decision analysis model, Sarasin and coworkers estimated that the cost-effectiveness ratios of surveillance ranged between USD 48,000 and USD 284,000 for each additional life-year gained (Sarasin et al., 1996). To lower the cost-effectiveness ratios to an acceptable level of USD 26,000 to USD 55,000 per life-year gained, the patients should have a predicted cirrhosis-related 5-year survival rate above 80% before HCC detection and a predicted 3-year survival rate 40% to 60% after curative surgery. In another cohort of Italian patients with liver cirrhosis (Child's B and C included), the cost per treatable HCC detected by surveillance program was USD 17,934, while the cost for each life-year gained was USD 112,993 (Bolondi et al., 1991). These figures were relatively high compared to other cancer surveillance programs.

To keep the HCC surveillance program reasonably cost-effective, vigilant risk stratification is needed. On the one hand, one should choose patients with higher risk of developing HCC. Including many patients with low risk of developing HCC not only drains resource to unnecessary surveillance tests but also increases the demand for further confirmatory tests due to false positive results. On the other hand, one should not include patients with poor premorbid state and little liver reserve into surveillance programs. These patients will unlikely tolerate liver resection or other curative procedures, and the clinical course will be dominated by liver failure and cirrhotic complications. In such cases, the detection of HCC may increase the patient's anxiety without altering the outcome. The only exception when patients with severe liver cirrhosis may benefit from HCC surveillance is in countries where liver transplantation is an accepted and readily available option for the treatment of early HCC.

Risk Factors of HCC

Clinical Factors

Older age and male gender are well established factors associated with increased risk of HCC. However, liver cirrhosis remains the most important risk factor of HCC. Over 90% of chronic HBV related HCC had histologic or clinical evidence of liver cirrhosis (Chan et al., 2004). The annual incidence of HCC increases from approximately zero percent in inactive HBV carriers (Villeneuve et al., 1994; De Francis et al., 1993), to approximately 1% among patients with chronic hepatitis (Liaw et al., 1986; Ideda et al., 1998) and 2-7% among patients with liver cirrhosis (Fattovich et al., 2000; Tsai et al., 1997). Liver cirrhosis is usually preceded by repeated cycles of necro-inflammation, degeneration and regeneration and increased hepatocyte turnover, which may facilitate spontaneous genomic mutation and hinder DNA repair. The release of reactive oxygen species on inflammation and distortion of liver architecture by hepatic fibrosis will also cause lost of control on cell growth, apoptosis and senescence. All these hepatic damages may explain the pathogenic mechanism of HCC development in a cirrhotic liver.

Viral Factors

HBV Genotype

Based on an inter-group divergence of 8 percent or more in the complete nucleotide sequence, HBV can be divided into 8 different genotypes (designated as A-H) (Norder et al., 1994; Stuyver et al., 2000). The prevalence of different HBV genotypes is strongly related to the geographical location and patient ethnicity (Lindh et al., 1997). Genotype A HBV is usually found in North America and Western Europe. Genotypes B and C are the predominant HBV genotypes in Asia. Genotype D is usually found in the Mediterranean area. Other HBV genotypes are less commonly found. The strongest evidence on the association between HBV genotypes and liver disease comes from Asian studies. Patients infected by genotype C HBV generally have more active liver inflammation and delayed HBeAg seroconversion as compared to those infected by genotype B HBV (Chan et al., 2003a; Chu et al., 2002). This finding is in line with the more severe necro-inflammation and advanced liver fibrosis on histology associated with genotype C HBV (Sumi et al., 2003; Chan et al., 2002). Higher prevalence of liver cirrhosis is also found among patients infected with genotype C HBV versus those infected with genotype B HBV (Kao et al., 2000). In all, the more active liver disease and advanced liver damage has laid the possible pathogenic mechanism for a higher risk of HCC among patients infected with genotype C HBV. However, conflicting results are yielded from various studies on the relationship between HBV genotypes and HCC. The first report comes from a case-control study in Taiwan that suggests genotype B HBV is associated with HCC among younger patients whereas genotype C HBV is associated with HCC in older patients (Kao et al., 2000). The higher risk of HCC among genotype C infected patients is supported by cross-sectional controlled studies in Japan and Taiwan as well as a prospective longitudinal study in Hong Kong (Kao et al., 2003; Yu et al., 2005; Fujie et al., 2001; Chan et al., 2004). However, there are reports from other cohort studies in which no relationship between HBV genotype and HCC can be demonstrated (Sumi et 2003; Yuen et al., 2003). There is not much data on the association of HBV genotypes A and D with HCC. The HCC risk of genotype B and C HBV as compared to other HBV genotypes is also rarely reported.

Subgroups of HBV can be classified within a specific HBV genotype based on a more than 4% but less than 8% difference in entire nucleotide sequence. Two subgroups have been identified in HBV genotype A: Ae, which is prevalent in Europe, and Aa, which is prevalent in African and Asian countries (Sugauchi et al., 2004). Higher prevalence of HBeAg and higher HBV DNA levels have been demonstrated among patients infected by HBV subgenotype Ae than those infected by HBV subgenotype Aa, but the relationship between genotype A HBV subgroups and HCC is not well studied (Tanaka et al., 2004). Two subgenotypes B HBV have been described; one almost exclusively found in Japan (Bj) and the other in the rest of Asia (Ba) (Sugauchi et al., 2003). Subgenotype Ba is associated with higher prevalence of HBeAg and basal core promoter mutations (A to T change at nucleotide 1762 and G to A change at nucleotide 1764) than subgenotype Bj. However, there is no difference in the prevalence of HCC between patients infected by HBV genotypes Ba and Bj (Kobayashi et al., 2005). Two major subgroups of genotype C HBV are Cs, which is predominant in Southeast Asian countries and Southern China, and Ce, which is predominant in the East Asia and Northern part of China (Chan et al., 2005a). One HBV strain with T at nucleotide 1858 (i.e. TCC at codon 15 of the precore region), which belongs to subgroup Cs, is associated with more aggressive liver disease but its relationship with HCC warrants further investigation (Chan et al., 2006).

HBV Mutations

Basal core promoter mutations have been reported to associate with higher risk of HCC in both black Africans and Asians (Baptistia et al. 1999; Kao et al., 2003; Kuang et al., 2004). The higher prevalence of basal core promoter mutation among patients infected by genotype C HBV may account for the higher risk of HCC among these patients (Kao et al., 2003; Chan et al., 2004). Basal core promoter mutations are translated to amino acid mutations K130M and V131I at the HBx region. These mutations increase the replication of HBV and downregulate the production of hepatitis B e antigen (HBeAg) in experimental models (Buckwold et al., 1996; Scaglioni et al., 1997). However, in the clinical setting, no increase in HBV DNA or biochemical activity can be demonstrated among patients infected by HBV harboring these mutations (Chan et al., 2000; Chan et al., 2002; Sung et al., 2002). In a study using laser capture microdissection of hepatocytes from patients with HBV-related HCC, no difference in the mutation profile at the basal core promoter region between tumor and non-tumor cells can be observed (Iavarone et al., 2003). As basal core promoter mutations are also commonly found among chronic hepatitis B patients without HCC, the use of these mutations as a marker for HCC surveillance may not be cost-effective (Chan et al., 2000).

Viral Load

In a large-scaled, longitudinal Taiwanese study, chronic hepatitis B patients who have positive HBeAg were found to have higher incidence of hepatocellular carcinoma as compared to those who have negative HBeAg and non-HBV infected controls over a follow-up of 10 years (Yang et al., 2002). This is probably related to the higher HBV DNA levels associated with HBeAg-positive patients. Patients who have persistently elevated HBV DNA have a higher risk of HCC regardless of the HBeAg status and the ALT level (Chen et al., 2006). Several long-term follow-up studies have also demonstrated that active liver disease and fluctuating HBeAg status after HBeAg seroconversion is associated with higher risk of HCC (Hsu et al., 2002; Di Marco et al., 1999; McMahon et al., 2001). Among HBeAg-negative patients, HBV DNA levels higher than 10,000 copies/ml is associated with active liver disease (Chan et al., 2003b; Manesis et al., 2002; Martinot-Peignoux et al., 2002). In a case-control study, HBV DNA higher than 10,000 copies/ml and genotype C HBV are the two independent risk factors associated with HCC among Taiwanese men (Yu et al., 2005).

Prevention of HCC

Prevention is better than cure. This is particularly important for a disease like HCC, where curative therapy is not efficacious or feasible in most of the cases. For HCC related to chronic hepatitis B, there are two strategies for cancer prevention. First, the general population can be prevented from getting HBV infection by universal vaccination program. Second, therapies to suppress the virus may reduce liver inflammation and thus damage. Sustained suppression of viral replication and reduction of HBV DNA is a reasonable strategy given the importance of viral load in hepatocarcinogenesis. The ultimate goals are to reduce liver-related complications and HCC.

Vaccination

The ultimate goal in the management of HBV is to eliminate the virus by universal vaccination. Nowadays, HBV vaccination is included in the neonatal vaccination programs in many countries. HBV vaccine is highly effective, and the long-term efficacy beyond 15 years has been demonstrated in areas with high endemicity (Lin et al., 2003; McMahon et al., 2005) and low endemicity (Boxall et al., 2004; Zanetti et al., 2005). In cases whose anti-hepatitis B surface antibody drop below 10 mIU/ml, persistence of immunological memory can still be detected in peripheral blood lymphocytes (Banatvala et al., 2000). The minimal cases of acute hepatitis B among vaccine recipients in long-term follow-up support the effectiveness of immunological memory (Ni et al., 2001).

Taiwan is one of the earliest areas to implement HBV vaccination programs. The HCC incidence decreased dramatically after HBV vaccine was available in 1984 (Chang, et al., 1997). Between 1981 and 1986, the average annual incidence of HCC in children 6 to 14 years of age was 0.7 per 100,000. Between 1990 and 1994, the average annual incidence dropped to 0.36 per 100,000. This was paralleled with a decline in HCC-related mortality.

Interferon

Interferon-alfa works by stimulating the host immune response against HBV and its direct antiviral effect. In a meta-analysis summarizing the data of 15 randomized controlled trials and 837 HBeAg-positive patients, patients receiving interferon-alfa had HBeAg seroconversion rate of 37%, compared to 17% in those receiving placebo (Wong et al., 1993). In 103 German patients treated with interferon-alfa and followed for 50 months, those with HBeAg seroconversion had significantly higher long-term survival (Niederau et al., 1996). In another study of 165 HBeAg positive chronic hepatitis B patients in a single institution in the Netherlands treated with interferon-alfa, 8 HCCs were found at a median follow-up of 8.8 years (Van Zonnevel et al., 2004). Six HCCs occurred in non-responders to interferon, one in relapser and one in a responder. The relative risk of developing HCC was 0.084 (95% confidence interval 0.09-0.75).

By the addition of polyethylene glycol to interferon-alfa, peginterferon-alfa has a longer half-life than convention interferon-alpha. A small-scaled study has suggested that peginterferon may be more effective than conventional interferon to induce HBeAg seroconversion, but more data is needed to confirm the superiority of peginterferon (Cooksley et al., 2003). The sustained virologic response, defined as HBeAg seroconversion and reduction of HBV DNA to below 5 log copies, 6 months after cessation of peginterferon occurred in 27% to 36% of the recipients (Chan et al., 2005b; Janssen et al., 2005; Lau et al., 2005). Peginterferon is also effective in reducing covalently closed circular DNA inside the hepatocytes (Sung et al., 2005). And patients who can achieve virological response at 6-month post-treatment tend to remain in remission in the long-term (Chan et al., 2005c). Similar benefit in terms of reduction in HCC as in the case of conventional interferon should be expected among sustained responders to peginterferon.

Nucleotide Analogs

As chronic hepatitis B is a chronic infection with complications often arising years to decades after the initial clinic visit, most treatment trials used surrogate markers such as normalization of alanine aminotransferase, HBeAg seroconversion, HBV DNA reduction and histologic improvement as endpoints. It is uncertain whether these are good surrogate markers for hard clinical endpoints like HCC and liver-related mortality. Currently, the only available evidence that nucleotide analogs prevent HCC is from a randomized controlled trial using lamivudine in chronic hepatitis B with severe fibrosis or early cirrhosis (Liaw et al., 2004). Over a median of 32 months, 436 patients received lamivudine and 215 received placebo. Child-Pugh score increased in 3.4% and 8.8% of patients receiving lamivudine and placebo, respectively. HCC occurred in 3.9% and 7.4% (P=0.047).

The major problem of nucleotide analogs is the emergence of drug-resistant mutants. After 5 years of treatment, 70% of patients receiving lamivudine developed drug resistant mutations (Lai et al., 2003). Once drug resistance develops, there may be biochemical flares, rebound of viral load, reversion of histologic benefits and worsened clinical outcome (Liaw et al., 2004; Leung et al., 2001). There was also a tendency of reduced benefit in terms of clinical complications among patients who developed viral breakthrough due to lamivudine resistance (Liaw et al., 2004). Newer anti-viral agents with fewer problem of drug resistance including adefovir dipivoxil and entecavir have been registered worldwide (Hadziyannis et al., 2005; Chang et al., 2006). Whether these agents can further reduce the risk of HCC requires further investigation.

Conclusion

The epidemiological link between HBV and HCC is unequivocally strong. Surveillance of HCC among HBV patients is getting increasingly important with the advances in the local ablative treatment for small early HCC. To enhance cost-effectiveness of the surveillance program, risk stratification of chronic hepatitis B patients is necessary. According to the latest recommendations by the American Association for the Study of Liver Diseases, the following chronic hepatitis B patients should undergo HCC surveillance (Bruix and Sherman, 2005): (1) Asian males above 40 years old; (2) Asian females above 50 years old; (3) cirrhotic patients; (4) patients with family history of HCC; and (5) Africans above 20 years old. However, patients with positive hepatitis B e-antigen, high HBV DNA are also at increased risk of developing HCC. Certain HBV genotypes and mutations may also increase the risk of HCC development and can be used as tumor markers in future. Further studies are warranted to integrate these factors into the decision algorithm of HCC surveillance. To prevent HCC, efforts to promote universal vaccination against HBV and to improve the treatment efficacy of anti-viral treatments are needed.

REFERENCES

Banatvala J, Van Damme P, Oehen S. Lifelong protection against hepatitis B: the role of vaccine imunogenicity in immune memory. *Vaccine* 2000;19:877-85.

Baptistia M, Kramvis A, Kew MC. High prevalence of 1762(T) 1764(A) mutations in the basic core promoter of hepatitis B virus isolated from black Africans with hepatocellular carcinoma compared with asymptomatic carriers. *Hepatology* 1999;29:946-53.

Beasley RP. Hepatitis B virus. The major etiology of hepatocellular carcinoma. *Cancer* 1988;61:1942-56.

Bisceglie AM, Hoofnagle JH. Elevations of serum alpha-fetoprotein levels in patients with chronic hepatitis B. *Cancer* 1989;64:2117-20.

Bolondi L, Sofia S, Siringo S, et al. Surveillance programme of cirrhotic patients for early diagnosis and treatment of hepatocellular carcinoma: a cost effectiveness analysis. *Gut* 2001;48:251-9.

Boxall EH, Sira JA, El-Shuhkri N, et al. Long-term persistence of immunity to hepatitis B after vaccination during infancy in a country where endemicity is low. *J Infect Dis* 2004;190:1264-9.

Bruix J, Sherman M. Management of hepatocellular carcinoma. Hepatology 2005;42:1208-36.

Buckwold VE, Xu Z, Chen M, et al. Effects of a naturally occurring mutation in the hepatitis virus basal core promoter on precore gene expression and viral replication. *J Virol* 1996;70: 5845-5851

Chan HLY, Leung NWY, Hussain M, et al. Hepatitis B e antigen-negative chronic hepatitis B in Hong Kong. *Hepatology* 2000;31:763-8.

Chan HLY, Tsang SWC, Liew CT, et al. Viral genotype and hepatitis B virus DNA levels are correlated with histological liver damage in HBeAg-negative chronic hepatitis B virus infection. *Am J Gastroenterol.* 2002;97:406-12.

Chan HLY, Wong ML, Hui AY, et al. Hepatitis B virus genotype C takes a more aggressive disease course than hepatitis B virus genotype B in hepatitis B e antigenpositive patients. *J Clin Microbiol* 2003;41:1277-79. [a]

Chan HLY, Wong ML, Hui AY, et al. The value of hepatitis B virus DNA quantitation to predict hepatitis B e antigen reversion in chronic hepatitis B. *J Clin Microbiol* 2003;41:4693-5. [b]

Chan HLY, Hui AY, Wong ML, et al. Genotype C Hepatitis B virus infection is associated with increased risk of hepatocellular carcinoma. *Gut* 2004;53:1494-8.

Chan HLY, Tsui SKW, Tse CH, et al. Epidemiological and virological characteristics of two subgroups of genotype C hepatitis C virus. *J Infect Dis* 2005;191:2022-32. [a]

Chan HLY, Leung NWY, Hui AY, et al. A randomized, controlled trial of combination therapy for chronic hepatitis B: comparing pegylated interferon-α2b and lamivudine with lamivudine alone. *Ann Intern Med* 2005;142:240-50. [b]

Chan HLY, Hui AY, Wong VWS, et al. Long-term follow-up of peginterferon and lamivudine combination treatment in HBeAg-positive chronic hepatitis B. *Hepatology* 2005;41:1357-64. [c]

Chan HLY, Tse CH, Ng YET, et al. Phylogenetic, virological and clinical characteristics of genotype C hepatitis B virus with TCC at codon 15 of the precore region. *J Clin Microbiol* 2006;44:681-7.

Chang MH, Chen CJ, Lai MS, et al. Universal hepatitis B vaccination in Taiwan and the incidence of hepatocellular carcinoma in children. *N Engl J Med* 1997;336:1855-9.

Chang TT, Gish RG, de Man R, et al. A comparison of entecavir and lamivudine for HBeAg-positive chronic hepatitis B. *N Engl J Med* 2006;354:1001-10.

Chen CJ, Yang HI, Su J, et al. Risk of hepatocellular carcinoma across a biological gradient of serum hepatitis B virus DNA level. *JAMA* 2006;295:65-73.

Chen JG, Parkin DM, Chen QG, et al. Screening for liver cancer: results of a randomized controlled trial in Qidong, China. *J Med Screen* 2003;10:204-9.

Chu CJ, Hussain M, Lok ASF. Hepatitis B virus genotype is associated with earlier HBeAg seroconversion compared with hepatitis B virus genotype C. *Gastroenterology* 2002;122:1756-62.

Cooksley WG, Piratvisuth T, Lee SD, et al. Peginterferon α-2a (40 KD): an advance in the treatment of hepatitis B e antigen-positive chronic hepatitis B. *J Viral Hepat* 2003;10:298-305.

De Franchis R, Meucci G, Vecchi M, et al. The natural history of asymptomatic hepatitis B surface antigen carriers. *Ann Intern Med* 1993;118:191-4.

Di Marco V, Iacono OL, Camma C, et al. The long-term course of chronic hepatitis B. *Hepatology* 1999;30:257-64.

El Serag HB, Mason AC. Rising incidence of hepatocellular carcinoma in the United States. *N Engl J Med* 1999;340:745-50.

Fattovich G, Giustina G, Christensen E, et al. Influence of hepatitis B delta virus infection on morbidity and mortality in compensated cirrhosis type B. *Gut* 2000;46:420-6.

Fujie H, Moriya K, Shintani Y, et al. Hepatitis B virus genotypes and hepatocellular carcinoma in Japan. *Gastroenterology* 2001;120:1564-5.

Hadziyannis SJ, Tassopoulos NC, Heathcote EJ, et al. Long-term therapy with adefovir dipivoxil for HBeAg-negative chronic hepatitis B. *N Engl J Med* 2005;352:2673-81.

Hsu YS, Chien RN, Yeh CT, et al. Long-term outcome after spontaneous HBeAg seroconversion in patients with chronic hepatitis B. *Hepatology* 2002;35:1522-7.

Hyams KC. Risks of chronicity following acute hepatitis B virus infection: a review. *Clin Infect Dis* 1995;20:992-1000.

Ideda K, Saitoh S, Suzuki Y, et al. Disease progression and hepatocellular carcinogenesis in patients with chronic viral hepatitis: a prospective observation of 2215 patients. *J Hepatol* 1998;28:930-8.

Iavarone M, Trabut JB, Delpuech O, et al. Characterisation of hepatitis B virus X protein mutants in tumor and non-tumor liver cells using laser capture microdissection. *J Hepatol* 2003;39:253-61.

Janssen HL, van Zonneveld M, Senturk H, et al. Pegylated interferon alfa-2b alone or in combination with lamivudine for HBeAg-positive chronic hepatitis B: a randomized trial. *Lancet* 2005;365:123-9.

Kao JH, Chen PJ, Lai MY, et al. Hepatitis B genotypes correlate with clinical outcomes in patients with chronic hepatitis B. *Gastroenterology* 2000;118:554-9.

Kao JH, Chen PJ, Lai MY, Chen DS. Basal core promoter mutations of hepatitis B virus increase the risk of hepatocellular carcinoma in hepatitis B carriers. *Gastroenterology* 2003;124:327-34.

Kobayashi M, Suzuki F, Akuta N, et al. Virological differences between patients infected with subtypes Ba and Bj of hepatitis B virus genotype B. *J Gastroenterol Hepatol* 2005;20:570-6.

Kuang SY, Jackson PE, Wang JB, et al. Specific mutations of hepatitis B virus in plasma predict liver cancer development. *Proc Natl Acad Sci USA* 2004;101:3575-80.

Lai CL, Dienstag J, Schiff E, et al. Prevalence and clinical correlates of YMDD variants during lamivudine therapy for patients with chronic hepatitis B. *Clin Infect Dis* 2003;36:687-96.

Lau GK, Piratvisuth T, Luo KX, et al. Peginterferon alfa-2a, lamivudine, and the combination for HBeAg-positive chronic hepatitis B. *N Engl J Med* 2005;352:2682-95.

Lee WM. Hepatitis B virus infection. *N Engl J Med* 1997;337:1733-45.

Leung NW, Lai CL, Chang TT, et al. Extended lamivudine treatment in patients with chronic hepatitis B enhances hepatitis B e antigen seroconversion rates: results after 3 years of therapy. *Hepatology* 2001;33:1527-32.

Liaw YF, Tai D, Chu CM, et al. Early detection of hepatocellular carcinoma in patients with chronic type B hepatitis. A prospective study. *Gastroenterology* 1986;90:263-7.

Liaw YF, Tai DI, Chu CM, et al. The development of cirrhosis in patients with chronic hepatitis B hepatitis: a prospective study. *Hepatology* 1988;8:493-6.

Liaw YF, Sung JJ, Chow WC, et al. Lamivudine for patients with chronic hepatitis B and advanced liver disease. *N Engl J Med* 2004;351:1521-31.

Lin YC, Chang MH, Ni YH, et al. Long-term immunogenicity and efficacy of universal hepatitis B virus vaccination in Taiwan. *J Infect Dis* 2003;187:134-8.

Lindh M, Andersson AS, Gusdal A. Genotypes, nt 1858 variants, and geographic origin of hepatitis B virus--large-scale analysis using a new genotyping method. *J Infect Dis* 1997;175:1285-93.

Manesis EL, Papatheodoridis GV, Hadziyannis SJ. Serum HBV-DNA levels in inactive hepatitis B virus carriers. *Gastroenterology* 2002;122:2092-3.

Martinot-Peignoux M, Boyer N, Colombat M, et al. Serum hepatitis B virus DNA levels and liver histology in inactive HBsAg carriers. *J Hepatol* 2002;36:543-6.

McMahon BJ, Alberts SR, Wainwright RB, et al. Hepatitis B-related sequelae. Prospective study in 1400 hepatitis B surface antigen-positive Alaska native carriers. *Arch Intern Med* 1990;150:1051-4.

McMahon BJ, Holck P, Bulkow L, et al. Serologic and clinical outcomes of 1536 Alaska natives chronically infected with hepatitis B virus. *Ann Intern Med* 2001;135:759-68.

McMahon BJ, Burden DL, Petersen KM, et al. Antibody levels and protection after hepatitis B vaccination: results of a 15-year follow-up. *Ann Intern Med* 2005;142:333-41.

Mok TS, Yeo W, Yu S, et al. An intensive surveillance program detected a high incidence of hepatocellular carcinoma among hepatitis B virus carriers with abnormal alpha-fetoprotein levels or abdominal ultrasonography results. *J Clin Oncol* 2005;23:8041-7.

Ni YH, Chang MH, Huang LM, et al. Hepatitis B virus infection in children and adolescents in a hyperendemic area: 15 years after mass hepatitis B vaccination. *Ann Intern Med* 2001;135:796-800.

Niederau C, Heintges T, Lange S, et al. Long-term follow-up of HBeAg-positive patients treated with interferon alfa for chronic hepatitis B. *N Engl J Med* 1996;334:1422-7.

Norder H, Courouce AM, Magnius LO. Complete genomes, phylogenetic relatedness, and structural proteins of six strains of the hepatitis B virus, four of which represent two new genotypes. *Virology* 1994;198:489-503

Oka H, Tamori A, Kuroki, et al. Prospective study of alpha-fetoprotein in cirrhotic patients monitored for development of hepatocellular carcinoma. *Hepatology* 1994;19:61-6.

Parkin DM, Bray F, Ferlay J, et al. Estimating the world cancer burden: GLOBOSCAN 2000. *Int J Cancer* 2001;94:153-6.

Pateron D, Ganne N, Trinchet JC, et al. Prospective study of screening for hepatocellular carcinoma in Caucasian patients with cirrhosis. *J Hepatol* 1994;20:65-71.

Sarasin FP, Giostra E, Hadengue A. Cost-effectiveness of screening for detection of small hepatocellular carcinoma in Western patients with Child-Pugh class A cirrhosis. *Am J Med* 1996;171:422-34.

Scaglioni PP, Melegari M, Wands JR. Biological properties of hepatitis B viral genomes with mutations in the precore promoter and precore open reading frame. *Virology* 1997;233: 374-381.

Sherman M, Peltekian KM, Lee C. Screening for hepatocellular carcinoma in chronic carriers of hepatitis B virus: incidence and prevalence of hepatocellular carcinoma in a North American urban population. *Hepatology* 1995;22:432-8.

Sheu JC, Sung JL, Chen DS, et al. Growth rates of asymptomatic hepatocellular carcinoma and its clinical implications. *Gastroenterology* 1985:89:259-66.

Sugauchi F, Orito E, Ichida T, et al. Epidemiology and virological characteristics of hepatitis B virus genotype B having the recombination with genotype C. *Gastroenterology* 2003;124:925-32.

Sugauchi F, Kumada H, Acharya S, et al. Epidemiology and sequence differences between two subtypes (Ae and Aa) of hepatitis B virus genotype A. *J Gen Virol* 2004;85:811-20.

Sumi H, Yokosuka O, Seki N, et al. Influence of hepatitis B virus genotypes on the progression of chronic type B liver disease. *Hepatology* 2003;37:19-26.

Sung JJY, Chan HLY, Wong ML, et al. Relationship of clinical and virological factors with hepatitis activity in hepatitis B e antigen-negative chronic hepatitis B virus-infected patients. *J Viral Hepat* 2002;9:229-34.

Sung JJY, Wong ML, Bowden S, et al. Intrahepatic hepatitis B virus covalently closed circular DNA can be a predictor of sustained response to therapy. *Gastroenterology* 2005;128:1890-7.

Stuyver L, De Gendt S, Van Geyt C, et al. A new genotype of hepatitis B virus: complete genome and phylogenetic relatedness. *J Gen Virol* 2000;81:67-74.

Tanaka Y, Hasegawa I, Kato T, et al. A case-control study for differences among hepatitis B virus infections of genotypes A (subtypes Aa and Ae) and D. *Gastroenterology* 2004;40:747-55.

Tsai JF, Jeng JE, Ho MS, et al. Effect of hepatitis C and B virus infection on risk of carcinoma: a prospective study. *Br J Cancer* 1997;76:968-74.

Van Zonneveld M, Honkoop P, Hansen BE, et al. Long-term follow-up of alpha-interferon treatment of patients with chronic hepatitis B. *Hepatology* 2004;39:804-10.

Villeneuve JP, Desronchers M, Infante-Rivard C, et al. A long-term follow-up study of asymptomatic hepatitis B surface antigen-positive carriers in Montreal. *Gastroenterology* 1994;106:1000-5.

Wong DK, Cheung AM, O'Rourke K, et al. Effect of alpha-interferon treatment in patients with hepatitis B e antigen-positive chronic hepatitis B. A meta-analysis. *Ann Intern Med* 1993;119:312-23.

Yang HI, Lu SN, Liaw YF, et al. Hepatitis B e antigen and the risk of hepatocellular carcinoma. *N Engl J Med* 2002;347:168-74.

Yu MW, Yeh SH, Chen PJ, Liaw YF et al. Hepatitis B virus genotype and DNA level and hepatocellular carcinoma: a prospective study in men. *J Natl Cancer Inst* 2005;97:265-72.

Yuen MF, Sablon E, Yuan HJ, et al. Significance of hepatitis B genotype in acute exacerbation, HBeAg seroconversion, cirrhosis-related complications, and hepatocellular carcinoma. *Hepatology* 2003;37:562-7.

Zanetti AR, Mariano A, Romano L, et al. Long-term immunogenicity of hepatitis B vaccination and policy for booster: an Italian multicentre study. *Lancet* 2005;366:1379-84.

Zhang B, Yang B. Combined α fetoprotein testing and ultrasonography as a screening test for primary liver cancer. *J Med Screen* 1999;6:108-10.

Zhang BH, Yang BH, Tang ZY. Randomized controlled trial of screening for hepatocellular carcinoma. *J Cancer Res Clin Oncol* 2004;130:417-22.

In: Hepatitis B Research Advances
Editor: Alicia P. Willis, pp. 187-199
ISBN: 978-1-60021-666-4

Chapter XI

Treatment Approaches for Chronic Hepatitis B with Respect to the Natural History of HBV Virus and Present Anti-Viral Therapies

Sabina Mahmood and Gotaro Yamada
Department of Internal Medicine, Center for Liver Disease, Kawasaki Hospital, Kawasaki Medical School, Okayama, Japan

Introduction

To discuss the treatment strategies for Hepatitis B virus (HBV) associated chronic liver disease, it is first necessary to review the natural course of HBV, from the geographical point of view, with respect to high endemic regions; factors commonly prevalent in those regions and main differences existing between high and low endemic areas. Depending on the above, disease progression is variable and with that comes the difference in approach to treatment. Besides viral and host factors which dually affect disease prognosis, the stable economic status of developed countries and the economic highs and lows of developing and under-developed countries, also play a major role in bringing about a treatment response, which aids in disease prevention or disease reduction. The clinical course of HBV is difficult to define due to it's benign course and lack of symptoms in the early stages and diversity in disease progression. Hepatitis B related liver disease stretches from a subclinical to acute symptomatic hepatitis state (rarely fulminant hepatitis) and from inactive carrier state to subsequent chronic hepatitis (CHB), cirrhosis (LC) and end-stage liver disease, sometimes culminating to Hepatocellular carcinoma (HCC). Host factors (age of infection, gender, immune status), viral factors (genotype, mutations, viral load) and exogenous factors (excessive alcohol consumption, cigarette smoking, aflatoxin B1, hepatotoxic drugs), all influence the course of the disease and henceforth it's outcome. Therefore, it is of great importance to know the natural history of HBV thoroughly and demarcate the main host & viral factors which influence the natural history of chronic hepatitis B and its treatment outcomes.

Epidemiology

The main difference in HBV associated liver disease is seen between 2 major regions worldwide. The endimicity of HBV can be broadly divided into:

1. Highly endemic areas (Southeast Asia, Africa, Pacific Islands).
2. Low Endemic areas (Western Countries).

In the Asia-Pacific region about 75% of the worlds HBV chronic carriers reside. Among which 45% are from the Western Pacific Regions of China, Mongolia, Taiwan and the Pacific Islands [1,2]. Marked variation is again observed among different sub regions and within different countries with Vietnam & the Western Pacific region having the highest prevalence (≧8%), Southeast Asia & South Korea with intermediate prevalence (2-8)% and low prevalence observed in Japan, Australia & New Zealand (≦2%) [3,4,5]. Western countries which are regarded as a region of low endimicity, HBV infection is found mainly in adolescents and adults, resulting from high risk sexual behavior and injection drug use. However, in the United States, though the prevalence is low, about 1.2 million people are affected [6]. In addition HBV infection is found to be high among certain populations such as the native Alaskans, Pacific Islanders and infants of first generation immigrant mothers coming from highly endemic areas [7].

Mode of Transmission

While vertical transmission (from infected mothers to newborns) and perinatal transmission (from infected family members during early childhood) are the predominant routes of infection in the highly endemic areas, in Western countries, horizontal transmission (high risk sexual partners; injection drug use) seems to account for most of the HBV infections [8]. Vertical transmissions have been found to be associated with increased risk of chronic HBV infection, while infections in late life are sometimes self limited may not always develop into chronic infection.

Natural Course of HBV

HBV infection which occurs perinatally usually undergoes three main phases:

1) *A long immunotolerant phase*: The patient tests positive for HBV e Antigen (HBeAg); has high HBV DNA in sera; has little or no symptoms; has normal alanine aminotransferase (ALT) and minimal histological activity in the liver) which may last for decades and render the patient highly infectious.
2) *An immune clearance phase* (patient has markedly decreased levels of HBV DNA, HBeAg undergoes seroconversion to anti-HBe) follows, which is preceded by an increase in ALT levels, as a result of immune mediated breakdown of infected hepatocytes. This second phase can last from months to years. If the patient's immune system is competent, this stage is self limiting and lasts for about 3-4 weeks, at the end of which the patient is usually cleared of the virus. However, if the patient's immune system is not properly functioning the second phase can persist leading to the development of HBeAg positive CHB.

   HBeAg positive CHB: Following seroconversion to anti-HBe, majority of patients undergo biochemical and histological disease remission. Seroconversion is usually preceded by marked ALT elevation and moderate or severe histological changes. At this time, the patient is usually asymptomatic but patients presenting with decompensated LC, may have liver failure or even death. The mean annual rate of spontaneous seroconversion, has been reported to be somewhere between (10-15)% [9-10], with as low as 2.7% and high as 25% being claimed by various studies [11,12]. Following seroconversion, the outcome of CHB depends mainly upon the initial liver damage and subsequent reactivation of HBV DNA and at times, on the patients age. While before the age of 3, the rate is less that 2%, after 3 years of age, the rate increases to about 5 % [13]. With pre-existing LC, disease progression may be severe due to complications of LC, while the absence of pre-existing LC may present with only slight fibrosis and a mild type of CHB. It is the duration and severity of liver injury during this phase that depicts the ultimate outcome of the patient.
3) *A low replicative phase*, where the hosts immune response clears most of the HBV infected hepatocytes, leading to cessation of active viral replication, seroconversion and normalization of ALT. However, HBV s Antigen (HBsAg) still persists in sera. Rarely seen in Asians, some patients may enter the immune phase 4 where, HBsAg is cleared, anti-HBs antibody appears in sera and HBV DNA becomes undetectable. At this stage the patient is free from the danger of re-infection or reactivation. Though reaching the stage 4 of the immune phase is the end point of HBV associated liver disease, it occurs rarely in patients naturally and in a minority of patient groups following treatment.

Reactivation of Viral DNA: Irrespective of HBeAg seroconversion to anti-HBe, reactivation of HBV viral DNA occurs at times either as a result of seroconversion or with the development of pre-core mutants, imposing a stop codon in the precore genomic region of HBV. This leads to the emergence of anti-HBe positive or HBeAg-negative mutants, and leads to the development of:

HBeAg negative chronic hepatitis: In this state, the patient tests positive for HBsAg, negative for HBeAg but with detectable HBV in sera along with raised ALT levels. Anti HBe may be either present or absent. Compared to HBeAg positive chronic hepatitis, HBeAg negative chronic liver disease is more severe and usually the patient has LC at the initial check-up. In addition the progression of liver disease follows a rapid course with very low rates of sustained spontaneous remission [9-17].

KEY VIRAL FACTORS

Viral Genotype: There is also a variation in the geographical distribution of the 8 HBV genotypes (A-H) and subgenotypes Aa, Ae, Bj, Ba and Ce, Cs [18-23], which seems to play an important role in the clinical manifestations of HBV disease and treatment response. HBV genotype C is predominantly found in Far Eastern Countries and is associated with delayed seroconversion, a more aggressive clinical course, increase resistance to IFN therapy and increased risk of HCC, compared to genotype B [24-30]. Whereas in India, genotype D is associated with more severe liver disease than genotype A [31]. In Japan, patients having genotype B's subgroup Bj, the severity of liver disease with higher prevelance of HCC is seems to be more compared to the subgroup Bj [23,25,32]. The prevalence of Genotype A is seen mostly in northwest Europe, North America and Central Africa, while Genotype E is common in Africa, Genotype F in American Natives, Polynesia, Central & South America and Genotype G in US and France [33].

Viral Mutaitons

HBV mutants emerge during the natural course of HBV infection.

Particularly the A to G mutation at nucleotide 1896 (A1896G) in the pre-core region(Pre-C) of the HBV genome and the A to T transversion at nucleotide 1762 (A1762T) in the basal core promoter (BCP) region, have been found to influence disease progression. Several studies have shown that BCP mutations are more prevalent in HBV genotype C and are associated with high viral load [34-36]. Pre-S deletions and mutations in BCP and Pre-core, have been found to occur more frequently in patients with progressive liver disease than chronic HBsAg carriers and combinations of mutations involving Pre-S deletions, rather than single mutations, contributed further to progressive disease [37].

Pre core mutations have been associated with HBeAg negative chronic hepatitis and may be partly related to older age and advanced liver disease on first presentation [38].

Viral Load

Unlike the geographic distribution of HBV genotypes and the prevalence of HBV mutants, the markers of HBV replication, namely HBeAg and HBV DNA are universal. Persistent HBeAg sero positivity or HBeAg reversion, in addition to HBV DNA levels > 10^4 - 10^5 copies/ml are associated with increased risk of LC and HCC [39-40]. Further studies have showed the dose-dependant relation between HBV DNA viral load and LC [41-42]. The role of HBV DNA viral load in HCC occurrence have also been documented [43-46].

KEY HOST FACTORS

Age at Infection: This seems to be the best determinant of chronicity, the younger the age at infection, the greater the probability of chronicity. Thus individuals infected perinatally or during infancy are at most risk in comparison to those infected in adulthood [47]. About 90% of infants born to highly infectious HBsAg- and HBeAg positive mothers become HBV carriers. Compared to 30% of children between ages 1to 5, only 1 to 5 % of adults infected become persistently infected after experiencing acute hepatitis [48-50]. HBV infection acquired in adulthood does not have the prolonged immuno tolerance phase, typical of early-life infection. A period of active disease leading to seroconversion occurs more rapidly in adults than in children, with subsequent histologic and biochemical remission of disease [51], with the exception of HBeAg negative chronic hepatitis B. The peak incidence of clinically evident LC and HCC is around 50 to 60 years of age [52].

Gender: Though there is no gender bias regarding the number of male/female infected with HBV, the ratio of male patients with CHB, progressing to LC is double that observed in females and the incidence of HCC is also 3 to 6 times more in men than women [52].

Host Immune Status: Disease progression in CHB patients is seen to be more rapid in immuno suppressed patients compared to immuno competent patients [53].

Treatment Basics

With knowledge of the natural course of HBV virus and the influence of different viral, host and exogenous factors on disease progression in mind, different treatment regimes may be adopted suitable for the patient. The target of every treatment is complete remission of disease with the emergence of antibodies against HBsAg accompanied by minimal or disappearance of symptoms of HBV disease. However, with reference to past and present long-term research data, the percentage of seroconversion to anti-HBs is low. So, he next approach is to define whether the patient has HBeAg positive or HBeAg negative CHB along with the presence of other host and other viral factors. Following that the best possible therapy can be chosen. If the patient presents with LC at the first visit, the degree of LC, compensated or decompensated LC needs to be assessed. While patients with compensated LC can be treated for prevention of further disease progression and development of HCC, those presenting with decompensated LC, require immediate treatment for ascites, variceal bleeding and hepatic encephalopathy, to prolong life. Once, such conditions are stabilized and brought under control, treatment to prevent further disease progression and HCC development can be implemented.

Anti-Viral Treatment Options

In most countries the present licensed anti-viral treatments for HBV related liver disease include:

a)Interferon α
b) Lamivudine
c) Adefovir
d) Entecavir
e) Peg interferon α-2a.

In addition some Asian countries have also licensed Thymosin α-1. The newest and effective drugs readily available are entecavir and Peg interferon α-2a which appear to be more favorable in terms of drug resistance and long term use, with minimal side effects.

Interferon α

Interferon α is a naturally occurring protein which exhibits antiviral, anti proliferative and immuno modulatory effects. When used for short term in HBeAg positiveCHB, it has been shown to induce loss of HBV DNA, HBeAg and HBsAg [54].

Those who lost HBeAg, seroconverted to anti HBe either during or soon after cessation of therapy. The long term effects of IFN in improving overall survival and preventing HCC, are conflicting and inconsistent [55-57]. Others have reported the efficacy of IFN in patients with pre-treatment LC compared to non-LC patients [58]. However, IFN use has some limiting factors related to its adverse side effects such as influenza like symptoms, irritability, headache and exacerbation of existing psychological disorders. Furthermore IFN is completely contraindicated in patients with uncontrolled seizures, autoimmune disorders and decompensated LC [59]. Expenses involved with prolonged continuation of IFN in countries lacking health insurance, also poses a major problem.

Lamivudine

Lamivudine is an oral dideoxy nucleoside inhibitor of DNA synthesis, which blocks DNA viral replication by terminating the nascent pro viral DNA chain. It has been shown to suppress viral replication of HBV DNA in CHB infection. With its good safety profile, oral administration, low cost it appears to be an effective medicine of choice for the treatment of chronic HBV infection. When administered on a short term-basis (1 year course), the primary outcome was histological improvement, with an end-of treatment histology showing significant decrease in inflammation and fibrosis by the Knodell HAI score. The overall HBeAg seroconversion rates at a dose of 100 mg were similar in studies from both North America and Asia, 17% and 16%, respectively [60-61]. Long-term lamivudine therapy evaluated in Asian studies reported marked increase in the serocoversion rates to 27% at 104 weeks [62]. Cumulative increases in the HBeAg seroconversion rate to 40% after 3 years with sustained histological improvements, have also been observed [63].

Predictors of response to lamivudine treatment, similar to IFN alpha include high baseline ALT levels and low baseline HBV DNA, though the importance of HBV DNA levels as a predictor is less, compared to IFN [64]. Though the tolerance, safety and cost of lamivudine therapy surpasses IFN, there are also a number of problems associated with long term therapy. The main being, the emergence of viral resistance to lamivudine with the appearance of YMDD mutants, which may appear as early as 2-3 months after initiation therapy [65]. In immuno competent patients, the significance of YMDD mutants following long-term treatment, in clinical disease, is less. However in immuno suppressed patients, moderate to severe complications have been observed. They include, exacerbation of hepatitis, decreased rate of seroconversion of HBeAg, rapid allograft re-infection with rapid disease progression in liver transplant patients [66]. In patients with LC or HIV co-infection, hepatic decompensation, sub massive hepatic necrosis and even death have been reported [67-68].

In HBeAg negative CHB infection, very high end-of treatment biochemical and virological response rates, ranging from 70% to 90% after 12 months, have been observed [69-72]. Nevertheless, relapse rates are high with overall low, sustained response rates. With the development of lamivudine resistant YMDD mutants resulting in increases in serum HBV DNA, elevated ALT levels and histological disease progression, the long term outcome in responders or the optimal duration of therapy, is not known. With the development of resistant mutants, cessation of lamivdine therapy is necessary, to avoid the adverse effects of YMDD mutants.

Adefovir

Adefovir dipivoxil is an oral nucleotide analogue for the treatment of chronic HBV infection. It is has been shown to be effective in lamivudine resistant patients following development of YMDD mutants, in addition to patients on immunosuppressive therapy after liver transplant [73-74]. The advantage of adefovir is that even after prolonged therapy, it does not develop drug resistance. With respect to HBeAg positive and HBeAg negative CHB, in HBeAg positive CHB, significantly higher rates of HBeAg seroconversion, improvements in necro inflammatory and fibrosis score, greater rates of serum ALT normalization and undetectable HBV DNA, (after a year on Adefovir) was seen in patients compared to controls [75]. A 48 week therapy of Adefovir in HBeAg negative patients, resulted in normalization of ALT, undetectable HBV DNA and significant histological improvement compared to controls. No resistance was observed [76]. The only disadvantage of prolonged Adevofir therapy is nephrotoxicity.

Entecavir

One of the promising new anti-HBV agents is entacavir. It is an oral guanosine nucleoside analogue with potent and selective inhibitory activity against HBV DNA replication. A 48 week long study has reported significant improvement in the primary endpoint of histological inflammation (≧2-point decrease in Knodell necroinflammatory score) in HBeAg positive, HBeAg negative and lamivudine resistant CHB patients with entecavir, compared to lamivudine. With respect to decrease in HBV viral load and normalization of ALT as endpoints of treatments, entecavir was found to be significantly better than lamivudine [77-79]. Regarding development of resistance to entecavir, it has been found that lamivudine resistance is a prerequisite for the emergence of resistance against entecavir, in comparison to entecavir naïve patients [80].

Peg interferon α-2a

Peginterferon α-2a is a recently approved licensed drug for the treatment of CHB. Studies comparing Peginterferon α-2a with lamivudine mono therapy and lamivudine plus Peginterferon α-2a combination therapy, showed after initial 48 weeks and a further 24 weeks of therapy, in HBeAg positive patients, more patients with combination therapy seroconverted and their HBV DNA was suppressed below 100,000 copies/ml. In HBeAg negative patients developed normalization of ALT and their HBV DNA was suppressed below 20, 000 copies/ml [81-82]. Addition of lamivudine to Peginterferon α-2a did not bring about any significant improvements in efficacy.

Treatment Approaches (based on the ACT-HBV Asia-Pacific Steering Committee recommendations and clinically practiced) [83]

An estimated 350 million persons worldwide are infected with HBV. Carriers of HBV are at risk for the development of cirrhosis and HCC. After briefly reviewing the natural history of HBV infection, it is clear that severity of disease, course and progression is variable. Chronically infected patients require life long monitoring to determine if, when and in whom disease intervention with the presently available anti-viral therapy is necessary, to prevent the development of end-stage disease, resulting in increased mortality.

Treatment regimes need to be adopted keeping in mind the host and viral factors which influence disease progression, response rates of anti-viral treatments and their side effects. In patients with compensated liver disease, in the absence of contraindications, the initial therapy can consist of Interferon α, lamivudine or adefovir. While IFN has the advantages of long duration of therapy, better response and lack of resistance, its disadvantages such as high cost and side effects cannot be overlooked. Lamivudine on the other hand is more economical, well tolerated but its long term therapy leads to the development of drug resistance. In worst cases, once resistance develops the state of liver disease may worsen further and override its initial benefits. Adefovir is effective in lamivudine resistant cases with a very low rate of adefovir resistance observed during initial therapy. However, in long term use, the risk of nephrotoxicity and also its high cost compared to lamivudine, are problems arise. The 2 newest licensed drugs namely entecavir and Peg interferon α-2a appear to be more promising with respect to minimal side effects, little or no drug resistance and ability to be used as a long term therapy. The first thing to decide in assessing patients for anti-viral therapy is whether the patient has HBeAg positive or HBeAg negative CHB.

Treatment Approaches in HBeAg Positive CHB Patients

1. HBV DNA $<10^5$ copies/ml, ALT normal = no treatment; monitoring of HBV DNA, HBeAg, ALT, every 3-6 months.
2. HBV DNA $\geqq 10^5$ copies/ml; ALT normal = no treatment; monitoring of HBV DNA, HBeAg, ALT, every 3 months. Liver biopsy for patients over 30-40 years old. If moderate or severe inflammation and fibrosis, treatment recommended.
3. HBV DNA $\geqq 10^5$ copies/ml; ALT 1-2 x ULN = no treatment; monitoring of HBV DNA, HBeAg, ALT, every 1-3 months.
4. HBV DNA $\geqq 10^5$ copies/ml; ALT 2-5 x ULN: Treatment indicated or treatment withheld for 3 months and observed for spontaneous seroconversion, provided there is no hepatic decompensation. Initial treatment options may include any one of the antiviral drugs.
5. HBV DNA $\geqq 10^5$ copies/ml; ALT > 5 x ULN: Treatment indicated or treatment withheld for 3 months and observed for spontaneous seroconversion, provided there is no hepatic decompensation. Initial treatment options may include lamivudine or entecavir due to greater suppressive effects and rapid onset of actions.
6. If response is achieved in steps 4 or 5, monitoring of HBV DNA, HBeAg, ALT, every 1-3 months, post therapy.
7. If anti-viral therapy results in non –response, OLT may be considered.

Treatment Approaches in HBeAg Negative CHB Patients

1. HBV DNA $<10^4$ copies/ml, ALT normal = no treatment (majority inactive carriers); monitoring of HBV DNA, ALT, every 6-12 months. Liver biopsy if any clinical indications.
2. HBV DNA $\geqq 10^4$ copies/ml; ALT normal = no treatment; monitoring of HBV DNA, ALT, every 1-3 months. Liver biopsy for patients over 30-40 years old. If moderate or severe inflammation and fibrosis, treatment recommended.
3. HBV DNA $\geqq 10^4$ copies/ml; ALT 2-5 x ULN: Treatment indicated usually long-term. Initial treatment options may include all 4 anti-viral drugs except Lamivudine, due to its high rate of drug resistance.
4. HBV DNA $\geqq 10^4$ copies/ml; ALT > 5 x ULN: Treatment indicated usually long-term. Initial treatment options may include lamivudine or entecavir due to their greater suppressive effects and rapid onset of actions. Entecavir preferred over lamivudine, due to its high rate of drug resistance.
5. If response is achieved in steps 4 or 5, monitoring of HBV DNA, HBeAg, ALT, every 1-3 months, post therapy.

6. If anti-viral therapy results in non–response, continued monitoring to recognize delayed response or other strategies may be considered.

Treatment Approaches in Compensated Cirrhosis (HBeAg Positive or HBeAg Negative) Patients

1. HBV DNA <10^4 copies/ml, monitoring of HBV DNA, ALT and HBeAg (in HBeAg positive patients) at least every 3 months.
2. HBV DNA $\geqq 10^4$ copies/ml, Treatment indicated usually long-term. Initial treatment options may include lamivudine adefovir, entecavir or interferon (infinitely). Adefovir or entecavir preferred over lamivudine, due to its high rate of drug resistance.
3. If response is achieved in steps 1 or 2, monitoring of HBV DNA, ALT and HBeAg (in HBeAg positive patients) every 1-3 months, post therapy.
4. If anti-viral therapy results in non –response, consider other strategies including OLT.

Treatment Approaches in Decompensated Cirrhosis (HBeAg Positive or HBeAg Negative) Patients

1. HBV DNA <10^4 copies/ml, observe/monitor closely; consider /refer for OLT.
2. HBV DNA $\geqq 10^4$ copies/ml, treatment indicated; consider /refer for OLT; entecavir, adefovir, lamivudine or combination therapy as first line options; Entecavir and adefovir preferred over lamivudine, due to its high rate of drug resistance.
3. If response is achieved in steps 1 or 2, close monitoring of hepatic function and HBV DNA; may delay OLT.
4. If anti-viral therapy results in non –response, OLT.

The main goal of anti-viral treatment for CHB is either elimination or permanent suppression of HBV DNA replication, to prevent progression of disease, prolong life and improve quality of life. Though there are already quite a few licensed antiviral drugs available and more are appearing, each comes with its advantages and disadvantages. Many detailed considerations are to be made by the physician which is both effective, safe and affordable by the patient. While in developed countries such as in Europe, or the US and Japan, both doctors and patients have the opportunity to undertake the best available treatments, in the poor or developing nations, a bigger challenge awaits, where poverty, poor communication and lack of knowledge stand in the way of disease prevention or it's ultimate elimination. Nevertheless, it is the duty of doctors, researchers and persons related to the medical and pharmaceutical fields, to thrive and achieve the best possible treatment for all patients worldwide.

REFERENCES

[1] Lok A S; Heatcote E J. Management of Hepatitis B:2000-summary of workshop. *Gastroenterology,* 2001 120,1828-53.

[2] Lavanchy D. Hepatitis B virus epidemiology, disease burden, treatement, and current and emerging prevention and control measures. *J Viral Hepat,* 2004 11, 97-107.

[3] Mohamed R; Desmond P. Practical difficulties in the management of hepatitis B in the Asia-Pacific region. *J Gastroenterol Hepatol,* 2004 19, 958-69.

[4] Park J W. Hepatocellular carcinoma in Korea: introduction and overview. *Korean J Gastroenterol,* 2005 45, 217-26.

[5] World Health Organization. Geographic pattern of Hepatitis B prevalence. Last update: July 7, 2004. Available at http://www.who.int/vaccines-surveillance/graphics/html/ hepbrev.htm. Accessed Feb 6, 2007

[6] Centers for Disease Control and Prevention (CDC). Incidence of acute hepatitis B-United States. *MMWR Morb Mortal Wkly Rep,* 2004 52 (51-52), 1252-4.

[7] [No authors listed]. Hepatitis B virus: a comprehensive strategy for eliminating transmission in the United States through universal childhood vaccination. Recommendations of the Immunization Practices Advisory Committee (ACIP). *MMWR Rrecomm Rep* 1991 40(RR-13), 1-25.

[8] Alter M J; Margolis H S. The emergence of hepatitis B as a sexually transmitted disease. *Med Clin North Am, 1*990 Nov 74(6), 1529-41.

[9] Liaw YF; Chu CM. Clinical and histological events preceding hepatitis Be antigen seroconversion in chronic type B hepatitis. *Gastroenterlogy,* 1983 84, 216-19.

[10] Lok ASF; Lai CL. Spontaneous hepatitis B e antigen to antibody seroconversion and reversion in Chinese patients with chronic hepatitis B e infection. *Gastroenterlogy,* 1987 92, 1839-43.

[11] Viola LA ; Barrison IG. The HBe antigen-antibody system and its relationship to clinical and laboratory findings in 100 chronic HBsAg carriers in Britain. *J Med Virol,* 1981 8, 169-75.

[12] Hoofnagle JH; Dsherko GM. Seroconversion from hepatitis Be antigen to antibody in chronic hepatitis type B hepatitis. *Ann. Intern. Med,* 1981 94, 744-8.

[13] Chang MH; Sung JL. Factors affecting clearance of hepatitis B e antigen in hepatitis B surface antigen in carrier children. *J Paeditr,* 1989 115, 385-90.

[14] Chu FV; Karayiannis P. Natural history of chronic hepatitis B infection in Taiwan: studies of HBV DNA in serum. *Hepatology,* 1985 5, 431-4.

[15] Hadziyannis SJ. Hepatitis B e antigen negative C hepatitis B: from clinical recognition to pathogenesis and treatment. *Viral Hep Rev,* 1995 1, 7-36.

[16] Fattovich G; Brollo L. Long-term follow-up of anti-HBe-positive chronic active hepatitis B. *Hepatology,* 1988 8, 1651-4.

[17] Fattovich G. Natural course and prognosis of chronic hepatitis type B. 1988 8, 1651-4. *Viral Hep Rev,* 1996 2, 263-76.

[18] Miyakawa Y; Mizokami M. Classifying hepatitis B virus genotypes. *Intervirology,* 2003 46, 329-38.

[19] Kao J H; Wu N H. Hepatitis B genotypes and the response to interferon therapy. *J Hepatol,* 2000 33, 998-1002.

[20] Kato H; Orito E. Characteristics of hepatitis B virus isolates of genotype G and their phylogenetic differences from the other six genotypes (A through F).*J Virol ,* 2002 76, 6131-7.

[21] Chan H L; Tsui S K. Epidemiological and virological characteristics of 2 subgroups of hepatitis B virus genotype C.*J Infect Dis,* 2005 191, 2022-32.

[22] Huy T T; Ushijima H. Genotype C of hepatitis B virus can be classified into at least two sub-groups.*J Gen Virol,* 2004 85, 283-92.

[23] Sugauchi F; Orito E. Epidemiologic and virological characteristics of hepatitis B virus genotype B having the recombination with genotype C. *Gastroenterlogy,* 2003 124, 925-32.

[24] Yu M W; Yeh S H. Hepatitis B virus genotype and DNA level and hepatocellular carcinoma: a prospective study in men.*J Natl Cancer Inst,* 2005 97,265-72.

[25] Orito E; Sugauchi F. Differences of hepatocellular carcinoma patients with hepatitis B virus genotypes of Ba, Bj or C in Japan. *Intervirology,* 2005 48, 239-45.

[26] Kao J H; Chen P J. Hepatitis B genotypes correlate with clinical outcomes in patients with chronic hepatitis B. *Gastroenterlogy,* 2000 118, 554-9.

[27] Sumi H; Yokosuka O. Influence of hepatitis B virus genotypes on the progression of chronic type B liver disease. *Hepatology,* 2003 37, 19-26.

[28] Yotsuyanagi H; Okuse C. Distinct geographic distributions of hepatitis B virus genotypes in patients with acute infection in Japan. *J Med Virol,* 2005 77, 39-46.

[29] Shina S; Fujino H. Relationship of HBsAg subtypes with HBeAg/anti-HBe status and chronic liver disease. Part I: analysis of 1744 HBsAg carriers. *Am J Gastroenterol,* 1991 86, 866-71.

[30] Chan H L; Hui A Y. Genotype C hepatitis B virus infection is associated with an increased risk of hepatocellular carcinoma. *Gut,* 2004 53, 1494-8.

[31] Thakur V; Guptan R C. Profile, spectrum and significance of HBV genotypes in chronic liver disease patients in the Indian subcontinent. *J Gastroenterol Hepatol,* 2002 17, 165-70.

[32] Sugauchi F; Orito E. Hepatitis B virus of genotype B with or without recombination with genotype C over the precore region plus the core gene. *J Virol,* 2002 76, 5985-92.

[33] Kidd-Ljunggren K; Miyakawa Y. Genetic vatiabilty in hepatitis B viruses. *J Gen Virol,* 2002Jun 83 (Pt6), 1267-80.

[34] Kao J H; Chen PJ. Hepatitis B genotypes correlate with clinical outcomes in patients with chronic hepatitis B. *Gastroenterology,* 2000 118, 554-9.

[35] Lindh M; Hannoun C. Core promoter mutations and genotypes in relation to viral replication and liver damage in East Asian hepatitis B virus carriers. *J Infect Dis,* 1999 179, 775-82.

[36] Orito E; Mizokami M. a case-control study for clinical and molecular biological differences between hepatitis B viruses of genotypes B and C. Japan HBV Genotype Research Group.*Hepatology,* 2001 33, 218-23.

[37] Chen B F; Liu C J. High prevalence and mapping of Pre-S deletion in hepatitis B virus carriers with progressive liver diseases. *Gastroenterology,* 2006 130, 1153-68.

[38] Brunetto M R; Oliveri F. Outcome of anti-HBe positive chronic hepatitis B in alpha interferon treated and untreated patients: a long term cohort study. *J Hepatol,* 2002 36,263-70.
[39] Liaw Y; Tai D I. The development of cirrhosis in patients with chronic type B hepatitis: a prospective study. *Hepatology,* 1998 8, 493-6.
[40] Hsu YS; Chien R N. Long-term outcome after spontaneous HBeAg seroconversion in patients with chronic hepatitis B. *Hepatology,* 2002 35, 1522-7.
[41] Iloeje U H; Yang HI. Predicting liver cirrhosis risk based on the level of circulating hepatitis B viral load. *Gastroenterology,* 2006 130, 678-86.
[42] Yuen M F; Yuan H J. Prognostic determinants for chronic hepatitis B in Asians: therapeutic implications. *Gut,* 2005 54, 1610-4.
[43] Tang B; Kruger WD. Hepatitis B viremia is associated with increased risk of hepatocellular carcinoma in chronic carriers.*J Med Virol,* 2004 72, 35-40.
[44] Evans A A, Fabre R E. Hepatitis B viral load is associated with the development of hepatocellular carcinoma.*Hepatology,* 2004 40 (Suppl.1),602A.
[45] Yu MW; Yeh S H. Hepatitis B virus genotype and DNA level and hepatocellular carcinoma: a prospective study in men. *J Natl Cancer Inst,* 2005 97, 265-72.
[46] Chen C J; Yang H I. Risk of hepatocellular carcinoma across biological gradient of serum hepatitis B virus DNA level. *JAMA*, 2006 295, 65-73.
[47] Hoofnagle J Y; Shafritz DA. Chronic type B hepatitis and the "healthy" HBsAg carrier state. *Hepatology,* 1987 7, 758-63.
[48] Mcmohan BJ; Alward WLM. Acute hepatitis B virus infection: relation of age to the clinical expression of disease and subsequent development of carrier state. *J Infect Dis,* 1985 151, 599-603.
[49] Chang MH. Natural history of hepatitis B infection in children. *J Gastroenterol Hepatol,* 2000 15 (Suppl) E11-E19.
[50] Tassopoulos NC; Papaevangelou GJ. Natural history of acute hepatitis B surface antigen-positive hepatitis in Greek adults. *Gastroenterology,* 1987 92, 1844-1850.
[51] Yuen MF; Lai CL. Natural history of chronic hepatitis B virus infections. *J Gastroenterol Hepatol,* 2000 15 (Suppl) E20-4.
[52] Fattovich G. Natural history and prognosis of hepatitis B.*Semin Liver Dis,* 2003 23, 47-58.
[53] Lee WM. Hepatitis B virus infection. *N Engl J Med,* 1997 337, 1733-45.
[54] Wong DK; Cheung AM. Effect of alpha-interferon treatment in patients with hepatitis B e antigen positive chronic hepatitis B: a meta-analysis. *Ann Intern Med,* 1993 119, 312-23.
[55] Lin SM; Sheen Is. Long-term beneficial effect of interferon therapy in patients with chronic hepatitis B virus infection. *Hepatology,* 1999 29, 971-5.
[56] Yuen MF; Hui CK. Long-term follow-up of interferon alfa treatment in Chinese patients with chronic hepatitis B infection: the effect on hepatitis B e antigen seroconversion and the development of cirrhosis-related complications. *Hepatology,* 2001 34, 139-45.
[57] Lau DT; Everhart J. Long-term follow-up of patients with chronic hepatitis B treated with interferon alpha. *Gastroenterology,* 1997 113, 1660-7.

[58] Fattovich G; Giustina G. Long-term outcome of hepatitis B e antigen-positive patients with compensated cirrhosis treated with interferon alpha. European Concerted Action on Viral Hepatitis (EUROHEP). *Hepatology,* 1997 26, 1338-42.

[59] Steven-Huy B. Han. Natural course, therapeutic options and economic evaluation of therapies for chronic hepatitis B. *Drugs,* 2006 66(14), 1831-1851.

[60] Dienstag JL; Schiff ER. Lamivudine as initial treatment for chronic hepatitis B in the United States. *N Engl J Med,* 1999 341, 1256-63.

[61] Lai CL; Chien RN. A one-year trial of lamivudine for chronic hepatitis B. Asia Hepatitis Lamivudine Study Group. *N Engl J Med,* 1998 339, 61-8.

[62] Liaw YF; Leung NW. Effects of extended lamivudine therapy in Asian patients with chronic hepatitis B. Asia Hepatitis Lamivudine Study Group. *Gastroenterology,* 2000 119, 172-80.

[63] Leung NW; Lai CL. Extended lamivudine treatment in patients with chronic hepatitis B enhances hepatitis B e antigen seroconversion rates: results after 3 years of therapy. *Hepatology,* 2001 33, 1527-32.

[64] Perrillo RP; Lai CL. Predictors of HBeAg loss after lamivudine treatment for chronic hepatitis B. *Hepatology,* 2002 36, 186-94.

[65] Nafa S, Ahmed S. Early detection of viral resistance by determination of hepatitis B virus polymerase mutations in patients treated by lamivudine for chronic hepatitis B. *Hepatology,* 2000 32, 1078-88.

[66] Yeh CT; Chien RN. Clearance of the original hepatitis B virus YMDD-motif mutants with emergence of distinct lamivudine-resistant mutants during prolonged lamivudine therapy. *Hepatology,* 2000 31, 1318-26.

[67] Bonancini M; Kurz A. Fulminant hepatitis B due to lamivudine-resistant mutant of HBV in a patient coinfected with HIV. *Gastroenterology,* 2002 122, 244-5.

[68] Kim JW; Lee HS. Fatal submassive hepatic necrosis associated with tyrosine-methionine-asparttate- motif mutation of hepatitis B virus after long-term lamivudine therapy. *Clin Infect Dis,* 2001 33, 403-5.

[69] Hadziyannis SJ; Papatheodis GV. Efficacy of long-term lamivudine mono therapy in patients with hepatitis B e antigen-negative chronic hepatitis B. *Hepatology,* 2000 32, 847-51.

[70] Papatheodoridis GV; Dimou E. Course of virological breakthroughs under long-term lamivudine in HBeAg-negative precore mutant HBV liver disease. *Hepatology,* 2002 36, 219-26.

[71] Santantanio T; Mazzola M. Long-term follow-up of patients with anti-HBe/HBV DNA positive chronic hepatitis B treated for 12 months with lamivudine. *J Hepatol,* 2000 32, 300-6.

[72] Tassopoulos NC; Volpes R. Efficacy of lamivudine in patients with hepatitis B e antigen-negative/hepatitis B virus DNA-positive (precore mutant) chronic hepatitis B. *Hepatology,* 1999 29, 889-96.

[73] Walsh KM; Woodall T. Successful treatment with adefovir dipivoxil in a patient with fibrosing cholestatic hepatitis and lamivudine resistant hepatitis B virus. *Gut,* 2001 49, 436-40.

[74] Peters MG; singer G. Fulminant hepatic failure resulting from lamivudine-resistant hepatitis B virus in a renal transplant recipient: durable response after orthotopic liver transplantation on adefovir dipivoxil and hepatitis B immune globulin. *Transplantation,* 1999 68, 1912-4.

[75] Marcellin P; Chang TT. Adefovir dipivoxil for the treatment of hepatitis B e antigen-negative chronic hepatitis B. *N Engl J Med,* 2003 348, 808-16.

[76] Angus P; Vaughan R. Resistance to adefovir dipivoxil therapy associated with the selection of a novel mutation in the HBV polymerase. *Gastroenterology,* 2003 125, 292-7.

[77] Hadziyannis SJ; Tassopoulos NC. Long-term therapy with adefovir dipivoxil for the HBeAg-negative chronic hepatitis B. *N Engl J Med,* 2005 352, 2673-81.

[78] Shouval D; Lai C-L. Entecavir demonstrates superior histologic an dvirologic efficacy over lamivudine in nucleoside-naïve HBeag(-) chronic hepatitis B: results of phase III trial ETV-027 [abstract no. LB07]. *Hepatology,* 2004 40, (4 Suppl. 1):728A.

[79] Sherman M; Yurdaydin C. Ecntecavir is superior to continued lamivudine for the treatment of lamivudine-refractory, HBeAg (+) chronic hepatitis B: results of phase III study ETV-026 [abstract no. 1152]. *Hepatology,* 2006 40(4 Suppl. 1): 664A.

[80] Colonno R J; Rose R E. Entecavir (ETV) resistance is not observed in nucleoside-naïve subjects and is observed infrequently by week 48 in lamivudine-rrefractory subjects with chronic hepatitis B infection, abstract 478. J *Hepatol,* 2005 42 (Suppl.2): 573A.

[81] Lau G K; Piratvisuth T. Peginterferon Alfa-2a, lamivudine, and the combination for HBeAg-positive chronic hepatitis B. *N Engl J Med,* 2005 352, 2682-95.

[82] Marcellin P; Lau G K. Peginterferon Alfa-2a alone, lamivudine alone, and the two in combination in patients with HBeAg-negative chronic hepatitis B. *N Engl J Med,* 2004 351, 1206-17.

[83] ACT-HBV Asia-Pacific Steering Committee Members. Chronic hepatitis B: treatment alert. *Liver International,* 2006 26, 47-58.

In: Hepatitis B Research Advances
Editor: Alicia P. Willis, pp. 201-213

ISBN: 978-1-60021-666-4

Chapter XII

PROPHYLAXIS OF RECURRENT HEPATITIS B AFTER LIVER TRANSPLANTATION

***Zhongyang Shen*[1,2], *Zifa Wang*[1,2,*], *Yunjin Zang*[1,2], *Yamin Zhang*[2] *and Zhijun Zhu*[2]**

[1]General Hospital of China People's Armed Police Force, Beijing 100039, China
[2]Orient Organ Transplantation Center, Tianjin First Central Hospital, Tianjin 300192, China

ABSTRACT

Approximately 2 billion people – one third of the world's population – have serologic evidence of past or present Hepatitis B virus (HBV) infection, and 350 million people are chronically infected. Each year over 1 million people die from HBV-related chronic liver disease. Liver transplantation is indicated in HBV-infected patients with end-stage diseases, such as, chronic encephalopathy, refractory ascites or recurrent variceal bleeding. However, in last century, liver transplantation for HBV related-liver diseases was a very controversial issue because the graft was inevitably recurrent after liver transplantation. HBV reinfection after liver transplantation results from HBV particles in circulation, or other extrahepatic sites. Significant progress has been made in the prophylaxis and treatment of recurrent hepatitis B after liver transplantation. Hepatitis B immune globulin (HBIG) was effective in reducing HBV reinfection and improving graft survival after liver transplantation. Lamivudine has also dramatically reduced the recurrence of HBV in the patient undergoing liver transplantation. Combination HBIG and lamivudine is the most effective porphylatic regimen. HBV-related liver disease is no longer a contraindication for liver transplantation. This article focuses on the mechanisms and prophylaxis of hepatitis B recurrent after liver transplantation.

* Correspondence concerning this article should be addressed to Zifa Wang, General Hospital of China People's Armed Police Force, 69 Yongding Road, Haidian Distract, Beijing 100039, China. Tel: 86-10-88276857; Fax: 86-10-68212585; Email: wangzf15213@yahoo.com.

Keywords: Liver transplantation; Hepatitis B; Prophylaxis; Recurrence

INTRODUCTION

Hepatitis B virus (HBV) infection is a major public health problem and cause of infectious disease mortality worldwide. Approximately 2 billion people – one third of the world's population – have serologic evidence of past or present HBV infection, and 350 million people are chronically infected. Each year over 1 million people die from HBV-related chronic liver disease [1]. The prevalence of HBV infection in China was around 60% and the proportion of chronic HBV carriage as high as 10% [2,3]. Orthotopic liver transplantation (OLT) is indicated in HBV-infected patients with a history of spontaneous bacterial peritonitis, chronic encephalopathy, refractory ascites or recurrent variceal bleeding [4]. In Europe and the United States, 5-10% of patients undergoing liver transplantation have HBV-associated liver diseases [5,6] . However, in China, HBV-associated liver diseases account for about 50% of patients undergoing liver transplantation. In 1990s liver transplantation for HBV related-liver diseases was a very controversial issue because the graft is inevitably reinfected, especially if the patient is HBV DNA positive [7]. In addition, the data from the University of Pittsburgh showed that the actuarial survival of patients undergoing liver transplantation for chronic hepatitis B was 45% to 50%, which was 25% to 30% less than survival following liver transplantation for other etiologies of advanced cirrhosis [8]. Therefore, patients with positive for hepatitis B surface antigen (HBsAg) had been regarded as poor candidates for liver transplantation. After Hepatitis B immuneglobulin (HBIG) and nucleoside analogues diminished the risk of HBV recurrence and led to improvement in patient and graft survival, liver transplantation is now considered to be the standard of care in patients with end-stage liver disease related to HBV [9-11]. The modern antiviral management improved the outcome of hepatitis B patients after liver transplantation. The results after OLT are nowadays reported to be as good or in a recent UNOS database report even better than in non-HBV patients. Now we summarize the mechanisms, prophylaxis, and treatment of HBV recurrent after liver transplantation.

Mechanisms of HBV Recurrent after Liver Transplant

After removal of the major source of HBV replication (i.e., the infected native liver), HBV reinfection is the consequence of either an immediate reinfection of the graft due to circulating HBV particles, of a reinfection of the graft from HBV particles coming from extrahepatic sites or both. The presence of active HBV replication before OLT is a reflection of a high circulating viral load with the ability to rapidly infect the graft. HBV-infected patients undergoing OLT without any prophylaxis developed HBV recurrence at a rate of more than 80% of patients 2 months after transplant [12]. HBV reinfection is characterized by appearance HBsAg in serum with high HBV replication. HBsAg may or may not disappear from serum in the first few weeks, but within 2 to 5 weeks after OLT, immunoperoxidase staining on liver biopsy can identify cytoplasmic expression of hepatitis B core antigen (HBcAg), typically without histologic features of hepatitis. In the subsequent several weeks, biochemical evidence of graft dysfunction is accompanied by biopsy features of acute viral hepatitis, although the inflammatory response may be somewhat attenuated, presumably because of immunosuppression. Within several months of OLT, features of chronic hepatitis emerge, with accelerated progression to cirrhosis and graft failure within an average of 2.5 years postoperatively. Most cases of HBV reinfection occurred during the first 3 years post-transplantation and rarely thereafter [13].

The more aggressive course of post-OLT HBV infection probably results from a number of factors, including enhanced viral replication and attenuated host response. In the absence of some form of antiviral prophylaxis, there is a logarithmic increase in serum HBV DNA levels as well as appearance of HBeAg even if this antigen was absent pretransplantation. The level of pre-OLT viral replication in determining the likelihood of HBV recurrence was highlighted in a large multicenter study involving more than 300 [14]. A unique form of severe graft injury resulting from HBV recurrence termed fibrosing cholestatic hepatitis (FCH) leads to rapid graft failure. The biopsy features of FCH are notable, in addition to cholestasis and fibrosis, for relatively little inflammation with periportal fibrosis and ballooning of pericentral hepatocytes. There is also abundant hepatocyte expression of HBsAg and HBcAg. In patients with FCH, there is increased transcription of HBV, presumably accentuating HBV protein accumulation in hepatocytes. This severe evolution is probably related to the high amount of HBV antigens suggesting a direct cytopathic effect. This high amount of virous particles within the graft is probably the consequence of the immunosuppressive therapy, which enhances HBV replication [15]. Hence, rapid reduction of corticosteroids in liver transplant recipients with HBV infection is a common practice. HBV recurrence can also rapidly progress to acute hepatocellular failure [14].

It has been reported that Asian race with presumed infancy-acquired or childhood-acquired HBV as a predictor of a poorer outcome resulting from aggressive recurrence of HBV after OLT [16]. It had been suggested that the apparent poorer outcome reflected more advanced liver disease at the time of OLT. However, a recent multicenter U.S. experience again has confirmed the observation that recurrent HBV is more lethal in Asian patients for reasons that remain to be elucidated [17].

HBV reinfection has a major impact on graft and patient survival. The outcome of patients undergoing transplantation in the United States from three major participating programs between 1990 and 1994 indicate that the survival of patients undergoing transplantation for HBV was significantly poorer not only when compared with the benchmark survival of cholestatic forms of cirrhosis (e.g., primary biliary cirrhosis and primary sclerosing cholangitis) but also when compared with the hepatitis C virus infected group [18]. In a retrospective multicenter U.S. experience of HBV recurrence, 1- and 5-year survival rates were significantly diminished, at 72% and 51%, respectively, compared with a control group undergoing transplantation for other forms of cirrhosis in which the corresponding survival rates were 84% and 74%, respectively. The decreased survival rates in patients undergoing transplantation for HBV were again predominantly related to recurrent allograft hepatitis [18]. Therefore, after initial graft failure resulting from recurrent HBV with a typically rapid infection of the new graft and progressive liver injury, the some patients had to undergoing retransplantation [19].

Related Factors of HBV Recurrence

1. Preoperative HBV Replication:

Pretransplant HBV DNA levels were significantly higher in patients with HBV reinfection than in those without it. Since HBV exists not only in the liver but also in circulation and other extrahepatic tissues, such as, the bone marrow, kidney, pancreas, and peripheral blood mononuclear cells, OLT could not completely eliminate virus replication outside the liver. Samuel, et al reported, the recurrence rate of HBV DNA and HBeAg-positive cirrhosis patients was 83%, but HBV DNA and HBeAg-negative was 58% [14]. In addition, The graft loss rates significantly increased in patients with preoperative positive HBV DNA [20]. The similar results also were confirmed by other doctors [21]. Therefore, most reports proposed to decrease preoperative viral replication and convert HBV DNA to negative before OLT using antiviral agents [22,23].

2. Immunosuppressants Protocol

Cyclosporin A, FK506 and prednisone are the most widely used immunosuppressive agents in OLT. The effect of immunosuppressive agents and glucocorticoid-responsive receptor on HBV genome also plays an important role in this process. Therapeutic immunosuppression is implicated in the enhanced viral replication by a series of observations. For example, the HBV genome contains a steroid-sensitive receptor with in vitro data from a hepatoma cell line of increased HBV DNA production upon exposure to steroids or azathioprine [15]. Corticosteroid may activate the glucocorticoid responsive element in the HBV genome to enhance HBV replication and gene expression [24,25]. Steroid-free immunosuppression in OLT patients was safe and effective [26]. Even though in an in vitro study in hepatocytes from patients with chronic HBV, acute tacrolimus (FK506) administration did not increase HBV replication, it is conceivable that longer immunosuppressants administration after OLT might promote the vigorous replication of HBV directly or through inhibiting the immune system. Immunosuppressants may also impair T cell function, thereby reducing immune-mediated hepatocytolysis and virus clearance. Therefore, when the use of immunosuppressive regimen is determined, it should be considered the balance between HBV recurrence in the graft and the immunosuppression of the host.

3. Drug Resistance and Mutation

HBV is a DNA virus, but its replication includes an RNA-intermediate requiring a step of reverse transcription. In addition, The HBV reverse transcriptase lacks a proofreading function. Therefore, the mutation rate of HBV is more than 10-fold increased compared to other DNA viruses. The mutation of YMDD locus and HBIG-resistant strains has become the major issue of concern. It was reported that YMDD mutation appeared in 20%-60% of liver transplant recipients treated with lamivudine [27,28]. Liver disease may be more clinically severe in the presence of naturally occurring precore mutant forms of HBV, which fail to secrete HBeAg [29], there had been concern that recurrence with this form of HBV would be also more severe after OLT. However, it appears that the presence of a precore mutant per se does not enhance the risk of HBV recurrence or graft loss in a recent European experience [30].

Hepatitis B Immune Globulin Prevent HBV Recurrence

Since Samuel's landmark study showed that the significant predictors of nonrecurrence were high-dose hepatitis B immune globulin (HBIG) for more than 6 months, absence of serum markers of active HBV replication, and acute HBV infection [12], there has been a rapid evolution in the understanding and management of hepatitis B infection in liver transplant recipients in the past decade. Effective modalities for prophylaxis of recurrent hepatitis B have significantly improved the graft and patient survival rates to a level comparable to those of other liver transplant recipients.

Passive immunoprophylaxis using parenteral HBIG was clinically effective in reducing HBV reinfection and improving graft survival after liver transplantation. It has been hypothesized that HBIG protects naive hepatocytes against HBV released from extrahepatic sites through blocking of a putative HBV receptor [17]. Alternatively, it may neutralize circulating virions through immune precipitation and immune complex formation [31]. Overall, the HBV reinfection rate was substantially lower (40%) than the historical rates observed in patients who did not receive HBIG immunoprophylaxis [12]. But under ongoing HBIG prophylaxis, about 15% to 50% of patients develop HBV recurrence, mostly due to escape mutations with alterations of the HBsAg structure. Factors associated with a decreased risk of HBV recurrence include HDV coinfection, acute liver failure, absence of viral replication before transplantation (HBV DNA negative, HBe antigen negative), and high-dose HBIg application [32]. Despite the evidence supporting the beneficial effect of HBIG prophylaxis, the optimal dosage and duration of HBIG therapy remain controversial. Administration of regular high-dose HBIG intravenously for more than 6 months postoperatively protected against HBV recurrence, but shorter-term administration did not [14]. In addition, the finding of HBV DNA in peripheral blood mononuclear cells beyond 12 months of HBIG prophylaxis suggests that the virus cannot be eradicated and there is an indefinite risk of reinfection [29]. Discontinuation of HBIG therapy, even years after transplantation, carries a high risk of graft reinfection and, therefore, there is a need for indefinite lifelong therapy with a high cost. Furthermore, breakthrough reinfection would still develop in 10% to 20% of patients receiving lifelong high-dose HBIG [30]. Sawyer et al. reported that 9 of 39 patients (23%) who received HBIG therapy to maintain an anti-HBs level greater than 500 IU/L for the first 6 months and greater than 150 IU/L thereafter developed recurrence [31]. In patients receiving HBIG, HBV reinfection may be the consequence of HBV overproduction coming from extrahepatic sites, of a too low protective titer of anti-HBs antibody, or of emergence of escape mutants. The majority of the HBIG failure can be attributed to the selection pressure on the surface antigen gene leading to the emergence of mutants that lack affinity for anti-HBs [32].

Lamivudine in Prophylaxis for Recurrence

Lamivudine, a cytosine analog, can inhibit reverse transcriptase of HBV by interfering with the synthesis of the proviral DNA chain from pre-genomic viral messenger RNA. It has been demonstrated efficacy against HBV after liver transplantation [33]. In patients awaiting liver transplantation, treatment with lamivudine results in stabilization of the disease as reflected by improvement in biochemical parameters and a greater survival rate without transplantation when compared with historic controls [34]. As with prophylaxis of recurrence, the availability of lamivudine has dramatically improved the management of established recurrent HBV in the patient undergoing OLT. A number of reports have described excellent suppression of HBV replication with lessening of allograft biochemical and histologic dysfunction. Perillo et al. [34] demonstrated that among 42 patients who underwent transplantation in the study by with more than 12 weeks of post-OLT follow-up, 25 (60%) did not have evidence of HBsAg. Six of the 17 reinfected patients remained persistently HBsAg positive after OLT, and 11 had transient loss of HBsAg. Lo et al [35]. reported that results of the initial experience with lamivudine monoprophylaxis in 31 patients. Twenty-three of 31 patients (74%) were positive for HBeAg or HBV DNA before lamivudine treatment. At a median follow-up of 16 months, breakthrough reinfection caused by YMDD mutant was detected in only one patient (3.8%), and the patient survival rate was 84%. Unfortunately, a proportion of patients develop mutations in the YMDD motif of the HBV polymerise gene, and the likelihood of emergence of mutants is related to duration of therapy. Mutimer et al. [36] reported that 11 of 17 patients (65%) survived at a median follow-up of 36 months after transplantation. The cause of death in two of the six patients who died during the observation period was graft failure from recurrent hepatitis B, and 2 of 11 survivors also developed breakthrough reinfection caused by the YMDD mutant. The optimal time to initiate therapy with a reasonable expectation of clinical response but without placing the recipient at greater risk of developing these mutations is undefined, although a recent case report describes a patient with a YMDD mutant who remained free of HBV recurrence 2.5 years after OLT with combination high-dose HBIG and lamivudine. In a recent report from Germany [37], two patients with YMDD mutants before OLT rapidly developed HBV reinfection despite combined prophylaxis. Although as with lamivudine use in other settings, there is ultimately frequent emergence of the YMDD mutation with an associated reduction in drug efficacy. The rates of emergence of lamivudine resistance in patients treated for recurrent HBV after OLT were13-45%. In the study with the longest duration of lamivudine treatment after OLT, Fontana et al. [37] demonstrated that 45% of patients developed evidence of virologic breakthrough. Moreover, although most data suggest that the YMDD mutant virus is not consistently associated with hepatic disease progression in the short term [38]. In a report from the Royal Free Hospital of 17 patients who received lamivudine without HBIG, 2 patients died at 19 and 23 months after OLT from graft failure [39]. Both patients had YMDD variants detected at 12 months after OLT; two additional patients developed YMDD variants but remain alive at 9 and 15 months. In addition, it was noted that some patients developed anti-HBs seroconversion. Cessation of lamivudine therapy in patients with such variants results in a reversion to wild-type HBV and may be associated with an increase in the levels of HBV DNA and ALT, so most authorities favor continuing lamivudine long term in an effort to prevent return of this potentially more virulent strain of HBV. A recent series of five patients with DNA polymerase mutant HBV (including four who had undergone liver transplantation) indicates that adefovir dipivoxil has potent inhibitory effects on both resistant and wild-type HBV, although nephrotoxicity was a concern [40]. In a patient with lamivudine-resistant YMDD mutant before transplantation, a combination of adefovir and high-dose HBIG had been used to prevent graft reinfection with success [41]. Lo et al. [42] reported five patients with YMDD mutants have undergone liver transplantation using a combination of adefovir and HBIG with excellent results. This combination appears to be an effective option for patients who require transplantation after the emergence of lamivudine-resistant strains. Other candidate nucleoside analogs such as entecavir may also prove useful but will require further study.

Combination Hepatitis B Immune Globulin and Lamivudine

Combination of lamivudine and high-dose HBIG as prophylaxis was first reported by Markowitz et al. [43]. As a result of the significant rate of failure with single-agent prophylaxis with either HBIG or lamivudine, combination therapy using both HBIG and lamivudine is increasingly regarded as a more effective approach. The rationale for combination therapy includes decreased likelihood of saturation of HBIG binding sites by a high viral burden, thus decreasing the pressure to select for HBIG mutants. In addition, HBIG binds viral particles and decreases the substrate available for lamivudine, theoretically reducing the risk for YMDD mutant development [44]. A recent survey of 19 liver transplant centers found that combination HBIG plus lamivudine was the most frequent prophylactic regimen [44]. The use of combination lamivudine and HBIG (high or low dose) has been reported in several hundred patients treated throughout the world, with recurrence rates consistently less than 10% [45]. Generally, patients with active HBV replication have been treated with lamivudine before OLT to diminish replication, with all patients receiving both lamivudine and HBIG after OLT. Substantially better results than with either lamivudine or HBIG prophylaxis alone have been reported by several groups, and the challenge has become the identification of the most cost-effective combination regimen given the expense of long-term intravenous HBIG either given as a fixed monthly dose or titrated to anti-HBs levels. Marzano et al. [46] in a recent report observed HBV recurrence in only 1 (4%) of 26 patients who had received lamivudine before OLT, followed by combination prophylaxis. Importantly, a number of studies have indicated that the total amount of HBIG necessary to maintain anti-HBs levels above 100 IU/L was lower in the combination prophylaxis group than historical controls who had received HBIG alone [45]. Angus et al. [47] used intramuscular HBIG given at a dose of 400 to 800 IU daily for a week after transplant and then monthly thereafter. At a median follow-up of 18 months, 31 of 32 patients remained HBsAg negative. Yao et al. [48] used a single dose of intravenous HBIG followed by intramuscular HBIG every 3 weeks in nonviremic patients, but selected viremic patients for additional intravenous administration of HBIG daily during the first week. During a mean follow-up of 15.6 months, 1 of 10 patients developed virologic and histologic evidence of recurrence. Such an approach seems to provide adequate allograft protection without the prohibitively high cost of high-dose HBIG and may become the prophylaxis of choice in the future. These reports, however, involve small samples with short follow-up and the low recurrence rate needs to be confirmed with long-term follow-up in large-scale studies.

We evaluate the efficacy of low-dose hepatitis B immune globulin (HBIG) and lamivudine in the prevention of recurrent HBV after liver transplantation. In our liver transplantation center, 202 patients who underwent liver transplantation were included in the study. All patients in the anhepatic phase were given 2000 IU of HBIG. Post-transplantation 1000 IU HBIG was administered intravenously daily for 7 days, and then 1000 IU intravenously once a week, or 400 IU intramuscularly daily or 2-3 times weekly, according to serum titer of antibodies to hepatitis B surface antigen (anti-HBs). Anti-HBs titer was 500 U/L within 6 months, 200 U/L within 12 months, and 100 U/L after 12 months post-transplantation. Lamivudine 100 mg/day was administered before and after transplantation and was administrated indefinitely. Median follow-up was 19 months (range 3-49 months). Recurrence of hepatitis B surface antigen (HBsAg)-positivity occurred in 13 out of 202 (6.4%) patients. Therefore, combined low-dose HBIG and lamivudine is effective in patients with controlled viral reinfection after liver transplantation. It is likely to be more cost-effective, and well tolerated.

In an attempt to reduce the financial burden of high-dose, lifelong HBIG, the use of sequential HBIG therapy for 2 years after transplantation followed by lamivudine monotherapy has been shown to be effective in preventing reinfection in patients with a low level of pretransplant viral replication [40].

Active Immunization

Although long-term combined hepatitis B immunoglobulins and lamivudine could be markedly reduced the reinfection rate and significantly improved survival rates, in immunosuppressed patients, a complete eradication of HBV is rarely possible. After liver transplantation in half of the patients HBV can be detected in extrahepatic reservoirs like peripheral white blood cells even 10 years of ongoing successful hepatitis B immunoglobulin (HBIg) prophylaxis [49]. Therefore, the recommended life long prophylaxis regimen against hepatitis B virus recurrence after liver transplantation is highly expensive. A recent study from Barcelona challenged the approach of most transplant centers-that is, HBIG administration on a life-long basis-by demonstrating the efficacy of a new prophylactic strategy consisting of the discontinuation of HBIG administration followed by active immunization with HBV vaccination [50]. Among highly selected group of 17 patients undergoing OLT with nonreplicative HBV who had received at least 18 months of HBIG, 14 (82%) developed protective serum titers of anti-HBs after HBV vaccination. By allowing discontinuation of HBIG prophylaxis, this strategy may be highly cost-effective. Bienzle et al. [51] used an intramuscular recombinant HBV vaccine combined with two immunostimulants under continuation of passive immunoprophylaxis: in 16 out of 20 patients (80%) protective antibody titers of more than 500 U/l were achieved and HBIg could be stopped subsequently. In contrast, a preliminary study from Italy demonstrated the vaccination starting 4 months after HBIG discontinuation (in conjunction with lamivudine treatment) with ineffective in yielding a protective anti-HBs titer in more than 90% of patients [52]. Whether the resultant antibody production will provide durable protection again HBV recurrence will need further follow-up, particularly as vaccine-induced anti-HBs declines even in the immune competent host over time. Seven male patients undergoing liver transplanted for hepatitis B virus-related cirrhosis were administrated a double reinforced course of S-recombinant hepatitis B virus vaccination. At the end of both the first and the second vaccination cycle none of the patients developed an anti-HBs titer greater than the basal anti-HBs titer [53]. Clearly, a vaccination-based strategy warrants further study in larger groups of patients, including those treated with other prophylactic regimens.

Treatment of the Reinfected Recipient

Because of the rapid viral replication in the immunocompromised host, emergence of lamivudine-resistant YMDD mutant is frequent. The significance of the development of lamivudine-resistant strains on the outcome of the liver graft is not fully understood. YMDD mutants have been said to have low replication competence [54], but breakthrough reinfection by mutants after liver transplantation has been associated with severe hepatitis, fibrosis, and graft failure [33,34]. Treatment of recurrent hepatitis B includes reduction of immunosuppression and alternative antiviral agents. There is little role for HBIG therapy in established recurrence. Reinfection by wild-type virus or surface mutants after failure of HBIG prophylaxis typically is characterized by an extremely high viral replication rate and histologic changes that may progress to severe fibrosis with cholestasis and hepatocyte ballooning, referred to as FCH [55].

Famciclovir, ganciclovir, or interferon alone is of limited efficacy. But lamivudine is the most effective treatment for suppressing the HBV replication [56]. Adefovir has been used successfully on a compassionate-use basis in the treatment of breakthrough reinfection caused by YMDD mutants and, so far, no adefovir-resistant strain has been identified [57]. The advent of adefovir and other antiviral agents, probably in combination, provides more effective therapeutic options in the treatment of HBV recurrence after liver transplantation.

Conclusion

End-stage liver disease related to HBV-infected is indicated liver transplantation. Hepatitis B immune globulin (HBIG) and lamivudine have dramatically reduced HBV reinfection and improving graft survival after liver transplantation. Combination of HBIG and lamivudine is the most effective porphylatic regimen. HBIG and lamivudine generally need to be administrated indefinitely. Recently the use of sequential HBIG therapy for 2 years after transplantation followed by lamivudine monotherapy has been shown to be effective in preventing reinfection in patients with a low level of pretransplant viral replication. Also, active immunization with HBV vaccination, a new prophylactic strategy by allowing discontinuation of HBIG prophylaxis may be highly cost-effective, although it is not confirmed by all researchers.

REFERENCES

[1] Alter MJ. Epidemiology and prevention of hepatitis B. *Semin Liver Dis*. 2003;23:39-46.

[2] Zhao S, Xu Z, Lu Y. A mathematical model of hepatitis B virus transmission and its application for vaccination strategy in China. *Int J Epidemiol*. 2000;29:744-752.

[3] Liu CB, Xu ZY, Cao HL. Sero-epidemiology of HBV infection in four provinces in China. *Chin J Virol* 1991;7(Suppl.):8–14.

[4] Lucey MR, Neuberger J, Shaked A. *Liver Transplantation*. Georgetown: Landes Bioscience, 2003:89

[5] European Liver Transplant Registry (ELTR) - Registry for the European liver transplant association, data analysis, 05/1968-6/2002, online: Available at http://www.eltr.org.

[6] Seaberg EC, Belle SH, Beringer KC, et al. Liver transplantation in the United States from 1987-1998: Updated results from the Pitt-UNOS liver transplant registry. In Cecka JM, Terasaki PI(eds): *Clinical Transplants 1998*, Los Angeles, UCLA Tissue Typing Laboratory,1999,p17-37)

[7] Lake JR. liver transplantation for chronic viral hepatitis. In Busattil RW, Klintmalm GB: *Transplantation of Liver*. Philadelphia: WB Saunders Company, 1996; 85-92

[8] Dodson SF, Issa S, Araya V, Gayowski T, Pinna A, Eghtesad B, et al. Infectivity of hepatic allografts with antibodies to hepatitis B virus. *Transplantation*. 1997;64:1582-1584.

[9] Shouval D and Samuel D. Hepatitis B immune globulin to prevent HBV graft reinfection following liver transplantation: a concise review. *Hepatology*, 2000;32 :1189–1195

[10] Anselmo DM, Ghobrial RM, Jung LC, Weaver M, Cao C, Saab S, et al. New era of liver transplantation for hepatitis B: a 17-year single-center experience. *Ann Surg*. 2002;235:611-619

[11] Sponseller CA, Ramrakhiani S. Treatment of hepatitis B and C following liver transplantation. *Curr Gastroenterol Rep* 2002;4:52-62

[12] Todo S, Demetris AJ, Van Thiel D, Teperman L, Fung JJ, Starzl TE. Orthotopic liver transplantation for patients with hepatitis B virus-related liver disease. *Hepatology* 1991, 13: 619-626

[13] Samuel D, Bismuth H, Marcellin P, Benhamou JP. Liver transplantation in the management of chronic viral hepatitis in: Zuckerman AJ, Thomas HC, eds. *Viral Hepatitis, 2nd Edition*. Churchill Livingstone: Harcourt Asia; 2001:237-244.

[14] Samuel D, Muller R, Alexander G, Fassati L, Ducot B, Benhamou JP, Bismuth H. Liver transplantation in European patients with the hepatitis B surface antigen. *N Engl J Med*, 1993;329(25):1842-7

[15] Demetris AJ, Todo S, Van Thiel DH, Fung JJ, Iwaki Y, Sysyn G, et al. Evolution of hepatitis B virus liver disease after hepatic replacement. Practical and theoretical considerations. *Am J Pathol*. 1990;137:667-676.

[16] Ho BM, So SK, Esquivel CO, Keeffe EB. Liver transplantation in Asian patients with chronic hepatitis B. *Hepatology*. 1997;25:223-225.

[17] Teo EK, Han SH, Terrault N, Luketic V, Jensen D, Keeffe EB, et al. Liver transplantation in patients with hepatitis B virus infection: outcome in Asian versus white patients. *Hepatology*. 2001;34:126-132.

[18] Charlton M, Seaberg E, Wiesner R, Everhart J, Zetterman R, Lake J, et al. Predictors of patient and graft survival following liver transplantation for hepatitis C. *Hepatology*. 1998;28:823-830.

[19] Wang ZF, Liu C. Liver Retransplantation: indications and outcome. *Hepatobiliary Pancreat Dis Int.* 2004;3:161-164

[20] Terrault NA, Zhou S, Combs C, Hahn JA, Lake JR, Roberts JP, Ascher NL, Wright TL. Prophylaxis in liver transplant recipients using a fixed dosing schedule of hepatitis B immunoglobulin. *Hepatology*, 1996;24(6):1327-33.

[21] Protzer-Knolle U, Naumann U, Bartenschlager R, et al. Hepatitis B virus with antigenically altered hepatitis B surface antigen is selected by high-dose hepatitis B immune globulin after liver transplantation. *Hepatology* 1998; 27: 254.

[22] Bramhall SR, Minford E, Gunson B, Buckels JA. Liver transplantation in the UK. *World J Gastroenterol* 2001;7:602-611. 25

[23] Seehofer D, Rayes N, Naumann U, Neuhaus R, Muller AR, Tullius SG, et al. Preoperative antiviral treatment and postopera-tive prophylaxis in HBV-DNA positive patients undergoing liver transplantation. *Transplantation* 2001;72:1381-1385.

[24] Liaw YF. Hepatitis viruses under immunosuppressive agents. *J Gastroenterol Hepatol* 1998;13:14-20.

[25] Shiota G, Harada K, Oyama K, Udagawa A, Nomi T, Tanaka K, et al. Severe exacerbation of hepatitis after short-term corticosteroid therapy in a patients with "latent" chronic hepatitis B. *Liver* 2000;20:415-420.

[26] Tisone G, Angelico M, Orlando G, Palmieri CP, Strati F, Di Paolo D, et al. Retrospective analysis of 30 patients who underwent liver transplantation without use of steroid. *Transplant Proc* 1999;31:2908-2909.

[27] Ben-Ari Z, Daudi N, Klein A, Sulkes J, Papo O, Mor E, et al. Genotypic and phenotypic resistance: longitudinal and sequential analysis of hepatitis B virus polymerase mutations in patients with lamivudine resistance after liver transplantation. *Am J Gastroenterol* 2003;98:151-159.

[28] Kim KH, Lee KH, Chang HY, Ahn SH, Tong S, Yoon YJ, et al. Evolution of hepatitis B virus sequence from a liver transplant recipient with rapid breakthrough despite hepatitis B immune globulin prophylaxis and lamivudine therapy. *J Med Virol* 2003;71:367-375.

[29] Feray C, Zignego AL, Samuel D, Bismuth A, Reynes M, Tiollais P, et al. Persistent hepatitis B virus infection of mononuclear blood cells without concomitant liver infection: The liver transplantation model. *Transplantation* 1990; 49: 1155-1158

[30] Naumann U, Protzer-Knolle U, Berg T, Leder K, Lobeck H, Bechstein WO, et al. A pretransplant infection with precore mutants of hepatitis B virus does not influence the outcome of orthotopic liver transplantation in patients on high dose anti-hepatitis B virus surface antigen immunoprophylaxis. *Hepatology*. 1997;26:478-484.

[31] Sawyer RG, McGory RW, Gaffey MJ, et al. Improved clinical outcome with liver transplantation for hepatitis B- induced chronic liver failure using passive Immunization. *Ann Surg* 1998; 227: 841-850.
[32] Protzer-Knolle U, Naumann U, Bartenschlager R, Berg T, Hopf U, Meyer zum Buschenfelde KH, et al. Hepatitis B virus with antigenically altered hepatitis B surface antigen is selected by high-dose hepatitis B immune globulin after liver transplantation. *Hepatology* 1998; 27: 254-263
[33] Lu SC, Yan LN, Li B, Wen TF, Zhao JC, Cheng NS, et al. Lamivudine prophylaxis of liver allograft HBV reinfection in HBV related cirrhotic patients after liver transplantation. *Hepatobiliary Pancreat Dis Int*. 2004;3:26-32.
[34] Perrillo RP, Wright T, Rakela J, Levy G, Schiff E, Gish R, et al. A multicenter United States-Canadian trial to assess lamivudine monotherapy before and after liver transplantation for chronic hepatitis B. *Hepatology*. 001;33:424-432
[35] Lo CM, Cheung ST, Lai CL, Liu CL, Ng IO, Yuen MF, et al. Liver transplantation in Asian patients with chronic hepatitis B using lamivudine prophylaxis. *Ann Surg* 2001; 233: 276-281
[36] Mutimer D, Dusheiko G, Barrett C, Grellier L, Ahmed M, Anschuetz G, et al. Lamivudine without HBIg for prevention of graft reinfection by hepatitis B: Long-term follow-up. *Transplantation* 2000; 70: 809-815.
[37] Saab S, Kim M, Wright TL, Han SH, Martin P, Busuttil RW. Successful orthotopic liver transplantation for lamivudine-associated YMDD mutant hepatitis B virus. *Gastroenterology*. 2000;119:1382-1384.
[38] Fontana RJ, Hann HW, Wright T, Everson G, Baker A, Schiff ER, et al. A multicenter study of lamivudine treatment in 33 patients with hepatitis B after liver transplantation. *Liver Transpl*. 2001;7:504-510.
[39] Perrillo R, Rakela J, Dienstag J, Levy G, Martin P, Wright T, et al. Multicenter study of lamivudine therapy for hepatitis B after liver transplantation.Lamivudine Transplant Group. *Hepatology*. 1999;29:1581-1586.
[40] Perrillo R, Schiff E, Yoshida E, Statler A, Hirsch K, Wright T, et al. Adefovir dipivoxil for the treatment of lamivudine-resistant hepatitis B mutants. *Hepatology*. 2000;32:129-134.
[41] Dodson SF, de Vera ME, Bonham CA, Geller DA, Rakela J, Fung JJ. Lamivudine after hepatitis B immune globulin is effective in preventing hepatitis B recurrence after liver transplantation. *Liver Transpl* 2000; 6: 434-439.
[42] Saab S, Kim M, Wright TL, Han SH, Martin P, Busuttil RW. Successful orthotopic liver transplantation for lamivudine-associated YMDD mutant hepatitis B virus. *Gastroenterology* 2000; 119: 1382.1384
[43] Lo CM, Fan ST, Liu CL, Lai CL, Wong J. Prophylaxis and treatment of recurrent hepatitis B after liver transplantation. *Transplantation*. 2003;75(3 Suppl):S41-44.
[44] Markowitz JS, Martin P, Conrad AJ, Markmann JF, Seu P, Yersiz H, et al. Prophylaxis against hepatitis B recurrence following liver transplantation using combination lamivudine and hepatitis B immune globulin. *Hepatology* 1998; 28: 585-589
[45] Han SH, Ofman J, Holt C, King K, Kunder G, Chen P, et al. An efficacy and cost-effectiveness analysis of combination hepatitis B immune globulin and lamivudine to

prevent recurrent hepatitis B after orthotopic liver transplantation compared with hepatitis B immune globulin monotherapy. *Liver Transpl.* 2000;6:741-748.

[46] Rizzetto M, Marzano A. Posttransplantation prevention and treatment of recurrent hepatitis B. *Liver Transpl.* 2000;6(6 Suppl 2):S47-51.

[47] Marzano A, Salizzoni , Wilma Debernardi-Venon, Antonina Smedile, Alessandro Franchello, Alessia Ciancio, et al. Prevention of hepatitis B virus recurrence after liver transplantation in cirrhotic patients treated with lamivudine and passive immunoprophylaxis. *Journal of Hepatology*, 2001,34: 903-910

[48] Angus PW, McCaughan GW, Gane EJ, Crawford DH, Harley H. Combination low-dose hepatitis B immune globulin and lamivudine therapy provides effective prophylaxis against post-transplantation hepatitis B. *Liver Transpl* 2000; 6: 429-433.

[49] Roche B, Feray C, Gigou M, et al. HBV DNA persistence 10 years after liver transplantation despite successful anti-HBS passive immunoprophylaxis. *Hepatology*, 2003;38:86

[50] Yao FY, Osorio RW, Roberts JP, Poordad FF, Briceno MN, Garcia-Kennedy R, et al. Intramuscular hepatitis B immune globulin combined with lamivudine for prophylaxis against hepatitis B recurrence after liver transplantation. *Liver Transpl Surg* 1999; 5: 491-496

[51] Sanchez-Fueyo A, Rimola A, Grande L, Costa J, Mas A, Navasa M, et al. Hepatitis B immunoglobulin discontinuation followed by hepatitis B virus vaccination: A new strategy in the prophylaxis of hepatitis B virus recurrence after liver transplantation. *Hepatology*, 2000;31:496-501.

[52] Bienzle U, Gunther M, Neuhaus R, et al. Immunization with an adjuvant hepatitis B vaccine after liver transplantation for hepatitis B-related disease. *Hepatology* 2003; 38: 811.

[53] Angelico M, Di Paolo D, Trinito MO, Petrolati A, Araco A, Zazza S, et al. Failure of a reinforced triple course of hepatitis B vaccination in patients transplanted for HBV-related cirrhosis. *Hepatology*. 2002;35:176-181.

[54] Di Paolo D, Lenci I, Trinito MO, Carbone M, Longhi C, Tisone G, Angelico M. Extended double-dosage HBV vaccination after liver transplantation is ineffective, in the absence of lamivudine and prior wash-out of human Hepatitis B immunoglobulins. *Dig Liver Dis*. 2006;38(10):749-54.

[55] Ling R, Mutimer D, Ahmed M, Boxall EH, Elias E, Dusheiko GM, et al. Selection of mutations in the hepatitis B virus polymerase during therapy of transplant recipients with lamivudine. *Hepatology* 1996; 24: 711-713

[56] Sanchez-Fueyo A, Rimola A, Grande L, Costa J, Mas A, Navasa M, et al. Hepatitis B immunoglobulin discontinuation followed by hepatitis B virus vaccination: A new strategy in the prophylaxis of hepatitis B virus recurrence after liver transplantation. *Hepatology* 2000; 31: 496-501

[57] Angelico M, Di Paolo D, Trinito MO, Petrolati A, Araco A, Zazza S, .et al. Failure of a reinforced triple course of hepatitis B vaccination in patients transplanted for HBV-related cirrhosis. *Hepatology* 2002; 35: 176-181.

In: Hepatitis B Research Advances
Editor: Alicia P. Willis, pp. 215-234
ISBN: 978-1-60021-666-4

Chapter XIII

HEPATITIS B VIRUS MUTANTS AND THEIR CLINICAL IMPLICATIONS

Beatriz María García-Montalvo *

Banco Central de Sangre, Centro Médico Nacional "Lic. Ignacio García Téllez", Instituto Mexicano del Seguro Social, Mérida, Yucatán, México

ABSTRACT

Hepatitis B (HBV) is the most important of the viruses that cause human hepatitis. Approximately 2 billion people worldwide have come into contact with HBV and over 350 million are chronic HBV carriers. HBV is a hepatotropic virus with a partial double-helix DNA genome within a central nucleocapsid covered by a coating containing the surface antigen (HBsAg). Its gene replication and expression is principally restricted to hepatocytes in the infectious process. Infection with HBV leads to a wide range of hepatic damage, including self-controlled hepatitis B, fulminant hepatitis, chronic hepatitis with progression to cirrhosis or acute exacerbation that can lead to hepatic failure, and a chronic asymptomatic carrier condition. There are numerous reports of mutations in all the viral genes and regulatory elements of the HBV genome, some of which arise during clearing of the infection by the immune system or after human interventions such as vaccination and antiviral therapy. Mutants that escape vaccination are characterized by mutations in the HBsAg antigen site and can cause mutations in other viral proteins implicated in acute or chronic hepatic disease. Given this phenomenon, epidemiological monitoring of HBV mutants is required to prevent their spread and possible hepatitis B outbreaks. This review focuses on regions of the viral genome that are frequently affected by mutations and the implications of these mutations in the pathogenesis of hepatic disease.

* Correspondence concerning this article should be addressed to Dr. Beatriz María García-Montalvo. Mailing address: Calle 19 No. 430 x 50, Fraccionamiento Jardines de Mérida, 97135 Mérida, Yucatán, México. Tel: +52 (999) 943 61 36; Fax: +52 (999) 943 22 84; E-mail: bgarciam04@yahoo.com.mx

Introduction

Hepatitis B virus (HBV) infection is a significant global public health concern. An estimated 2 billion people worldwide have come in contact with the virus and over 350 million people are chronic HBV carriers [1]. Of these, 75% live in South East Asia and the Western Pacific [2]. Approximately 400,000 new cases occur annually in Latin America alone, of which 25 to 67% become chronic [3]. The clinical course of HBV can vary from an unapparent, self-limiting infection to chronic hepatitis that can lead to severe complications such as cirrhosis and hepatocellular carcinoma [4]. Liver damage from HBV infection is caused by host response to the viral antigens expressed on the surface of liver cells; it is mediated by MCH Class-I and -II restricted cytotoxic T-lymphocytes. The virus's cytopathic effect may play a lesser role [5].

Of all the DNA viruses than can infect humans, HBV has the smallest genome (3.2 kb) and a unique replication strategy with a reverse transcription intermediate stage. Because the reverse transcriptase activity of the HBV polymerase protein lacks a proof- reading function, random misincorporation of base pairs in the replicating DNA strand can occur. Introduction of mutations leads to generation and formation of a quasispecies pool [6]. The genomic DNA of the HBV is located within a central nucleocapsid covered by an envelope consisting of a host cell-derived lipid bilayer and viral surface proteins. It has 4 partially-overlapping, open reading frames (ORFs) that code for the core antigen (HBcAg) and e antigen (HBeAg); surface proteins (HBsAg); polymerase proteins; and X protein [7]. The HBsAg is a complex antigen with an "a" group determinant that is common to all the HBV subtypes. Based on the HBsAg antigenic determinants, HBV can be classified into four main subtypes (adr, adw, ayw and ayr) the prevalence of which varies by geographic area [8,9]. In addition, the 8% (or more) intergroup divergence in HBV's complete nucleotide sequence allows it to be further classified into eight different genotypes: A to H [10-13].

Mutations in all the viral genes and regulatory elements of the HBV genome have been identified. Some of these have emerged after human interventions such as vaccination [14] and antiviral therapy [15]. Mutants that escape vaccination are characterized by having mutations in sites antigenic to HBsAg, whereas mutations in other viral proteins are associated with resistance to antiviral therapy or are implicated in acute or chronic hepatic disease. Molecular identification of these different mutants could reveal the mechanisms by which they escape, identify the cause of HBV viral resistance and provide useful data for more effective eradication measures.

This review is focused on regions of the viral genome that are frequently affected by these mutations and the implications of these mutations in the pathogenesis of the resulting liver disease.

HBsAg Mutants

The viral proteins that form part of the HBV envelope are codified by three overlapping envelope genes contained within the same ORF: pre-S1, pre-S2, and S. These proteins have a common carboxy-terminal end, and, depending on the translated initiation site, produce three proteins: large (LHBsAg); middle (MHBsAg); and small (SHBsAg) [16-19]. The LHBsAg has 400 amino acid residues, is codified by the Pre-S1 sequence and is found in the envelope of circulating infectious virions. It is essential to virion assembly and is not efficiently secreted from cultured mammal cells. This protein is involved in the attachment of HBV to hepatocytes (amino acids 21 to 47) [20-22], as well as in protective immunity, the result of its containing B-cell and T-cell epitopes [23,24]. The MHBsAg has 281 amino acid residues, is produced by Pre-S2 + S and is apparently not indispensable to HBV virion assembly [16-19]. The SHBsAg has 226 amino acid residues and is the most abundant protein in the viral envelope.

Antigenicity of the HBs depends mainly on the structure of the "a" determinant, which is located within the major hydrophilic region (MHR) of the HBsAg (residue 100-160 in SHBsAg) [25,26]. The "a" determinant in the 124-147 amino acid region is highly preserved and is believed to adopt a two-loop structure on the virus exterior. This region is highly immunogenic and subject to selective pressure from the immune system. Antibodies against the "a" determinant protect against HBV infection, but amino acids substitutions within this determinant can lead to structural changes that can then affect the binding of neutralizing antibodies [27-29].

It has been proposed that "a" determinant mutations that occur during the natural course of infection are mainly observed in the first loop (amino acids 107 to 138) [27,30], whereas those induced under immune pressure from active and/or passive immunization are more frequently observed in the second loop (amino acids 139 to 147) [31-33].

Mutations in HBsAg have been reported in chronic infection [34] and fulminant hepatitis patients [35], after lamivudine treatment [36] and after liver transplants [37]. The most frequent of the HBsAg mutations is a simple substitution of glycine by arginine in the 145 position amino acid [29,38]. This mutation has been reported repeatedly in children actively and passively immunized immediately after birth, and born of HBsAg- and HBeAg-positive mothers, as well as in HBV carriers who received a liver transplant and were given immunoglobulin against hepatitis B to prevent transplant reinfection [29,38,39]. Some of these mutants cannot be detected by the reagents currently used in HBsAg screening, with significant clinical and epidemiological implications [40,41].

Seddigh-Tonekaboni et al. reported that Chinese blood donors positive only for antibodies against the central HBV antigen (anti-HBc) had an amino acid substitution in position 131 (I for T); none of the commercial screening kits detected HBsAg in these donors [42]. Amino acid substitutions (Q for R in position 129, and M for T in position 133) were also reported by Jongerius et al. in a blood donor with undetected HBsAg [43]. These variants may be acquired by blood transfusion or propagated by other means. Post-transfusion HBV infection from blood units that are HBsAg-negative, anti-HBc positive and HBV DNA-positive has been reported in a number of countries [44,45]. This is important because HBsAg-negative/anti-HBc-positive blood units are currently used in countries where anti-HBc screening is not required. Carman et al. reported two cases of T131I variants in patients from Papua New Guinea who were HBsAg-negative, but positive for both anti-HBc and antibodies against HBsAg (anti-HBs) [46]. The presence of HBV DNA in the blood of patients who are HBsAg-negative but anti-HBs positive may be due to a circulating

HBsAg/anti-HBs immune complex that prevents routine methods from detecting both the antigen and the antibody.

Coexistence of HBsAg and anti-HBs in chronic HBV carriers has been reported in a number of studies, even though these antibodies are usually protectors (i.e. neutralizing antibodies) [47-49]. Despite the presence of viral replication, the mechanism underlying the presence of both HBsAg and anti-HBs remains unclear, although one possible explanation is selection of HBsAg immune escape variants. Another contributing factor may be cumulative changes in T-helper-cell epitopes in chronic hepatitis patients. This may alter immune response efficiency and could facilitate virus persistence, as documented by Bauer et al. [50]. Some amino acid substitutions reported in chronic carriers that were HBsAg- and anti-HBs-positive are: G145R; I/T126N/S; Q129N; D144A; C107R; S45A; and I213L [48,49]. The S45A substitution is located at both a T- and B-cell epitope (positions 44 to 49), suggesting that this replacement may be crucial to immune escape [49].

Mutations in the Pre-S2 start codon prevent synthesis of this protein. Also, infection with a virus defective for Pre-S2 has been reported as frequently associated with fulminant hepatitis, suggesting that this variant may play a pathogenetic role in cases of acute liver failure [25]. Other researchers have associated mutants exhibiting deletions of 39-60 nucleotides in the Pre-S2 region with chronic HBV infections [51]. In an effort to determine the prevalence of the HBV variant with the pre-S mutant in countries with low and high endemic HBV infection levels, Huy et al. analyzed blood samples from patients with acute hepatitis, fulminant hepatitis, chronic hepatitis, liver cirrhosis and hepatocellular carcinoma, as well as asymptomatic carriers. They identified four Pre-S mutant patterns: a Pre-S1 in-frame deletion; a Pre-S2 in-frame deletion; both Pre-S1 and Pre-S2 deletions; and a point mutation in the Pre-S2 start codon. Nearly 35% of the HBV Pre-S mutants were identified in hepatocellular carcinoma patients. Moreover, their results show a high prevalence of the Pre-S mutant in patients infected with the B and C genotypes, which are major HBV genotypes in Asian countries [34]. *In vitro* research has shown that Pre-S1 mutants may cause a decrease in HBsAg secretion [52]. Overproduction and accumulation of LHBsAg may lead to severe, prolonged hepatocellular injury.

Mutations in different positions of the "a" determinant have been reported in vaccinated children: G145R; D144A; M133L; Q129H; and I/T126A [26]. Mutations within the "a" determinant often lead to emergence of mutants that escape vaccine-induced neutralizing antibodies. But mutations (N116T, V118A, P120S, A159V, F183C and V184A) have also been found outside the "a" determinant in Singaporean patients and vaccines that were HBsAg-negative. These mutants had altered binding affinity to anti-HBs [32,36].

Mutations in the S gene have been documented in patients given hyperimmune globulin against HBV as a prophylaxis to prevent reinfection after receiving a liver transplant. These mutations were induced or selected for due to the immune pressure applied by the immunoglobulin. HBV S gene mutations can play a role in reinfection of liver transplant recipients administered passive immune prophylaxis [53,54].

Circulation of some HBsAg mutants can pose a public health risk since neither current hepatitis B vaccines nor hyperimmune hepatitis B immune globulin effectively prevents the associated liver disease.

PRECORE/CORE MUTANTS

Hepatitis B virus precore/core (Pre-C/C) ORF codifies for two closely-related proteins: HBcAg and HBeAg. HBcAg is involved in capsid formation, packaging of the pregenome reverse transcriptase complex and capsid traffic in the cell and envelope. HBeAg is found in the blood and probably on the surface of hepatocytes, but does not form part of viral particles [55,56]. It is found in patient blood during active HBV replication. Both of these proteins are targets for both cytotoxic T-lymphocyte and antibody-dependent cellular cytotoxicity [55].

Core promoter and precore region mutations interfere with mRNA transcription and translation, causing HBeAg down-regulation. These mutations have been reported as associated with chronic hepatitis, cirrhosis, fulminant hepatitis and hepatocellular carcinoma [57-59].

Seroconversion of HBeAg is widely recognized as a sign that active virus replication has notably declined. However, core gene mutations that impede HBeAg production are frequently found in chronic HBV carriers who develop antibodies against HBeAg (anti-HBe) [60]. Persistence of viral replication has also been reported after anti-HBe seroconversion induced by interferon, lamivudine or famciclovir [61].

Almost all chronic HBV patients in Asian countries have been perinatally infected by HBeAg-positive mothers [62]. In 10-20% of these cases, however, perinatal HBV transmission is by anti-HBe-positive mothers, and these children are more likely to develop severe acute or fulminant hepatitis [63]. Previous studies have associated presence of the G1896A precore stop codon mutation with HBeAg-negative serology. This variant consists of a G to A mutation in the position 1896 nucleotide that converts precore region codon 28 from tryptophan (TGG) to a stop codon (TGA). This premature stop codon prevents synthesis of HBeAg, a viral protein normally secreted by HBV-infected hepatocytes. This mutation also increases the stability of the encapsidation signal for pregenomic encapsidation and initiation of HBV DNA synthesis [64,65]. The G1896A mutation has also been associated with fulminant hepatitis and more severe hepatitis B evolution [58,64,66,67]. This has been linked to absence of the HBeAg immune response modulator and alterations in ε signal binding, both of which lead to more efficient viral replication.

Different HBV genotypes have been associated with different core promoter and precore region mutations. Chan et al. reported that 92% of studied chronic HBV infection patients experienced core promoter or precore mutation after HBeAg seroconversion. Core promoter changes were significantly more common in patients infected with HBV genotypes having C in nucleotide 1858, whereas the precore stop codon mutation was found only in patients infected with HBV genotypes having T in nucleotide 1858 [68]. Cytosine in position 1858 precludes the G1896A mutation, since this nucleotide pairs with nt 1896 in the secondary structure of the ε encapsidation signal and would thus destabilize the RNA encapsidation signal stem-loop structure. Interaction between this encapsidation signal and the viral DNA polymerase is an essential step in the viral replication cycle. The increased strength of the G-to-A base pairing present in precore mutants is thought to imply a stronger ε encapsidation signal, thus allowing more efficient replication of these strains [69]. Variant C1858 is characteristic of HBV genotype A and is frequently found in genotypes C and F, but does not occur in genotypes B, D or E [70]. Because genotype distribution is not globally uniform, neither is precore mutant distribution. It is rare in North America, Europe and Southern Africa, where genotype A predominates, but more common and frequent in Asia and the Mediterranean Basin, where genotypes B, C and D predominate [71-73]. In Brazil, precore mutants have been reported as more common in patients with genotype D and core promoter mutants as more common in those with genotype F [74].

Owiredu et al. reported on HBV isolated from the serum of black African patients with fulminant hepatitis B [72]. Genotype A is predominant in HBV isolates from Southern Africa, and therefore the G1896A stop-codon mutation (the most frequently reported in fulminant hepatitis B patients) was not observed in the genotype A isolates. One patient did, however, have the mutation that substitutes T for A at nucleotide 1762 and A for G at 1764 in the core promoter region, which is also commonly described in fulminant hepatitis B patients [58,75]. As is to be expected, the HBeAg titer was low in this patient since this mutation reduces HBeAg expression and increases HBV replication [76].

The G1896A mutation frequently co-occurs with the A1762T and G1764A mutations [58,75]. Because it is a single mutation, G1764A is reported less frequently in fulminant hepatitis B cases [58]. In addition to blocking transcription of precore RNAs, the A1762T and G1764A mutations induce two amino acid changes, K130M and V131I, that may affect X gene transcriptional activity [75].

Lindh et al. analyzed blood from chronic HBV carriers of East Asian origin and compared liver damage between genotype B and C carriers [73]. They found that the AGG to TGA mutation at 1762-1764 was most common in the core promoter region and that this mutant was more frequent in genotype C carriers than in genotype B carriers. Presence of the TGA mutant was associated with more severe inflammation and fibrosis, but no association was observed between the TGA mutation and HBeAg status (in both HBeAg-positive and -negative subjects). The G1896A mutation was more common in genotype B carriers. Its presence was associated with HBeAg negativity and lower HBV DNA levels. Regardless of genotype, the TGA precore mutation (i.e. G1896A) tended to produce less severe inflammation, but not less fibrosis, than associated with wild type infection. Other core promoter mutations, such as C-1752, were observed in relatively few cases, were always next to TGA at 1762-1764 and were associated with liver damage. The lack of association between presence of the TGA mutation and HBeAg status reported by Lindh et al. is consistent with the results of Davidson et al. [77] in Scottish blood donors. It contrasts, however, with other reports suggesting that the effects on HBeAg expression are the principal mechanism for emergence of this mutant [78,79].

Vietnam has one of the highest HBV infection endemicities in the world, and the double core promoter mutation (1762/1764) here is most frequent in patients with hepatocellular carcinoma. Other core promoter mutation points in this region include G1766A and T1773C, although their role in HBV pathogenesis remains unclear [80]. This coincides with recent data reported by Tong et al. showing that HBV genome precore (G1896A) and core promoter (T1762/A1764) mutations are more predictive for development of hepatocellular carcinoma [81].

Nucleotide mutations associated with HBeAg negativity, as well as mutations in the precore or core promoter regions, have been reported by Sun et al. in Chinese patients infected with HBV genotype C. They identified six mutations (G529A, C934A, A1053G,

G1915T/A, T2005C/A and C3027T) which were significantly more common in anti-HBe-positive patients (who had neither precore nor core promoter mutations) than in HBeAg-positive patients. Based on these results the authors suggested that these six mutations are associated with HBeAg negativity, although their actual significance and clinical relevance remain unclear [82].

Other researchers have suggested that precore variant HBV can be transmitted to children as a primary infection and undergo subsequent reactivation after treatment with steroids like methylprednisolone [83]. Recent research also suggests that the mutation in the core promoter region (T1762/A1764) may be involved in HBV reactivation in patients that develop fulminant hepatitis after allogenic bone marrow transplantation [84].

HBV DNA Polymerase Mutants

HBV DNA polymerase consists of 832 amino acids and is composed of four domains: the amino-terminal region (residue 1-178), involved in priming the viral template; the spacer region (residues 179-336), the function of which is unknown; the HBV DNA polymerase (residues 337-680), which contains signals for viral pregenome encapsidation and possesses dual RNA- and DNA-dependent polymerase activity; and the RNase H. The active DNA polymerase site has been defined as containing the five functional motifs of A-E [85], and is therefore an ideal action site for antiviral agents. Antiviral treatment of chronic hepatitis B is limited by selection of antiviral-resistant mutations.

Lamivudine is a nucleoside analogue that suppresses HBV replication through inhibition of the RNA-dependent DNA polymerase, and is the first approved oral therapy for HBV infection treatment [86]. Clinical trials have shown that lamivudine reduces HBV DNA levels in blood, normalizes alanine aminotransferase levels and is effective in preventing the progression of chronic liver disease [87-89]. Nonetheless, although complete suppression of viral prereplication may be achieved in most patients, clearance of HBsAg through anti-HBe seroconversion has been observed in only a small proportion of patients [87,88,90]. Seroconversion rates in HBeAg-positive patients range from 16-22% after one year and 35-40% after three years of lamivudine treatment [87,90-92]. Long-term use of lamivudine, however, has been associated with increased emergence of lamivudine-resistant HBV, with rates varying from 17% after one year to 67% after 4 years of treatment [91].

The most common mutations in the lamivudine-resistant virus are in the conserved tyrosine-methionine-aspartate-aspartate (YM552DD) motif located in the C domain of the viral DNA polymerase [36,85,93]. The YMDD motif comprises a portion of the reverse transcriptase action site where lamivudine binds and terminates DNA chain elongation [85]. Mutations in the highly conserved YMDD motif sequence, such as methionine 552 to isoleucine or valine (M552I or M552V), have been associated with loss of lamivudine inhibitory activity [94]. Breakthrough hepatitis induced by lamivudine-resistant mutations can be difficult to treat and even fatal, and is one of the main problems in chronic hepatitis B patients treated with lamivudine.

Substitution of amino acids within domain B of the reverse transcriptase, including V521L and L528M, has been described in patients receiving famciclovir [95]. The L528M mutation has been described as accompanying the M552I or M552V mutations in patients receiving lamivudine; it has also been described in patients receiving famciclovir, although without mutation the YMDD motif [93,96]. The double mutants L528M/M552I and L528/M552V increase nucleoside analogue resistance [97].

The clinical course of patients with lamivudine-resistant mutants is variable. Emergence of these mutants can be accompanied by exacerbations of liver disease in some patients [94,98]. Exacerbation of liver dysfunction has also been observed after emergence of mutants such as M204I, L180M/M204I and L180M/M204V in the HBV polymerase region [99]. Lamivudine-resistant HBV can also lead to severe hepatitis in patients with HIV/HBV coinfection [100].

Given the high rate of lamivudine resistance upon prolonged treatment, the nucleotide analogue adefovir dipivoxil has been proposed as an antiviral treatment for chronic HBV infection. Viral resistance to adefovir dipivoxil, however, has been shown to develop and increase over time, from 1-2% after one year to 18% after four years of treatment. Two of the mutations that have been identified in these resistant strains are substitution of threonine for aspargine at residue 236 (N236T) in domain D of the HBV DNA polymerase, and of valine for alanine at residue 181 (A181V) in domain B [101,102].

The S gene ORF is completely overlapped by the P gene ORF; therefore, changes in the S gene can produce changes in the overlapping polymerase gene and mutations in the P gene can cause consecutive changes in the S gene. The major antigenic "a" determinant in HBsAg is located in the variable linker region between domains A and B of the DNA polymerase [85]. Torresi et al. reported that changes in the polymerase associated with lamivudine resistance produce consequent changes in the overlapping S gene and its HBsAg envelope protein, resulting in decreased binding of the anti-HBs antibody [103]. Other researchers have observed substitution of cystein for serine in codon 132 (S132C) located in the HBsAg "a" determinant during lamivudine treatment, although it is still unknown if the S132C mutation influences anti-HBs binding capacity [104].

Primary infection with lamivudine-resistant HBV has been documented [105]. This suggests that distribution of the lamivudine-resistant strain with reduced antigenicity could cause serious epidemiological problems by undermining the effectiveness of current vaccines. The presence of mutations in the precore and core promoter regions that enhance replication efficacy of lamivudine-resistant mutants could worsen this situation [106].

HBx Mutants

The X-ORF codifies for HBx, a protein with 154 amino acids, a N-terminal negative regulatory domain and a C-terminal transactivation or coactivation domain [107]. Using mutagenesis studies, Tang et al. demonstrated that the amino acids regions 52-65 and 88-154 of the C-terminal transactivation domain are important for the augmentation function of HBx in HBV replication [108]. HBx is a multifunctional protein associated with a wide variety of biological functions such as gene transcription, cellular cycle control, protein degradation, signal pathways, cellular proliferation, genotoxic stress responses and apoptosis

[107,109,110]. As a transcriptional transactivator, it can regulate transcription of a wide variety of viral and cellular promoters [110-112].

Infection with HBV is known to be a main cause of hepatocellular carcinoma, but the mechanism by which HBV causes transformation of hepatocytes is unknown. Some studies suggest that HBx plays a significant role in the molecular pathogenesis of HBV-related hepatocellular carcinoma [113,114]. Chen et al. identified a total of 54 different mutations in the HBx gene, and these same mutations were found in 95.2% of tumor tissue samples from hepatocellular carcinoma patients. The most frequently observed HBx mutation pattern in these patients is an insert mutation at position 204AGGCCC and point mutations at 260 (G to A) and 264 (G/C/T to A). HBx with this specific mutation pattern appears to be associated with this protein's location inside the nucleus of tumor tissue hepatocytes. Development of multiple HBx mutation types in the same patient may contribute to the process of multiple steps in hepatocarcinogenesis [115].

In a study done in Taiwan, the HBx mutant involving a change from serine to alanine at position 31 (HBx-A31) was most frequently detected in hepatocellular carcinoma and liver cirrhosis patients. Development of HBx-A31 may be a viral strategy intended to escape immune surveillance and thus contribute to the carcinogenesis process [116]. This coincides with Song et al., who reported that HBx-A31 frequency was significantly higher in hepatocellular carcinoma patients than in asymptomatic HBV carriers. They also identified mutations predicted to result in truncated HBx in hepatocellular carcinoma patients. One of these mutations affected nt 1607-1611 (CATGG to ATATT), leading to a frameshift mutation of amino acids followed by a new stop codon at position 78, and resulting in an X protein truncated to 76 amino acids shorter than the full-length X protein. Another mutation was observed at nt 1603-1606 (GTTG to TGAA), leading to a frameshift and a new stop codon at position 104, and resulting in an X protein truncated to 50 amino acids shorter than the full-length X protein. Finally, the insertion and/or mutation of 6 nucleotides at positions 1604-1622, leads to a frameshift mutation generating a new stop codon at position 134, and results in an X protein 20 amino acids shorter than the full-length X protein [80].

Changes in the HBx amino acids sequence at positions 130 and 131 (M130K and V131I) produced by T-A point mutations at the nucleic level have been associated with severe liver damage and hepatocellular carcinoma in patients from China and Africa [117,118]. In Costa Rica, T-A mutations have been observed more frequently in chronic HBV carriers with moderate to severe liver damage, but not in acute recovered patients [119]. Other studies have shown a correlation between T-A mutation presence and patients with fulminant hepatitis, severe exacerbation [120] or liver cirrhosis [121].

A high correlation has also been reported between the presence of antibodies against HBX (anti-HBx) and HBx positivity in HCC tissues. These data indicate that HBx plays a role in the development of HBV-related hepatocellular carcinoma [122].

Mutations in amino acids positions 26-45 in the N-terminal, and positions 87, 88, 116, 118, 119 and 127 are reported to coincide with B-cell epitopes (positions 29-48), particularly in the HBx proline- and serine-rich domain, and the T-cell epitopes regions (positions 116-127). This suggests that these HBV variants could be involved in immune system escape [123].

The X-ORF overlaps with regions that are important to viral replication, including the direct repeat sequences DR1 and DR2, the N-terminal of the Pre-C/C gene and the enhancer II region. There are several mutational hotspots, some of which seem to relate to the HBx immunological epitopes. One clinically-important mutation is the deletion of eight nucleotides between nt 1770 and 1777, which truncates 20 amino acids from the HBx C-terminal. This deletion leads to suppression of HBV DNA replication and expression, resulting in immunoserological marker (HBsAg) negativity. This silent HBV infection is responsible for the majority of non-A to non-E hepatitis. Substitutions of T for C at nucleotide 1655, T for A at nucleotide 1764 and A for G at nucleotide 1766 seem to be associated with fulminant hepatitis [124].

Shiota et al. demonstrated that the HBV genome is present in hepatocellular carcinoma patients who are HBsAg-negative but anti-HBc- and/or anti-HBs-positive. The HBx expression rates in these patients were comparable to those in hepatocellular carcinoma patients positive for HBsAg, suggesting that HBx could play a significant role in hepatocarcinogenesis [125]. Other researchers have suggested that occult HBV infection may play an important role in hepatocarcinogenesis [126,127].

Conclusion

A number of mutations along the HBV genome have been described over the last twenty years. However, their real meaning, the mechanisms by which they affect HBV replication capacity and their clinical relevance are still not completely understood. Contradictory study results may reflect differences between study populations such as genotype distribution, clinical stages of patients or the use of immunotherapy or antiviral treatment. Efficient prophylactic mechanisms and potent antiviral agents are currently in use, but, as is the case with many other viruses, this places HBV under constant selective pressure. Consequently, mutant forms emerge that can cause serologically undetectable (i.e. silent) viral infections. This highlights the need to maintain epidemiological monitoring systems aimed at detecting these mutants, preventing their spread and stopping new hepatitis B outbreaks. An important first step in this effort would be to increase the sensibility of commercial HBV assays to detect a wider range of mutations. Incorporation of additional antigen components into current HBV vaccines needs to be considered so as to induce production of antibodies that protect against the HBsAg mutants that escape HBV hyperimmune globulin and conventional HBV vaccine. Further research is also needed on the role different mutants play in the natural history of hepatitis B infections. Studies including molecular characterization of HBV mutants could provide relevant data to aid in developing better detection systems as well as new prophylactic and therapeutic treatments against these mutants.

References

[1] Zuckerman, JN; Zuckerman, AJ. Current topics in hepatitis B. *J Infect* 2000; 41(2): 130-136.

[2] Gust, ID. Epidemiology of hepatitis B infection in the Western Pacific and South East Asia. *Gut* 1996; 38 Suppl 2: S18-S23.

[3] Tanaka, J. Hepatitis B epidemiology in Latin America. *Vaccine* 2000; 18 Suppl 1: S17-S19.

[4] Lai, CL; Ratziu, V; Yuen, MF; Poynard, T. Viral hepatitis B. *Lancet* 2003; 362(9401): 2089-2094.

[5] Chisari, FV; Ferrari, C. Hepatitis B virus immunopathogenesis. *Annu Rev Immunol* 1995; 13: 29-60.

[6] Ngui, SL; Hallet, R; Teo, CG. Natural and iatrogenic variation in hepatitis B virus. *Rev Med Virol* 1999; 9(3): 183-209.

[7] Tiollais, P; Pourcel, C; Dejean, A. The hepatitis B virus. *Nature* 1985; 317(6037): 489-495.

[8] Le Bouvier, GL. The heterogeneity of Australia antigen. *J Infect Dis* 1971; 123(6): 671-675.

[9] Bancroft, WH; Mundon, FK; Russell, PK. Detection of additional antigenic determinants of hepatitis B antigen. *J Immunol* 1972; 109(4): 842-848.

[10] Okamoto, H; Tsuda, F; Sakugawa, H; Sastrosoewignjo, R; Imai, M; Miyakawa, Y; Mayumi, M. Typing of hepatitis B virus by homology in nucleotide sequence: Comparison of surface antigen subtypes. *J Gen Virol* 1988; 69(Pt 10): 2575-2583.

[11] Norder, H; Couroucé, AM; Magnius, LO. Complete genomes, phylogenetic relatedness, and structural proteins of six strains of the hepatitis B virus, four of which represent two new genotypes. *Virology* 1994; 198(2): 489-503.

[12] Stuyver, L; de Gendt, S; van Geyt, C; Zoulim, F; Fried, M; Schinazi, RF. A new genotype of hepatitis B virus: Complete genome and phylogenetic relatedness. *J Gen Virol* 2000; 81(Pt 1): 67-74.

[13] Arauz-Ruiz, P; Norder, H; Robertson, BH; Magnius, LO. Genotype H. A new Amerindian genotype of hepatitis B virus revealed in Central America. *J Gen Virol* 2002; 83(Pt 8): 2059-2073.

[14] Fortuin, M; Karthigesu, V; Allison, L; Howard, C; Hoare, S; Mendy, M; Whittle, HC. Breakthrough infections and identification of a viral variant in Gambian children immunized with hepatitis B vaccine. *J Infect Dis* 1994; 169(6): 1374-1376.

[15] Niesters, HG; Honkoop, P; Haagsma, EB; de Man, RA; Schalman, SW; Osterhaus, AD. Identification of more than one mutation in the hepatitis B virus polymerase gene arising during prolonged lamivudine treatment. *J Infect Dis* 1998; 177(5): 1382-1385.

[16] Persing, DH; Varmus, HE; Ganem, D. The preS1 protein of hepatitis B virus is acylated at its amino terminus with myristic acid. *J Virol* 1987; 61(5): 1672-1677.

[17] Persing, DH; Varmus, HE; Ganem, D. A frameshift mutation in the pre-S region of the human hepatitis B virus genome allows production of surface antigen particles but eliminates binding to polymerized albumin. *Proc Natl Acad Sci USA* 1985; 82(4): 3440-3444.

[18] Pontisso, P; Petit, MA; Bankowski, MJ; Peeples, ME. Human liver plasma membranes contain receptors for the hepatitis B virus pre-S1 region and, via polymerized human serum albumin, for the pre-S2 region. *J Virol* 1989; 63(5): 1981-1988.

[19] Bruss, V; Thomssen, R. Mapping a region of the large envelope protein required for hepatitis B viron maturation. *J Virol* 1994; 68(3): 1643-1650.

[20] Berthelot, P; Neurath, R; Courouce, AM; Brechot, C; Degos, F; Tron, F; Girad, M. Hepatitis B vaccines with pre-S gene product. *Lancet* 1986; 1(8490): 1150.

[21] Neurath, AR; Adamowicz, P; Kent, SB; Riottot, MM; Strick, N; Parker, K; Offensperger, W; Petit, MA; Wahl, S; Budkowska, A; et al. Characterization of monoclonal antibodies specific for the pre-S2 region of the hepatitis B virus envelope protein. *Mol Immunol* 1986; 23(9): 991-997.

[22] Neurath, AR; Kent, SB; Parker, K; Prince, AM; Strick, N; Brotman, B; Sproul, P. Antibodies to a synthetic peptide from the preS 120-145 region of the hepatitis B virus envelope are virus neutralizing. *Vaccine* 1986; 4(1): 35-37.

[23] Milich, DR; McNamara, MK; McLachlan, A; Thornton, GB; Chisari, FV. Distinct H-2-linked regulation of T-cell responses to the pre-S and S region of the same hepatitis B surface antigen polypeptide allows circumvention of nonresponsiveness to the S region. *Proc Natl Acad Sci USA* 1985; 82(23): 8168-8172.

[24] Milich, DR; Thornton, GB; Neurath, AR; Kent, SB; Michel, ML; Tiollais, P; Chisari, FV. Enhanced immunogenicity of the pre-S region of hepatitis B surface antigen. *Science* 1985; 228(4704): 1195-1199.

[25] Pollicino, T; Zanetti, AR; Cacciola, I; Petit, MA; Smedile, A; Campo, S; Sagliocca, L; Pasquali, M; Tanzi, E; Longo, G; Raimondo, G. Pre-S2 defective hepatitis B virus infection in patients with fulminant hepatitis. *Hepatology* 1997; 26(2): 495-499.

[26] Oon, CJ; Lim, GK; Ye, Z; Goh, KT; Tan, KL; Yo, SL; Hopes, E; Harrison, TJ; Zuckerman, AJ. Molecular epidemiology of hepatitis B variants in Singapore. *Vaccine* 1995; 13(8): 699-702.

[27] Carman, WF; Owsianka, A; Wallace, LA; Dow, BC; Multimer, DJ. Antigenic characterization of pre- and post-liver transplant hepatitis B surface antigen sequences from patients treated with hepatitis B immune globulin. *J Hepatol* 1999; 31(2): 195-201.

[28] Ni, F; Fang, D; Gan, R; Li, Z; Duan, S; Xu, Z. A new immune escape mutant of hepatitis B virus with an Asp to Ala substitution in aa 144 of the envelope major protein. *Res Virol* 1995; 146(6): 397-407.

[29] Seddigh-Tonekaboni, S; Waters, JA; Jeffers, S; Gehrke, R; Ofenloch, B; Horsch, A; Hess, G; Thomas, HC; Karayiannis, P. Effect of variation in the common "a" determinant on the antigenicity of hepatitis B surface antigen. *J Med Virol* 2000; 60(2): 113-121.

[30] Song, BC; Kim, SH; Kim, H; Ying, YH; Kim, HJ; Kim, YJ; Yoon, JH; Lee, HS; Cha, CY; Hook, YH; Kim, BJ. Prevalence of naturally occurring surface antigen variants of hepatitis B virus in Korean patients infected chronically. *J Med Virol* 2005; 76(2): 194-202.

[31] Hino, K; Katoh, Y; Vardas, E; Sim, J; Okita, K; Carman, WF. The effect of introduction of universal childhood hepatitis B immunization in South Africa on the prevalence of serologically negative hepatitis B virus infection and the selection of immune escape variants. *Vaccine* 2001; 19(28-29): 3912-3918.

[32] Oon, CJ; Chen, WN; Koh, S; Lim, GK. Identification of hepatitis B surface antigen variants with alterations outside the "a" determinant in immunized Singapore infants. *J Infect Dis* 1999; 179(1): 259-263.

[33] Protzer-Knolle, U; Naumann, U; Bartenschlager, R; Berg, T; Hopf, U; Meyer zum Buschenfelde, KH; Neuhaus, P; Gerken, G. Hepatitis B virus with antigenically altered hepatitis B surface antigen is selected by high-dose hepatitis B immune globulin after liver transplantation. *Hepatology* 1998; 27(1): 254-263.

[34] Huy, TT; Ushijima, H; Win, KM; Luengrojanakul, P; Shrestha, PK; Zhong, ZH; Smirnov, AV; Taltavull, TC; Sata, T; Abe, K. High prevalence of hepatitis B virus pre-S mutant in countries where it is endemic and its relationship with genotype and chronicity. *J Clin Microbiol* 2003; 41(12): 5449-5455.

[35] Owiredu, WK; Kramvis, A; Kew, MC. Molecular analysis of hepatitis B virus genomes isolated from black African patients with fulminant hepatitis B. *J Med Virol* 2001; 65(3): 485-492.

[36] Melegari, M; Scaglioni, PP; Wands, JR. Hepatitis B virus mutants associated with 3TC and famciclovir administration are replication defective. *Hepatology* 1998; 27(2): 628-633.

[37] Trautwein, C; Schrem, H; Tillmann, HL; Kubicka, S; Walker, D; Boker, KH; Maschek, HJ; Pichlmayr, R; Manns, MP. Hepatitis B virus mutations in the pre-S genome before and after liver transplantation. *Hepatology* 1996; 24(3): 482-488.

[38] Weinberger, KM; Zoulek, G; Bauer, T; Bohm, S; Jilg, W. A novel deletion mutant of hepatitis B virus surface antigen. *J Med Virol* 1999; 58(2): 105-110.

[39] Carman, WF; Zanetti, AR; Karayiannis, P; Waters, J; Manzillo, G; Tanzi, E; Zuckerman, AJ; Thomas, HC. Vaccine-induced escape mutant of hepatitis B virus. *Lancet* 1990; 336(8711): 325-329.

[40] Wang, JT; Lee, CZ; Chen, PJ; Wang, TH; Chen, DS. Transfusion-transmitted HBV infection in an endemic area: the necessity of more sensitive screening for HBV carriers. *Transfusion* 2002; 42(12): 1592-1597.

[41] Ireland, JH; O'Donnell, BO; Basuni, AA; Kean, J; Wallace, LA; Lau, GK; Carman, WF. Reactivity of 13 in vitro expressed hepatitis B surface antigen variants in 7 commercial diagnostic assays. *Hepatology* 2000; 31(5): 1176-1182.

[42] Seddigh-Tonekaboni, S; Lim, WL; Young, B; Hou, JL; Waters, J; Luo, KX; Thomas HC; Karayiannis, P. Hepatitis B surface antigen variants in vaccines, blood donors and an interferon-treated patient. *J Viral Hepat* 2001; 8(2): 154-158.

[43] Jongerius, JM; Wester, M; Cuypers, HT; van Oostendorp, WR; Lelie, PN; van der Poel, CL; van Leeuwen, EF. New hepatitis B virus mutant form in a blood donor that is undetectable in several hepatitis B surface antigen screening assays. *Transfusion* 1998; 38(1): 56-9.

[44] Saraswat, S; Banerjee, K; Chaudhury, N; Mahant, T; Khandekar, P; Gupta, RK; Naik, S. Post-transfusion hepatitis type B following multiple transfusions of HBsAg-negative blood. *J Hepatol* 1996; 25(5): 639-643.

[45] Larsen, J; Hetland, G; Skaug, K. Post-transfusion hepatitis B transmitted by blood from a hepatitis B surface antigen-negative hepatitis B virus carrier. *Transfusion* 1990; 30(5): 431-432.

[46] Carman, WF; van-Deursen, FJ; Mimms, LT; Hardie, D; Coppola, R; Decker, R; Sanders, R. The prevalence of surface antigen variants of hepatitis B virus in Papua New Guinea, South Africa, and Sardinia. *Hepatology* 1997; 26(6): 1658-1666.

[47] Kohno, H; Inoue, T; Tsuda, F; Okamoto, H; Akahane, Y. Mutations in the envelope gene of hepatitis B virus variants co-curring with antibody to surface antigen in sera from patients with chronic hepatitis B. *J Gen Virol* 1996; 77(Pt 8): 1825-1831.

[48] Lada, O; Benhamou, Y; Poynard, T; Thibault, V. Coexistence of hepatitis B surface antigen (HBs Ag) and anti-HBs antibodies in chronic hepatitis B virus carriers: Influence of "a" determinant variants. *J Virol* 2006; 80(6): 2968-2975.

[49] Cuestas, ML; Mathet, VL; Ruiz, V; Minassian, ML; Rivero, C; Sala, A; Corach, D; Alessio, A; Pozzati, M; Frider, B; Oubiña, JR. Unusual naturally occurring humoral and cellular mutated epitopes of hepatitis B virus in a chronically infected Argentine patient with anti-HBs antibodies. *J Clin Microbiol* 2006; 44(6): 2191-2198.

[50] Bauer, T; Weinberger, K; Jilg, W. Variants of two major T cell epitopes within the hepatitis B surface antigen are not recognized by specific T helper cells of vaccinated individuals. *Hepatology* 2002; 35(2): 455-465.

[51] Santantonio, T; Jung, MC; Schneider, R; Fernholz, D; Milella, M; Monno, L; Pastore; G; Pape, GR; Will, H. Hepatitis B virus genomes that cannot synthesize pre-S2 proteins occur frequently and as dominant virus populations in chronic carriers in Italy. *Virology* 1992; 188(2): 948-952.

[52] Melegari, M; Scaglioni, PP; Wands, JR. The small envelope protein is required for secretion of a naturally occurring hepatitis B virus mutant with pre-S1 deleted. *J Virol* 1997; 71(7): 5449-5454.

[53] Ghany, MG; Ayola, B; Villamil, FG; Gish, RG; Rojter, S; Vierling, JM; Lok, AS. Hepatitis B virus S mutants in liver transplant recipients who were reinfected despite hepatitis B immune globulin prophylaxis. *Hepatology* 1998; 27(1): 213-222.

[54] Rodriguez-Frias, F; Buti, M; Jardi, R; Vargas, V; Quer, J; Cotrina, M; Martell, M; Esteban, R; Guardia, J. Genetic alterations in the S gene of hepatitis B virus in patients with acute hepatitis B, chronic hepatitis B and hepatitis B liver cirrhosis before and after liver transplantation. *Liver* 1999; 19(3): 177-182.

[55] Schlicht, J; Wasenauer, G; Köck, J. Molecular basis of the diversity of hepatitis B virus core-gene products. *Arch Virol* 1993; Suppl 8: 43-52.

[56] Koschel, M; Thomssen, R; Bruss, V. Extensive mutagenesis of hepatitis B virus core gene and mapping of mutations that allow capsid formation. *J Virol* 1999; 73(3): 2153-2160.

[57] Takahashi, K; Ohta, Y; Kanai, K; Akahane, Y; Iwasa, Y; Hino, K; Ohno, N; Yoshizawa, H; Mishiro, S. Clinical implications of mutations C-to-T1653 and T-to-C/A/G1753 of hepatitis B virus genotype C genome in chronic liver disease. *Arch Virol* 1999; 144(7): 1299-1308.

[58] Friedt, M; Gerner, P; Lausch, E; Trubel, H; Zabel, B; Wirth, S. Mutations in the basic core promoter and the precore region of hepatitis B virus and their selection in children with fulminant and chronic hepatitis B. *Hepatology* 1999; 29(4): 1252-1258.

[59] Ehata, T; Omata, M; Chuang, WL; Yokosuka, O; Ito, Y; Hosoda, K; Ohto, M. Mutations in core nucleotide sequence of hepatitis B virus correlate with fulminant and severe hepatitis. *J Clin Invest* 1993; 91(3): 1206-1213.

[60] Hamasaki, K; Nakata, K; Nagayama, Y; Ohtsuru, A; Daikoku, M; Taniguchi, K; Tsutsumi, T; Sato, Y; Kato, Y; Nagataki, S. Changes in the prevalence of HBeAg-negative mutant hepatitis B virus during the course of chronic hepatitis B. *Hepatology* 1994; 20(1 Pt 1): 8-14.

[61] Pichoud, C; Berby, F; Stuyver, L; Petit, MA; Trepo, C; Zoulim, F. Persistence of viral replication after anti-HBe seroconversion during antiviral therapy for chronic hepatitis B. *J Hepatol* 2000; 32(2): 307-316.

[62] Okada, K; Kamiyama, I; Inomata, M; Imai, M; Miyakawa, Y. E antigen and anti-e in the serum of asymptomatic carrier mothers as indicator of positive and negative transmission of hepatitis B virus to their infants. *N Engl J Med* 1976; 294(14): 746-749.

[63] Chang, MH; Lee, CY; Chen, DS; Hsu, HC; Lai, MY. Fulminant hepatitis in children in Taiwan: the important role of hepatitis B virus. *J Pediatr* 1987; 111(1):34-39.

[64] Carman, WF; Jacyna, MR; Hadziyannis, S; Karayiannis, P; McGarvey, MJ; Makris, A; Thomas, HC. Mutation preventing formation of hepatitis B e antigen in patients with chronic hepatitis B infection. *Lancet* 1989; 2(8663): 588-591.

[65] Scaglioni, PP; Melegari, M; Wands, JR. Biologic properties of hepatitis B viral genomes with mutations in the precore promoter and precore open reading frame. *Virology* 1997; 233(2): 374-381.

[66] Omata, M; Ehate, T; Yokosuka, O; Hosoda, K; Ohto, M. Mutations in the precore region of hepatitis B vírus DNA in patients with fulminant and severe hepatitis. *N Engl J Med* 1991; 324(24): 1699-1704.

[67] Hou, J; Lau, GK; Cheng, CC; Luo, K; Carman, WF. T1762/A1764 variants of the basal core promoter of hepatitis B virus; serological and clinical correlations in Chinese patients. *Liver* 1999; 19(5): 411-417.

[68] Chan, HL; Hussain, M; Lok, AS. Different hepatitis B virus genotypes are associated with different mutations in the core promoter and precore regions during hepatitis B e antigen seroconversion. *Hepatology* 1999; 29(3): 976-984.

[69] Lok, AS; Akarca, U; Greene, S. Mutations in the pre-core region of hepatitis B virus serve to enhance the stability of the secondary structure of the pre-genome encapsidation signal. *Proc Natl Acad Sci USA* 1994; 91(9): 4077-4081.

[70] Lopez, JL; Mbayed, VA; Telenta, PF; Gonzalez, JE; Campos, RH. "HBe minus" mutants of hepatitis B virus. Molecular characterization and its relation to viral genotypes. *Virus Res* 2002; 87(1): 41-49.

[71] Lindth, M; Andersson, AS; Gusdal, A. Genotypes, nt1858 variants, and geographic origin of hepatitis B virus: large-scale analysis using a new genotyping method. *J Infect Dis* 1997; 175(6): 1285-1293.

[72] Owiredu, WK; Kramvis, A; Kew, MC. Molecular analysis of hepatitis B virus genomes isolated from black African patients with fulminant hepatitis B. *J Med Virol* 2001; 65(3): 485-492.

[73] Lindh, M; Hannoun, C; Dhillon, AP; Norkrans, G; Horal, P. Core promoter mutations and genotypes in relation to viral replication and liver damage in East Asian hepatitis B virus carriers. *J Infect Dis* 1999; 179(4): 775-782.

[74] Sitnik, R; Pinho, JR; Bertolini, DA; Bernardini, AP; Da Silva, LC; Carrillo, FJ. Hepatitis B virus genotypes and precore and core mutants in Brazilian Patients. *J Clin Microbiol* 2004; 42(6): 2455-2460.

[75] Stuyver, L; De Gendt, S; Cadranel, JF; Van Geyt, C; Van Reybroeck, G; Dorent, R; Gandjbachkh, I; Rosenheim, M; Charlotte, F; Opolon, P; Huraux, JM; Lunel, F. Three cases of severe sub-fulminant hepatitis in heart transplanted patients after nosocomial transmission of a mutant hepatitis B virus. *Hepatology* 1999; 29(6): 1876-1883.

[76] Buckwold, VE; Xu, Z; Chen, M; Yen, TS; Ou, JH. Effects of a naturally occurring mutation in the hepatitis B virus basal core promoter on precore gene expression and viral replication. *J Virol* 1996; 70(9): 5845-5851.

[77] Davidson, F; Lycett, C; Sablon, E; Petrik, J; Dow, BC. Hepatitis B virus genotypes and precore mutations in Scottish blood donors. *Vox Sang* 2005; 88(2): 87-92.

[78] Grandjacques, C; Pradat, P; Stuyver, L; Chevallier, M; Chevallier, P; Pichoud, C; Maisonnas, M; Trepo, C; Zoulim, F. Rapid detection of genotypes and mutations in the pre-core promoter and the precore region of hepatitis B virus genome: correlation with viral persistence and disease severity. *J Hepatol* 2000; 33(3): 430-439.

[79] Lin, CL; Liao, LY; Liu, CJ; Chen, PJ; Lai, MY; Kao, JH; Chen, DS. Hepatitis B genotypes and precore/basal core promoter mutants in HBeAg-negative chronic hepatitis B. *J Gastroenterol* 2002; 37(4): 283-287.

[80] Song, LH; Duy, DN; Binh, VQ; Luty, AJF; Kremsner, PG; Bock, CT. Low frequency of mutations in the X gene, core promoter and precore region of hepatitis B virus infected Vietnamese. *J Viral Hepat* 2005; 12(2): 160-167.

[81] Tong, MJ; Blatt, LM; Kao, HJ; Cheng, JT; Corey, WG. Precore/basal core promoter mutants and hepatitis B viral DNA levels as predictors for liver deaths and hepatocellular carcinoma. *World J Gastroenterol* 2006; 12(41): 6620-6626.

[82] Sun, X; Rokuhara, A; Tanaka, E; Glad, A; Mutou, H; Matsumoto, A; Yoshizawa, K; Kiyosawa, K. Nucleotide mutations associated with hepatitis B e antigen negativity. *J Med Virol* 2005; 76(2): 170-175.

[83] Smith, PR; Zampino, R; Gutteeridge, C; Karayiannis, P; Aitken, C. Reactivation of precore variant hepatitis B virus in a child with severe aplastic anaemia. *J Med Virol* 2001; 65(3): 470-472.

[84] Kitano, K; Kobayashi, H; Hanamura, M; Furuta, K; Ueno, M; Rokuhara, A; Tanaka, E; Umemura, T; Kiyosawa, K. Fulminant hepatitis alter allogenic bone marrow transplantation caused by reactivation of hepatitis B virus with gene mutations in the core promotor region. *Eur J Haematol* 2006; 77(3): 255-258.

[85] Poch, O; Sauvager, I; Delarue, M; Tordo, N. Identification of four conserved motif among the RNA-dependent polymerase encoding elements. *EMBO J* 1989; 8(12): 3867-3874.

[86] Gordon, D; Walsh, JH. Hepatitis drugs win approval. *Gastroenterology* 1998; 116: 235-236.

[87] Lai, CL; Chien, RN; Leung, NW; Chang, TT; Guan, R; Tai, DI; Ng, KY; Wu, PC; Dent, JC; Barber, J; Stephenson, SL; Gray, DF. A one-year trial of lamivudine for chronic hepatitis B. *N Engl J Med* 1998; 339(2): 61-68.
[88] Jonas, MM; Mizerski, J; Badia, IB; Areias, JA; Schwarz, KB; Little, NR; Greensmith, MJ; Gardner, SD; Bell, MS; Sokal, EM; International Pedriatric Lamivudine Investigator Group. Clinical trial of lamivudine in children with chronic hepatitis B. *N Engl J Med* 2002; 346(22): 1706-1713.
[89] Liaw, YF; Sung, JJ; Chow, WC; Farrell, G; Lee, CZ; Yuen, H; Tanwandee, T; Tao, QM; Shue, K; Keene, ON; Dixon, JS; Gray, DF; Sabbat, J; Cirrhosis Asian Lamivudine Multicentre Study Group. Lamivudine for patients with chronic hepatitis B and advanced liver disease. *N Engl J Med* 2004; 351(15): 1521-1531.
[90] Dienstag, JL; Schiff, ER; Wright, TL; Perrillo, RP; Hann, HW; Goodman, Z; Crowther, L; Condreay, LD; Woessner, M; Rubin, M; Brown, NA. Lamivudine as initial treatment for chronic hepatitis B in the United States. *N Engl J Med* 1999; 341(17): 1256-1263.
[91] Chang, TT; Lai, CL; Liaw, YF; Guan, R. Incremental increases in HBeAg seroconversion and continued ALT normalization in Asian chronic HBV patients treated with lamivudine for four years. *Antiviral Ther* 2000; 5 Suppl 1: 44.
[92] Leung, NW; Lai, CL; Chang, TT; Guan, R; Lee, CM; Ng, KY; Lim, SG; Wu, PC; Dent, JC; Edmundson, S; Condreay, LD; Chien, RN; On behalf of the Asia Hepatitis Lamivudine Study Group. Extended lamivudine treatment in patients with chronic hepatitis B enhances hepatitis e antigen seroconversion rates: results after 3 years of therapy. *Hepatology* 2001; 33(6): 1527-1532.
[93] Allen, MI; Deslauriers, M; Andrews, CW; Tipples, GA; Walters, KA; Tyrrell, DL; Brown, N; Condreay, LD. Identification and characterization of mutations in hepatitis B virus resistant to lamivudine. Lamivudine Clinical Investigation Group. *Hepatology* 1998; 27(6): 1670-1677.
[94] Bartholomew, MM; Jansen, RW; Jeffers, LJ; Reddy, KR; Johnson, LC; Bunzendahl, H; Condreay, LD; Tzakis, AG; Schiff, ER; Brown, NA. Hepatitis B-virus resistance to lamivudine given for recurrent infection after orthotopic liver transplantation. *Lancet* 1997; 349(9044): 20-22.
[95] Aye, TT; Bartholomeusz, A; Shaw, T; Bowden, S; Breschkin, A; McMillan, J; Angus, P; Locarnini, S. Hepatitis B virus polymerase mutation during antiviral therapy in a patient following liver transplantation. *J Hepatol* 1997; 26(5): 1148-1153.
[96] Seigneres, B; Pichoud, C; Ahmed, SS; Hantz, O; Trepo, C; Zoulim, F. Evolution of hepatitis B virus polymerase gene sequence during famciclovir therapy for chronic hepatitis B. *J Infect Dis* 2000; 181(4): 1221-1233.
[97] Ono, SK; Kato, N; Shiratori, Y; Kato, J; Goto, T; Schinazi, RF; Carrilho, FJ; Omata, M. The polymerase L528M mutation cooperates with nucleotide binding-site mutations, increasing hepatitis B virus replication and drug resistance. *J Clin Invest* 2001; 107(4): 449-455.
[98] Liaw, YF; Chien, RN; Yeh, CT; Tsai, SL; Chu, CM. Acute exacerbation and hepatitis B virus clearance after emergence of YMDD motif mutation during lamivudine therapy. *Hepatology* 1999; 30(2): 567-572.

[99] Natsuizaka, M; Hige, S; Ono, Y; Ogawa, K; Nakanishi, M; Chuma, M; Yoshida, S; Asaka, M. Long-term follow-up of chronic hepatitis B after the emergence of mutations in the hepatitis B virus polymerase region. *J Viral Hepat* 2005; 12(2): 154-159.

[100] Bessesen, M; Ives, D; Condreay, L; Lawrence, S; Sherman, KE. Chronic active hepatitis B exacerbations in human immunodeficiency virus-infected patients following development of resistance to or withdrawal of lamivudine. *Clin Infect Dis* 1999; 28(5): 1032-1035.

[101] Angus, P; Vaughan, R; Xiong, S; Yang, H; Delaney, WE; Gibbs, CS; Brosgart, CL; Colledge, D; Edwards, R; Ayres, A; Bartholomeusz, A; Locarnini, S. Resistance to adefovir dipivoxil therapy associated with the selection of a novel mutation in the HBV polymerase. *Gastroenterology* 2003; 125(2): 292-297.

[102] Hadziyannis, SJ; Tassopoulos, NC; Heathcote, J; Chang, TT; Kitis, G; Rizzetto, M; Marcellin, P; Lim, SG; Goodman, Z; Arterburn, HMS; Xiong, S; Currie, G; Brosgart, CL. Long-term theraphy with adefovir dipivoxil for HBeAg-hegative chronic hepatitis B. *N Engl J Med* 2005; 352(26): 2673-2681.

[103] Torresi, J; Earnest-Silveira, L; Deliyannis, G; Edgtton, K; Zhuang, H; Locarnini, SA; Fyfe, J; Sozzi, T; Jackson, DC. Reduced antigenicity of the hepatitis B virus HBsAg protein arising as a consequence of sequence changes in the overlapping polymerase gene that are selected by lamivudine therapy. *Virology* 2002; 293(2): 305-313.

[104] Conzelmann, I; Wintermeyer, P; Wirth, S; Radke, R; Gerner, P. Complete hepatitis B virus genome analysis in chronically infected children before and during lamivudine treatment. *J Med Virol* 2005; 77(2): 194-202.

[105] Thibault, V; Aubron-Oliver, C; Agut, H; Katlama, C. Primary infection with a lamivudine- resistant hepatitis B virus. *AIDS* 2002; 16(1): 131-133.

[106] Tacke, F; Gehrke, C; Luedde, T; Heim, A; Manns, MP; Trautwein, C. Basal core promoter and precore mutation in the hepatitis B virus genome enhance replication efficacy of lamivudine-resistant mutants. *J Virol* 2004; 78(16): 8524-8535.

[107] Murakami, S. Hepatitis B virus X protein: structure, function and biology. *Intervirology* 1999; 42(2-3): 81-99.

[108] Tang, H; Delgermaa, L; Huang, F; Oishi, N; Liu, L; He, F; Zhao, L; Murakami, S. The transcriptional transactivation function of HBx protein is important for its augmentation role in hepatitis B virus replication. *J Virol* 2005; 79(9): 5548-5556.

[109] Murakami, S. Hepatitis B virus X protein: multifunctional viral regulator. *J Gastroenterol* 2001; 36(10): 651-660.

[110] Lee, H; Yun, Y. HBx protein of hepatitis B virus activates Jakl-STAT signaling. *J Biol Chem* 1998; 273(39): 25510-25515.

[111] Nakatake, H; Chisaka, O; Yamamoto, S; Matsubara, K; Koshy, R. Effect of X protein on transactivation of hepatitis B virus promoters and on viral replication. *Virology* 1993; 195(2): 305-314.

[112] Kumar, V; Jayasuryan, N; Kumar, R. A truncated mutant (residues 58-140) of the hepatitis B virus X protein retains transactivation function. *Proc Natl Acad Sci USA* 1996; 93(11): 5647-5652.

[113] Kim, CM; Koike, K; Saito, I; Miyamura, T; Jay, G. HBx gene of hepatitis B virus induces liver cancer in transgenic mice. *Nature* 1991; 351(6324): 317-320.

[114] Yu, DY; Moon, HB; Son, JK; Jeong, S; Yu, SL; Yoon, H; Han, YM; Lee, CS; Park, JS; Lee, CH; Hyun, BH; Murakami, S; Lee, KK. Incidence of hepatocellular carcinoma in transgenic mice expressing the hepatitis B virus X-protein. *J Hepatol* 1999; 31(1): 123-132.

[115] Chen, GG; Li, MY; Ho, RL; Chak, EC; Lau, WY; Lai, PB. Identification of hepatitis B virus X mutation in Hong Kong patients with hepatocellular carcinoma. *J Clin Virol* 2005; 34(1): 7-12.

[116] Yeh, CT; Shen, CH; Tai, DI; Chu, CM; Liaw, YF. Identification and characterization of a prevalent hepatitis B virus X protein mutant in Taiwanese patients with hepatocellular carcinoma. *Oncogene* 2000; 19(46): 5213-5220.

[117] Fang, ZL; Ling, R; Wang, SS; Nong, J; Huang, CS; Harrison, TJ. HBV core promoter mutations prevail in patients with hepatocellular carcinoma in Guangxi, China. *J Med Virol* 1998; 56(1): 18-24.

[118] Batista, M; Kramvis, A; Kew, M. High prevalence of 1762(T) 1764(A) mutations in the basic core promoter of hepatitis B virus isolated from black Africans with hepatocellular carcinoma compared with asymptomatic carriers. *Hepatology* 1999; 29(3): 946-953.

[119] León, B; Taylor, L; Vargas, M; Luftig, RB; Albertazzi, F; Herrero, L; Visona, K. HBx M130K and V131I (T-A) mutations in HBV genotype F during a follow-up study in chronic carriers. *Virol J* 2005; 2: 60.

[120] Honda, A; Yokusaka, O; Suzuki, K; Saisho, H. Detection of mutations in hepatitis B virus enhancer 2/core promoter and x protein regions in patients with fatal hepatitis B virus infection. *J Med Virol* 2000; 62(2): 167-176.

[121] Cho, SW; Shin, YJ; Hahm, KB; Jin, JH; Kim, YS. Analysis of the precore and core promoter DNA sequences in liver tissues from patients with hepatocellular carcinoma. *J Korean Med Sci* 1999; 14(4): 424-430.

[122] Hwang, GY; Lin, CY; Huang, LM; Wang, YH; Wang, JC; Hsu, CT; Yang, SS; Wu, CC. Detection of the hepatitis B virus x protein (HBx) antigen and anti-HBx antibodies in cases of human hepatocellular carcinoma. *J Clin Microbiol* 2003; 41(12): 5598-5603.

[123] Hwang, GY; Huang, CJ; Lin, CY; Wu, CC. Dominant mutations of hepatitis B virus variants in hepatoma accumulate in B-cell and T-cell epitopes of the HBx antigen. *Virus Res* 2003; 92(2): 157-164.

[124] Uchida, T; Saitoh, T; Shinzawa, H. Mutations of the X region of hepatitis B virus and their clinical implications. *Pathol Int* 1997; 47(4): 183-193.

[125] Shiota, G; Oyama, K; Udagawa, A; Tanaka, K; Nomi, T; Kitamura, A; Tsutsumi, A; Noguchi, N; Takano, Y; Yashima, K; Kishimoto, Y; Suou, T; Kawasaki, H. Occult hepatitis B virus infection in HBs antigen-negative hepatocellular carcinoma in a Japanese population: involvement of HBx and p53. *J Med Virol* 2000; 62(2): 151-158.

[126] Higashi, Y; Tada, S; Miyase, S; Hirota, K; Imamura, H; Kamio, T; Suko, H. Correlation of clinical characteristics with detection of hepatitis B virus X gene in liver tissue in HBsAg-negative, and HCV-negative hepatocellular carcinoma patients. *Liver.* 2002; 22(5): 374-379.

[127] Tamori, A; Nishiguchi, S; Kubo, S; Narimatsu, T; Habu, D; Takeda, T; Hirohashi, K; Shiomi, S. HBV DNA integration and HBV-transcript expression in non B, non-C hepatocellular carcinoma in Japan. *J Med Virol.* 2003; 71(4): 492-498.

In: Hepatitis B Research Advances
Editor: Alicia P. Willis, pp. 235-252

ISBN: 978-1-60021-666-4

Chapter XIV

Radiation-Induced Mucositis in Head and Neck Cancer: Protective Effect of Alpha-Tocopherol (Vitamin E)

Paulo Renato Figueiredo Ferreira and Caroline Sartori
Department of Radiation Oncology, Hospital de Clinicas de Porto Alegre,
Universidade Federal do Rio Grande do Sul (UFRGS), Porto Alegre, RS, Brazil

Abstract

The fundamental principle of radiotherapy is to destroy malignant cells while minimizing damage to normal tissues. Almost all patients who receive radiotherapy to the head and neck area develop some grade of acute mucositis, which is not only painful, but may compromise tumor control by determining decrease in dose intensity and interruptions of the treatment. The term 'oral mucositis' describes the adverse effect of chemotherapy or radiation induced inflammation of the oral mucosa. Symptoms of mucositis vary from pain and discomfort to an inability to tolerate food or fluids. The degree and duration of mucositis in patients receiving radiotherapy are related to radiation source, cumulative dose, dose intensity, volume of irradiated mucosa, smoking/alcohol consumption and oral hygiene conditions. To our knowledge, there is no other controlled study which has evaluated vitamin E as a single radioprotective agent in patients with head and neck tumors treated with radiation therapy alone or post-operative. For this reason, we conducted a double-blind, randomized trial with the objective to investigate the potential mucosal protection of vitamin E in irradiated patients with head and neck cancer, motivated by its simplicity of administration, no severe toxicity in conventional doses, low cost and easy availability.

The fundamental principle of radiotherapy is to destroy malignant cells while minimizing damage to normal tissues. Almost all patients who receive radiotherapy to the head and neck area develop some grade of acute mucositis [1], which is not only painful, but may compromise tumor control by determining decrease in dose intensity and interruptions of the treatment [2]. The term 'oral mucositis' describes the adverse effect of chemotherapy or radiation induced inflammation of the oral mucosa [3]. Symptoms of mucositis vary from pain and discomfort to an inability to tolerate food or fluids. The degree and duration of mucositis in patients receiving radiotherapy are related to radiation source, cumulative dose, dose intensity, volume of irradiated mucosa, smoking/alcohol consumption and oral hygiene conditions [4,5]. The pathogenesis of oral mucositis is thought to involve direct and indirect mechanisms. It is generally believed that oral mucositis is consequent to the direct inhibitory effects of therapy on DNA replication and mucosal cell proliferation [6]. Indirect effects result from release of inflammatory mediators, loss of protective salivary constituents, therapy-induced neutropenia, and the emergence of microorganisms on damaged mucosa [7]. Sonys et al [8] proposed a four phase hypothesis as to the mechanisms of the development of mucositis: 1) inflammatory or vascular phase, induced by toxic cytokines released from epithelial cells after chemotherapy or radiotherapy administration; 2) epithelial phase, characterized by atrophy and ulceration due to reduced renewal of the oral basal epithelium; 3) ulcerative or bacteriological phase, during which some areas of erosion become covered with a fibrinous pseudomembrane. Bacterial colonization occurs, producing endotoxins which contribute to further cytokines release; and 4) healing phase, with epithelial renewal and reestablishment of the local flora. Histopathologically, edema and vascular changes such as thickening of the tunica intima, reduction in the size of the lumen and destruction of the elastic and muscle fibers of the vessel walls are noted [9]. A number of agents with potentially mucosal protection capabilities and different mechanisms of action in radioinduced mucositis has been investigated in randomized trials. Most of them have reduced number of patients, and their efficacy and safety have not been clearly established [1,10,11]. Consequently, there is no standard intervention for oral radioinduced mucositis [7].

Prevention and Treatment of Radioinduced Mucositis

General Measures

Adequate mouth and dental hygiene during the radiotherapy period is one of the most effective measure to prevent mucositis [11,12]. Abrasive toothpastes, oral irritating solutions, smoking, alcohol, acid or excessively hot or cold foods should be avoided [13]. In a consensus conference, the National Institute of Health of the USA [14] recommended some previous measures for head and neck patients candidates to radiotherapy, such as patient and family counseling about side effects of therapy, treatment of preexisting dental cavities at least 14 days before treatment commencement, and intensive use of toothpaste, dental floss and frequent mouth washes with oral fluoride.

Oral Antiseptics, Antibiotics and Antiinflamatories

The oropharyngeal bacterial flora is composed mainly of anaerobics, streptococci and neisseria sp. Necrotic tumors are an adequate medium for many microorganisms, and radiotherapy may predispose to bacterial overgrowth by damaging dividing cells leading to colonization by abnormal bacteria and by reducing saliva. Oral antiseptics such as chlorhexidine, have been tested as mucosal protectants, but no significant effect has been observed [15,16,17]. By the other hand, iodine povidone was reported to decrease incidence, intensity and duration of oral mucositis when compared with placebo [18]. The antibiotic association of polimyxin E, tobramycin and anfotericin B was evaluated by three trials, which found different conclusions. Spijkervet *et al.* [15] conducted a three arm trial comparing polimixin E, tobramycin and anfotericin B versus chlorhexidine versus placebo in patients with head and neck tumors treated with radiotherapy alone. There was a significant reduction in mucositis intensity in the first arm. In a similar larger trial, Symonds *et al.* [19] confirmed these results. However, Okuno *et al.* [20] found no differences favouring these antibiotics association. In a trial conducted by Leborgne et al [21], prednisone reduced interruptions in radiotherapy necessary for recovering of oral toxicity, but it had no effect on intensity and duration of mucositis. Two additional pilot studies confirmed the efficacy of corticosteroids versus placebo [22,23].

Anti-Ulcer Agents

Because ulceration of the oral epithelium is part of the mucositis process, the preventive role of anti- peptic ulcer agents has been evaluated. Sucralfate has been the most investigated agent in randomized trials, but results are conflicting. Lievens *et al.* [24], Barker *et al.* [25], Epstein *et al.* [26], Makkonen *et al.* [27] and Ferreira [28] have found no significant differences between sucralfate and placebo, whereas Scherlacher *et al.* [29], Valls *et al.* [30] and Franzén *et al.* [31] found significant mucosal protection. In a literature review, Belka *et al.* [32] concluded that, except in pelvic tumors, sucralfate has limited benefit in radiation induced mucositis of the head and neck.

Prostaglandins and Antiprostaglandins

Prostaglandins are radioprotective drugs, especially of the gastrointestinal tract [11]. Some small trials found reduction in mucositis intensity with prostaglandin E (PGE_2) in irradiated patients with head and neck tumors [33,34,35]. The role of prostaglandins in the infammatory process envolved in mucositis was investigated by Pillsbury *et al.* [36]. Compared to placebo, indometacin, an anti-prostaglandin agent, reduced intensity and postponed the onset of mucositis in irradiated patients with head and neck tumors.

Colony Stimulating Factors

Granulocytes colony stimulating factor (G-CSF) and granulocytes and macrophages colony stimulating factor (GM-CSF) are glycoproteins related to neutrophille and monocytes/macrophages proliferation and differentiation [11]. GM-CSF may also stimulate proliferation and migration of oral mucosal cells [37,38]. Two phase II studies showed that GM-CSF reduced the incidence of mucositis in patiens undergoing total body irradiation (TBI) [39,40] and radiotherapy for head and neck cancer [41,42,43]. Keratinocyte growth factor-2 (KGF-2) is an new class of agent that has no in vitro or in vivo proliferative effects on human epithelial-like tumor, but it selectively induces epithelial cell proliferation, differentiation and migration. This failure to stimulate tumor cell growth characterizes the ability of this drug to specifficaly target normal epithelial cells [44,45]

Amifostine

Amifostine, an aminothyol with radioprotective capabilities in normal tissues, was tested in some trials with patients with head and neck tumors. Büntzel *et al.* [46] evaluated 39 patients treated with radiotherapy and chemotherapy and found that amifostine reduced significantly the frequency of grade 3 and 4 mucositis, with apparently no interference on the therapeutic effect of therapy. Similar results were observed in a small trial conducted by Wagner *et al.* [47], where amifostine reduced both intensity and duration of oral mucositis. However, data for protection of mucositis are considered marginal and insufficient to recommend amifostine at this time [48].

Other Agents

Other agents with different mechanisms of action have been used as potential radioprotectants. Capsaicin, an agent which has been used in neuropathic syndroms, was topically employed in the oral mucosa of 11 patients with head and neck tumors undergoing chemoradiotherapy [49]. There was a significant reduction in pain intensity. Silver nitrate at 2% was investigated in 16 patients with head and neck tumors submitted to a split- course hiperfractionated radiotherapy. In the 5 days before and the 2 days after the onset of radiotherapy, left oral mucosa was topically treated with silver nitrate 3 times a day. The right size was kept as control without medication. Duration and intesity of mucositis were significantly reduced.

Vitamins

Several vitamins have shown radioprotective activity in animal and human models. Ascorbic acid (vitamin C) protected mouse spermatogonies against irradiation of ^{125}I [50]. In a randomized clinical trial, β-caroten, a vitamin A precursor, significantly reduced grades 3 and 4 oral mucositis in patients with head and neck tumors treated by radiotherapy and chemotherapy [51]. Although one study reported no radioprotective effect of vitamin E in rats by the criteria of chromosomal aberrations [52], many authors found significant evidence of intestinal [53,54,55,56] and oral mucosal protection [57] in irradiated rodents receiving systemic or topic vitamin E. Some phase III clinical trials also found significant oral mucosal protection when vitamin E was used alone in chemotherapy studies or combined to other protective agents in a chemoradiation study. In a randomized, double-blind trial with 18 evaluable patients treated with chemotherapy alone for several malignancies, Wadleigh et al [58] found that daily doses of 400 mg of vitamin E topically applied significantly speeded the healing of oral mucositis. The duration of mucositis (median of 3 days) was significantly shorter in the vitamin E group comparing to placebo group (only 1 among 9 patients had healing of mucosal lesions on the five days of observation). No toxicity was observed. The authors concluded that topical use of vitamin E is safe in preventing oral mucositis induced by chemotherapy.

One trial evaluated vitamin E and other similar drugs as radioprotective agents, in which vitamin E was not the experimental drug. Osaki et al. [59] randomized 63 patients with head and neck tumors treated with radiotherapy and concomitant chemotherapy. The experimental group received daily doses of azelastine, a histamin H1 antagonist with antioxidant activity, vitamin C, vitamin E and gluthation. The control group received identical treatment, but no azelastine. The study showed that 21 patients of the experimental group had grades 1 and 2 oral mucositis, and 16 had lesions grades 3 and 4. In the control group, only 5 patients had grades 1 and 2 oral mucositis, but 21 had lesions grades 3 and 4. The authors conclude that azelastine may be useful in the prevention of grades 3 and 4 oral mucositis induced by chemoradiotherapy.

In another randomized trial, Lopez et al [60] evaluated 19 patients with acute myelogenous leukemia treated with either induction or intensive chemotherapy followed by autologous bone marrow transplant. The duration of grades 3-4 of oral mucositis was significantly shorter in patients receiving 2 ml of topical vitamin E over the oral mucosa in the arm treated with induction chemotherapy. The plasmatic concentration of vitamin E was unexpectedly lower in patients receiving vitamin E than in patients receiving placebo. Their data suggested that the intestinal absorption of vitamin E does not seem significant, and that the mucosal protective action is mainly due to a local effect.

Rational for the Preventive Effect of Vitamin E in Radioinduced Mucositis

As experimentally demonstrated in the intestinal mucosa of rodents, there is substantial data to support that radiation induced oxygen free radicals act as mediators of cell injury following ionizing irradiation [53,54,61]. Free radicals induce DNA structural modifications which are incompatible with cell survival, if not repaired [62]. They also remove hydrogen atoms from cell membrane fatty acids, a reaction called lipidic peroxidation, which results in alterations of membrane permeability and, ultimately, in cell death [63].

Under physiological conditions, some protective mechanisms are important natural defensive agents against the oxidative action caused by free radicals, such as cytoprotective enzymes (superoxide dismutase, catalase, glutathione peroxidase) and antioxidants (tocopherols, carotenes, ascorbic acid, reduced glutathione) [64]. Providing ionizing radiation and many cytotoxic drugs are known to produce free radicals, and because they are implicated in the process of cell killing, mutagenesis, transformation and carcinogenesis, it is reasonable to assume that scavenging free radicals agents would play a significant role in modulating these processes [55].

Alpha-tocopherol, the main constituent of vitamin E, is the most important natural antioxidant present in the human blood [63]. Its main biological function is to scavenge peroxil free radicals (HO_2) in the cell membrane. Vitamin E has been reported as capable to stabilize cellular membranes and to improve herpetic gengivitis, possibly through its antioxidant activity [65,66,67]. According to Köstler et al [68], the rational for the topical use of vitamin E as a mucosal protective agent is based upon its antioxidant and membrane stabilizing action, which interferes with the inflammatory damage caused by reactive oxygen free radicals created in the course of chemotherapy or radiotherapy. Consequently, because vitamin E is inexpensive, readily available and well tolerated, confirmatory and prophylactic trials would be of great interest.

A Double-Blind, Randomized Trial on the Protective Effect of Vitamin E on Radioinduced Mucositis in Head and Neck Cancer

To our knowledge, there is no other controlled study which has evaluated vitamin E as a single radioprotective agent in patients with head and neck tumors treated with radiation therapy alone or post-operative. For this reason, we conducted a double-blind, randomized trial with the objective to investigate the potential mucosal protection of vitamin E in irradiated patients with head and neck cancer, motivated by its simplicity of administration, no severe toxicity in conventional doses, low cost and easy availability [69,70]. Our study admitted patients with confirmed histological diagnosis of cancer of the oral cavity and oropharynx referred to radiotherapy. They were evaluated at Hospital de Clinicas de Porto Alegre – Universidade Federal do Rio Grande do Sul (UFRGS) and received irradiation alone or post-operative at Hospital Sao Lucas da PUCRS - Pontificia Universidade Catolica do Rio Grande do Sul (HSL-PUCRS) in Porto Alegre, Southern Brazil. The trial was approved by the Scientific and Bioethics Committees of both institutions in accordance with the precepts established by the Helsinki Declaration. An informed consent was obtained from all patients. Admission requirements consisted of: 1) a minimal irradiated buccal mucosal area $\geq$ 12,2 cm^2. The limits of this area, measured on verification films, were the hard palate (superior), the floor of the mouth (inferior), the anterior border of the vertical portion of the mandible (posterior) and the distal border of the irradiation field (anterior); 2) age ≥ 21; 3) Zubrod [71] performance status grade 2 or lower, 4) tolerance of solid food at study entry, and 5) no trismus, concomitant use of oral anticoagulants, previous or current history of other cancers, previous history of radiotherapy in the head and neck area nor previous or concomitant chemotherapy. The initial evaluation consisted in history, physical/ otolaryngological/dental examination, computed tomography of the head and neck, chest x-ray study and complete blood count. Patients were staged according to the UICC (International Union Against Cancer) -TNM classification [72].

Randomization process was conducted by coworkers not directly involved in this study. Patient's names were picked out by lot and allocated in a grid with 5 blanks per line, according to the group of treatment: vitamin E or placebo. Intermittently, the line sequences were changed in order to improve the randomization. Neither the authors nor patients were aware of the identification of the prescribed drugs. Patients were given either 400 mg of vitamin E (Ephynal©, Produtos Roche Quimicos e Farmaceuticos, Sao Paulo, SP, Brazil) or 500 mg of placebo (Efamol Pure Evening Primrose Oil©, Kentville, NS, Canada). The drugs were available as an oil solution enclosed in capsules. Patients were taught to dissolve it in saliva, rinse it all over the oral cavity during 5 minutes, and then swallow it immediately before every session of irradiation, Monday through Friday, from the first to the last day of radiotherapy. A second capsule was similarly administered at patient's home after 8-12 hours. Both vitamin E and placebo capsules had the same size, shape, color and texture and were given to the patients in vials supplied weekly. The drug used as placebo is a combination of fatty acids (oleic, linoleic, gama-linoleic, palmitic, stearic and others), but also contains 2.5 % of vitamin E in its formula (13 I.U. per capsule of 500 mg). Prescribed analgesics were paracetamol/codeine or dipyrone whenever necessary.

Radiotherapy was provided by a Cobalt 60 unit (Theratron Phoenix) operating at 80 cm target-skin distance. Two parallel opposed fields were designed with customized alloy shielding blocks to include the tumor within a 2 cm safe margin and the upper cervical lymph nodes bilaterally. Anterior supraclavicular fields were added whether metastatic cervical lymph nodes were present or the primary tumor was located in tonsils or tongue. A daily dose of 2 Gy/section/5 days a week was calculated at the midline up to a cumulative dose of 44 Gy/4.5 weeks. A first field reduction was made for spinal cord sparing up to the dose of 60 Gy/6 weeks. A second reduction was made to encompass only the tumor within 1 cm margins up to the final dose of 70 Gy/7 weeks. Patients previously treated with complete or incomplete resections were planned to receive total doses of 50 or 60 Gy in 5 and 6 weeks, respectively, with a similar technique. Check films were obtained during patient set up and weekly for subsequent quality control, throughout radiotherapy. Protocol violations were established when patients: 1) did not receive the prescribed dose of irradiation, 2) interrupted radiotherapy more than 3 consecutive fractions, or 3) did not take the protocol medications adequately.

A comprehensive dentistry evaluation was made in order to assure adequate balancing of pre-treatment conditions related to secondary factors associated with mucositis severity. Patients had their weight recorded and oral mucositis evaluated and graded by the same investigator on the first day of radiotherapy, and then subsequently once a week until the last fraction. The RTOG/EORTC [73] (Radiation Therapy Oncology Group/European Organization for Research and Treatment of Cancer) objective grading system was used: grade 0- no changes over baseline; grade 1- Injection. May experience mild pain. No analgesics required; grade 2- patchy mucositis may produce inflammatory serosanguinous discharge. May experience moderate pain requiring analgesia; grade 3- confluent fibrinous mucositis. May experience severe pain requiring narcotic; grade 4-ulceration, hemorrhage or necrosis. For the purposes of this study, symptomatic mucositis was considered as grade ≥2. To evaluate the impact on quality of life, at the end of the treatment patients filled out a questionnaire based on the World Health Organization Grading of Mucositis/Stomatitis [7], where they informed the occurrence of pain and oral intake difficulty during radiotherapy. This subjective grading system consisted in the following scale: grade 0- no pain; grade 1- painful mucositis did not require modifications in oral intake; grade 2- painful mucositis, can eat but did require decrease in liquids intake any time during radiotherapy; grade 3- painful mucositis prevented oral intake; 4-painful mucositis required parenteral or enteral support any time during radiotherapy.

The main endpoint was the severity of oral mucositis. All randomized patients were counted for the analysis, according to the intention to treat principle. Not all the patients completed 7 weeks of radiotherapy because some had been submitted to previous surgery and required lower doses of irradiation. "Patients-week" were defined as the number of patients at risk who were in the study in every week of radiotherapy. For every patient-week, each record of symptomatic buccal mucositis was considered as a single event. The number of events of symptomatic mucositis was correlated with the number of patients-week, aiming to take into account the duration of time the patient suffered the toxicity. A density of incidences of symptomatic mucositis was calculated as a coefficient obtained by the number of symptomatic mucositis events divided by the number of patients-week in every week of radiotherapy. The study was designed to test a moderate to large effect. The expected sample size was estimated based on a 15% difference in the scores of symptomatic mucositis between vitamin E and placebo groups from a previous pilot study carried out with 28 patients reported elsewhere [74]. One hundred fifty-one patients-week were estimated as necessary in each arm. A significant level of 5% and a statistical power of 80% were adopted in order to test a minimal incidence difference of at least 15 events for every 100 patients-week. Secondary endpoints were duration of mucositis and weight loss. For the same significance level, statistical power and sample size, the estimated differences required for the duration of symptomatic mucositis and weight loss between both groups were at least 10 days and 11 kg, respectively.

Pre-treatment characteristics, as well as differences in the intensity of mucositis and complications, were analyzed by the Pearson's Chi-square test with a confidence interval of 95% (CI95%). Student's t test and Mann-Whitney test were utilized to compare differences between means and medians, respectively. Survival estimates were obtained by the Kaplan-Meier test [75], and the differences between survival curves by the Log Rank Test. All P values were two-tailed.

From December 1997 to December 1999, fifty-four patients were randomized. Twenty-eight were accrued to vitamin E group and 26 to the placebo group. Frequencies of gender, age, histological type, tumor location, stage, previous surgery, oral and dental evaluation, smoking and alcohol consumption were similar in both arms (table 1). Most of the patients were male. The mean age was 55.4 years (standard deviation [SD]=12.5). The most frequent histology and anatomical site were squamous cell carcinoma and oral cavity, respectively. Forty patients had stages III and IV disease: 24/28 (85.7%) belonged to the vitamin E group and 16/26 (61.5%) to the placebo group (RR [relative risk]=1.39; CI95%=0.99-1.96; P=0.086). Around 2/3 of the patients had been submitted to previous surgery. Most of them had some type of oral or dental alteration (23/28 and 16/26 patients in vitamin E and placebo groups, respectively), and history of cigarette and alcohol consumption. Three patients from the vitamin E group did not receive the prescribed doses: two due to intense mucositis and one due to death assigned to tumor progression. The median follow-up of the 54 patients was 12 months (range:2-24 months).

Table 1. Patient characteristics

	Number of patients per treatment group (%)				
Characteristics	**Vitamin E**		**Placebo**		**P**
GENDER					0.999
Male	25	(89.3)	23	(88.5)	
Female	3	(10.7)	3	(11.5)	
AGE					0.268
Mean (standard deviation)	53.5 (9.1)		57.3 (15.3)		
HISTOLOGY					0.347
Squamous cell carcinoma	26	(92.8)	21	(80.8)	
Undifferentiated Carcinoma	1	(3.6)	4	(15.4)	
Adenoid cystic carcinoma	0	(0)	1	(3.8)	
Fibrossarcoma	1	(3.6)	0	(0)	
ANATOMICAL SITE					0.789
Tonsil	3	(10.7)	5	(19.2)	
Base of the tongue	4	(14.3)	2	(7.7)	
Retromolar trigone	3	(10.7)	2	(7.7)	
Soft palate	0	(0)	1	(3.8)	
Oral tongue	10	(35.7)	9	(34.6)	
Floor of the mouth	8	(28.6)	7	(26.9)	
STAGE					0.142
I	0	(0)	3	(11.5)	
II	4	(14.3)	7	(26.9)	
III	5	(17.8)	4	(15.4)	
IV	19	(67.9)	12	(46.2)	
PREVIOUS SURGERY					0.840
Yes	18	(64.3)	17	(65.4)	
No	10	(35.7)	9	(34.6)	
ORAL AND DENTAL EVALUATION					0.610
Normal teeth and oral mucosa	5	(17.8)	10	(38.5)	
Single alterations					
Periodontal disease	5	(17.8)	4	(15.4)	
Increased coating of the tongue	3	(10.7)	1	(3.8)	
Fibrous hyperplasia	2	(7.1)	1	(3.8)	
Gingivitis	1	(3.6)	1	(3.8)	
Multiple alterations					
Periodontal disease, cavities, pericoronitis, fibrous hyperplasia, increased coating of the tongue	8	(28.6)	4	(15.4)	
No evaluation	4	(14.3)	5	(19.2)	

Table 1. (Continued)

	Number of patients per treatment group (%)				
Characteristics	**Vitamin E**		**Placebo**		**P**
CIGARRETTE SMOKING HISTORY	27	(96.4)	24	(92.3)	0.603
Yes					
No	1	(3.6)	2	(7.7)	
ALCOHOL HISTORY					0.878
Yes	21	(75.0)	20	(77.0)	
No	7	(25.0)	6	(23.0)	

At twenty-four months, the estimated overall and median survivals for all patients were 44.8% and 9.5 months (range: 2-24) respectively. For patients of the vitamin E and placebo groups, these figures were 32.2% and 8.5 months (range: 2-24) and 62.9% and 12.5 months (range: 2-23) respectively (P=0.126).

Table 2. Events of symptomatic mucositis according to the radiotherapy week and the number of patients-week

	Events of symptomatic mucositis						
	***Vitamin E group* (28 patients)**				**Placebo group (26 patients)**		
Week	Patients-week	Number of events	(%)		Patients-week	Number of events	(%)
1	28	1	(3.6)		26	0	(0)
2	28	4	(14.3)		26	7	(27.0)
3	28	8	(28.6)		26	10	(38.5)
4	27	8	(29.6)		26	11	(42.3)
5	25	5	(20.0)		26	13	(50.0)
6	23	8	(34.8)		21	9	(42.9)
7	8	2	(25.0)		10	4	(40.0)
TOTAL	167 (100)	36	(21.6)		161 (100)	54	(33.5)

All the patients developed varying degrees of mucositis during radiotherapy (table 2). Symptomatic mucositis was more frequent in the placebo group than in the vitamin E group: 36 events of symptomatic mucositis were observed in 167 patients-week (21.6%) of the vitamin E group, whereas 54 events of symptomatic mucositis were observed in 161 patients-week (33.5%) of the placebo group. These data were computed in the calculation of a density of incidences (RR= 0.643, 95CI%= 0.42-0.98, P= 0.038) (table 3). Accordingly, 8.3 patients-week were required for vitamin E avoiding one event of symptomatic mucositis. Maximum peaks of symptomatic mucositis occurred at the 6th week and 5th week for the vitamin E and placebo groups, respectively (figure 1). As shown in table 4, an analysis of the questionnaires answered by patients at the end of the treatment also revealed that vitamin E decreased pain and restriction in oral intake (grades 2-3) during radiotherapy (3/28 patients= 10.7% vs. 14/26 patients= 53.8%) (P=0.0001).

Table 3. Density of incidences of symptomatic mucositis

Group	Number of events: Symptomatic mucositis	Patients-week	Incidence per 100 patients-week
Vitamin E	36	167	21.6
Placebo	54	161	33.5

*RR= 0.643, 95CI%= 0.42-0.98, P= 0.038.

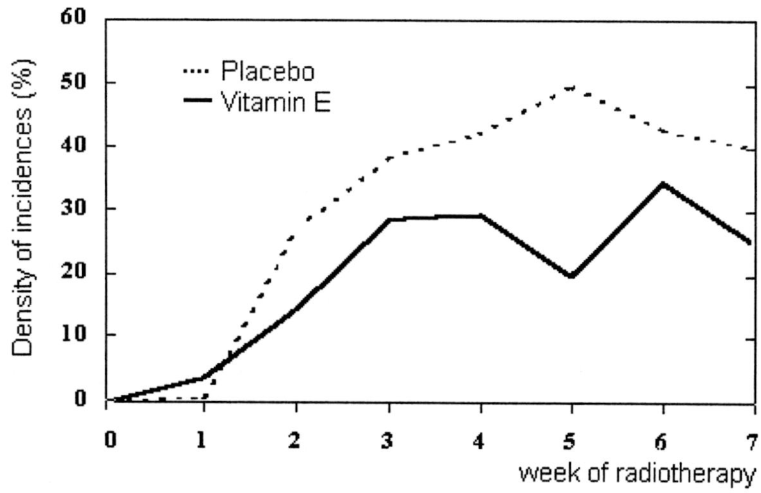

Figure 1. Density of incidences of symptomatic mucositis according to the week of radiotherapy.

Table 4. Pain and oral intake restriction based on subjective data provided by patients at the end of the treatment*

Grade	Vitamin E Number of patients (%)		Placebo Number of patients (%)	
0	13	(46.4)	3	(11.5)
1	12	(42.8)	9	(34.6)
2	3	(10.7)	9	(34.6)
3	0	(0)	5	(19.2)
4	0	(0)	0	(0)
Total	28	(100)	26	(100)

*P= 0.0001.

Total doses of radiotherapy were similarly distributed in both arms (table 5). There was no dose-response relationship or mucosal area-dependence with the severity of mucositis. Mean doses at the primary site for the vitamin E and placebo groups were 61 Gy and 62 Gy (P=0.664) and mean durations of radiotherapy were 5.9 and 6.1 weeks, respectively

(P=0.520). The median area of buccal mucosal irradiation for the vitamin E and placebo groups were 20.7 cm^2 (range:12.2-33.8) and 22.9 cm^2 (range:12.5-35.0), respectively (P=0.176).

Table 5. Frequency of the total doses of radiotherapy according to the treatment group*

	Vitamin E	**Placebo**
Total dose (Gy)	**Number of patients (%)**	**Number of patients (%)**
50	5 (17.8)	5 (19.2)
60	15 (53.5)	11 (42.3)
70	8 (28.6)	10 (38.4)
Total	28 (100)	26 (100)

* P=0.68.

The median duration of symptomatic mucositis in patients of the vitamin E and placebo groups was one week (range: 0-5) and two weeks (range: 0-5), respectively (P=0.102). The initial mean weight in patients of the vitamin E and placebo groups (60.4 kg [SD= 10.4] and 66.2 kg [SD= 14.0], respectively) was compared to the mean weight during radiotherapy (55.5 kg [SD=20.8] and 60.7 kg [SD=22.1], respectively). The observed differences in weight were 4.9 kg and 5.5 kg, respectively (P=0.249).

Two thirds of the patients presented acute complications during the treatment (table 6). Mild nausea was the most frequent, but the majority of them may be related to the disease's natural history or to irradiation itself. Their frequencies in both treatment arms were similar (P=0.216). No late reactions were observed.

Table 6. Frequency of acute complications according to treatment group*

	Treatment group§			
Complication	**Vitamin E 28 patients (%)**		**Placebo 26 patients (%)**	
None	10	(35.7)	9	(34.6)
Mild nausea	12	(42.8)	10	(38.5)
Vomit	4	(14.3)	5	(19.2)
Fever	4	(14.3)	1	(3.8)
Candidiasis	2	(7.1)	4	(15.4)
Bleeding	2	(7.1)	9	(34.6)

*P=0.216.
§Some patients had more than one complication simultaneously.

In the vitamin E treated group, 6/9 patients had complete resolution of their mucositis within 4 days of initiating therapy, whereas in the placebo group only one patient had resolution of the lesions during the same time.

The proper assessment of the oral mucosa is of great importance before initiating therapy and throughout a treatment course. A variety of protocols and grading systems has been established and at least two of them incorporate both subjective and objective criteria: the RTOG/EORTC and the Wold Health Organization Grading of Mucositis/Stomatitis [7]. We used both scales based on their simplicity. Some studies define grade 3 and 4 as severe mucositis. No conventions for such reporting have been published. Many studies only report the incidence of severe reactions, whereas others combine "grade 2-3" reactions [76]. We considered RTOG grade 2 as symptomatic mucositis because it also expresses impairment in quality of life as consequence of inflammatory reaction, moderate to significant pain and necessity of analgesics. The frequency of symptomatic mucositis in the experimental arm was 64% of that observed in the placebo arm, which means that vitamin E reduced the risk of symptomatic mucositis development by 36%. By the other hand, since the differences in duration of mucositis and weight loss were lower than the minimal differences detectable by the sample size, our study had no sufficient statistical power to, conclusively, define whether vitamin E was capable or not to significantly influence these secondary endpoints.

The concentration of vitamin E in our placebo was considered acceptable for the purpose of this study because it corresponds to only 3.1% of drug concentration present in the active drug. The presence of vitamin E in placebo capsules has been reported in similar studies [58].

Although there was a trend of poorer survival in the experimental arm, it is unlikely that vitamin E has influenced short term survival, since the differences between both curves were non significant. We attribute this trend to the higher frequency of stages III and IV prevailing in the vitamin E arm, although these differences were also non significant. Mild nausea was more frequently reported by patients in the vitamin E group, whereas bleeding was more frequent in the placebo group. However, many of these symptoms may be attributable to radiotherapy and the tumor itself. Differences in complications between both groups were non significant, suggesting that vitamin E did not induce relevant toxicity.

We conclude that patients of the vitamin E group had lower frequencies of symptomatic mucositis than patients of the placebo group. On the other hand, our study had no sufficient statistical power to conclusively assess differences in the duration of symptomatic mucositis and weight loss. The administration of vitamin E was simple, side effects had low toxicity and no significant influence in survival was observed. We consider that vitamin E has a potential protective effect on the oral mucosa of irradiated patients with tumors of the oral cavity and oropharynx. The most effective dose, frequency of administration, and synergistic role of other natural antioxidants with vitamin E are issues still to be investigated. New studies are necessary to confirm our results and address further questions.

REFERENCES

[1] Loprinzi CL, Gastineau DA, Foote RL: Oral complications. In: Abeloff M, Armitage JO, Lichter AS, Niederhuber JE, editors. *Clinical Oncology*. 2nd ed. New York: Churchill Livingstone; 2000. pp. 965-979.

[2] Parsons J: the effect of radiation on normal tissues of the head and neck. In: Million R, Cassisi N, editors. *Management of the head and neck cancer: A multidisciplinary approach*. 2nd ed. Philadelphia: JB Lippincott; 1994, pp. 245-289.

[3] Naidu MU, Ramana GV, Rani PU, Mohan IK et al: Chemotherapy-induced and/or radiation therapy-induced oral mucositis-complicating the treatment of cancer. *Neoplasia.* 2004;6:423-431.

[4] Franzen L, Funegard U, Ericson T, and Henriksson R (1992). Parotid gland function during and following radiotherapy of malignancies in the head and neck. *Eur J Cancer* 1992:28, 457– 462.

[5] Verdi CJ: Cancer therapy and oral mucositis—an approval of drug prophylaxis. *Drug Saf* 1993:9: 185 – 195.

[6] Lockhart PB, Sonis ST: Alterations in the oral mucosa caused by chemotherapeutic agents. *J Dermatol Surg* 1981;7:1019-1025.

[7] Wilkes JD: Prevention and treatment of oral mucositis following cancer chemotherapy. *Semin Oncol* 1998;5:538-551.

[8] Sonis ST: Mucositis as a biological process: a new hypothesis for the development of chemotherapy-induced stomatotoxicity. *Oral Oncol* 1998;34: 39-43.

[9] Berger A, Kilroy T: Oral complications. In: De Vita VT, Hellman S, Rosenberg SA, editors. *Cancer, Principles and Practice of Oncology.* 5th ed. Philadelphia: JB Lippincott; 2001. pp. 2714-2725.

[10] Berger A, Kilroy T: Oral complications. In: De Vita VT, Hellman S, Rosenberg SA, editors. *Cancer, Principles and Practice of Oncology.* 6th ed. Philadelphia: JB Lippincott; 2001. pp. 2881.

[11] Symonds RP: Treatment-induced mucositis: An old problem with new remedies. *Br J Cancer* 1998;77:1689-1695.

[12] Feber T. Management of mucositis in oral irradiation. *Clin. Oncol* (R. Coll. Radiol.) 1996;8: 106-111.

[13] Loprinzi CL.; Gastineau DA; Foote RL: Oral complications. In: Abeloff M., Armitage JO; Lichter AS; Niederhuber JE; (ed.) . *Clinical Oncology.* 2.ed. New York. Churchill Livingstone; 2000. p. 965-979.

[14] NIH Consens Statement Online - 1989 April 17-19. Oral complications of cancer therapy. *Diagnosis, prevention and treatment.* National Institutes of Health Consensus Development Conference Statement 1989;7: 1-11.

[15] Spijkervet FL; Van Saene HK; Panders AK et al: Effect of chlorhexidine rinsing on the oropharyngeal ecology in patients with head and neck cancer who have irradiation mucositis. *Oral Surg. Oral Med. Oral Path* 1989;67: 154-158.

[16] Foote RL; Loprinzi CL; Frank R et al: Randomized trial of a chlorhexidine mouthwash for the alleviation of radiation induced mucositis. *J Clin. Oncol* 1994;12: 2630, 2633.

[17] Samaranayake LP; Robertson AG; Macfarlane TW et al: The effect of chlorhexidine and benzydamine on mucositis induced by therapeutic irradiation. *Clin. Radiat* 1988;39: 291-294.

[18] Adamietz I; Rahn R; Böttcher H et al: revention of radiochemotherapy-induced mucositis: Value of the prophylactic mouth rinsing with PVP-iodine solution. *Strahlenther Onkol* 1998; 174:149-155.

[19] Symonds RP, McIlroy P, Khorrami J et al: The reduction of radiation mucositis by selective decontamination antibiotic pastilles: a placebo-controlled double-blind trial. *Br J Cancer* 1996;74:312-317.

[20] Okuno S; Foote R; Loprinzi C et al: A randomized trial of nonabsorbable antibiotic lozenge given to alleviate radiation-induced mucositis. *Cancer* 1997;79: 2193-2199.

[21] Leborgne J; Leborgne F; Zubizarreta E et al: Corticosteroids and radiation mucositis in head and neck cancer. A double-bind placebo controlled randomized trial. Radiother. *Oncol* 1998; 47: 145-148.

[22] Rothwell BR; Speltor WS: Palliation of radiation-related mucositis. *Special Care Dentistry* 1990;10: 21-25.

[23] Abdelaal A; Barker D; Fergusson M. Treatment for irradiation-induced mucositis. *Lancet,* 1987;1:97-102.

[24] Lievens Y; Haustemans K; Van den Weyngaert D *et al:* Does sucralfate reduce the acute side effects in head and neck cancer treated with radiotherapy? A double-bind randomized trial. *Radiother Oncol* 1998;47: 149-153.

[25] Barker G; Loftus L; C et al: The effects of sucralfate suspension and diphenhydramine syrup plus kaolin-pectin on radiotherapy-induced mucositis. *Oral Surg. Oral Méd. Oral Pathol* 1991; 71:288-293.

[26] Epstein JB; Wong FL: The efficacy of sucralfate suspension in the prevention of oral mucositis due to radiation therapy. *Int J. Radiat Oncol Biol Phys* 1994;28: 693-698.

[27] Makkonen T; Böstrom P; Vilja P et al: Sucralfate mouth washing in the prevention of radiation-induced mucositis: a placebo-controlled double-bind randomized study. *Int J Radiat Oncol Biol. Phys* 1994;30:177-182,.

[28] Ferreira PR: Utilização de sucralfato para a prevenção de mucosite na radioterapia dos tumores da cabeça e pescoço: um estudo randomizado. *Radiol Bras* 1993; 26: 71-80.

[29] Scherlacher A; Beufort-Spontin E: Radiotherapy of head and neck neoplasms: prevention of the inflamation of the mucosa by sucralfate treatment. *HNO* 1990;38: 24-28.

[30] Valls A; Algara M; Domènech M et al: Efficacy of sucralfate in the prophylaxis of diarrhea secondary to acute radiation-induced enteritis. Preliminary results of a double-bind randomized trial. *Med Clin (Barc.)* 1991;96: 449-452.

[31] Franzén L; Henriksson R; Littbrand B et al: Effects of sucralfate on mucositis during and following radiotherapy of malignancies in the head and neck region. A double-blind placebo-controlled study. *Acta Oncol* 1995;34: 2, 219-223.

[32] Belka C; Hoffmann W; Paulsen F et al: The use of sucralfate in radiation oncology. *Strahlenter Onkol* 1997;173:247-2525 (abst).

[33] Matejka M; Nell A; Kment G et al: Local benefit of prostaglandin E2 in radiochemotherapy-induced oral mucositis. *Br J Oral Maxillofac Surg* 1990;28: 89-94.

[34] Sinzinger H; Porterder H; Matejka M et al: Prostaglandins in irradiation induced mucositis. *Lancet* 1989;1:556-558.

[35] Porteder H; Rausch E; Kment G et al: Local prostaglandin E_2 in patients with oral malignancies undergoing chemo and radiotherapy. *J. Craniomaxillo Surg* 1988;16: 371.

[36] Pillsbury H; Webster W; Rosenman J: Prostaglandin inhibitor and radiotherapy in advanced head and neck cancers. *Arch. Otolaryngol. Head Neck Surg* 1986;112:552-553.

[37] Dinarello C: Interleukin 1 and interleukin antagonism. *Blood* 1991;77:1627-1652.

[38] Zaghloul MS; DORIE M; KALLMAN RF: Interleukin 1 increases thymidine labeling index of normal tissues of mice but not the tumor. *Int J Radiat Oncol Biol Phys* 1994;29: 805-811.

[39] Troussard X; Macro M.; Vie B et al: Human recombinant granulocyte macrophage colony stimulating factor (hr GM-CSF) improves double hemibody irradiation (DHBI) tolerance in patients with stage III multiple myeloma. a pilot study. *Br J Hematol* 1995;89: 191-195.

[40] Taylor K; Jagannath S; Spitzer G et al: Recombinant human granulocyte colony stimulating factor hastens granulocyte recovery after high dose chemotherapy and autologous bone marrow transplantation in Hodgkin's disease. *J Clin Oncol* 1989;7: 791-1799.

[41] Kannan V; Bapsy P; Anantha N et al: Efficacy and safety of granulocyte macrophage colony stimulating factor (GM-CSF) on the frequency and severity of radiation mucositis in patients with head and neck carcinoma. *Int. J. Radiat. Biol. Phys* 1997;37:1005-1010.

[42] Rosso M; Blasi G; Gherlone E et al: Effect of of granulocyte macrophage colony stimulating factor (GM-CSF) on prevention of mucositis in head and neck cancer patients treated with chemo-radiotherapy. *J. Chemother* 1997;9:382-385.

[43] Throuvalas M; Antonadou D; Pulizzi M et al: Evaluation of the efficacy and safety of GM-CSF in the prophylaxis of patients with head and neck cancer treated by RT. *Apresentado na European Conference of Clinical Oncology* (ECCO), p. 593. Federation of European Cancer Societies, Paris, 1995 (abst 431).

[44] Meropol NJ, Somer RA, Gutheil J et al: Randomized phase I trial of recombinant keratinocyte growth factor plus chemotherapy: potential role as mucosal protectant. *J Clin Oncol* 2003;1452 – 1458.

[45] Alderson R, Gohari-Fritsch S, Olsen H et al: In vitro and in vivo effects of repifermin (keratinocyte growth factor-2, KGF-2) on human carcinoma cells. *Cancer Chemother Pharmacol* 2002;50,202 – 212.

[46] Büntzel J; Küttner K; Fröhlich D et al: Selective radioprotection with amifostine in concurrent radiochemotherapy for head and neck cancer. *Annals Onco* 1998;9: 505-509.

[47] Wagner W; Prott F; Schonekas K:. Amifostine: a radioprotector in locally advanced head and neck tumors. *Oncol. Rep* 1998;5:1255-1257.

[48] Wasserman T, Chapman J: Radiation response modulator. In: *Principles and practice of radiation oncology*. Perez C, Brady L, Halperin E, Schmidt-Ullrich R (eds.). Philadelphia: Lippincott Williams and Wilkins, 2004. P. 679.

[49] Berger A; Ederson M; Madoolman W et al: Oral capsaicin provides temporary relief for oral mucositis pain secondary to chemotherapy/radiation therapy. *J. Pain Symptom Manage* 1995;10: 243-248.

[50] Narra V Harpanhalli R; HOWELL R et al: Vitamins as radioprotectants in vivo. I. Protection by vitamin C against internal radionuclides in mouse testes: implications to the mechanisms of the Auger effect *Radiat Res* 1994;137: 394-399.

[51] Mills E: The modifying effect of beta-carotene on radiation and chemotherapy induced oral mucositis. *Br J Cancer* 1988;57: 416-42.

[52] El-Nahas SM, Mattar FE, Mohamed AA: Radioprotective effect of vitamins C and E. *Mutat Res* 1993;301:143-147.

[53] Felemovicius I, Bonsak ME, Baptista ML: Intestinal radioprotection by vitamin E (alpha tocopherol). *Ann Surg* 1995;222: 4,504-508.

[54] Delaney JP, Bonsak M, Hall P: Intestinal radioprotection by two new agents applied topically. *Ann Surg* 1992;216: 417-421,

[55] Empey LR, Papp JD, Jewell LD, et al: Mucosal protective effects of vitamin E and misoprostol during acute radiation-induced enteritis in rats. *Dig Dis Sci* 1992;37:205-214.

[56] Blumenthal RD, Lew W, Reising A, et al: Anti-oxidant vitamins reduce normal tissue toxicity induced by radio-immunotherapy. *Int J Cancer* 2000;86:276-280.

[57] Shaheen AA, Hassan SM: Radioprotection of whole body gamma-irradiation-induced alteration in some haematological parameters by cysteine, vitamin E, and their combination in rats. *Strahlenther Onkol* 1991;167:498-501.

[58] Wadleigh RG, Redman RS, Graham ML, et al: Vitamin E in the treatment of chemotherapy-induced mucositis. *Am J Med* 1992;92: 481-484.

[59] Osaki T, Ueta E, Yoneda K, et al: Prophylaxis of oral mucositis associated with chemoradiotherapy for oral carcinoma by Azelastine hydrochloride (Azelastine) with other antioxidants. *Head Neck* 1994;16:331-339.

[60] Lopez I, Goudou C, Ribrag V, et al: Traitement des mucines par la vitamine E lors de l'administration d'anti-neoplastiques neutropéniants. *Ann Med Interne* 1994;145: 405-408.

[61] Schofield FF, Holden D, Carr HD: Bowel disease after radiotherapy. *J R Soc Med* 1983;76:463-466.

[62] Brock WA: Kinectis of micronucleus expression in synchronized irradiated Chinese hamster ovary cells. *Cell Tissue Kinet* 1985;18: 247-252.

[63] Van Acker SA, Hoyman L, Bast A: Molecular pharmacology of vitamin E: Structural aspects of antioxidant activity. *Free Radic Biol Med* 1993;15: 311-328.

[64] Ward R, Peters T: Free radicals. In: Marshal W, Bangert S, editors. *Clinical Biochemistry – Metabolic and Clinic Aspects*. London: Church Livingstone; 1995. pp. 765-777.

[65] Regan V.; Servinova E.; Packer L: Antioxidant effects of ubiquinones in microsomes and mitochondria are mediated by tocopherol recycling. *Biochem Biophys Res Commun* 1990;169: 851-856.

[66] Tampo Y, Yonaha M: Vitamin E and gluthatione are required for preservation of microsomal gluthatione S-transferase from oxidative stress in microsomes. *Pharmacology* 66:259, 1990.

[67] Starasoler S, Haber GS: Use of vitamin E oil in primary herpes gingivostomatitis in an adult. NY State Dentristy 1978;44:382.

[68] Köstler WJ, Hejna M, Wenzel C, et al: Oral Mucositis Complicating Chemotherapy and/or Radiotherapy: Options for Prevention and Treatment. *CA Cancer J Clin* 2001;51: 290-315.

[69] Ferreira PR, Fleck JF, Diehl A et al: Protective effect of vitamin E (VE) in head and neck cancer radiation induced mucositis: a double-blind randomized trial. *Presented in the annual meeting of American Society of clinical Oncology*, 2002 (abstr 909).

[70] Ferreira PR, Fleck JF, Diehl A et al: Protective effect of alpha-tocopherol in head and neck cancer radiation-induced mucositis: a double-blind randomized trial. *Head Neck* 2004;26:313-21.

[71] Zubrod CG, Scheiderman M: Appraisal of methods for the study of chemotherapy of cancer in man. *J Chronic Dis* 1960;11:7-33.

[72] UICC, *International Union Against Cancer. TNM Classification of Malignant Tumours*. 5th ed. Wiley-Liss Inc. 1997. p. 19.

[73] Cox JD, Stetz J, Pajak TF: Toxicity criteria of the Radiation Therapy Oncology Group (RTOG) and the European Organization for Research and Treatment of Cancer (EORTC). *Int J Radiat Oncol Biol Phys* 1995;31: 1341-1346.

[74] Ferreira PR, Fleck JF, Diehl AS, et al: Vitamin E preventing radiation-induced mucositis in head and neck cancer: Interim analysis of a randomized, double-blind clinical trial. Proceedings of the 29th Paulista Meeting of Radiology, Sao Paulo, Brazil. *Rev Imagem* 1999, p. 22 (suppl).

[75] Kaplan G, Meier P: Non-parametric estimation from incomplete observations. *J Am Stat* 1958;53: 457-481.

[76] Trotti A: Toxicity in head and neck cancer: A review of trends and issues. *Int J Radiat Oncol Biol Phys* 2000;47:1-12.

In: Hepatitis B Research Advances
Editor: Alicia P. Willis, pp. 253-293
ISBN: 978-1-60021-666-4

Chapter XV

Essential Immune Responses to Hepatitis B Virus Infection

***Ali A. Al-Jabri*[1,*] *and Abdullah A. Balkhair*[2]**
Department of Microbiology and Immunology[1], Infectious Diseases Unit[2],
Department of Medicine, College of Medicine and Health Sciences,
Sultan Qaboos University, Muscat, Oman

Abstract

Although a vaccine is available for the prevention of hepatitis B virus (HBV) infection, HBV infects nearly two billion people around the world and mainly in the underdeveloped countries. The liver is the primary target of HBV. The virus infects the hepatocytes leading to the release of infectious virions and non-infectious particles into the blood. HBV infection can be either acute, which may last for several months or chronic which is a life long infection.

The immune system both innate and acquired (humoral and cell mediated) responses, play essential roles in HBV infection. It is known that neutralizing antibodies play an important role during HBV infection and can reduce the spread of infection. Cellular immune mechanisms are also important for the clearance of HBV and disease pathogenesis. The different structural forms of the hepatitis B viral proteins, can elicit different T helper cell subsets with different cytokines being produced. Cytokines are very important proteins in the defense against viral infections including HBV.

In this chapter, we will discuss our current knowledge of the immunology of the HBV infection and factors that make this infection more common in the underdeveloped countries, especially the middle-eastern countries. We will discuss in detail the essential role played by the immune system innate and acquired responses and we will briefly

* Correspondence concerning this article should be addressed to Dr. Ali A. Al-Jabri, Associate Professor of Immunology, Department of Microbiology and Immunology, College of Medicine and Health Sciences, Sultan Qaboos University, P.O. Box 35, Al Khod, Muscat, Sultanate of Oman. Tel: 00968-2415186 Tel: 00968-2415170 Fax: 00968-2413419, e.mail: aaljabri@squ.edu.om.

discuss the ways of controlling HBV infection in general and in particular to this part of the world.

1. Introduction

Hepatitis B is a disease of the liver caused by the Hepatitis B virus (HBV), a member of the *Hepadnavirus* family and one of several unrelated viral species which cause viral hepatitis. Since the discovery of hepatitis B virus in 1966, our understanding of its details has continued to unfold (Purcell, 1993). It was originally known as "serum hepatitis" and has caused current epidemics in parts of Africa and Asia. Hepatitis B is recognized as endemic in China and various other parts of Asia. The proportion of the world's population currently infected with the virus is estimated at 3 to 6%. Symptoms of the acute illness caused by the virus include liver inflammation, vomiting, jaundice, and rarely, death. Chronic hepatitis B may cause liver cirrhosis which may then lead to liver cancer (Echevarra *et al.,* 1995). The Hepatitis B virus is the second most prevalent cause of cancer in humans after Tobacco smoke.

Hepatitis B virus infection can either be acute (self-limited) or chronic (long-standing). Individuals with self-limited infection clear the infection spontaneously within weeks to months. More than 95% of individuals who become infected as adults or older children will stage a full recovery and develop protective immunity to the virus. However, only 5% of new-borns that acquire the infection from their mother at birth will clear the infection. Usually of those infected between the ages of one to six, 70% will clear the infection. When the infection is not cleared, one becomes a chronic carrier of the virus (Desmet *et al.,* 1999).

Acute infection with hepatitis B virus is associated with acute viral hepatitis - an illness that begins with general ill-health, loss of appetite, nausea, vomiting, body-aches, mild fever, dark urine, and then progresses to development of jaundice. It has also been noted that itchy skin all over the body, has been an indication as a possible symptom of all hepatitis virus types. The illness lasts for a few weeks and then gradually improves in most of the affected people. A few patients may have more severe liver disease (fulminant hepatic failure), and may die as a result of it. The infection may also be entirely asymptomatic and may go unrecognized (Echevarra *et al.,* 1995).

Chronic infection with hepatitis B virus may be either asymptomatic or may be associated with a chronic inflammation of the liver (chronic hepatitis), leading to cirrhosis over a period of several years (Maruyama *et al.,* 1994). This type of infection dramatically increases the incidence of liver cancer (Echevarra *et al.,* 1995). Although potent antiviral agents have now emerged, the virus itself and the diseases it causes continue to evolve. The availability of new treatments coupled with effective vaccines and risk avoidance should begin to diminish the burden of chronic hepatitis B in the near future (Jung and Pape, 2002; Jung *et al.,* 2002).

1.1. Occurrence of HBV in the Underdeveloped Countries

It is estimated that over two billion people worldwide have evidence of hepatitis B virus exposure (Mast *et al.,* 1998) and 5% of the world population have chronic infection with hepatitis B virus and between 300 to 400 million carriers (Maddrey, 2001). The estimates of WHO for hepatitis B virus is that there are over five million cases of acute hepatitis B infection every year (Kane *et al.,* 1999). Infection with HBV results in 0.5 to 1.2 million deaths per year due mainly to chronic hepatitis, cirrhosis and hepatocellular carcinoma (HCC) making hepatitis B the 10th leading cause of death worldwide (WHO, 1997, 2000). The incidence of HBV infection and patterns of transmission vary greatly throughout the world and in different populations (WHO, 1996).

Worldwide, the prevalence of hepatitis B virus varies greatly. In hyperendemic areas, such as China, Southeast Asia, Western Pacific, and sub-Saharan Africa, the carrier rate exceeds 8% and transmission occurs mainly from mother to child at time of parturition, as well as by horizontal transmission among children less than five years of age, and to a lesser extent between sexually active adults. In North America and Europe less than 1% are chronically infected, as a result of injection drug use, sexual transmission, nosocomial infection, or emigration from endemic areas (McQuillan *et al.,* 1999).

Although the world can be broadly classified into regions of high, intermediate and low HBV endemicity, there are substantial differences between countries in the same continent. South-East Asia has previously been classified as a high endemicity area, but China is now the only country in Asia that remains in this category, with 7–20% prevalence of HBV surface antigen (HBsAg) (Tandon and Tandon, 1997). This is because the epidemiological picture changes with time, as hepatitis B prevention programmes become effective. Probably half of the world's chronic carriers reside in China and India, though the latter is an intermediate endemicity area. The other intermediate endemicity countries are Korea, Thailand and the Philippines. The low endemicity countries in this area include Japan, Pakistan, Bangladesh and Sri Lanka, with 0.2–1.9% prevalence of HBsAg and 4–10% prevalence of antibodies to HBV core antigen (anti-HBc) (Tandon and Tandon, 1997). Singapore and Malaysia now also have low endemicity of HBV, as their very successful vaccination programmes have greatly reduced the incidence of infection.

Although overall Africa is an area of high HBV endemicity, Tunisia and Morocco fall into the intermediate category, with current infection rates of less than 7%, whereas most of West and East Africa are indeed high endemicity areas, with current chronic infection rates of 7–26% (Kew, 1997). In some countries, e.g. Senegal, over 90% of the population will be exposed in the course of their lives to HBV and become infected. All of central and southern Africa is also in the high endemicity category, with the possible exception of Zambia, which has borderline intermediate endemicity with current chronic infection rates of 6.5–7.5% (Kew, 1997)

In the Middle East, Bahrain, Iran and Kuwait, which all reach over 80% of the population with hepatitis B vaccination as part of their Expanded Programme on Immunization (EPI), are also areas of low endemicity, with HBsAg carrier rates of under 2% (Toukan, 1997). The areas of intermediate endemicity include Cyprus, Iraq and the United Arab Emirates, all of which include hepatitis B vaccination in their EPI and reach 68–90% of the population. The carrier rates in these countries are 2–5% (Toukan, 1997). The areas of high endemicity in this region include Egypt, Jordan, Oman, Palestine, Yemen and Saudi Arabia, in which carrier rates range from 2 to 18.5%. All of these countries include hepatitis B vaccination in their EPI.

The epidemiological picture of hepatitis B infection changes with time, as hepatitis B prevention programmes become effective. The potential impact of vaccination programmes can be illustrated by the experience of two countries: Saudi Arabia and Taiwan. In Saudi Arabia, the prevalence of HBsAg in children has decreased from 6.7% to 0.3% within 8 years of starting a mass vaccination programme (Al-Faleh, 1998). Similarly, the prevalence of anti-HBc decreased from about 4.2% to under 0.5%. In Taiwan, The vaccination program has also greatly reduced the HBV infection rate producing a dramatic decrease in the incidence of hepatocellular carcinoma in birth cohorts born after implementation of the vaccination programme (Chang *et al.,* 1997)

The long-term objective of a hepatitis B vaccination programme is to prevent virus transmission in all age groups (newborns, children, adolescents and at-risk adults), with the ultimate aim eventually of eliminating the infection, and even more long-term, of eradicating the virus. This is likely to prove much more difficult than the eradication of smallpox and polio, because of the pool of chronic carriers. The short- and medium-term goals are to prevent chronic and acute symptomatic infection and to reduce healthcare costs. The long-term goals are to prevent the chronic complications, i.e. cirrhosis and hepatocellular carcinoma (Francis, 2000).

Most countries in South-East Asia and the Middle East have now started hepatitis B prevention programmes, though in Africa only a few countries have started infant vaccination programmes (Thompson and Ruff, 1995). Although eradication of hepatitis B is theoretically possible, it will be very difficult to achieve with the current tools, because of the 350 million carriers of this virus in the world. In the next 20–30 years, the objective should be to convert the high endemicity and the intermediate endemicity countries into low endemicity countries, which can be practically achieved with vaccination programmes. (Francis, 2000)

HBV genotypes have distinct geographical distribution. In general, genotype A is pandemic, but most prevalent in North West Europe, North America, Central Africa (Stuyver et al., 2000) and India (Kao, 2002). Genotypes B and C are prevalent in Asia (Kao, 2002; Kao *et al.,* 2002; Huy and Abe, 2004), especially in populations of Eastern Asia and the far East origin (Yalcin *et al.,* 2004). Genotype D is also more or less pandemic, but is predominant in the Mediterranean area and the Middle East (Francis, 2000; Yalcin *et al.,* 2004). Genotype E is restricted to Africa and genotype F is found in Central and South America (Kao, 2002; Kao et al., 2002). Genotype G has been recently identified in France and North America (Kao, 2002; Kao *et al.,* 2002). It has been reported that there are remarkable differences in the clinical and virologic characteristics between the patients with different genotypes (Chan *et al.,* 2003; Lin *et al.,* 2002).

1.2. The Human Hepatitis B Virus

Hepatitis B virus is an enveloped doubled-stranded DNA virus of 3.2 kb genome which exists in circular construct. It is a member of the family *Hepadnaviridae* and is a non-cytopathic DNA virus.

1.2.1. Hepatitis B Virus Modes of Transmission

Hepatitis B is mainly transmitted by exposure to bodily fluids containing the HBV. This includes unprotected sexual contact, blood transfusions, re-use of contaminated needles and syringes, vertical transmission from mother to child during childbirth, etc (Lee, 1997). The primary method of transmission depends on the prevalence of the disease in a given area. In low prevalence areas, intravenous drug abuse and unprotected sex are the primary methods of getting the virus. In moderate prevalence areas, the disease is predominantly spread among children. In high prevalence areas, such as South East Asia, vertical transmission is very common. Without intervention, a mother who is positive for the hepatitis B surface antigen confers a 20% risk of passing the infection to her offspring at the time of birth. This risk is as high as 90% if the mother is also positive for the hepatitis B "e" antigen (Kane, 1995). Roughly 16-40% of unimmunized sexual partners of individuals with hepatitis B will be infected through sexual contact. The risk of transmission is closely related to the rate of viral replication in the infected individual at the time of exposure.

The large quantities of hepatitis B virus in serum and other body fluids ($\sim 10^8$ copies/mL) allow spread by mucosal and percutaneous routes with greater efficiency than is observed with hepatitis C virus (10^6 copies/mL) or human immunodeficiency virus (HIV; 10^4 copies/mL).

1.2.2. Virus Structure and Classification

Hepatitis B virus has been classified into 8 genotypes, A to H, based on genetic sequence variability between genotypes of more than 8% (Ljunggren *et al.,* 2002). Certain genotypes predominate within different geographic, regional, and racial groups. Different genotypes are associated with somewhat different clinical outcomes, treatment responses, and mutations. The role of genotypes in the clinical management of chronic hepatitis B virus is still not completely understood (Fung & Lok, 2004).

Electron microscopy of sera from patients with hepatitis B infection reveals the presence of three distinct morphologic entities (Figure 1). The more numerous forms (by a factor of 10^4 to 10^6) are small, hepatitis B surface antigen (HBsAg)–positive, pleomorphic spherical particles measuring 17 to 25 nm in diameter (mean of 20 nm). Tubular or filamentous forms of various lengths, but with a diameter similar to that of the smaller particles, also are observed. Neither of these forms contains viral-specific nucleic acid, which is found in a complex, double-shelled particle with a diameter of 42 nm that comprises the hepatitis B virion. It consists of a 27 nm core surrounded by a 7 to 8 nm viral protein coat called HBsAg. This protein is identical to that detected on the smaller particles and the filaments. It contains three related glycoproteins designated S or major, M or middle (pre-S1+ S), and L or large (pre-S1+ pre-S2 + S). These proteins are not distributed uniformly between the various HBV particles that circulate in the blood. For example, the more numerous 20 nm particles (by a factor of 10,000 to 1 million) are composed primarily of the S protein, with variable amounts of the M polypeptide and essentially none of the L chains. Conversely, the HBV virion contains relatively large amounts of the L chains to M or S chains. The L chains are believed to contain the recognition site for binding to hepatocytes and are important for viral assembly and infectivity.

a. Electron microscopy of HBV

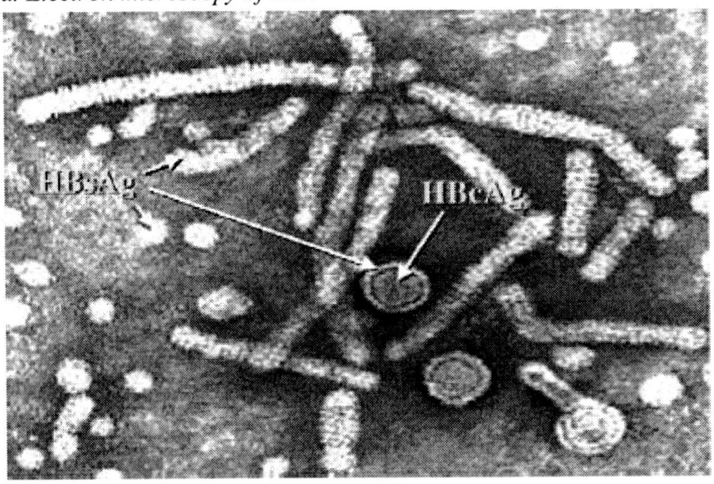

Obtained from Hollinger & Lau, 2006

b. Simple diagram illustrating the basic components of HBV

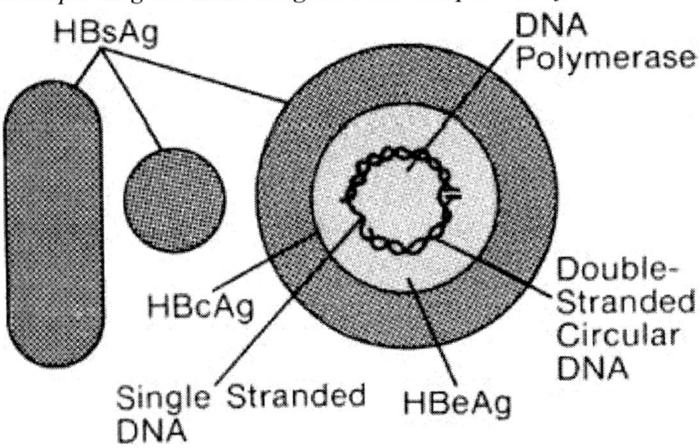

Schematic illustration of the hepatitis B virus and its antigens: hepatitis B surface antigen (HBsAg), hepatitis B core antigen (HBcAg), and hepatitis B e antigen (HBeAg). (Source: Gershon: Krugman's, Infectious Diseases of Children, 11th Ed).

Figure 1. Structure of HBV.

The nucleocapsid of the virion contains a single capsid protein called hepatitis B core antigen (HBcAg). The HBV DNA is encapsidated within the nucleocapsid as a relaxed circular, partially double-stranded DNA molecule. The viral genome has four partially overlapping open reading frames: S (surface or envelope, hepatitis B surface antigen [HBsAg]) gene, C (core, hepatitis B core antigen [HBcAg], structural protein of the nucleocapsid) gene, X gene, a complex regulatory protein that is required for infectivity and the P (polymerase) gene (Seeger & Mason, 2000). Infected individuals develop antibodies to HBsAg (anti-HBs) and HBcAg (anti-HBc) and some also generate an antibody response to the X protein. The open reading frame, that code for the core protein also codes for another protein known serologically as the hepatitis B "e" antigen (HBeAg) (Maruyama *et al.,* 1993). This product is not a part of the virion, and is secreted from the cell. Its accumulation in the serum is usually indicative of highly active replication of the virus. It often evokes its own antibody response (anti-HBe), which can signify a return to a less active state of viral replication. Mutant viruses with lesions in the pre-C or core promoter region of the HBV genome, however, can prevent the expression of HBeAg (Hadziyannis and Vassilopulos, 2001).

1.2.3. Hepatitis B Virus (HBV) Replication (Life Cycle)

When the virus enters the body of a new host its initial response, if it's gets past the immune system, is to infect a liver cell. To do this the virus attaches to a liver cells membrane and the core particle enters the liver cell. The core particle then releases its contents of DNA and DNA polymerase into the liver cell nucleus. From within the cell nucleus the hepatitis B DNA causes the liver cell to produce, via messenger RNA; surface (HBs) proteins, the core (HBc) protein, DNA polymerase, the HBe protein, HBx protein and possibly other as yet undetected proteins and enzymes (Maruyama *et al.,* 1993).

DNA polymerase causes the liver cell to make copies of hepatitis-B-DNA. It is believed that the replication of HBV-DNA does not go via RNA. Via the above process, versions of the hepatitis B virus are constructed by the liver cell. These copies of the virus are released from the liver cell membrane into the blood stream and from there can infect other liver cells and thus replicate effectively. However, when reproducing, mistakes may be made in copying viral DNA and this may results in different strains and mutant strains of hepatitis B virus occurring.

The incubation of the Hepatitis B Virus is about 6 to 25 weeks (i.e. before physical and generally detectable histological or physical symptoms occur), however, there are several biochemical and histological changes that occur in stages after infection with the hepatitis B virus.

HBV initiates infection by binding to its receptor on the hepatocytes, penetrating the cellular membrane, followed by uncoating of the virion (Ganem *et al.,* 2001). The nucleocapsid is translocated through nuclear pores into the nucleus of the cell where the genomic DNA is matured to the **c**ovalently **c**losed **c**ircular DNA [CCCDNA]. The CCCDNA is the power source for continuing replication of the virus and is amplified during the replicative cycle. The DNA is transcribed and the resulting RNAs translated in the cytoplasm to the various viral proteins. Pregenomic RNAs are encapsidated within sub-viral core particles in the cytoplasm along with a viral DNA polymerase enzyme for viral DNA synthesis. Unlike most DNA viruses, it replicates by reverse transcription of the genomic RNA template. This process includes polymerization of the minus-strand DNA, degradation of the RNA intermediate and incomplete synthesis of the plus-strand. Progeny cores bud into the endoplasmic reticulum where they acquire their envelope before undergoing vesicular transport out of the cell. During this process, HBV production may approach 10^{11} molecules per day.

Ordinarily, DNA polymerases have excellent fidelity in reading DNA templates. Fidelity is defined as the frequency of correct nucleotide insertions per incorrect insertion. In contrast to that observed with other DNA viruses, the HBV-DNA-polymerase lacks either fidelity or proofreading function partly because exonuclease activity is either absent or deficient in HBV. As a result, the genome, and especially the envelope gene, is mutated with unusually high frequency during replication. The mutation rate of HBV lies somewhere between the RNA-containing retroviruses, such as HIV, and other DNA viruses, that lack requirements for reverse transcriptase activity. The reasons for this are not entirely clear, but may be caused by the fact that mutations in HBV are not well tolerated because over 50% of the open reading frames in the HBV genome are overlapping. Therefore, any mutation that occurs during replication can affect more than one open reading frame.

1.3. Clinical Outcome of HBV Infection

The clinical and serologic changes that occur following infection represent a complex interaction between the virus and the host associated immune response to the viral infection (Hollinger *et al.*, 2001). In addition to the in apparent or sub clinical cases, patients may develop anicteric or icteric hepatitis. The term ''anicteric hepatitis'' should be reserved for those patients who develop clinical symptoms but who are not jaundiced. Patients with in apparent (sub-clinical) hepatitis have neither symptoms nor jaundice. Symptoms ranging from mild and transient to severe and prolonged may accompany clinical hepatitis. Patients may recover completely, progress to chronic hepatitis, or develop fulminant hepatitis and die. It is important to recognize that the frequency of clinical disease increases with age, whereas the percentage of carriers decreases (McMahon *et al.*, 1985). In endemic regions, asymptomatic perinatal acquisition of disease from HBeAg-positive mothers results in a high carrier rate of 85% to 90%. In contrast, symptomatic acute infection occurs in approximately 40% of the adult-acquired infection, but the carrier rate is only approximately 2% to 5% in the absence of immunodeficiency.

The incubation period for hepatitis B virus ranges from 45 to 120 days. Incubation periods of less than 35 days or more than 150 days are unusual. A short prodromal or preicteric phase, varying from several days to more than a week, precedes the onset of jaundice in over 85% of the HBV cases. Fever, if present, usually subsides after the first few days of jaundice. Occasionally, more extensive necrosis of the liver occurs. This entity, designated fulminant hepatitis B if it occurs during the first 8 weeks of illness, is characterized by the sudden onset of high fever, marked abdominal pain, vomiting, and jaundice, followed by the development of hepatic encephalopathy associated with deep coma and seizures and accompanied by severe impairment of hepatic synthetic processes, excretory functions, and detoxifying mechanisms. Although fulminant hepatitis is uncommon when compared with overall infection rates, it is observed in up to 4% of the hospitalized cases and leads to death in 70% to 90% of the patients in the absence of transplantation (Papaevangelou *et al.,* 1984). At least one prospective study (McMahon *et al.,* 1985) indicates that higher proportions of individuals with sub-clinical hepatitis B are more likely to progress to chronic hepatitis (14.8% of 162) than are those who develop clinical hepatitis B (3.8% of 26). In general, chronic disease occurs in 2% to 5% of immuno-competent adults who are infected, whereas a higher rate is observed in immuno-compromised patients.

1.3.1. Clinical Phases of Chronic Hepatitis B Virus Infection

Chronic HBV (CHB) infection is defined by the persistence of HBsAg for six months or longer. It can be classified into three major forms: (1) HBsAg carriers with inactive disease, (2) HBeAg-positive CHB, and (3) HBeAg-negative CHB. Most patients with chronic infection remain asymptomatic for many years. Some of these patients may have no clinical or biochemical evidence of liver disease. To distinguish this group from patients with chronic hepatitis, they are often categorized as asymptomatic hepatitis B carriers or simply HBsAg carriers. De Franchis and coworkers (de Franchis *et al.,* 1993) have studied the natural history of chronic HBV infection in a cohort of these patients. At baseline, 96% of 92 patients were anti-HBe positive and histologic abnormalities were normal or minimal in all but five who had only mild chronic hepatitis. During a mean follow up of approximately ten years, liver enzymes remained normal in 85% of 68 patients who were extensively followed, and 13% of these patients cleared their HBsAg. Among 21 HBsAg carriers who showed no biochemical changes during 10 years of follow-up, there were no histologic changes; spontaneous reactivation was a rare event (4% of 68 patients); and no hepatocellular carcinoma was detected.

CHB is the term used to describe HBeAg-positive or HBeAg-negative patients with significant chronic necroinflammatory disease of the liver associated with moderate to advanced fibrosis or cirrhosis caused by persistent HBV infection as found on liver biopsy. This is to distinguish them from the inactive (healthy) HBsAg carrier state described previously in which chronic HBV infection is present without significant ongoing necroinflammatory disease and no or minimal fibrosis on a biopsy. HBeAg negative CHB is common in Asia and the Middle East, accounting for about 70% to 80% of the chronic HBV cases in those regions (Schalm *et al.,* 1990). In contrast, an overall low prevalence of HBeAg-negative chronic HBV infection (24%) was reported in the USA in 1996 (Margolis *et al.,* 1991).

Patients with moderate to severe chronic hepatitis may have no symptoms, or they may be significantly incapacitated. At the time of the initial diagnosis, jaundice is uncommon, ascites and pedal edema are seen in approximately 20%, whereas fewer than 5% present with endogenous encephalopathy or variceal bleeding. Aminotransferases, bilirubin, and gamma globulin levels are mild to markedly elevate. During follow-up, there may be a series of remissions and relapses. Remissions may last a few months to several years. During a relapse, aminotransferases may be markedly elevated and jaundice may be present. Predictors of progression to cirrhosis include hepatic decompensation; repeated episodes of severe acute exacerbation with bridging hepatic necrosis or high alpha fetoprotein levels (>100 ng/mL); acute exacerbations without HBeAg clearance; and HBV reactivation with the reappearance of HBeAg (Liaw *et al.,* 1988).

Patients with HBeAg-negative CHB display markedly different patterns of serum aminotransferase elevations: (1) continuous elevation of ALT level in approximately 24%, (2) fluctuating ALT levels in 48%, and (3) intermittent or relapsing activities in 28% (Brunetto *et al.*, 2002). Those patients with intermittent ALT elevations could be misdiagnosed as inactive HBV carriers in between flares of hepatitis. These observations underscore the importance of regular assessments of HBsAg-positive patients over time to confirm the diagnosis of HBeAg-negative CHB versus the inactive HBV carrier. In most cases, patients require a liver biopsy. Both HBeAg-positive and HBeAg-negative CHB with persistent or intermittent elevation of aminotransferases and HBV-DNA levels, associated with histologic evidence of active hepatitis, should be considered for antiviral therapy.

1.3.2. Hepatocellular Carcinoma (HCC)

Among other causative factors, chronic hepatitis B virus appears responsible for a large number of hepatocellular carcinoma (HCC) cases worldwide. HCC is the third highest cause of death from cancer in the world, the fifth most common malignancy in males, and the eighth in females. Untreated, it yields a dismal 5-year survival between 2% and 6%.

A proportion of hepatitis B patients, especially those who acquire the disease perinatally, are at risk of developing HCC, a tumor that is relatively slow growing with a median doubling time of 4 months (range of 1–14 months) (Sheu *et al.*, 1985). Metastatic spread is uncommon, with the most frequent sites being the lung (36%); direct extension through the hepatic or portal venous systems (12%); adrenal glands (10%); skeletal tissue (10%); and brain (6%) (Ihde *et al.*, 1974).

Persons at high risk of developing HCC include adult male CHB patients with cirrhosis who contracted their disease in early childhood and who display serologic or histologic evidence of active HBV replication (HBV-DNA, HBeAg, IgM anti-HBc) (Di Bisceglie *et al.*, 1988).

Approximately 55% to 85% of hepatitis B patients with HCC have cirrhosis at the time of diagnosis. Conversely, only about 5% of patients with cirrhosis develop HCC. The cumulative 5-year probability of developing HCC in HBV-infected patients with compensated cirrhosis is 9%; the incidence per 100 person-years is 2.2 (Fattovich *et al.*, 2002 & Fattovich, 2003). Crockett and Keeffe (2005) reviewed the relationship between various serologic patterns and the cumulative risk of HCC. The highest adjusted relative risk was found in HBsAg/HBeAg–positive patients with additional risk observed when these patients were found to be co-infected with HCV.

Recently, a great deal of interest has been generated concerning the relationship between a patient's HBV-DNA level and the longer-term risk of liver cancer that is independent of HBeAg status, ALT level, and the presence of liver damage or cirrhosis (Chen *et al.*, 2006). Another study implied that HBV replication, as manifested by the presence of HBeAg, is hazardous in terms of disease progression and HCC development (Yang *et al.*, 2002). Critical analyses that take into account the other known risk factors for the development of HCC (age >40 years, male gender, HBeAg positivity, excessive alcohol consumption, elevated ALT level, increased fibrosis) are necessary to establish treatment decisions, especially in adult-acquired CHB patients who have persistently normal aminotransferases and mild histology.

Resolution of chronic hepatitis B significantly diminishes the risk of subsequent hepatocellular carcinoma, as does seroconversion to HBeAg negativity.

2. IMMUNE RESPONSE TO HBV INFECTION

The immune system is a complex network of specialized organs, glands and cells which when working properly protect the body from pathogens such as viruses, bacteria, fungi and parasites. The immune system is divided into innate immunity and acquired or specific immunity. The acquired immunity is mainly composed of two basic sub-systems, the Humoral and the Cellular or Cell Mediated. These two sub-systems have different ways of defending the body from disease. The Humoral side uses mainly antibodies to defeat invading pathogens whereas Cell Mediated Immunity employs an army of cells, and their products, to attack and kill invaders.

B-lymphocytes (B-cells) and T-lymphocytes (T-cells) are sub-populations of white blood cells and are the main cells used by the immune system. B-cells differentiate into plasma cells upon antigen stimulation and produce antibodis used in Humoral Immunity; T-cells are used in Cell Medicated Immunity. They are all born in the bone marrow, but they mature differently. B-cells mature in the bone marrow, hence the "B" for bone marrow. T-cells are matured by proteins produced by the thymus gland, hence the "T" for thymus. Both sides of the Immune System must function properly in order for the body to have an optimum Immune Response to invading pathogens. In fact, B-cells will react quicker, proliferate, expand clonally and produce an antibody response more efficiently in the presence of a T-cell response (help).

Central to beginning the immune response is the activation of the helper lymphocyte (CD4 cells). This activation takes place when the CD4 cell recognizes the antigen displayed by an invading pathogen. Once the CD4 is activated, it produces Interleukin and Interferon proteins also called lymphokines or cytokines (see later), but more simply defined as immune proteins. These immune proteins in turn activate or program killer T lymphocytes (CD8 cells) to find and kill the specific antigen producing pathogen. Additionally, the activated CD4 cell causes B-cells to produce antibodies more efficiently.

The immune system, both innate and acquired plays important roles during HBV infection. Usually more than 90% of infected people will recover from Hepatitis B virus infection and around half of these will have had no symptoms. Recovery means that no hepatitis B surface antigen (HBsAg) is found in their blood and the Hepatitis B Antibody to surface antigens (HBsAb) is present. Antibodies to HBsAg, usually persists for life after recovery (Innacone *et al.,* 2006).

Following HBV infection, HBV-DNA and DNA-polymerase appear in the blood stream. Several weeks later HB "c" Ag and HB "e" Ag are detectable. Thereafter, HB "s" Ag is detected in the blood stream and usually after one to six weeks symptoms may appear on the patient (Chisari and Ferrari, 1995). HB "c" Ab is the first detectable antibody in the blood. In the majority of cases, as the immune system continues it's fight, HB "e" Ag disappears from the blood stream and a few weeks later HB "e" Ab's appear. The level of liver enzymes (see below) in the blood then starts to fall and HB "s" Ag disappears from serum at about the same time as HB "s" Ab's are first detected (Juszczyk, 2000).

Alanine aminotransferase (ALT) and aspartate aminotransferase (AST) are enzymes produced in liver cells that can be detected in the blood stream. When liver cells are damaged these enzymes are released and elevated levels can be detected in serum. The value of ALT in the blood stream is generally taken as an indicator of the damage that hepatitis causing to liver cells. However, damage may be occurring with little or no elevation of ALT. ALT and AST and other substances are measured when a liver function test is taken.

After an initial infection and at around the same time as HB "c" Ab appears in the blood stream the level of ALT starts to rise sharply. The rise in ALT is because of damage to the liver cells as indicated earlier. It is believed that the damage to liver cells is not caused directly by the virus, i.e. the virus does not kill liver cells, but by the human bodies own immune system killing infected and surrounding cells. In patients with compromised immune systems and/or with HIV infection there is an increased risk of the infection becoming chronic but damage done by the chronic infection appears mild in comparison to people not infected with HIV (Chisari and Ferrari, 1995). In cases of acute infection, ALT starts to drop at around the same time as when the 'e' antigen is no longer detectable and is down to normal levels when antibodies to the surface antigen appear (Chisari and Ferrari, 1995).

If the immune system is strong, it will eliminate or clear the HBV within a few weeks, from the time first symptoms appeared, and full recovery from acute hepatitis B will occur. To overcome the infection, the immune system will produce antibodies to vanquish each of the antigens or foreign proteins that make up the hepatitis B virus. These antigens include the surface antigen, the core antigen, and the "e" antigen. Once enough antibodies are produced to neutralize each of these antigens, the patient is considered cured. The immune system will also unleash special cells to kill the liver cells infected with the virus. By this, the immune system eradicates the virus and viral antigens, and clears the infection in the liver (Huang *et al.,* 2006). The stronger the immune response, the greater the chance of eliminating the virus and, therefore, recovering from infection.

If, however, the immune system is weak and unable to eradicate all the antigens and the infection in the liver, this can lead to a chronic hepatitis B. Chronic hepatitis B infection occurs in approximately 90% of infants, 30% of children between the ages of one and five years, and 6% of persons older than age five who are infected with HBV. Young children are especially vulnerable to infection because of their developing immune systems that do not effectively fight the virus. Adults with weak immune systems can also develop chronic hepatitis B. Viral clearance depends on the age and the immune status of the individual, and most infections of the immuno-compromised adults are self-limiting (Visvanathan and Lewin, 2006). Persistence or chronic infection is more likely to occur following transmission from mother to child or in immuno-compromised adults (Visvanathan and Lewin, 2006).

The study of the immuno-pathogenesis of HBV has been limited by the lack of available animal models (Dandri *et al.,* 2006) and also in vitro cell lines that can support the HBV infection (Zoulim, 2006). Below we describe our current knowledge of the essentials of the immune responses dealing with HBV infection.

3. Innate Immune Responses to HBV Infection

Immune response to viruses, in general, relies on a complex interaction of several cells; the cells of the innate immune system: the dendritic cells, which are key cells in priming and directing the virus-specific T-cell response; and the T cells, which are the main antiviral effectors. The innate immune responses involves the phagocytic cells (neutrophils, monocytes, and macrophages), cells that are important during inflammation (mast cells, basophils, and eosinophils), natural killer (NK) cells, NKT cells, and proteins of the complement system and acute phase proteins and different cytokines (Biron, 1999).

Following infection of the hepatocyte various humoral and cellular responses occur aiming at eliminating the virus (Figure 2). The earliest responses are the non-specific and include the interferon, natural killer (NK) cells, and non-specific activation of Kupffer cells in the liver. In acute HBV infection, the clearance of HBV-DNA is mediated mainly by antiviral cytokines (especially interferon-gamma (IFN-γ) and tumor necrosis factor-alpha (TNF-α) and interferon-alpha/beta (IFN-α/β) produced by cells of the innate and acquired immune responses (Murray *et al.*, 2005).

The precise role of several of these innate mechanisms is not completely understood in HBV infection. However, it is known that the innate immune response uses conserved recognition receptors, of which, the Toll like receptors (or TLR) family are recently recognized as important molecules for fighting viruses.

3.1. Toll Like Receptors and HBV Infection

Toll like receptors were shown originally to confer resistance to fungus. Toll like receptors-4 (TLR-4) was the first TLR to be shown to play a role in innate immunity. There are now ten TLRs been identified in humans and most of them have been shown to play important roles in innate immunity. These molecules are expressed on many antigen presenting cells (such as dendritic cells, macrophages and monocytes) and during innate immunity these molecules bind to their legends on effector cells and immediately unleash their functions rather than following cellular proliferation which takes time for the effector cell to perform its appropriate function. Binding of the TLR to their ligands initiates the activation of complex networks of intracellular signal transduction pathways to coordinate the ensuing inflammatory response. This is important for the acquired immune responses and the activation of T cells. It has been shown that the specific immune response only respond to a pathogen after it has been recognized and processed by the innate immune system. For the T cell to be activated, the T cell receptor (TCR) requires co-stimulatory molecules such as CD80 and CD86 to be expressed on the cell surface of the APC in association with the MHC molecules. The expression of CD80 and CD86 and the MHC is controlled partly by TLRs (Visvanathan and Lewin, 2006).

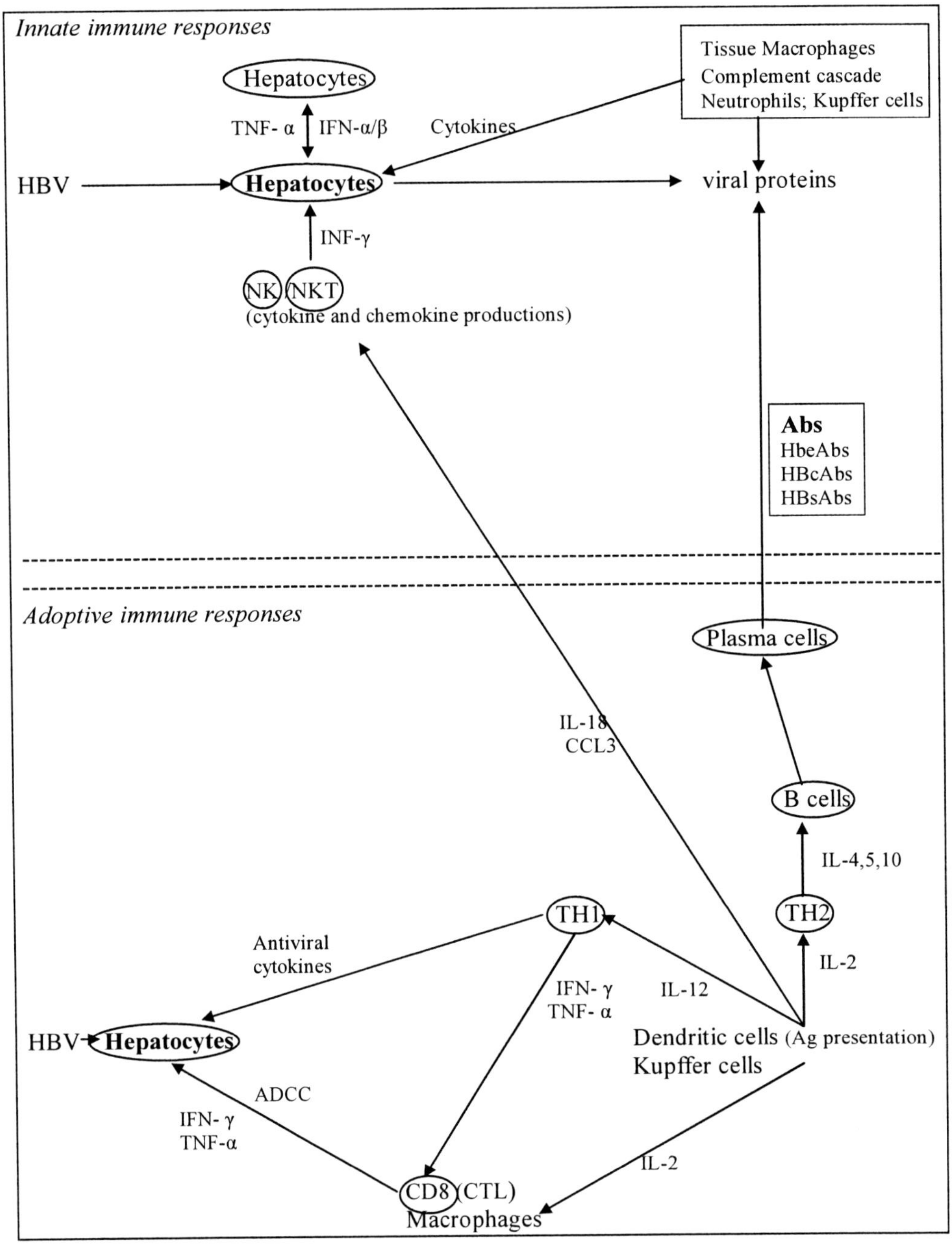

Figure 2. Diagrammatic summary of immune responses to hepatitis B virus infection.

Abberviations: HBV= hepatitis B virus; IL-= Interleukin; ADCC= Antibody dependent cell mediated cytotoxicity; IFN=interferon; TNF= Tumour necrosis factor, TH= T helper CD4 cells; CTL=Cytotoxic T lymphocytes; NK= Natural killer cells. The above diagram summarizes the main parts of the immune response during hepatitis B virus infection. The innate mechanisms include the tissue macrophages and the complement cascade which represent the first line of son-specific defense. Activated neutrophils, NK cells, inflammatory cells all can secrete cytokines that affects the HBV. The second line of defense is composed of both humoral and cell mediated immune mechanisms (see text for details).

The host immune response to viruses involves the induction of type-1 interferon (Joklik, 1991). The TLR are important for the induction of type-1 interferon. In addition, the initial recognition of HBV infection may be mediated by TLRs following recognition of the pathogen associated molecular patterns.

The epression of TLR2 and TLR4 on hepatocytes have been reported in humans and recent studies have shown that the hepatocytes can respond directly to microbial products including LPS independent of kupffer cells and therefore hepatocytes may be considered as immune cells (Herkel *et al.,* 2003).

3.2. Natural Killer (NK) Cells Responses to HBV Infection

Natural Killer (NK) cells are considered as the first immunological barrier against infection and cancer (Chen *et al.,* 2005) and important cells in innate immunity. Upon activation they show strong cytotoxic ability and produce important chemokines and cytokines. Up to date, the specific target recognition molecule for NK cells is not known. However, it is well known that NK cells display at least two important functions to control infection, they can kill infected cell directly by cell to cell contact and they produce cytokines and lymphokines that have direct antiviral activity (such as IFN-γ and TNF-α) and immuno-regulatory effects (such as IL-3 and granulocyte-macrophage-colony-stimulating factor, GM-CSF) (Chen *et al.,* 2005). Activated NK cells play an important role in the regulation of the adoptive immune responses by interacting with other lymphocytes and may contribute to the lymphocyte liver injury during HBV infection (Chen *et al.,* 2005).

A lot of natural killer cells are detected in the normal liver, accounting for approximately one third of intra hepatic lymphocytes. These cells are important for the defense against HBV infection as part of the innate immunity. Recently, there is increased evidence to support that the liver is actually a lymphoid organ with a unique immunological properties (Herkel *et al.,* 2003).

In chronic HBV infection, recent evidence show that the numbers of hepatic NK cells are decreased and also their natural activation ability is also declined, this is in addition to their ability to function as cytotoxic cells (Chen *et al.,* 2005).

3.3. NK T Cells Responses to HBV Infection

NK T cells account for one third of the intrahepatic lymphocytes with conventional T cell markers (CD3 + CD56). It has been suggested that the therapeutic activation of NK T cells may represent the innate immune response, like the adoptive immune response and has the potential to control viral replication during the natural HBV infection (Kazuhiro *et al.,* 2000; Baron *et al.,* 2002).

It has been demonstrated that NK T cells directly inhibit HBV replication via INF-γ (Kakimi *et al.,* 2000). The activity of NK and NKT cells may be an important anti-HBV response and possibly precedes the upregulation of human leukocyte antigens (HLA-class-I) on hepatocytes. Upregulation of HLA class-I molecules expression is essential for presentation and recognition of foreign antigen by T cells during the acquired element of the immune response.

3.4. Kupffer Cells Immune Responses to HBV Infection

Kupffer cells are important for mediating early immune response and also participate in the acquired immune responses (Biron, 1999). The activation of Kupffer cells during viral infection can lead to cytokine production to control and clear HBV infection. In addition, these cells coordinate the recruitment and maturation of HBV-specific T cells by producing cytokines and lymphokines such as IFN-γ, CXCL-9 and CXCL-10 (Kakimi *et al.,* 2001).

3.5. Other Cells and Molecules Involved in HBV Infection

In addition to the cells mentioned above, HBV causes an inflammatory hepatic illness characterized by mononuclear (monocytes) and polymorphonuclear (neutrophils, eosinophils, mast cells and basophils) cellular infiltrates with evidence of hepatic macrophage activation (Gilles *et al.,* 1992). These inflammatory cells produce such cytokines as TNF-α, IFN-γ, IFN-α, IL-1α, and IL-6 (Andus *et al.,* 1991), which mediate the inflammatory process and which contribute to the successful clearance of the virus, avoiding the mechanisms of the immune response or the progression of infection and persistence of the virus (Biron, 1994). In addition, other molecules are considered important during the innate immune response for HBV, and these include proteins of the complement system, the acute phase proteins and cytokines (see later). Serum levels of acute phase proteins (APP) have been used to diagnose and follow up treatment of liver diseases (Thio *et al.,* 2005). Mannose binding lectin (MBL) plays a central role in the innate immune response (Turner, 2003) and the functional MBL plays a central role in the pathogenesis of acute hepatitis B (Thio *et al.,* 2005).

4. Acquired Immune Responses to HBV Infection

4.1. Humoral Immune Responses

Humoral and cell-mediated immune responses to various types of antigens are induced during viral infection. However, these do not always seem to be protective and, in some instances, may cause autoimmune phenomena that contribute to disease pathogenesis. The immune response to infection with hepatitis B virus is directed toward at least the three main antigens: hepatitis B "surface" antigen, the "core" antigen, and the "e" antigen.

The surface antigen appears in the sera of most patients during the incubation period, before biochemical evidence of liver damage or onset of jaundice. The antigen persists during the acute illness and usually clears from the circulation during convalescence. Next to appear in the circulation is the virus-associated DNA polymerase activity, which correlates in time with damage to liver cells as indicated by elevated serum transaminases. The polymerase activity persists for days or weeks in acute cases and for months or years in some persistent carriers (Echevarra and Leon, 1995). Antibody to the core antigen is found in the serum after the surface antigen appears, and it is frequently detectable for many years after recovery. The titer of core antibody appears to correlate with the amount and duration of virus replication. Finally, antibody to the surface antigen component appears (Echevarra and Leon, 1995).

During an acute HBV infection, symptoms may last from ten to twenty weeks after infection. Before symptoms appear HBsAg and HBeAg are detectable in the bloodstream. Antibodies against HBeAg are detectable usually few months after infection. Initially, anti-HBcAg antibodies are IgM but this wanes although total anti-HBcAg continues at a high level. HBsAg is detectable in the bloodstream from one to six months after infection, but anti-HBsAg is only detectable from about eight months. Thus, there is a "window" in which neither HBsAg nor anti-HBsAg antibodies can be detected. As a result of the immune response, the disease resolves in most patients. In a chronic infection, HBsAg and HBeAg are detectable throughout the course of the infection. Anti-HBcAg (initially IgM) and anti-HBeAg are also detectable (Maruyama *et al.,* 1993).

During the incubation period and during the acute phase of the illness, surface antigen-antibody complexes may be found in the sera of some patients. Immune complexes have been found by electron microscopy in the sera of all patients with fulminant hepatitis, but are seen only infrequently in non-fulminant infection. Immune complexes are important in the pathogenesis of other disease syndromes characterized by severe damage of blood vessels (for example, polyarteritis nodosa, some forms of chronic glomerulonephritits, and infantile papular acrodermatitis) (Jung and Pape, 2002).

Immune complexes have been identified in variable proportions of patients with virtually all the recognized chronic sequelae of acute hepatitis. Deposits of such immune complexes have also been shown in the cytoplasm and plasma membrane of hepatocytes and on or in the nuclei; why only a small proportion of patients with circulating complexes develop vasculitis or polyarteritis is, however, not completely clear at present (Chisari and Ferrari, 1995; Czaja *et al.,* 1999). These immune complexes may be critical pathogenic factors only if they have a particular size and of a certain antigen-to-antibody ratio. It is thought that in persistently HBV infected individuals, specific humoral immune response is too weak to eliminate HBV from all infected hepatocytes, but strong enough to continuously destroy HBV infected hepatocytes and to induce chronic inflammatory liver disease (Huang *et al.,* 2006).

The humoral immune response as indicated earlier is essential for the long term clearance of HBV and protection from infection with HBV (Figure 2). In patients who recover from acute HBV infection, activated Th2 CD4 cells induce B cell production and differentiation into plasma cells and the synthesis of antibodies to HBcAg, HBsAg and HBeAg.

4.1.1. Antibodies to the Hepatitis B "Core" Antigen (HBcAg)

The first detectable antibody to appear, around eight weeks after infection with HBV are antibodies to the HBV "core" protein. Hepatitis B core antibody (Anti-HBc) is usually detected within two weeks of the appearance of hepatitis B surface antigen. These antibodies to HBcAg (HBcAb) do not neutralize the virus. HBcAb's persist in serum after an infection with HBV has been defeated and testing for this antibody has been used to detect previous exposure to the live virus. Antibodies to HBcAg are detected in the sera of patients with chronic HBV infection and these antibodies are usually unable to neutralize viral infectivity (Wilson *et al.,* 1994). In patients with persistent HBV infection, antibodies to HBcAg can be detected throughout the course of infection (Borzi *et al.,* 1992). The core protein (HBc) is not detectable in the blood stream, however it can be detected in the sample of liver cells taken after a liver biopsy is performed. Generally, the HBc proteins link together, to form the hepatitis B core that encapsulates HBV-DNA and DNA-polymerase.

4.1.2. Antibodies to the Hepatitis B "Surface" Antigen (HBsAg)

Humoral immune responses, in terms of antibody production, to each of the virus particles have been reported following transient HBV infection. For example, antibodies to HBsAg are used as marker of resolution of transient HBV infection. It is well known that anti-HBsAg antibodies play a key role during the recovery of HBV infection by neutralizing virus particles and containing the spread of infection. These antibodies may also prevent re-infection by blocking the ability of virus particles to bind to their receptors on target cells (Brown *et al.,* 1990).

Hepatitis B surface antigen (HBsAg) represents the first viral marker present in blood tests after the patient is infected. It usually disappears from the blood in two months. Hepatitis B surface antibody (Anti-HBs) is found both in those who have been immunized and those who have recovered from hepatitis infection. Both hepatitis B surface antibody and core antibody persist indefinitely in the blood of patients who have recovered from hepatitis B.

In up to 10% of people infected with hepatitis B the HBsAg persists and HBsAb do not appear. If this persists for six months or more after acute infection then the condition is termed chronic. Of the 10% who develop chronic HB most are asymptotic carriers of the virus. People with HBsAg, HBeAg, with no HBsAb and no HBeAb are generally termed as having "chronic active HB" and around 50% of chronic cases are of the active form. People with HBsAg, no HBeAg or have HBeAb are generally termed as having "chronic persistent HB" or "sub clinical carriers".

It is thought that excess HBs proteins produced may allow infectious viral particles to escape the immune system by mopping up any low levels of surface antibodies that may be produced by the immune response (Maruyama *et al.,* 1993). These are generally the last antibodies to appear. HBsAb can neutralize the hepatitis B virus and there appearance taken as an indicator that an initial infection has been defeated. HBsAb can also be induced to appear by vaccination and so provide protection against hepatitis B (Maruyama *et al.,* 1993). However, the immune response produced by vaccination may not be 100% protective. Although very rare, hepatitis B infection has occurred in vaccinated individuals. It is believed that this may be due to mutant virus strains that express different surface proteins to those used in the genetically engineered vaccine (Maruyama *et al.,* 1993).

4.1.3. Antibodies to the Hepatitis B "e" Antigen (HBeAg)

A correlation seems to exist between the presences or not of Hepatitis 'e' antigen (HBeAg) in serum and liver damage in patients with persistent HBV infection (Niederau *et al.,* 1996). The HBeAg is a peptide and normally detectable in the bloodstream when the hepatitis B virus is actively reproducing, this in turn leads to the person being much more infectious and at a greater risk of progression to liver disease. The exact function of this non structural protein is unknown however it is thought that HB "e" may be influential in suppressing the immune systems response to HBV infection (Tsai *et al.,* 1992). HBeAg is generally detectable at the same time as HBsAg and disappears before HBsAg disappears. The presence of HBeAg in chronic infection is generally taken to indicate that HBV is actively reproducing and there is a higher probability of liver damage. In acute infection HBeAg is generally only transiently present. However, mutant strains of HBV exist that replicate without producing HBeAg (Tsai *et al.,* 1992). In many cases infection with these mutant strains is more aggressive than HBe producing strains. Antibodies to the 'e' antigen (HBeAb), normally appears a few weeks after HBeAg is no longer detectable. The presence of HBeAb is generally taken to be a good sign and indicates a favorable prognosis.

4.1.4. Antibodies to the Hepatitis B"x" Protein (HBxAg)

Hepatitis B "x" protein is known to modify several cellular pathways including NF-kB and this may subsequently affect antigen presentation and the immune response (Fischer *et al.,* 1995; Murakami, 2001). It is also known that expression of HBxAg can lead to increase expression of HLA class I molecules on hepatocytes and usually class I molecules are present in low levels on hepatocytes. It is belived that an increase in HLA class I expression on hepatocytes leads to recognition of foreign antigens by T cells and during HBV infection could recruit T cells to the liver and cause liver damage. Although it can be detected, current tests are not very reliable as other proteins interfere with the results. The functions, of antibodies to this protein, are not known for details at the present time.

4.1.5. Classes and IgG Subclasses Patterns to HBV

Differences in the secreted antibodies, manifested in classes, subclasses and subclass patterns could be the result of the conformational binding of different antigenic structures to the MHC class I or class II antigens (Wilson, *et al.,* 1994). The specific role of each of the antibodies plays in the clearance of HBV is not very clear at the present time. It is documented that the different proteins of HBV can evoke the production of different IgG subclasses. The different subclasses patterns to the different antigens of HBV may reflect the difference between antigens, immune response and the stage of viral disease (Huang *et al.,* 2006). In persons who are naturally infected with HBV, the antibody to HBsAg is mainly of IgG1 and IgG3 (Morell *et al.,* 1983). For persons immunized with cDNA HBsAg, the IgG antibodies are mainly of IgG1 and IgG2 (Brozi *et al.,* 1992). The IgG subclass pattern for antibodies to HBcAg is mainly of IgG1 followed by IgG3, then IgG4 in chronic carriers and in recovered individuals IgG3 mainly followed by IgG1 then IgG4 (Yang *et al.,* 2001; Yang *et al.,* 2002). For anti HBeAg, the subclass pattern is mainly IgG1 followed by IgG4 and then IgG3 in chronic carriers and IgG1 followed by IgG3 and then IgG4 in recovered individuals (Huang *et al.,* 2006).

5. Cell Mediated Immune Responses

Cellular immune responses are known to be particularly important in determining the clinical features and course of viral infections. The occurrence of cell-mediated immune responses to hepatitis B antigens has been demonstrated in most patients during the acute phase of hepatitis B and in a significant proportion of patients with surface-antigen-positive chronic active hepatitis, but not in asymptomatic persistent hepatitis B carriers (Thomas *et al.,* 1982). These observations have suggested that cell-mediated immunity may be important in terminating the infection and, under certain circumstances, in promoting immune-mediated liver damage and possibly in the genesis of autoimmunity. Evidence suggests that progressive liver damage may result from an autoimmune reaction directed against antigens of hepatocyte membrane, initiated in many cases by infection with hepatitis B virus (Guidotti and Chisari, 1999 and 2001).

The immune response to HBV-encoded antigens is responsible for clearance of virus and for disease pathogenesis during this infection. While the humoral antibody response to viral envelope antigens contributes to the clearance of circulating virus particles, the cellular immune response, the CD4 T cell immune responses and in particular the cytotoxic T cell response, to the envelope, nucleocapsid, and polymerase antigens destroys and eliminates infected cells (Figure 2).

5.1. Antigen Presenting Cells (Dendritic cells) Responses to HBV Infection

Antigen presenting cells (APC) especially dendritic cells and kupffer cells are essential for antigen processing and presentation and the maturation of HBV-specific T cells. They present foreign antigens to CD4 and CD8 T cells and produce cytokines (e.g. IL-12 and TNF-α).

Dendritic cells are excellent antigen presenting cells and play an important role for T cell activation. It has been reported that a simultaneous decrease numbers of circulating CD8 T cells and NK cells in HBV infected cirrhotic patients (Duan *et al.,* 2003). The decline of host immune response was suggested to partially contribute to the disease progression of HBV infection (Duan *et al.,* 2003).

Dendritic cells constitute a heterogeneous group of unique antigen-presenting cells that builds the bridge between pathogens and the T-cell system. The full effect of this system in viral disease has only recently been appreciated, as well as the means for first-time identification, separation, and functional analysis of these cells (e.g. the recognition of the plasmacytoid dendritic cells as the principal type-I-interferon-producing cells). Our knowledge is limited of the dendritic cell system in viral infection and, in particular, in HBV infection. A precise definition of its function, however, is needed for understanding the host's antiviral immune response, and for the design and development of therapeutic strategies in which dendritic cells are used as vectors and targets (Jung and Pape, 2002).

5.2. CD4+ T Cell Response to HBV Infection

In the direct elimination performed by CTL, the cell mediated immune response, requires the assistance from CD4 cells. CD4 T helper cells works in two ways; first, the Th1 cells stimulate macrophages, which in turn clear virus particles. Second, the Th2 cells stimulate B cells to generate antibodies, which adhere to the surface of the virus particles and induce opsonization and neutralization (Barrios *et al.,* 1996; Marinos *et al.,* 1995). It is documented that low doses of virus were able to induce a protective CTL response (Th1-mediated) whereas high doses of virus failed to do so and induced a non-protective humoral (Th2-mediated) response (Ridge *et al.,* 1996). This suggests that the initial viral dose may be critical in determining whether hosts develop protective or non-protective immune response. The viral Ag is presented and the dose may determine whether immunological tolerance or a vigorous immune response is the final outcome and this may serve to explain the outcome of HBV infection (Ridge *et al.,* 1996).

During acute self-limited HBV infection, there is a vigorous CD4+ response directed against multiple epitopes within HBcAg, HBeAg, and HBsAg (Lohr *et al.,* 1995; Missale *et al.,* 1993; Nayersina *et al.,* 1993). HBeAg has been shown to induce a Th2 immune response in mice, whereas HBcAg induced a Th1 response (Milich *et al.,* 1997; Milich *et al.,* 1998). The Th2 response to the HBeAg was shown to be dominant over the Th1 response to HBcAg resulting in the depletion of HBcAg- specific Th1 cells in vivo (Milich *et al.,* 1997).

The development of a vigorous CD4, MHC class-II-restricted response to core is temporally associated with the clearance of HBV from the serum, and is probably essential for efficient control of viraemia through several mechanisms (Ando, *et al.,* 1994; Jung, *et al.,* 1995). These CD4 responses exert their effect by production of cytokines. The cytokine profile secreted by core-specific $CD4^+$ T lymphocytes in self-limited acute hepatitis B showed production of Th1 cytokines dominated by the production of IFN-γ, which suggests that Th1-mediated effects could contribute to liver cell injury and recovery from disease (Penna *et al.,* 1997). In acute HBV infection, HBV-specific CD4 T cells are detected at the time of elevated HBV-DNA (i.e. before the peak of liver damage) and persist long after recovery from HBV infection.

During chronic HBV infection, the peripheral blood HLA class-II-restricted T-cell response to all viral antigens, including HBcAg and HBeAg, is much less vigorous than in patients with acute hepatitis (Jung *et al.,* 1991). It has been noted that the affinity of HLA-class-II molecules for HBV antigens is stronger with ligands from the core proteins and weaker with ligands from the envelope (Godkin *et al.,* 2005). This may explain the fact that increase frequency of HBcAg-specific T cells are observed following acute HBV clearance as it is known that peptides with high affinity are likely to act as epitopes as the case with the core protein in HBV (Godkin *et al.,* 2005).

5.3. The Cytotoxic T Cell Response to HBV

The T cell response to HBV is strong, with a vigorous T cell response to all viral proteins, and broadly specific in acutely infected patients (Chisari and Ferrari, 1995; Chisari,

1997), and these T cells typically secrete type-1 antiviral cytokines such as IFN-γ and TNF-α upon antigen stimulation (Kakumu *et al.*, 1994). In chronically infected patients, the T cell response to HBV is weak, with a markedly diminished HBV-specific T cell response, and narrowly focused (Chisari and Ferrari, 1995), except during exacerbations of liver disease or after viral clearance, and the cytokine profile of the intra-hepatic HBV-specific T cells is variable (Inoue *et al.*, 1989; Barnaba *et al.*, 1994). These observations have suggested a scenario in which viral clearance from organs like the liver that contain a large numbers of infected cells depends on the development of a vigorous CTL response, the destruction of some of the infected cells, the production of antiviral cytokines, and the susceptibility of the infecting virus to cytokine mediated control. If the CTL response is strong and rapid, the number of infected cells is low, and the virus is susceptible to cytokine-mediated control, viral clearance should occur while only a fraction of the infected cells are actually killed, resulting in a self-limited inflammatory liver disease. This is compatible with the course of events during acute hepatitis B.

The pathogenesis and antiviral potential of the CTL response to HBV has been demonstrated by the induction of a severe necro-inflammatory liver disease following the adoptive transfer of HBsAg-specific CTL into HBV transgenic mice, and by the non-cytolytic suppression of viral gene expression and replication in the same animals by a posttranscriptional mechanism mediated by IFN-γ, TNF-α, and interleukin-2 (IL-2) (Wieland *et al.*, 2000). The dominant cause of viral persistence during HBV infection is the development of a weak antiviral immune response to the viral antigens.

Although the HBV nucleoprotein has been suggested to be a major target antigen for CTL (Ando *et al.*, 1993), it is entirely possible that selected regions of the viral envelope and other nonstructural proteins such as the polymerase may serve as target structure for HLA class I- or class II-restricted CTL recognition, as has been shown in other viral systems. CTL might in turn be negatively modulated by antibody masking of target antigen(s) (Reherman *et al.*, 1995) and by specific intra-hepatic suppressor T cells which have been demonstrated to be active in chronic HBV infection (Maim *et al.*, 1999). In addition, helper T lymphocytes may exert an indirect cytotoxic effect through the release of cytokines such as tumor necrosis factor. This circuit can be potentially amplified by soluble factor(s) secreted by auto-reactive cells. Moreover, antibody-dependent cell-mediated cytotoxicity (ADCC) may also be a determinant of liver cell necrosis (Jung *et al.*, 1991).

As indicated earlier the CTL response to HBV is vigorous, polyclonal, and multi-specific in patients with acute hepatitis who ultimately clear the virus, and it is weak or barely detectable in patients with chronic hepatitis (Bertoletti *et al.*, 1991), except during acute exacerbations of chronic disease or after spontaneous or IFN-α-induced viral clearance (Rehermann *et al.*, 1996a). Despite the vigor of the T cell response to HBV during acute viral hepatitis, very low levels of virus persist in the circulation for several decades after complete clinical and serological resolution of disease (Rehermann *et al.*, 1996b). Long-term persistence of trace amounts of viral DNA is associated with equally long term persistence of HBV-specific CTL that display recent activation markers. This suggests that transcriptionally active virions can apparently maintain the CTL response indefinitely after recovery, perhaps for life (Rehermann *et al.*, 1996b). This indicates that small quantities of HBV persist in immunologically privileged sites after sero-conversion and that spread of the infection is controlled by CTL. This also raise questions about the site of persistent infection, the basis for incomplete clearance, the chance of viral reactivation during immunosuppression, and the possibility that individuals or their organs may be infectious for others.

While the strong association between liver disease and the CTL response during acute HBV infection suggests an important role for CTL in the pathogenesis of acute viral hepatitis, proof of this hypothesis required the development of transgenic mice that express and replicate HBV in their hepatocytes and the demonstration that these animals develop an acute necro-inflammatory liver disease after adoptive transfer of hepatitis B surface antigen-specific CTL lines and clones (Moriyama *et al.,* 1990). Importantly, the number of CTL injected into the mice, and the intrinsic cytopathic activity of these CTL can be easily manipulated such that the severity of the ensuing liver disease can be tightly controlled. It has been shown that HBV gene expression and replication can be completely abolished in all of the hepatocytes in the liver by a non-cytopathic antiviral process in which the viral nucleocapsids disappear from the cytoplasm and the viral RNAs are degraded in the nucleus of the hepatocytes under conditions in which < 1% of the hepatocytes is destroyed (Guidotti *et al.,* 1996). As a result, all of the viral gene products and virions disappear from the liver and the serum in the absence of serum transaminase elevations or histological evidence of liver disease (Guidotti *et al.,* 1996). Viral clearance in this model is completely blocked when antibodies to IFN-γ and TNF-α are injected before the CTL, indicating that these cytokines are responsible for the antiviral effect. These results illustrate a new principle in viral immunology, i.e., CTL can activate HBV-infected cells to participate in the antiviral response by triggering them to produce cellular proteins that interrupt the viral life cycle.

It might be predicted that super-infection of the liver by other hepato-tropic viruses might lead to the clearance of HBV if they induce the production of antiviral cytokines to which HBV is susceptible. Indeed, precisely these events have been shown to occur in the HBV transgenic mice during lymphocytic choriomeningitis virus infection (Guidotti *et al.,* 1996) as well as during adenovirus- and cytomegalovirus-induced hepatitis. Intriguingly, isolated case reports have been published suggesting that super-infection by HAV is sometimes associated with clearance of HBV in chronically infected patients (Davis *et al.,* 1984). These results suggest that a strong intra-hepatic CTL response to HBV during acute viral hepatitis can suppress HBV gene expression and replication and perhaps even "cure" infected hepatocytes of the virus in addition to killing them. Conversely, the data suggest that a weak immune response, such as that which occurs in chronically infected patients, could contribute to viral persistence and chronic liver disease by reducing the expression of viral antigens sufficiently for the infected cells to escape immune recognition but not enough for the virus to be eliminated. Therefore, the ability of CTL derived cytokines to inhibit HBV replication could represent a survival strategy by the virus, contributing to persistence, or a tissue-sparing antiviral strategy by the host, contributing to viral elimination (McClary *et al.,* 2000).

Following antigen activation, CTL deliver an apoptotic signal to their target cells, killing them. CTL also secrete IFN-γ and TNF-α, cytokines that have been shown to abolish HBV gene expression and viral replication in vivo, curing them. The curative effect of the CTL response is several orders of magnitude more efficient than its destructive effect. The outcome of an infection may depend on the relative balance of these two effects with a predominantly curative response leading to viral clearance, and a predominantly destructive response leading to viral persistence and chronic liver disease (Bertoletti *et al.,* 1994; Bertoletti *et al.,* 2000). Importantly, if the curative process abolishes viral gene expression and replication but does not eliminate the viral cDNA from the hepatocyte, it could paradoxically lead to viral persistence by rendering the virus immunologically invisible without removing its transcriptional template. However, if the T cell response is quantitatively suboptimal, the virus may persist even if the appropriate antiviral cytokines are present since they are produced in limited quantities that are likely to suppress viral gene expression without completely clearing the virus, thus causing it to be less visible to the immune system and leading to persistent infection. This may be the case in patients with chronic hepatitis B. Even a strong CTL response may not be able to clear a massive viral infection unless the cytokine-mediated curative part of the response is called into play since the cytopathic function of the immune response may simply not be able to destroy all of the infected cells, thus leading to persistent infection and chronic liver disease. This can occur either if the CTL fail to produce the appropriate antiviral cytokines, or if the virus is not susceptible to cytokine-mediated control. If this hypothesis is correct, strategies designed to boost the CTL response (e.g., virus-specific immunotherapy) or to enhance or mimic the regulatory functions of the CTL response in the liver (e.g., intra-hepatic cytokine induction therapy) could help to terminate chronic HBV infection.

While neonatal tolerance may plays important roles in viral persistence in patients infected at birth, the basis for poor responsiveness in adult-onset infection is not well understood and requires further investigations. Additional factors that may contribute to viral persistence are viral inhibition of immunological antigen processing and or presentation, infection of immunologically privileged sites, modulation of the immune response to cytotoxic mediators and viral mutations (Guidottiti *et al.,* 1996; Barrios *et al.,* 1996a & b).

6. Affect of Cytokines on HBV Infection

Cytokines are essential molecules in the defense against viral infections, both directly by inhibition of viral replication and indirectly by determination of the predominant Th1/Th2 patterns of immune response (Paul and Seder, 1994). In HBV infection, cytokines may further lead to the liver damage (de Lalla *et al.,* 2004). Cytokines have a central role in influencing the type of immune response needed for optimum protection against particular types of infectious agents. For example, the release of interleukin-12 (IL-12) by antigen-presenting cells stimulates the production of IFN-γ by Th1 cells (Bertagonalli *et al.,* 1992; Trinchieri, 1995). This cytokine efficiently activates macrophages, enabling them to kill intracellular organisms. In general, the production of cytokines by Th1 cells facilitates cell-mediated immunity, including the activation of macrophages and T-cell-mediated cytotoxicity; Th2 cells help B cells produce antibodies (Delves and Roitt, 2000).

Chemokines are another group of proteins that has a large effect on immunologic responses. They are important for activation or chemoattraction of leukocytes. Each chemokine contains 65 ~ 120 amino acids, with molecular weight of 8 ~ 10 kD. Since the discovery of their essential roles in the entry of HIV into host cells they have gain a lot of interest and the chemokine receptors, their antagonists are being developed to treat AIDS.

The interaction of chemokines with their respective receptors on lymphocytes is a prerequisite to attract these cells to the liver. So far, the chemokine repertoire expressed on HBV-infected liver compared with uninfected liver is not completely clear. However, it is believed that IFN-γ, required for recruitment of HBV specific T cells and also for non-cytopathic clearance of HBV, is also responsible for increasing susceptibility of hepatocytes to TNF-α-induced apoptosis and mediating macrophage recruitment of more necroinflammatory cells. IFN-γ inducible chemokines including macrophage inflammatory protein-1 (MIP-1-α), MIP-1-β, and regulated on activation normal T expressed and secreted (RANTES) are up-regulated and together with CXCL-9 and CXCL-10 bind chemokine co-receptor CCR5, which activate lymphocytes regardless of their specificity (Bonecchi *et al.,* 1998).

During acute HBV infection a vigorous polyclonal cellular immune response occurs and Th1 cytokine profile is essential to initiate an effective immune response. Although cytotoxic T cell functions certainly contribute to viral clearance, non-cytotoxic T cell functions also play a role by a non-cytopathic interferon (e.g. IFN-γ) mediated mechanism (Boehm *et al.,* 1993). It is well known that interferon can modulate the immune system, alter cell membranes to reduce infection of surrounding uninfected cells and also causes many changes. This naturally produced interferon assists the body in fighting hepatitis B. However, it was discovered that the interferon response was deficient in some people and also infants/children with immature immune systems. This findings lead to interferon being considered as a treatment.

The cytokines released by CD4 and CD8 cells play important roles in down regulating HBV replication, indicating that the immune system is able to control viral infection without destroying infected cells (Jung & Pape, 2002). However, HBV seems to have specific mechanisms to inhibit cytokine production, and therefore the virus is winning. In addition, the virus have some evasion strategies such as antagonism of immune function through the use of homologous of cytokine receptors, expression of viral proteins which interact with cytokine signal transduction and expression of cytokine mimics and host proteins that influence the Th1 and/or Th2 cytokine responses. These immunomodulatory strategies can protect the host from the lethal inflammatory effects as well as inhibit the local inflammatory response elicited to kill the HBV. In addition, the HBV may adopt alterations in cytokine expression which can inhibit interferon gene expression (Ilan, 2002)

Activation of macrophage represents one of the first events of innate resistance against intracellular infection. In response to pathogens, macrophages and other inflammatory cells secrete cytokines; IFN-γ, Interleukins 1, 6, & 8, TNF-α and IFN-β. Some of these cytokines lead to activities against pathogens, activate effecter cells involved in the cellular interactions that occur during inflammation, and are part of the acute and chronic stages of viral hepatitis (Heinzel *et al.,* 1989; Trinchieri, 1997). The antibody response in patients with HBV infection plays a critical role in viral clearance through the formation of complexes with viral particles and their removal from the circulation (Bocher *et al.,* 2000; Chisari and Ferrari 1995; Machado *et al.,* 1997).

The specific cellular immune response plays a main role in the hepatic necrosis that occurs with HBV infection and in the persistence or lack of persistence of viral infection. Certain cytokines can contribute to this process by efficiently inhibiting viral replication when the subtype Th1 cytokine secretion pattern is predominant or by facilitating the propagation of the pathogens in the patient if the subtype Th2 cytokine secretion pattern is predominant (Lee *et al.,* 1999).

Many studies carried out with cultures of peripheral blood mononuclear cells from patients with acute HBV infection showed a Th1-like cytokine pattern with increased levels of production of IFN-γ and TNF-α (Al-Wabel *et al.,* 1993; Bocher *et al.,* 2000). This high level of cytokine production stimulates the immune response, allowing the cure of HBV disease (Guidotti *et al.,* 1996). On the other hand, decreases in the levels of IL-2 and TNF-α synthesis and increases in the levels of IL-1 and the soluble form of the IL-2 receptor in serum have been observed in patients with chronic HBV infection (Missale *et al.,* 1995), while high levels of IL-4 and IL-6 were found in patients with autoimmune chronic hepatitis (Al-Wabel *et al.,* 1993).

During the convalescent phase, the decrease in serum IFN-γ levels coincides with the increase in the levels of IL-10, which inhibits IFN-γ synthesis (Raynor, 1996). This decrease would be related to the decrease in the levels of production of cytokines secreted by macrophages (IL-1, IL-6, IL-8, and TNF-α), which, if increased, would exacerbate the hepatic damage (Trinchieri, 1997). Increased levels of these cytokines have been observed in patients with chronic hepatitis caused by HBV whose condition later evolved to a cirrhotic state (Lohr *et al.,* 1994).

Both IFN-γ and TNF-α can be inhibited by IL-10 (Raynor, 1996), who's levels remained high during the acute and convalescent phases. Besides the regulation possibly carried out by the inhibitory cytokine, an increase in the number of TNF-α soluble receptors (sRTNF-α) could be responsible for the maintenance of the control levels of TNF-α and for the decrease in the levels of TNF-α during the convalescent phase. Increased concentrations of sRTNF-α in serum, which seem to modulate the endogenous effects of TNF-α, have been detected in patients with chronic HBV infection (Tilg *et al.,* 1992).

IL-10 is one of the key cytokines in the Th2 response. It is a pleiotropic cytokine able to inhibit the synthesis of other cytokines secreted by the Th1 subpopulation and the functions of the cell antigen bearers. IL-10 increases the levels of sRTNF-α released, inducing B-lymphocyte differentiation into plasmocytes and immunoglobulin synthesis (Raynor, 1996). Therefore, IL-10 has as an important role, acting like a general suppressor of the cell-mediated response and increasing the level of humoral immunity. The increment of IL-10 in the two phases might modulate the levels of IFN-γ and TNF-α since an exaggerated immune response by these cytokines to a viral antigen load would be responsible for the death of large numbers of hepatocytes, producing a lethal hepatitis. The persistence of high IL-10 levels in the convalescent phase is important in the secretion of surface antibodies against HBV and the development of immunity. Antibodies to HBsAg block the adherence of viral particles to non-infected cells and remove from the circulation the free antigenic particles, protecting the individual against re-infection (Machado *et al.,* 1997).

It was determined that the serum IL-4 concentrations are decreased during the acute and convalescent phases (Mansour *et al.,* 1994). Increased levels of this cytokine have been reported in patients with several parasitic and autoimmune diseases (Heinzel *et al.,* 1989; Kelso, 1995). The decrease in IL-4 levels in patients with HBV infection could be due to the fact that this cytokine is preferentially stimulated by parasitic antigens but not by viral antigens, which mainly induce IL-10. The type of stimulus could determine the production profile for each cytokine. Also, the decrease in IL-4 levels would be a consequence of the auto-regulatory mechanisms of IL-10 (Borish, 1998).

The increased levels of IL-2 during the acute phase and until the total resolution of the HBV infection could allow for higher levels of T-lymphocyte activation during this period. IL-2 could be a stimulus for the activation of NK cells and CD8+ lymphocytes participating in the development of immunity. Investigations carried out with IL-2 report decreases in the levels of its production in patients with chronic HBV infections (Anastassakos *et al.*, 1998). The increase in IL-2 levels in the acute phase of HBV infection is necessary to stimulate the activities of the NK cells and the CD8+ lymphocytes and to achieve remission. It has been demonstrated that a positive correlation between natural cytotoxicity and IL-2 levels is needed to control HBV infection before the specific cytotoxic mechanisms settle down totally (Echevarría *et al.*, 1991). The sustained increases in IL-2 levels during the convalescent phase suggest that, despite the resolution of the infection indicated by normal ALT values and the presence of anti-HBs, an increase in hepatic damage would not be determined by the high concentrations of this cytokine. In addition, anti-HBs mask tissue surface antigens, forming immune complexes that induce a trans-membrane signal able to suppress the synthesis of intracellular viral antigens (Fujinami and Oldstone, 1979). This would then preclude the cytotoxic actions of the CD8+ lymphocytes.

The circulating profile of cytokine in chronic hepatitis B is related to the replication level of the virus and the activity of liver disease (Bozkaya *et al.*, 2000). It was reported that IL-18 can inhibit the hepatitis B virus replication in the livers of transgenic mice (Lynch *et al.*, 1995).

Although the magnitude of the cellular immune response in acute, resolved HBV and non-resolving HBV is quite different, the functional characterization of these cells with respect to the polarization of cytokine response has been studied. A type 1 response is present among CD4+ T cells of persons who ultimately recover from acute HBV (Al-Wabel *et al.*, 1993), whereas T-cell clones from persons with chronic HBV produce a predominantly type 2 response (Al-Wabel *et al.*, 1993). Moreover, among chronic carriers, those with a response to interferon therapy had substantial increases in IL-12 and type-1 cytokines as compared with IFN non-responders. This finding is consistent with the observation that robust CD4+ and CD8+ HBV-specific cellular immune responses are critical to the resolution of acute HBV. However, it is unclear why this polarization occurs in some persons but not in others. This may be secondary to the host genetic background, as certain murine haplotypes preferentially express a type-1 or -2 response when immunized with HBc. Several groups have reported an association between a particular MHC class II allele, DRB*1302, and a resistance to chronic HBV in Gambian and Caucasian persons (Thursz *et al.*, 1995). However, the reason for this resistance to chronic infection has not been linked to either a particular T-cell response or pattern of cytokine response in humans, although it is tempting to speculate that this underlies this genetic pattern. Alternatively, the relative amounts of different HBV antigens may drive different immune responses. In mice, HBcAg preferentially elicits type-1-like cells and HBeAg preferentially elicits type "0" or type-2-like cells, so it might be that persons who express relatively larger amount of HBeAg early in infection develop a type-2 response.

Both in vitro and in vivo evidence indicates that certain cytokines directly inhibit HBV replication. In vitro, recombinant TNF-α inhibits HBV replication (Hohler *et al.,* 1998), through a posttranslational mechanism that accelerates the degradation of HBV mRNA. In addition, the core promoter element is sensitive to TNF-α, IFN-γ, and IFN-α. Guidotti and Chisari and colleagues have performed a series of elegant experiments designed to test the hypothesis that cytokines produced by CTL mediate control of HBV infection in vivo. After adoptive transfer of cloned HBV-specific CTL into transgenic mice expressing a full-length replicative form of HBV, liver inflammation and down regulation of HBV gene expression occur. Production of IFN-γ and TNF-α by the virus-specific CTL amplifies the ability of the CTL to clear viral infection in this model (Guidotti and Chisari, 1996 & 1999). Blockade of the cascade of events occurs when animals are pretreated with antibodies to IFN-γ and TNF-α before adoptive transfer of HBV-specific CTL. This inhibition of viral replication occurs even when using CTL from perforin-knockout mice, which are unable to lyse target cells, suggesting that apoptotic cell death and production of cytokines are separate events in controlling viral replication.

Cell-mediated immune responses directed against infected liver cells have been considered to be the main inducer of hepatic injury and mediators of HBV clearance (Chisari and Ferrari, 1995; Curry and Koziel, 2000). On the other hand, evidence also suggests that antiviral cytokines, such as TNF-α and IFN-γ, released by the activated effecter cells of innate and adoptive immune systems in the region of their targets, can induce the noncytolytic suppression of HBV expression and replication in the liver (Guidotti and Chisari 1996; Guidotti, *et al.,* 1996; Guidotti *et al.,* 1999). TNF-α inhibits the transcriptional activity of the HBV core promoter in vitro (Romero and Lavine, 1996). In an HBV transgenic mouse model and acutely infected chimpanzees, only a minority of infected hepatocytes were eliminated by direct contact with cytotoxic T cells (Guidotti and Chisari, 1996; Guidotti *et al.,* 1999). In the vast majority of infected cells, HBV appears to be suppressed and eliminated by antigen-non-specific cytokines (Guidotti *et al.,* 1996; Guidotti, 1999).

7. Immunogenetic Aspects of HBV Infection

Many factors can influence the probability of developing a chronic HBV infection. Age is important and transmission from mother to infant at birth or infection while very young nearly always results in chronic infection. In children the rate is lower and in healthy adults the risk of developing chronic infection is much reduced. Other risk factors for developing chronic hepatitis include: being of the male gender; homosexual sexual orientation; having an altered immune system; there may also be genetic component with certain racial groups having a higher risk of cronicity.

The variations in the immune response are often associated with polymorphism in the human genome. Differences in host susceptibility to infections and disease severity can not be attributed solely to the virulence of viral agents. Several recent advances concerning the influence of human genes on HBV infection are briefly discussed below:

7.1. Major Histocompatibility Complex (MHC)

The major histocompatibility complex (MHC) molecules in human are called human leukocyte antigens (HLA) and consists of class I (A, B and C) and class II (DR-B1, DQA1, DPA1 and DPB1) alleles. HLA are glyco-proteins which are encoded by the MHC found, on the short arm of chromosome 6. HLA class I molecules are found on all nucleated cells whereas class II molecules are restricted to immune cells like antigen presenting cells and activated T cells. HLA are essential in presenting antigens to both CD4 and CD8 cells. Generally class I molecules present endogenous antigens including epitopes from viruses and class II molecules present exogenous antigens including viral peptides.

The DRB1*1302, A0301, DR2, DR6 and DR13 alleles are correlated with better outcome of HBV infection (Thursz *et al.,* 1995; Hohler *et al.,* 1997; Ahn *et al.,* 2000). On the other hand, persistence of HBV infection seems to correlate with B08, B44, Cw0501, Cw1601 DQA1*0501 and DQB1*0301alleles (Thio *et al.,* 1999) and HLA-DR7 was shown to be a risk factor for HBV infection (Aikawa *et al.,* 1996).

7.2. Tumor Necrosis Factor Alpha (TNF-α) Gene

The gene, that code for the TNF-α has been shown to play a role in HBV pathogenesis. High levels of TNF-α have been detected in patients with HBV and high levels of TNF-α receptors (Hohler *et al.,* 1998). It has been suggested that TNF-α gene polymorphism may influence HBV persistence (Hohler *et al.,* 1998).

7.3. Mannose Binding Protein (MBP) Gene

Mutations in the gene coding for mannose binding protein (MBP) result in low concentration of MBP in the serum and preventing its important functions in activating the complement system and acting as an opsonin (Thomas *et al.,* 1996). The HBV has an envelope which is rich in mannose oligosaccharide to which MBP could bind. Therefore, mutations in the MBP gene may be important for the pathogenesis of HBV (Thomas et al., 1996). Recently it has been shown that polymorphism in the gene coding for MBP (MBP-2) lead to a decrease expression of MBP and this was associated with HBV persistence (Thio *et al.,* 2005).

7.4. Active Form of Vitamin D Gene

In addition to its function in the regulation of calcium, the active form of vitamin D is immunomodulatory hormone that inhibits Th1 response and activates Th2 response. The polymorphism of the gene for vitamin D receptor was suggested to play a role in the clearance of HBV (Bellmy *et al.,* 1999).

8. Methods of Controlling HBV Infection

Screening of all donated blood has reduced the likelihood of contracting hepatitis B from a blood transfusion. As an initial screen, blood donors are now required to fill out a questionnaire about their sexual and drug use activities. The blood of those who are in high-risk groups is not used.

Mandatory reporting of the disease allows state health care workers to track people who have been exposed and to immunize contacts that have not yet developed the disease. Formerly, hepatitis B vaccine was made from human blood products, so it was not received well by the public. Now hepatitis B vaccine is entirely artificial, with no human products, and therefore cannot transmit hepatitis B virus. The new vaccine is both safe and effective. Those receiving the vaccine require three vaccinations administered within a six month period to achieve full immunity.

Sexual contact with a person who has acute or chronic hepatitis B should be avoided. Condoms, if used consistently and properly, may also reduce transmission through sexual contact. However, immunization provides the only definitive protection against the virus. Vaccination of those at high risk has been of only limited success.

Infants born of mothers who either currently have acute hepatitis B or who have had the infection receive a special immunization series to prevent viral transmission. This includes administering hepatitis B immunoglobulin and a hepatitis B immunization within 12 hours of birth.

If an unvaccinated individual is exposed to the virus accidentally, hepatitis B immunoglobulin can be given. Ideally within 24 hours of exposure and no later than a week after exposure, a repeat dose is necessary 28 - 30 days later. Hepatitis B immunoglobulin is generally given where there is a known risk of infection, e.g. via needle stick injury or to new born infants born to HBsAg positive mothers. In many cases hepatitis B immunoglobulin can prevent initial infection with hepatitis B but there are also a significant number of cases where it has not prevented infection after exposure.

Several vaccines have been developed for the prevention of hepatitis B virus infection. These rely on the use of one of the viral proteins (HBsAg). The vaccine was originally prepared from plasma obtained from patients who had long-standing hepatitis B virus infection. However, currently, these are more often made using recombinant technology, though plasma-derived vaccines continue to be used; the two types of vaccines are equally effective and safe.

Many countries now routinely vaccinate infants against hepatitis B. In many areas, vaccination against hepatitis B is also required for all health-care workers. Some college campus housing units now require proof of vaccination as a prerequisite. Booster doses are not needed for low-risk general population. Some recommend such doses every five to ten years for health-care workers, though the evidence supporting such doses is quite limited. The vaccine is highly effective. In endemic countries with high rates of hepatitis B infection, vaccination of newborns has not only reduced the risk of infection, but has also led to marked reduction in liver cancer. This was reported in Taiwan where a nationwide hepatitis B vaccination program was implemented in 1984 was associated with a decline in the incidence of childhood hepatocellular carcinoma.

Patients with HIV appear to have inferior antibody responses to hepatitis B vaccination. Safe and effective genetically engineered vaccine for hepatitis B is available. It is given in 3 subcutaneous injections generally over a period of 6 months and conveys immunity in approximately 95% of people treated. For the 5% of people who do not respond some new research has shown that a repeat course of injections given intramuscularly can create an immune response in up to 98% of those who did not respond or whose response did not last when given subcutaneously. Once vaccinated present it is important to be periodically tested to ensure that the body has sufficient levels of antibodies to prevent infection and a single booster dose may be required every 5 to 10 years to ensure immunity from infection. At present vaccines are ineffective for those already infected with the hepatitis B virus. New vaccines are being developed and some of these promise increased response rates, only require a single injection and some may be effective for people with chronic hepatitis B.

The current vaccines are subunit vaccines made in yeast that has been transfected with a plasmid that contains the S gene (that codes for HBsAg). The HBV vaccines go under the names of Recombivax-HB (Merke) and Energix-B (Glaxo). In addition, there is an approved vaccine against both HAV and HBV (Twinrix – Glaxo). Another formulation for infants (Pediarix – Glaxo) contains vaccines against diphtheria, tetanus, pertussis (whooping cough), polio and HBV. For vaccination of infants, there are several options depending on whether the mother is HBsAg positive. In the latter case, the vaccine is given along with HBV immunoglobulin. If the mother is seronegative, the vaccine alone is given.

9. Conclusion

We have shown in this chapter that during HBV infection, innate immunity plays an important role and antibodies provide a defense against cell free virions while T cells are the primary mechanisms to clear virus infected cells. When MHC restricted T cells enter the liver and recognize antigen, they kill some of the infected cells and secrete IFN-γ which induces the expression of a large number of genes that enhance antigen processing and presentation; recruit macrophages, NK cells, dendritic cells and T cells that also produce IFN-γ and amplify the process. These important cellular and molecular events continue until HBV infection is terminated and thereafter they rapidly subside.

The full understanding of how the immune system works against infection with HBV, with no doubt, will help us to dissect the immune response to HBV. This will permit us to identify the function, phenotype, HLA restriction and antigenic fine specificity of HBV-specific CTL in HBV infection with the hope that such knowledge may ultimately be translated into more specific and effective therapeutic strategies for eradication of persistent HBV infection and associated liver disease in the future. Elucidation of the immunological and virological basis for HBV persistence may yield immunotherapeutic and antiviral strategies to terminate chronic HBV infection and reduce the risk of its life-threatening sequellae.

ACKNOWLEDGEMENTS

We would like to acknowledge the help of Mr. Shabbir Ahmed during the preparation of this chapter.

REFERENCES

Ahn SH, Han KH, Park JY, Lee CK, Kang SW, Chon CY, Kim YS, Park K, Kim DK, Moon YM. (2000). Association between hepatitis B virus infection and HLA-DR type in Korea. *Hepatology 31*: 1371–1373.

Aikawa T, Kojima M, Onishi H, et al. (1996). HLA DRBI and DQB1alleles and haplotypes influencing the progression of hepatitis C. *J Med Virol. 49*:274-278.

Al-Faleh FZ. (1998). Integration of hepatitis B vaccine into the EPI: the Saudi Arabian experience. *Abstract Vaccines Today — Protecting the Future*, Kuala Lumpur, P19.

Al-Wabel A, Al-Janadi M, Raziuddin S. (1993). Cytokine profile of viral and auto immune chronic active hepatitis. *J. Allergy Clin. Immunol.* 92:902-908.

Anastassakos A, Wolstencroft A, Portman P, De Dumon E, Roge W. (1998). Interleukin-1 and interleukin-2 activity in chronic hepatitis B virus infection. *Gastroenterology 94*: 999-1005

Ando K, Guidotti LG, Wirth S, Ishikawa T, Missale G, Moriyama T, Schreiber RD, Schlicht HJ, Huang S, Chisari FV. (1994). Class I restricted cytotoxic T lymphocytes are directly cytopathic for their target cells in vivo. *J. Immunol. 152*: 3245-3253.

Ando K, Moriyama T, Guidotti LG, Wirth S, Schreiber RD, Schlicht HJ, Huang S, and Chisari FV. (1993) Mechanisms of class I restricted immunopathology. A transgenic mouse model of fulminant hepatitis. *J. Exp. Med. 178*: 1541-1554.

Andus T, Bauer J, and Gerok W. (1991). Effects of cytokines on the liver. *Hepatology 13*: 364-375.

Barnaba V, Franco A, Paroli M, Benvenuto R, De Petrillo G, Burgio VL, Santilio I, Balsano C, Bonavita MS, Cappelli G, et al. (1994). Selective expansion of cytotoxic T lymphocytes with a $CD4^+CD56^+$ surface phenotype and a T helper type 1 profile of cytokine secretion in the liver of patients chronically infected with hepatitis B virus. *J. Immunol. 152*: 3074-3087.

Baron JL, Gardiner L, Nishimura S, ShinkaiK, Locksley R, Ganem D. (2002). Activation of nonclassical NKT cell subset in a transgenci mouse model of hepatitis B virus infection. *Immunity 16*: 583-594.

Barrios C, Brandt C, Berney M, Lambert PH, Siegrist CA. (1996a). Partial correction of the TH2/TH1 imbalance in neonatal murine responses to vaccine antigens through selective adjuvant effects. *Eur. J. Immunol. 26*: 2666-70.

Barrios C, Brawand P, Berney M, Brandt C, Lambert PH, Siegrist CA. (1996b). Neonatal and early life immune responses to various forms of vaccine antigens qualitatively differ from adult responses: predominance of a Th2-biased pattern which persists after adult boosting. *Eur. J. Immunol. 26*:1489-96.

Bellamy R, Ruwende C, Corrah T, et al. (1999). Tuberculosis and chronic hepatitis B virus infection in Africans and variation in the vitamin D receptor gene. *J. infect. Dis. 179*: 721-724.

Bertagnolli MM, Lin BY, Young D, Herrmann SH. (1992). IL-12 augments antigen-dependent proliferation of activated T lymphocytes. *J Immunol. 149*: 3778–3783.

Bertoletti A, Ferrari C, Fiaccadori F, Penna A, Margolskee R, Schlicht HJ, Fowler P, Guilhot S, Chisari FV. (1991). HLA class I-restricted human cytotoxic T cells recognize endogenously synthesized hepatitis B virus nucleocapsid antigen. *Proc. Natl. Acad. Sci. USA. 88*: 10445-10449.

Bertoletti A, Maim K. (2000). Protection of damage: a dual role for the virus specific cytotoxic T lymphocyte response in hepatitis B and C infection? *Curr. Opin. Immunol. 12*: 403–408.

Bertoletti AA, Sette FV, Chisari A, Penna, M, Levrero M, DeCarli F, Fiaccadori, and Ferrari C. (1994). Natural variants of cytotoxic epitopes are T cell receptor antagonists for antiviral cytotoxic T cells. *Nature (Lond.). 369*: 407-410.

Biron C. (1999). Initial and innate responses to viral infection — pattern setting in immunity or disease, *Curr. Opin. Microbiol. 2*: 374–381.

Biron CA. (1994). Cytokines in the generation of immune response to, and resolution of virus infection. *Curr. Opin. Immunol. 6*: 530-538.

Bocher WO, Galun E, Marcus H, Daudi N, Terkieltaub D, Shouval D, Lhor HF, Reisner Y. (2000). Reduced hepatitis B virus surface antigen-specific Th1 helper cell frequency of chronic HBV carriers is associated with a failure to produce antigen-specific antibodies in the trinera mouse. *Hepatology 31*: 480-487.

Boehm U, Klamp T, Groot M, Howard JC. (1993). Cellular responses to interferon-y and its receptor. *Annu Rev. Immunol. 11*: 571-611.

Bonecchi R, Binachi G, Bordignon PP, et al., (1998). Differential expression of chemokine receptors on chemotactic responsiveness of type-1 T helper cells (Th1s) and Th2s. *J. Exp. Med. 187*:129-134.

Borish L. (1998). Updates on cell and cytokine. *J. Allergy Clin. Immunol. 101*: 293-297.

Borzi RM, Dal Monte P, Honorati MC, Facchini A. (1992). IgG subclass distribution of anti-HBs antibodies following vaccination with cDNA HBsAg. *J. Immunol. Meth. 21*:146: 17-23.

Borzi RM, Dal Monte P, Honorati MC, Facchini A. (1992). IgG subclass distribution of anit-HBs antibodies following vaccination with cDNA HbsAg. *J. Immunol Meth. 146*:17-23.

Bozkaya H, Bozdayi M, Turkyilmaz R et al., (2000). Circulating IL-2, IL-10, and TNF-α in chronic hepatitis B: their relations to HBeAg status and the activity of liver disease. *Hepatogastroenterology 47*:1675-1679.

Brown JL, Carman WF, Thomas HC. (1990). The hepatitis virus Baillieres Clin. *Gasteroenterol. 4*: 721-747.

Brunetto MR, Oliveri F, Coco B, et al. (2002). Outcome of anti-HBe positive chronic hepatitis B in alpha-interferon treated and untreated patients: a long term cohort study. *J. Hepatol. 36*: 263–70.

Chan HL, Wong ML, Hui AY, Hung LC, Chan FK, Sung JJ. (2003). Hepatitis B virus genotype C takes a more aggressive disease course than hepatitis B virus genotype B in hepatitis B e antigen-positive patients. *J. Clin. Microbiol. 41*:1277-1279.

Chang MH, Chen CJ, Lai MS, et al., (1997). Universal hepatitis B vaccination in Taiwan and the incidence of hepatocellular carcinoma in children. Taiwan Childhood Hepatoma Study Group. *New. Engl. J. Med. 336*:1855–1859.

Chen CJ, Yang HI, Su J, et al. (2006). Risk of hepatocellular carcinoma across a biological gradient of serum hepatitis B virus DNA level. *JAMA 295*: 65–73.

Chen Y, Wei H, Sun R, Tian Z. (2005). Impaired function of hepatic natural killer cells from murine chronic HBsAg carriers. *Int. Immunopharmacol. 5*: 1839-1852.

Chisari FV, Ferrari C. (1995). Hepatitis B virus immunopathogenesis. *Ann. Rev. Immunol. 13*: 29-60

Chisari FV. (1997). Cytotoxic T cells and viral hepatitis. *J. Clin. Invest. 99*: 1472–1477.

Crockett SD, Keeffe EB. (2005). Natural history and treatment of hepatitis B virus and hepatitis C virus coinfection. *Ann. Clin. Microbiol. Antimicrob. 4*: 13.

Curry M.P, Koziel M. (2000). The dynamics of the immune response in acute hepatitis B: new lessons using new techniques. *Hepatology 32*: 1177–1179.

Czaja AJ, Cookson S, Constantini PK, Clare M, Underhill JA, Donaldson PT. (1999). Cytokine polymorphisms associated with clinical features and treatment outcome in type 1 autoimmune hepatitis. *Gastroenterology 117*: 645–652.

Dandri M, Lutgehetmann M, Volz T, Petersen J. (2006). Small animal models for studying hepatitis B virus replication and pathogenesis. *Semin. Liver Dis. 26*: 181-191.

Davis GL, Hoofnagle JH, Waggoner JG. (1984). Acute type A hepatitis during chronic hepatitis B virus infection: association of depressed hepatitis B virus replication with appearance of endogenous alpha interferon. *J. Med. Virol. 14*: 141-147.

de Franchis R, Meucci G, Vecchi M, et al. (1993). The natural history of asymptomatic hepatitis B surface antigen carriers. *Ann. Intern. Med. 118*:191–4.

De Lalla C, Galli G, Aldrighetti L, et al. (2004). Production of profibrotic cytokines by invariant NKT cells characterizes cirrhosis progresion in chronic viral hepatitis. *J. Immunol. 173*: 1417-1425.

Delves PJ, Roitt IM. (2000). Advances in immunology: the immune system. *New Engl. J Med. 343*: 108–117.

Desmet VJ, Gerber M, Hoofnagle JH, Manns M, Scheuer PJ. (1999). Classification of chronic hepatitis: diagnosis, grading and staging. *Hepatology 19*:1513–1520.

Di Bisceglie AM, Rustgi VK, Hoofnagle JH, et al. (1988). NIH conference: hepatocellular carcinoma. *Ann. Intern. Med. 108*:390–401.

Duan XZ, Wang FS, Wang M, et al. (2003). Identification of phenotype and interferon-α-producing capability of circulating type II dendritic cells and its clinical implication in HBV-infected patients. *Zhonghua Yi Xue Za Zhi. 83*:548-552.

Echevarría S, Casafont F, Miera JL, De La Cruz F, San Miguel G, Romero FP. (1991). Interleukin-2 and natural killer activity in acute type B hepatitis. *Hepatogastroenterology 4*:307-310.

Echevarría, JM Leon P. (1995). Hepatitis B virus: biology, natural history, and diagnosis of the infection. *Enferm. Infec. Microbiol. Clin. 13*:22-30.

Fattovich G, Pantalena M, Zagni I, et al. (2002). Effect of hepatitis B and C virus infections on the natural history of compensated cirrhosis: a cohort study of 297 patients. *Am. J. Gastroenterol. 97*:2886–95.

Fattovich G. (2003). Natural history and prognosis of hepatitis B. Semin. Liver Dis. 23:47–58.

Fischer M, Runkel L, Schaller H. (1995). HBx protein of hepatitis B virus interacts with the C-terminal portion of a novel human proteasome alpha-subunit. *Virus Genes. 10*: 99-102.

Francis A. (2000). Hepatitis B epidemiology in Asia, the Middle East and Africa. *Vaccine 18*: S20-S22.

Fujinami RS, Oldstone MA. (1979). Antiviral antibody reacting on the plasma membrane alters measles virus expression inside the cell. *Nature 279*:529-530.

Fung SK, Lok AS. (2004). Hepatitis B genotypes: do they play a role in the outcome of HBV infection? *Hepatology 40*:790-792.

Ganem D, Schneider RJ. (2001). Hepadnaviridae: the viruses and their replication. In: Fields BN, Knipe DM, Howley PM, et al, editors. *Field Virology, 4th edition*. Philadelphia: Lippincott Williams & Wilkins. pp. 2923–69.

Gilles P, Fey G, Chisari FV. (1992). Tumor necrosis factor alpha negatively regulates hepatitis B virus gene expression in transgenic mice. *J. Virol. 66*:3955-3960.

Godkin A, Davenport M, Hill AV. (2005). Molecular analysis of HLA class II associations with hepatitis B virus clearance and vaccine nonresponsiveness. *Hepatology 41*:1383-1390.

Guidotti LG, Borrow P, Hobbs MV, Matzke B, Gresser I, Oldstone MBA, Chisari FV. (1996). Viral cross talk: intracellular inactivation of the hepatitis B virus during an unrelated viral infection of the liver. *Proc. Natl. Acad. Sci. USA. 93*: 4589-4594.

Guidotti LG, Chisari FV. (1996). To kill or to cure option in host defense against viral infection. *Curr. Opin. Immunol. 8*: 478-483.

Guidotti LG, Chisari FV. (1999). Cytokine induced viral purging — role in viral pathogenesis, *Curr. Opin. Microbiol. 2*: 388–391.

Guidotti LG, Chisari FV. (2001). Non-cytolytic control of viral infections by the innate and adaptive immune response. *Annu. Rev. Immunol. 19*: 65–91.

Guidotti LG, Ishikawa T, Hobbs MV, Matzke B, Schreiber R, Chisari FV. (1996). Intracellular inactivation of the hepatitis B virus by cytotoxic T Lymphocytes. *Immunity 4*: 25-36.

Guidotti LG, Ishikawa T, Hobbs MV, Matzke B, Schreiber R, Chisari. FV. (1996). Intracellular inactivation of the hepatitis B virus by cytotoxic T lymphocytes. *Immunity 1*: 25-36.

Guidotti LG, Matzke B, Pasquinelli C, Shoenberger JM, Rogler C, Chisari FV. (1996). The hepatitis B virus (HBV) precore protein inhibits HBV replication in transgenic mice. *J. Virol. 70*: 7056-7061.

Guidotti LG, Rochford R, Chung J, Shapiro M, Purcell R, Chisari FV (1999). Viral clearance without destruction of infected cells during acute HBV infection. *Science 284*: 825–829.

Hadziyannis SJ, Vassilopoulos D. (2001). Hepatitis B e antigen-negative chronic hepatitis B. *Hepatology 34*:617–24.

Heinzel FP, Sadick MD, Holaday BJ, Coffman RL, Locksley RM (1989). Reciprocal expression of interferon γ or interleukin 4 during the resolution or progression of murine leishmaniasis. Evidence for expression of distinct helper T cell subset. *J. Exp. Med. 169*:59-72.

Herkel J, Jagemann B, Wiegard C, et al. (2003). MHC class II-expressing hepatocytes function as antigen-presenting cells and activate specific CD4 T lymphocytes. *Hepatology 37*:1079-1085.

Hohler T, Gerken G, Notghi A., Lubjuhn R., Taheri H, Protzer U, Lohr HF, Schneider PM, Meyer zum Buschenfelde KH, Rittner C. (1997). HLA-DRB1*1301 and *1302 protect against chronic hepatitis. *Bri. J. Hepatol. 26*: 503–507.

Hohler T, Kruger A., Gerken G, Schneider PM, Meyer zum Buschenefelde KH, Rittner C. (1998). A tumor necrosis factor-alpha (TNF-alpha) promoter polymorphism is associated with chronic hepatitis B infection. *Clin. Exp. Immunol. 111*: 579–582.

Hollinger FB, Lau D. (2006). Hepatitis B: the pathway to recovery through treatment. Gastroenterol. *Clin. North Am. 35*: 425-461

Hollinger FB, Liang JT. (2001). Hepatitis B virus. In: Fields BN, Knipe DM, Howley PM, et al, editors. *Fields Virology, 4th edition*. Philadelphia: Lippincott Williams & Wilkins. pp. 2971–3036.

Huang CF, Lin SS, Ho YC, Chen FL, Yang CC. (2006). The immune response induced by hepatitis B virus principal antigens. *Cell Mol Immunol. 3*: 97-106.

Huy TT, Abe K. (2004). Molecular epidemiology of hepatitis B and C virus infections in Asia. *Pediatr. Int. 46*:223-230.

Iannacone M, et al (2006). "Pathogenetic and antiviral immune responses against hepatitis B virus". *Future Virology 1*: 189-196.

Ihde DC, Sherlock P, Winawer SJ, et al. (1974). Clinical manifestations of hepatoma: a review of 6 years' experience at a cancer hospital. *Am. J. Med. 56*:83–91.

Ilan Y. (2002). Immune downregulation leads to upregulation of an antiviral response: a lesson from the hepatitis B virus. *Microb. Infect. 4*:1317-1326.

Inoue M, Kakumu S, Yoshioka K, Tsutsumi Y, Wakita T, Arao M. (1989). Hepatitis B core antigen specific IFN-gamma production of peripheral blood mononuclear cells in patients with chronic hepatitis B virus infection. *J. Immunol. 142*: 4006-4011.

Joklik WK (1991). Interferons, In B. N. Fields, D. M. Knipe, et al. (ed.), *Fundamental virology, 2nd ed.* Raven Press, New York, N.Y. pp. 343-361.

Jung MC, Gruner N, Zachoval R, Schraut W, Gerlach T, Diepolder H, Schirren CA, Page M, Bailey J, Birtles E, Whitehead E, Trojan J, Zeuzem S, Pape GR. (2002). Immunological monitoring during therapeutic vaccination as a prerequisite for the design of new effective therapies: induction of a vaccine-specific CD4+ T-cell proliferative response in chronic hepatitis B carriers. *Vaccine 20*:3598-612.

Jung MC, Pape GR. (2002). Immunology of hepatitis B infection. Lancet Infect. Dis. 2: 43-50.

Jung MC, Spengler U, Schraut W, Hoffmann R, Zachoval R, Eisenburg J, Eichenlaub D, Riethmüller G, Paumgartner G, Ziegler-Heitbrock HW, et al. (1991). Hepatitis B virus antigen-specific T-cell activation in patients with acute and chronic hepatitis. *Bri. J. Hepatol. 13*: 310–317.

Jung, M.C., Diepolder HM, Spengler U, Wierenga EA, Zachoval R, Hoffmann RM, Eichenlaub D, Frosner G, Will H, Pape GR (1995). Activation of a heterogenous hepatitis B (HB) core and e antigen-specific $CD4^+$ T-cell population during seroconversion to anti-HBe and anti-HBs in hepatitis B virus infection. *J. Virol. 69*: 3358-3368.

Juszczyk J. (2000). Clinical course and consequences of hepatitis B infection. *Vaccine 1*:S23-S25.

Kakimi K, Guidotti LG, Koezuka Y, Chisari FV. (2000). Natural killer T cell activation inhibits hepatitis B virus replication in vivo. *J. Exp. Med. 192*: 921–930.

Kakimi K, Lane TE, Chisari FV, Guidotti LG. (2001). Cutting edge: inhibition of hepatitis B virus replication by activated NK T cells does not require inflammatory cell recruitment to the liver. *J. Immunol. 167*: 6701–6705.

Kakumu S, Ishikawa T, Wakita T, Yoshioka K, Takayanagi M, Tahara H,. Kusakabe A. (1994). Interferon-gamma production specific for hepatitis B virus antigen by intrahepatic T lymphocytes in patients with acute and chronic hepatitis B. *Am. J. Gastroenterol. 89*: 92-96.

Kane A, Lloyd J, Zaffran M, Simonsen L, Kane M. (1999). Transmission of hepatitis B, hepatitis C and human immunodeficiency viruses through unsafe injections in the developing world: model-based regional estimates. *Bull World Health Organ 77*: 801–817.

Kane M. (1995). Global programme for control of hepatitis B infection. *Vaccine 13*: 47-49.

Kao JH, Chen PJ, Lai MY, Chen DS. (2002). Genotypes and clinical phenotypes of hepatitis B virus in patients with chronic hepatitis B virus infection. *J. Clin. Microbiol. 40*:1207-1209.

Kao JH. (2002). Hepatitis B viral genotypes: clinical relevance and molecular characteristics. *J. Gastroenterol. Hepatol. 17*: 643-650.

Kazuhiro K, Guidotti LC, Yasuhiko K, Chisari FV. (2000). Natural killer T cell activation inhibits hepatitis B virus replication in vivo. *J. Exp. Med. 192*: 921–930.

Kelso A. (1995). Th1 and Th2 subsets: paradigms lost? *Immunol. Today 8*:374-379.

Kew M.C. (1997). Current epidemiological trends of viral hepatitis in Africa. In: M. Rizetto et al. *Viral hepatitis and liver diseases*. Minerva Medica, Turin, pp562–566.

Lee M, Lee M,. Lee SK, Son M, Sho SW, Park S, Kim HI. (1999). Expression of Th1 and Th2 type cytokines responding to HbsAg and HbxAg in chronic hepatitis B patients. *J. Korean Med. Sci. 2*:175-181.

Lee WM. (1997). Hepatitis B virus infection. *New Engl. J. Med. 337*: 1733-1745.

Liaw YF, Tai DI, Chu CM, et al. (1988). The development of cirrhosis in patients with chronic type B hepatitis: a prospective study. *Hepatology 8*:493-6.

Lin CL, Liao LY, Liu CJ, Chen PJ, Lai MY, Kao JH, Chen DS. (2002). Hepatitis B genotypes and precore/basal core promotore mutants in HBeAg-negative chronic hepatitis B. *J. Gastroenterol. 37*:283-287.

Ljunggren KK, Miyakawa Y, Kidd AH. (2002). Genetic variability in hepatitis B viruses. *J. Gen. Virol. 83*:1267-1280.

Lohr HF, Schlaak JF, Gerken G, Fleischer B, Dienes HP, Meyer ZB. (1994). Phenotypical analysis and cytokine release of liver infiltrating and peripheral blood T lymphocytes from patients with chronic hepatitis of different etiology. *Liver 3*:161-166.

Löhr HF, Weber W, Schlaak J, Goergen B, Meyer zum Buschenfelde KH, Gerken G. (1995). Proliferative response of CD4+ T cells and hepatitis B virus clearance in chronic hepatitis with or without hepatitis B e-minus hepatitis B virus mutants. *Hepatology 22*: 61–68.

Lynch DH, Ramdell F, Alderson MR. (1995). Fas and FasL in the homeostatic regulation of immune responses. *Immunol. Today 16*:569-574.

Machado, B. I., L. Deibis, and F. Toro. (1997). Respuesta inmunológica en hepatitis viral. *Gen. 2*:85-93.

Maddrey WC. (2001). Hepatitis B: an important public health issue. *Clin. Lab. 47*:51–5.

Maim K., Boni C, Ogg GS, et al. (1999). Direct ex vivo analysis of hepatitis B virus specific CD8+ T cells associated with control of infection. *Gastroenterology 117*: 1386-1396.

Mansour AJ, Abdulhamid A.W, and. Syed R. (1994). Soluble CD23 and interleukin-4 levels in autoimmune chronic active hepatitis and systemic lupus erythematosus. *Clin. Immunol. Immunopathol. 1*:33-37.

Margolis HS, Alter MJ, Hadler SC. (1991). Hepatitis B: evolving epidemiology and implications for control. Semin. *Liver Dis. 11*: 84–92.

Marinos G, Torre F, Chokshi S, Hussain M, Clarke BE, Rowlands DJ, Eddleston AL, Naoumov NV, Williams R. (1995). Induction of T-helper cell response to hepatitis B core antigen in chronic hepatitis B: a major factor in activation of the host immune response to the hepatitis B virus. *Hepatology (4 Pt 1)*:1040–1049.

Maruyama T, Iino S, Koike K, Yasuda K, Milich DR. (1993). Serology of acute exacerbation in chronic hepatitis B virus infection. *Gastroenterology 105*: 1141-1151.

Maruyama T, McLachlan A, Iino S, Koike K, Kurokawa K, Milich DR. (1993). The serology of chronic hepatitis B infection revisited. *J. Clin. Invest. 91*: 2586–2595.

Maruyama T, Schödel F, Iino S, Koike K, Yasuda K, Peterson D, Milich DR. (1994). Distinguishing between acute and symptomatic chronic hepatitis B virus infection. *Gastroenterology 106*:1006-1015.

Mast EE, Mahoney FJ, Alter MJ, Margolis HS. (1998). Progress toward elimination of Hepatitis B transmission in the United States. *Vaccine 16*: 48-51

McClary H, Koch R, Chisari FV, Guidotti LG. (2000). Relative sensitivity of hepatitis B virus and other hepatotropic viruses to the antiviral effects of cytokines. *J. Virol. 74*: 2255-2264.

McMahon BJ, Alward WL, Hall DB, et al. (1985). Acute hepatitis B virus infection: relation of age to the clinical expression of disease and subsequent development of the carrier state. *J. Infect. Dis. 151*:599-603.

McMahon BJ, Alward WL, Hall DB, et al. (1985). Acute hepatitis B virus infection: relation of age to the clinical expression of disease and subsequent development of the carrier state. *J. Infect. Dis. 151*:599-603.

McQuillan GM, Coleman PJ, Kruszon-Moran D, Moyer LA, LambertSB, Margolis HS. (1999). Prevalence of hepatitis B virus infection in theUnited States: the National Health and Nutrition Examination Surveys, 1976 through 1994. *Am. J. Public. Health 89*:14-18.

Milich DR, Chen MK, Hughes JL, Jones JE. (1998). The secreted hepatitis B precore antigen can modulate the immune response to the nucleocapsid: a mechanism for persistence. *J. Immunol. 160*:2013-2021.

Milich DR, Schodel F, Hughes JL, Jones JE, Peterson DL. (1997). The Hepatitis B virus core and e antigens elicit different Th cell subsets: sntigen structure can be affect Th cell phenotype. *J. Virol. 71*: 2191-2201.

Missale G, Ferrari C, Fiaccadori F. (1995). Cytokines mediators in acute inflammation and chronic course of viral hepatitis. *Ann. Ital. Med. Int. 1*:14-18.

Missale G, Redeker A., Person J, Fowler P, Guilhot S, Schlicht HJ, Ferrari C, Chisari FV. (1993). HLA-A31 and HLA-Aw68 restricted cytotoxic T cell responses to a single hepatitis B virus nucleocapsid epitope during acute viral hepatitis. *J. Exp. Med. 177*: 751-762.

Morell A, Roth-Wicky B, Skvaril F. (1983). Immunoglobulin G subclass restriction of antibodies against hepatitis B surface antigen. *Infect. Immun. 39*:565-568.

Moriyama T, Guilhot S, Klopchin K, Moss B, Pinkert CA., Palmiter RD, Brinster RL, Kanagawa O, Chisari FV (1990). Immunobiology and pathogenesis of hepatocellular injury in hepatitis B virus transgenic mice. *Science (Wash. DC) 248*: 361-364.

Murakami S. (2001). Hepatitis B virus X protein: a multifunctional viral regulator. *J. Gastroenterol. 36*:651-660.

Murray JM, Wieland SF, Purcell RH, Chisari FV. (2005). Dynamics of hepatitis B virus clearance in chimpanzees. *Proc. Natl. Acad.. Sci. (USA) 102*:17780-17785.

Nayersina R, Folwer P, Guilhot S, Missale G, Cerny A, Schlicht HJ, Vitiello A, Chesnut R, Person JL, Redeker AG, Chisari FV. (1993). HLA A2 restricted cytotoxic T lymphocyte responses to multiple hepatitis B surface antigen epitopes during hepatitis B virus infection. *J. Immunol. 150*: 4659-4671.

Niederau C, Heintges T, Lange S, Goldmann G, Niederau CM, Mohr L, Haussinger D. (1996). Long-term follow-up of HBeAg-positive patients treated with interferon alfa for chronic hepatitis *Bri. N. Engl. J. Med. 334*:1422-7.

Papaevangelou G, Tassopoulos N, Roumeliotou-Karayannis A, Richardson C. (1984). Etiology of fulminant viral hepatitis in Greece. *Hepatology. 4*:369-72.

Paul WE, Seder RA. (1994). Lymphocyte responses and cytokines. *Cell. 76*:241–251.

Penna A., Del Prete G, Cavalli A, Bertoleti A, D'elios M, Sarmiento R. (1997). Predominant T-helper 1 cytokine profile of hepatitis B virus nucleocapsid-specific T cell in acute self-limited hepatitis B. *Hepatitis 4*:1022-1027.

Purcell RH. (1993). The discovery of the hepatitis viruses. *Gastroenterology 104*:955–963.

Raynor BD. (1996). Cytokines. *Adv. Obstet. Gynecol. 3*:27-46.

Rehermann B, Ferrari C, Pasquinelli C, Chisari FV. (1996a) The hepatitis B virus persists for decades after recovery from acute viral hepatitis despite active maintenance of a cytotoxic T lymphocyte response. *Nat. Med. 2*: 1104-1108.

Rehermann B, Lau D, Hoofnagle JH, Chisari FV. (1996b). Cytotoxic T lymphocyte responsiveness after resolution of chronic hepatitis B virus infection. *J. Clin. Invest. 97*: 1655-1665.

Rehermann B, Person J, Redeker A, Fowler P, Brown M, Moss B, Sette A, Chisari FV. (1995). The cytotoxic T lymphocyte response to multiple hepatitis B virus polymerase epitopes during and after acute viral hepatitis. *J. Exp. Med. 181*: 1047-1058.

Ridge JP, Fuchs EJ, Matzinger P. (1996). Neonatal tolerance revisited: turning on new born cells with dendritic cells. *Science 271*:1723-1726.

Romero, R, Lavine JE. (1996). Cytokine inhibition of the hepatitis B virus core promoter. *Hepatology 23*: 17–23.

Schalm SW, Thomas HC, Hadziyannis SJ. (1990). Chronic hepatitis B. In: Popper H, Schaffner F, Editors. *Progress in liver disease*. New York: WB Saunders. pp 443–62.

Seeger C, Mason WS. (2000). Hepatitis B virus biology. *Microbiol. Mol. Biol. Rev. 64*:51-68.

Sheu JC, Sung JL, Chen DS, et al. (1985). Growth rate of asymptomatic hepatocellular carcinoma and its clinical implications. *Gastroenterology 89*:259–66.

Stuyver L, De Gendt S, Van Geyt C, Zoulim F, Fried M, Schinazi RF, Rossau R. (2000). A new genotype of hepatitis B virus: complete genome and phylogenetic relatedness. *J. Gen. Virol. 81*:67-74.

Tandon BN, Tandon (1997). A. Epidemiological trends of viral hepatitis in Asia. In: M. Rizetto et al. *Viral hepatitis and liver diseases Minerva Medica*, Turin, pp. 559–561.

Thio CL, Carrington M, Marti D, et al. (1999). Class II HLA alleles and hepatitis B virus persistence in African Americans. *J. Infect. Dis. 179*:1004-1006.

Thio CL, Mosbruger T, Astemborski J, Greer S, Kirk GD, O'Brien SJ, Thomas DL. (2005). Mannose Binding Lectin Genotypes Influence Recovery from Hepatitis B Virus Infection. *J. Virol. 79*: 9192–9196.

Thomas HC, Foster GR, Sumiya M, et al. (1996). Mutation of gene of mannosebinding protein associated with chronic hepatitis B viral infection. *Lancet 348*:1417-1419.

Thomas HC, Montano L, Goodall A, DeKoning R, Oladapo J, Weidman KH. (1982). Immunological mechanism in chronic hepatitis B virus infection, *Hepatology 2*: 116S–121S.

Thomas HC, Pignatelli M, Scully LJ. (1985). Viruses and immune reactions in the liver. *Scand. J. Gastroenterol. (Suppl.) 114*:105-117.

Thompson SC, Ruff TA. (1995). Hepatitis B vaccination. What are the current international recommendations? *Clin. Immunother. 3*:15–26.

Thursz MR, Kwiatkowski D, Allospp CEM, et al. (1995). Association between an MHC class II allele and clearance of hepatitis B virus in the Gambia. *New Engl. J. Med. 332*:1065-1069.

Tilg H, Wilmer A, Vogel W, Herold M, Nolchen B, Julmaier G, Huber C. (1992). Serum levels of cytokines in chronic liver disease. *Gastroenterology 103*:264-274.

Toukan AU. (1997). Control of hepatitis B in the Middle East. In: M. Rizetto et al. *Viral hepatitis and liver diseases*. Minerva Medica, Turin, pp 678–680.

Trinchieri G. (1995). a Interleukin-12: proinflammatory cytokine with immunoregulatory functions that bridge innate resistance and antigen-specific adaptive immunity. *Annu. Rev. Immunol. 13*:251–276.

Trinchieri G. (1997). Cytokines acting on or secreted by macrophages during intracellular infection (IL-10, IL-12, IFNg). *Curr. Opin. Immunol. 9*:17-23.

Tsai SL, Chen PJ, Lai MY, Yang PM, Sung JL, Huang JH, Hwang LH, Chang TH, Chen DS. (1992). Acute exacerbations of chronic type B hepatitis are accompanied by increased T cell responses to hepatitis B core and e antigens. Implications for hepatitis B e antigen seroconversion. *J. Clin. Invest. 89*: 87–96.

Turner MW. (2003). The role of mannose-binding lectin in health and disease. *Mol. Immunol. 40*:423-429.

Visvanathan K, Lewin SR. (2006). Immunopathogenesis: role of innate and adaptive immune responses. *Semin. Liver Dis. 26*:104-15.

WHO. (2000). Hepatitis B Fact Sheet No. 204 Web site. *WHO.*

WHO. (1996). Hepatitis B Vaccine-making global progress. Update, Expanded Programme on Immunization, *WHO.*

WHO. (1997). The World Health Report, *WHO.*

Wieland SF, Guidotti LG, Chisari FV. (2000). Intrahepatic induction of IFN-α/β eliminates viral RNA containing capsids in HBV transgenic mice. *J. Virol 74*: 4165–4173.

Wilson IA, Stanfield RL, Jewell DA, Ghiara JB, Fremont DH, Stura EA. (1994). Immune recognition of viral antigen. Infect. *Agents Dis. 3*:155-161.

Yalcin K, Degertekin H, Bahcecioglu IH, Demir A, Aladag M, Yildirim B, Horasanli S, Ciftci S, Badur S. (2004). Hepatitis B virus genotype D prevails in patients with persistently elevated or normal ALT levels in Turkey. *Infection 32*:24-29.

Yang CC, Lin CC, Wang L, Ku CS, Chen CK. (2001). Anti-HBc IgG subclasses in different populations by comparing a variety of ELISA plates. *J. Immunoassay Immunochem. 22*:33-45.

Yang HI, Lu SN, Liaw YF, et al. (2002). Hepatitis B e antigen and the risk of hepatocellular carcinoma. *New Engl. J. Med. 347*:168–74.

Zoulim F. (2006). In vitro models for studying hepatitis B virus drug resistance. Semin. *Liver Dis*. 26:171-80.

INDEX

A

B

C

D

E

F

G

H

I

J

K

L

M

N

Q

R

S

T

U

V

W

Y

Biomimetic Technologies

Related titles

Large, *Optical biomimetics: Materials and applications*
9781845698027, £140

Anton-Haro and Dohler, *Machine-to-machine (M2M) communications: Architecture, performance and applications*
9781782421023, £190

Nihtianov and Luque, *Smart sensors and MEMS: Intelligent devices and microsystems for industrial applications*
9780857095022, £170

Woodhead Publishing Series in Electronic and Optical Materials: Number 82

Biomimetic Technologies

Principles and applications

Edited by

Trung Dung Ngo

ELSEVIER

AMSTERDAM • BOSTON • CAMBRIDGE • HEIDELBERG
LONDON • NEW YORK • OXFORD • PARIS • SAN DIEGO
SAN FRANCISCO • SINGAPORE • SYDNEY • TOKYO
Woodhead Publishing is an imprint of Elsevier

WP
WOODHEAD
PUBLISHING

Woodhead Publishing Limited is an imprint of Elsevier
80 High Street, Sawston, Cambridge, CB22 3HJ, UK
225 Wyman Street, Waltham, MA 02451, USA
Langford Lane, Kidlington, OX5 1GB, UK

ISBN: 978-0-08-100249-0 (print)

British Library Cataloguing in Publication Data
A catalogue record for this book is available from the British Library

Library of Congress Control Number: 2015942343

Contents

Contributors

M. Akcakaya University of Pittsburgh, Pittsburgh, PA, USA

S. Alers Maastricht University, Maastricht, The Netherlands

M. Ambroise IMS Laboratory, University of Bordeaux, Talence, France

H. Araki Faculty of Information Science, Osaka Institute of Technology, Hirakata City, Japan

L. Brandão BioMark-Cintesis/ISEP, Instituto Superior de Engenharia do Porto, Porto, Portugal

B. Broeker University of Liverpool, Liverpool, UK

I. Caliskanelli University of Liverpool, Liverpool, UK

C. Chevrot Laboratoire de Physicochimie des Polymères et des Interfaces, Université de Cergy-Pontoise, Cergy-Pontoise, France

D. Claes University of Liverpool, Liverpool, UK

R. Dahiya Electronics and Nanoscale Engineering, University of Glasgow, Glasgow, UK

M.J. de Boer MESA$^+$ Institute for Nanotechnology, University of Twente, Enschede, The Netherlands

H. Droogendijk MESA$^+$ Institute for Nanotechnology, University of Twente, Enschede, The Netherlands

A. Ellery Space Exploration Engineering Group, Carleton University, Ottawa, ON, Canada

N. Festin University of Nottingham Ningbo China (UNNC), Ningbo, China

D.J. Frankel University of Newcastle, Newcastle upon Tyne, UK

J.R.L. Guerreiro BioMark-Cintesis/ISEP, Instituto Superior de Engenharia do Porto, Porto, Portugal

Y. Ikeda College of Science and Technology, Nihon University, Funabashi-shi, Japan

H. Jörntell Lund University, Lund, Sweden

S. Kim Exergy Devices Ltd., Cambridge, UK

G.J.M. Krijnen MESA$^+$ Institute for Nanotechnology, University of Twente, Enschede, The Netherlands

T. Levi IMS Laboratory, University of Bordeaux, Talence, France

A. Mazzoni The Biorobotics Institute, Scuola Superiore Sant'Anna, Pisa, Italy

F.T.C. Moreira BioMark-Cintesis/ISEP, Instituto Superior de Engenharia do Porto, Porto, Portugal

C. Muravchik LEICI, Universidad Nacional de La Plata, La Plata, Argentina

A. Nehorai Washington University in St. Louis, St. Louis, MO, USA

F. Nicolas Laboratoire de Physicochimie des Polymères et des Interfaces, Université de Cergy-Pontoise, Cergy-Pontoise, France Brain Vision Systems (BVS), Paris, France

C. Oddo The Biorobotics Institute, Scuola Superiore Sant'Anna, Pisa, Italy

S. Omatu Faculty of Engineering, Osaka Institute of Technology, Osaka, Japan

P. Pirim Brain Vision Systems (BVS), Paris, France

C. Plesse Laboratoire de Physicochimie des Polymères et des Interfaces, Université de Cergy-Pontoise, Cergy-Pontoise, France

B. Ranjbar-Sahraei Maastricht University, Maastricht, The Netherlands

K. Saito College of Science and Technology, Nihon University, Funabashi-shi, Japan

S. Saïghi IMS Laboratory, University of Bordeaux, Talence, France

M.G.F. Sales BioMark-Cintesis/ISEP, Instituto Superior de Engenharia do Porto, Porto, Portugal

R.G.P. Sanders MESA$^+$ Institute for Nanotechnology, University of Twente, Enschede, The Netherlands

C. Santulli School of Architecture and Design, Università di Camerino, Ascoli Piceno, Italy

M. Takato College of Science and Technology, Nihon University, Funabashi-shi, Japan

M. Tavakoli Institute of Systems and Robotics, University of Coimbra, Coimbra, Portugal

K. Tuyls University of Liverpool, Liverpool, UK

F. Uchikoba College of Science and Technology, Nihon University, Funabashi-shi, Japan

F. Vidal Laboratoire de Physicochimie des Polymères et des Interfaces, Université de Cergy-Pontoise, Cergy-Pontoise, France

C. Viegas Institute of Systems and Robotics, University of Coimbra, Coimbra, Portugal

G. Weiss Maastricht University, Maastricht, The Netherlands

O. Yarkoni University of Cambridge, Cambridge, UK

R. Yoshida School of Engineering, The University of Tokyo, Tokyo, Japan

Woodhead Publishing Series in Electronic and Optical Materials

1 **Circuit analysis**
J. E. Whitehouse

2 **Signal processing in electronic communications: For engineers and mathematicians**
M. J. Chapman, D. P. Goodall and N. C. Steele

3 **Pattern recognition and image processing**
D. Luo

4 **Digital filters and signal processing in electronic engineering: Theory, applications, architecture, code**
S. M. Bozic and R. J. Chance

5 **Cable engineering for local area networks**
B. J. Elliott

6 **Designing a structured cabling system to ISO 11801: Cross-referenced to European CENELEC and American Standards**
Second edition
B. J. Elliott

7 **Microscopy techniques for materials science**
A. Clarke and C. Eberhardt

8 **Materials for energy conversion devices**
Edited by C. C. Sorrell, J. Nowotny and S. Sugihara

9 **Digital image processing: Mathematical and computational methods**
Second edition
J. M. Blackledge

10 **Nanolithography and patterning techniques in microelectronics**
Edited by D. Bucknall

11 **Digital signal processing: Mathematical and computational methods, software development and applications**
Second edition
J. M. Blackledge

12 **Handbook of advanced dielectric, piezoelectric and ferroelectric materials: Synthesis, properties and applications**
Edited by Z.-G. Ye

13 **Materials for fuel cells**
Edited by M. Gasik

14 **Solid-state hydrogen storage: Materials and chemistry**
Edited by G. Walker

15 **Laser cooling of solids**
S. V. Petrushkin and V. V. Samartsev

16 **Polymer electrolytes: Fundamentals and applications**
Edited by C. A. C. Sequeira and D. A. F. Santos

17 **Advanced piezoelectric materials: Science and technology**
Edited by K. Uchino

18 **Optical switches: Materials and design**
Edited by S. J. Chua and B. Li

19 **Advanced adhesives in electronics: Materials, properties and applications**
Edited by M. O. Alam and C. Bailey

20 **Thin film growth: Physics, materials science and applications**
Edited by Z. Cao

21 **Electromigration in thin films and electronic devices: Materials and reliability**
Edited by C.-U. Kim

22 ***In situ* characterization of thin film growth**
Edited by G. Koster and G. Rijnders

23 **Silicon-germanium (SiGe) nanostructures: Production, properties and applications in electronics**
Edited by Y. Shiraki and N. Usami

24 **High-temperature superconductors**
Edited by X. G. Qiu

25 **Introduction to the physics of nanoelectronics**
S. G. Tan and M. B. A. Jalil

26 **Printed films: Materials science and applications in sensors, electronics and photonics**
Edited by M. Prudenziati and J. Hormadaly

27 **Laser growth and processing of photonic devices**
Edited by N. A. Vainos

28 **Quantum optics with semiconductor nanostructures**
Edited by F. Jahnke

29 **Ultrasonic transducers: Materials and design for sensors, actuators and medical applications**
Edited by K. Nakamura

30 **Waste electrical and electronic equipment (WEEE) handbook**
Edited by V. Goodship and A. Stevels

31 **Applications of ATILA FEM software to smart materials: Case studies in designing devices**
Edited by K. Uchino and J.-C. Debus

32 **MEMS for automotive and aerospace applications**
Edited by M. Kraft and N. M. White

33 **Semiconductor lasers: Fundamentals and applications**
Edited by A. Baranov and E. Tournie

34 **Handbook of terahertz technology for imaging, sensing and communications**
Edited by D. Saeedkia

35 **Handbook of solid-state lasers: Materials, systems and applications**
Edited by B. Denker and E. Shklovsky

36 **Organic light-emitting diodes (OLEDs): Materials, devices and applications**
Edited by A. Buckley

37 **Lasers for medical applications: Diagnostics, therapy and surgery**
Edited by H. Jelínková

38 **Semiconductor gas sensors**
Edited by R. Jaaniso and O. K. Tan

39 **Handbook of organic materials for optical and (opto)electronic devices: Properties and applications**
Edited by O. Ostroverkhova

40 **Metallic films for electronic, optical and magnetic applications: Structure, processing and properties**
Edited by K. Barmak and K. Coffey

41 **Handbook of laser welding technologies**
Edited by S. Katayama

42 **Nanolithography: The art of fabricating nanoelectronic and nanophotonic devices and systems**
Edited by M. Feldman

43 **Laser spectroscopy for sensing: Fundamentals, techniques and applications**
Edited by M. Baudelet

44 **Chalcogenide glasses: Preparation, properties and applications**
Edited by J.-L. Adam and X. Zhang

45 **Handbook of MEMS for wireless and mobile applications**
Edited by D. Uttamchandani

46 **Subsea optics and imaging**
Edited by J. Watson and O. Zielinski

47 **Carbon nanotubes and graphene for photonic applications**
Edited by S. Yamashita, Y. Saito and J. H. Choi

48 **Optical biomimetics: Materials and applications**
Edited by M. Large

49 **Optical thin films and coatings**
Edited by A. Piegari and F. Flory

50 **Computer design of diffractive optics**
Edited by V. A. Soifer

51 **Smart sensors and MEMS: Intelligent devices and microsystems for industrial applications**
Edited by S. Nihtianov and A. Luque

52 **Fundamentals of femtosecond optics**
S. A. Kozlov and V. V. Samartsev

53 **Nanostructured semiconductor oxides for the next generation of electronics and functional devices: Properties and applications**
S. Zhuiykov

54 **Nitride semiconductor light-emitting diodes (LEDs): Materials, technologies and applications**
Edited by J. J. Huang, H. C. Kuo and S. C. Shen

55 **Sensor technologies for civil infrastructures**
Volume 1: Sensing hardware and data collection methods for performance assessment
Edited by M. Wang, J. Lynch and H. Sohn

56 **Sensor technologies for civil infrastructures**
Volume 2: Applications in structural health monitoring
Edited by M. Wang, J. Lynch and H. Sohn

57 **Graphene: Properties, preparation, characterisation and devices**
Edited by V. Skákalová and A. B. Kaiser

58 **Silicon-on-insulator (SOI) technology**
Edited by O. Kononchuk and B.-Y. Nguyen

59 **Biological identification: DNA amplification and sequencing, optical sensing, lab-on-chip and portable systems**
Edited by R. P. Schaudies

60 **High performance silicon imaging: Fundamentals and applications of CMOS and CCD sensors**
Edited by D. Durini

61 **Nanosensors for chemical and biological applications: Sensing with nanotubes, nanowires and nanoparticles**
Edited by K. C. Honeychurch

62 **Composite magnetoelectrics: Materials, structures, and applications**
G. Srinivasan, S. Priya and N. Sun

63 **Quantum information processing with diamond: Principles and applications**
Edited by S. Prawer and I. Aharonovich

64 **Advances in non-volatile memory and storage technology**
Edited by Y. Nishi

65 **Laser surface engineering: Processes and applications**
Edited by J. Lawrence, C. Dowding, D. Waugh and J. Griffiths

66 **Power ultrasonics: Applications of high-intensity ultrasound**
Edited by J. A. Gallego-Juárez and K. F. Graff

67 **Advances in delay-tolerant networks (DTNs): Architectures, routing and challenges**
Edited by J. J. P. C. Rodrigues

68 **Handbook of flexible organic electronics: Materials, manufacturing and applications**
Edited by S. Logothetidis

69 **Machine-to-machine (M2M) communications: Architecture, performance and applications**
Edited by C. Anton-Haro and M. Dohler

70 **Ecological design of smart home networks: Technologies, social impact and sustainability**
Edited by N. Saito and D. Menga

71 **Industrial tomography: Systems and applications**
Edited by M. Wang

72 **Vehicular communications and networks: Architectures, protocols, operation and deployment**
Edited by W. Chen

73 **Modeling, characterization and production of nanomaterials: Electronics, photonics and energy applications**
Edited by V. Tewary and Y. Zhang

74 **Reliability characterisation of electrical and electronic systems**
Edited by J. Swingler

75 **Handbook of industrial wireless sensor networks: Monitoring, control and automation**
Edited by R. Budampati and S. Kolavennu

76 **Epitaxial growth of complex metal oxides: Techniques, properties and applications**
Edited by G. Koster, G. Rijnders and M. Huijben

77 **Semiconductor nanowires: Materials, synthesis, characterization and applications**
Edited by J. Arbiol and Q. Xiong

78 **Superconductors in the Power Grid**
Edited by C. Rey

79 **Optofluidics, sensors and actuators in microstructured optical fibres**
Edited by S. Pissadakis

80 **Magnetic Nano- and Microwires: Design, Synthesis, Properties and Applications**
Edited by M. Vázquez

Preface

Nature has been an unlimited source of inspiration for scientists, technologists, and business men to develop new scientific research methods and innovative technologies and applications that are far from what the human mind could have imagined and simulated. Through billions of years of natural selection, living organisms have evolved to adapt to their living environments. As a result, natural materials and structures over the test of time provide highly efficient and nontolerant solutions for technological development of man-made products.

Over half a century, biomimetics has been emerged to become the research discipline of studying biological characteristics and operational principles of living organisms for refining our knowledge in designing complex real-world systems. The formal method in biomimetics is usually conducted through three approaches of mimicry, replication, and imitation to transfer lessons learned from the biological science to technological solutions. New findings from this research field have successfully promoted technological development of innovative materials, sensors, actuators, and system integrations such as Velcro mimicked from burdock plant, shark skin mimicked nanotechnology materials, self-cleaning materials replicated from the surface of lotus plant, aircraft wings imitated from birds, or neural network-inspired cybernetics, and DaimlerChrysler concept vehicles with high fuel efficiency imitated from the shape of boxfish.

The goal of this edited book is to bring the current state of the art in the biomimetics field to light. The book is organized into 4 parts including 16 chapters. Part One focuses on biomimetic materials with emphases on synthetic methods of molecular biomimetics, fiber composites, and biomachine interface. In Part Two, the latest research results of biomimetic sensor technologies embracing tactile sensors, hair-based inertial sensors, gas sensing systems, and bat-inspired sonar system are extendedly presented. Part Three is dedicated to biomimetic actuators with the development of interpenetrating polymer networks-based actuators for the biological vision system, self-oscillating polymers and gels as materials for soft-actuators, and fabrication of biomimetic artificial muscles for dynamic agile robots. Part Four starts with the comprehensive review of artificial intelligence themes through symbolic connectionism and then extends with a specific example of central pattern generators for the robotic applications. The part is enriched a wide range of bio-inspired applications including biologically inspired coordination of multi-robot systems, up-to-date technologies of climbing robots, and biological rhythm generation of micro-quadruped robot locomotion, and Ormia-inspired antenna array design.

Although this book is only a small collection of the up-to-date research activities on biomimetic technologies, it certainly covers the important portion of what have been recently done in the field. As such, this book can serve as a valuable source for students, researchers, and scientists interested in the emerging interdisciplinary research area.

This book is suitable for graduate students and researchers who have general interests in biomimetic technologies including robotics, cybernetics, design of sensors and actuators, complex system integration, and artificial intelligence. For researchers with some experiences in the field, you can read each chapter mostly independently. However, graduate students are recommended to read through the book to obtain the overview of this growing research field.

This book would not have been done without great contributions of all authors and the well-organized plan of the editorial project management board of Woodhead Publishing Ltd. I would like to express my special thanks to all authors for high-quality chapters contributed to this book. I would like to extend my sincere thanks to all members of the editorial management board involved in this project.

Trung Dung Ngo

Part One

Principles and Materials for Biomimetic Technologies

Synthesis of molecular biomimetics

1

F.T.C. Moreira, J.R.L. Guerreiro, L. Brandão, M.G.F. Sales

1.1 Introduction

Scientists have been exploring approaches and mechanisms adopted by nature to create functional structures for technical applications. This is usually referred to as biomimetics (Seeman and Belcher, 2002). Thus, biomimetics refers to general approaches/processes mimicking biology or nature, including herein the synthesis of nanomaterials/nanostructures that imitate physicochemical, mechanical, and biological properties of natural materials, either in nano- or macroscale dimensions. Such nanomaterials/nanostructures can be used in various applications, including (i) chemical and biochemical sensors; (ii) wiring matrices; (iii) chemical reactors; (iv) modular positioners; (v) light-emitting diodes; (vi) optical storage; (vii) drug delivery; (viii) biomedical devices; and (ix) as scaffolds for tissue regeneration.

But the synthesis of biomimetic materials is in practice a difficult task, because it is at the cross-point of biology, biochemistry, physics, chemistry, physiology, and material sciences, requiring a profound understanding of biological functions, structures, and principles of various objects found in nature. In essence, the synthesis of biomimetic materials emerges from bio-inspired approaches.

1.1.1 Bio-inspiration

Nature has been the great model for imitation, copying, and learning, thereby acting as an ideal inspiration for new materials and technologies (Bar-Cohen, 2006). The first bio-inspired approaches looked for a direct match of the natural materials. Flying using human-developed capabilities was inspired by birds and the invention of the solar cell may have been inspired by photosynthesis in leafs, among many other examples of technology in our society. But recent developments in nanotechnology have emerged in nanoscale engineering advances and lead biomimetics into the molecular scale, where biomolecules and their supra-molecular organization play the leading role.

1.1.2 Bio-nanomaterials

Nature combines few elementary building pieces into a wide range of biomolecules that are arranged in nanomaterials of nano- or macro-scale dimensions to provide specific properties of biological interest. This includes molecular scale devices, superhydrophobicity, self-cleaning, energy conversion, energy conservation, high adhesion, reversible adhesion, aerodynamic lift, materials, and fibers with high mechanical strength, biological self-assembly, antireflection, structural coloration, thermal insulation, self-healing, and sensory-aid mechanisms (Bhushan, 2009), among many others.

The most recent advances in nanotechnology and nanosciences have lead biomimeticists to reproduce those properties. A wide range of new functional materials have been produced in this context, including carbon nanotubes (CNTs), graphene, fullerenes, polymeric nanoparticles, metal organic nanomaterials, self-assembled and supramolecular nanostructures, and their derivatives, among others. These materials display unique physicochemical properties such as catalytic, dielectric, optical and mechanical, giving rise to distinctive applications ranging from biomedical to environmental engineering and high-energy storage (Bhattacharya et al., 2014).

Nature uses simple organic compounds as building blocks in a suitably organized manner, while biomimetics may employ eventually any bio or artificial molecules of interest. Although this may seem an advantage compared to Nature, Nature is certainly much more effective than man in developing effective and functional nanomaterials. Either way, the core of synthetic biomimetics is the main building blocks used as the elementary pieces of the final material.

1.2 Building blocks

Life on Earth is formed by four essential building blocks (amino acids, nucleic acids, carbohydrates, and lipids) in which their self-assembly and interaction are vital. Each building block has specific function(s): nucleic acids are responsible for transferring genetic information and eventually controlling the cell; carbohydrates store energy, reconstitute recognition systems, and provide building materials; lipids create membranes and accumulate energy; and amino acids are combined into proteins to act as structural elements and execute cell functions (Paltauf, 1994).

Along with biological building blocks, artificial building blocks may be employed in the synthesis of biomimetic materials (Figure 1.1). In general, this includes oligonucleotides, amino acids, sugars, proteins, peptides, dendrimers, CNTs, fullerenes, and so on. The use of biological elements is widely selected regarding their similarity

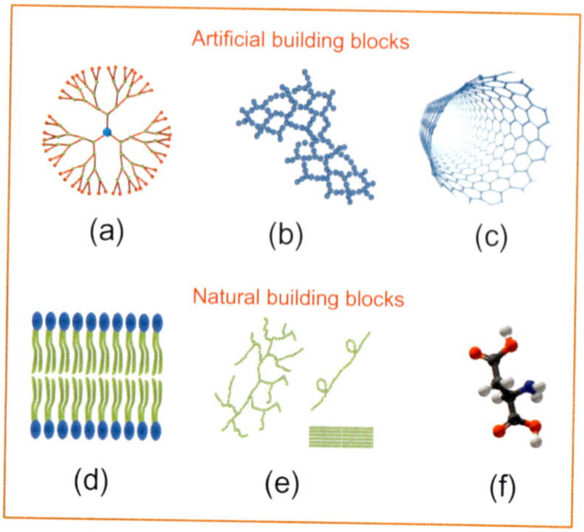

Figure 1.1 Synthetic and natural building blocks. (a) Dendrimers; (b) organosilane; (c) carbon nanotube; (d) phospholipid; (e) carbohydrate; and (f) amino acid.

with biological systems and high specific molecular affinity. But biological elements often present poor stability and are typically linked to complex and expensive production processes (the production of some biological elements may not be even available). Some artificial elements may overcome these disadvantages, offering higher physical robustness and high resistance to temperatures and pressures, assembled at a lower cost.

1.2.1 Amino acids

Amino acids are natural compounds composed of amine ($-NH_2$) and carboxylic acid ($-COOH$) functional groups, linked to the same carbon atom (Figure 1.1). Different amino acids have a different and specific side chain linked to this exact carbon. There are more than 500 amino acids identified, some of which occurring free in nature and some as intermediates in metabolism (Wagner and Musso, 1983), but the assembly of proteins within the same species depends on a very small number. Amino acids are mainly proteinogenic (protein-building amino acids) but can also be linked to other nonprotein biological roles. Several examples exist, such as glutamic acid being involved in the excitatory neurotransmission in the human brain; proline being used to synthesize hydroxyproline, which is a major component of the connective tissue collagen; and glycine being involved in the synthesizes of porphyrins of the red blood cells.

Proteins often perform a specific task million-fold with high reliability, in which their stability is crucial (Pompe et al., 2013). Proteins also exhibit high specificity of interaction and functional diversity, self-organization in higher ordered networks, and high sensitivity with respect to external signals (Pompe et al., 2013). High specificity and diverse functionality can be realized by a combination of rigid subunits that can be arranged with high flexibility.

Biomimetics of proteins may include new structures acting as the natural protein as well as biomimetic surfaces that interact with the proteins. Recent works in the field include the development of biomimetic protein nanoparticles that promote dendritic cell activation and cross-presentation (Molino et al., 2013) or the development of biomimetic surface for selective protein recognition (Moreira et al., 2013). Proteins may also be employed to full the biological system at the cell delivery of specific compounds (McMahon et al., 2011).

1.2.2 Lipids

Lipids are the major source of amphiphilic structures within the cells that contain a polar head group linked to a hydrophobic hydrocarbon chain. These amphiphilic structures act mainly as membrane barriers as they are arranged in double layer (Figure 1.1). The polar ends point outward and the nonpolar ends point inward, thereby forming a "lipid bilayer." The membrane lipids belong to three major classes of membrane lipids: phospholipids, glycolipids, and cholesterol.

Phospholipids are the predominant forms of amphiphilic lipids within the cells. In these, the polar head includes a negatively charged phosphate group, with nitrogen containing alcohol and a backbone of glycerol (glycerophospholipids) or sphingosine (sphingomyelin). They may be neutral (phosphatidyl choline or lecithin and phosphatidyl ethanolamine or cephalin) or negatively charged (phosphatidyl inositol, phosphatidyl serine, and bisphosphatidyl glycerol or cardiolipin). Overall, phospholipids play an important role as building materials and structural elements. Besides acting as important barrier function in cell membranes, phospholipids contribute to the stabilization and function of native membrane-bound proteins (Sandermann, 1978), acting as receptors and channel pores in the membrane.

The great importance of lipid-based membranes in biotechnology applications, such as medicine, diagnostics, sensor systems, environmental monitoring, and energy storage (Jackman et al., 2012; Shen et al., 2014; Sleytr et al., 2014), has promoted the development of biomimetic model membranes, where mono or bilayers of lipids are of utmost importance (Schuster and Sleytr, 2014). These model membranes are obtained by the immobilization of planar lipid membranes on a solid support and have been able to mimic fundamental properties of natural cell membranes, including fluidity, electrical sealing, and hosting integral membrane proteins (Schuster and Sleytr, 2014). Overall, biomimetic membranes incorporate biological elements or borrow concepts, ideas, or inspiration from biological systems (Shen et al., 2014).

1.2.3 Carbohydrates

Carbohydrates are a large group of organic compounds made with monomeric units named monosaccharides. According to the number of combined monosaccharide units, sugars are usually subdivided into the following groups: monosaccharides, disaccharides, oligosaccharides, and polysaccharides. A typical polysaccharide is shown in Figure 1.1.

Monosaccharides contain a backbone of carbon to which hydroxyl groups and hydrogen atoms are attached. One of these carbons has a carbonyl bond (C=O), and it can be located at the first (aldose) or the second (ketose) position at the backbone. Hydroxyl groups are attached to all other carbon atoms. In aqueous solution, monosaccharides are found preferentially under cyclic forms, resulting from the intramolecular nucleophilic addition of the hydroxyl group to the carbonyl function. Disaccharides (such as maltose, lactose, or sucrose) consist of two monosaccharides covalently bonded by means of an *O*-glycosidic, oligosaccharides join more than 2 and up to 20 monosaccharide monomeric units, and polysaccharides more than 20 monosaccharide units.

The most important monosaccharides in biological systems include D-Glucose and D-Fructose, both with a 6-carbon backbone, but glucose is an aldose while fructose is a ketose. Cyclodextrins (CDs) are among glucose-based sugars, one of the most important in biomimetics. They are inclusion compounds made with cyclic oligosaccharides, which form a tunnel that may accommodate different species. Natural CDs are α, β, or γ when the ring member contains six, seven, and eight glucose units, respectively, and display noticeable association constant for different compounds (Jaime et al., 1991). CDs and other monosaccharides may also be used to create biomimetic surfaces for target biomolecules, provided that the appropriate polymerization conditions are selected.

N-Acetylglucosamine is another monosaccharide of great relevance in biological systems. It is an acetylated derivate of glucosamine with several functions. It is a member of cell walls in bacteria and fungi; a member of chitin in insects and crustaceans; and it is a part of hyaluronan present in the extracellular matrix of cells. It is the second most abundant biopolymer, but its application in many fields is hindered by its low solubility in most solvents, being most often deacetylated to produce Chitosan. Chitosan, in turn, has been used in many medical applications. It serves as biomimetic material of anti-hemoglobin antibodies, by using it to create an imprinted recognition surface of hemoglobin on beads (Guo et al., 2005).

Several sugars have also been involved in mimicking the highly hydrated glycocalyx coatings of cells to create antifouling surfaces (Knoll, 2012). In this approach, polymeric structures are composed of specific carbohydrates, which may constitute a biomimetic alternative to other polymeric structures currently acting as antifouling coatings.

1.2.4 Nucleic acids

Nucleic acids are linear polymers incorporating four nucleotide repeating units (Hu and Li, 2011). Each nucleotide has in common a phosphate bridge and a sugar residue. The phosphate of one nucleotide (in position 3′) bonds to the hydroxyl of the sugar of the following nucleotide (in 5′) and ensures the propagation of a polynucleotide strand from the 5′ to the 3′ end by means of phosphodiester bonds (Nelson and Cox, n.d.). Every single nucleotide carries one of four heterocyclic bases: adenine (A), thymine (T, in DNA) or uracil (U, in RNA), guanine (G), and cytosine (C). They are appended to the main backbone and sustain hydrogen bonding and [π–π] stacking interactions. Hydrogen bonds, formed between [N–H] donors and either N or O acceptors, support the pairing of A with T (or U) and of G with C. The stacking interactions involve attractive contacts between the extended π-surfaces of heterocyclic bases.

Oligonucleotides may be used to create biomimetic surfaces of molecular recognition. This is done mostly by placing complementary oligonucleotide sequences and the target deoxyribonucleic acid (DNA) or ribonucleic acid (RNA) biomolecules are further recognized by hybridization (Jayasena, 1999; Strehlitz et al., 2008). Oligonucleotides may also be employed to establish stable and selective complexes with other biomolecules than nucleic acids (Spolar and Record, 1994). These specific sequences are named aptamers and are typically DNA or RNA single-stranded chains. Their interaction with the target molecule relies on the phosphodiester charged backbone (leading to nonspecific binding by electrostatic interaction) (Demchenko, 2001) and to the specific sequence recognition (leading to stacking interactions, shape complementary, electrostatic interactions, and hydrogen bonding) (Strehlitz et al., 2008). Typically, the binding affinities are comparable to antibodies (Collett et al., 2005), after proper *in vitro* selection process by Systematic Evolution of Ligands by EXponential enrichment (SELEX) or Cell-SELEX (Pan et al., 2010).

1.2.5 Carbon allotropes

The family of carbon allotropes included for many years the classic forms of graphite and diamond until it became enriched by fullerenes. In contrast to graphite and diamond, with extended solid state structures, fullerenes are spherical molecules and are soluble in a variety of organic solvents, an important requirement for chemical manipulations (Hirsch, 1994). Fullerenes are graphitic cage structures incorporating pentagons (absent in graphite) that provide the curvature to the overall structure. Different forms of fullerenes exist, such as buckyballs and nanotubes, among others. Buckyballs are spheres that may comprise from 20 to 60 carbon atoms, and nanotubes are hollow tubes of very small dimensions, organized in single or multiple walls (Figure 1.1) (Singh and Singh, 2013). CNTs have several promising features, including their large length-to-diameter aspect ratios, providing high surface-to-volume ratios (Merkoci et al., 2005; Rivas et al., 2007; Yang et al., 2007). The recent awareness of graphene (exfoliated from graphite) and its unique optical and electronic properties has lead carbon allotropes into a new era.

Several carbon allotropes have been employed with success in biomimetic technologies, including graphite (Almeida et al., 2012), graphene (Rebelo et al., 2014, Truta et al., 2014), and CNTs (Moreira et al., 2011a,b; Queiros et al., 2012). Graphite is an inexpensive material with reasonable electrical features to be applied in electrical-based strategies. It has been used as simple support to assemble biomimetic surfaces for antimicrobial drugs (Almeida et al., 2012) or protein biomarkers (Rebelo et al., 2014; Truta et al., 2014). In these, carbon nanostructures are modified with a suitable polymeric layer after covalent binding of the biomolecule to be targeted. The overall procedure is simple, because carbon can be chemically modified by covalent and noncovalent attachment of the molecules on its surface (Ajayan, 1999). Covalent functionalization implicates the elimination of the C double bonds, where carbon atoms change from sp^2 to sp^3 hybridization, leaving "holes" in the structure and, thus, modifying both their mechanical and electrical properties (Bacsa et al., 2003).

1.2.6 Dendrimers

Dendrimers are hyperbranched globular architectures of nanoscopic size (Figure 1.1) with three distinct domains: the *core*, a central part that is either a single atom or an atomic group having at least two identical chemical functions; the *dendron*, branches emanating from the core, constituted of repeat units having at least one branch junction, whose repetition is organized in a geometrical progression that results in a series of radially concentric layers called generations; and the *terminal functional groups*, generally located in the exterior of the macromolecule, which play a key role of their properties (Caminade et al., 2005). Typically, dendrimers have a spherical three-dimensional morphology with symmetry around the core and cavities in the interior, offering the possibility of introducing chromophores, redox active species, catalytic sites, etc. at defined locations, making these unique building blocks for the construction of novel and exploitable materials.

In general, the preparation of dendrimers is made in a stepwise fashion using either convergent or divergent strategies (Lee et al., 2005). In divergent methods, the dendrimer grows outward from a multifunctional core molecule. The core molecule reacts with monomer molecules containing one reactive and two dormant groups giving the first-generation dendrimer. Then, the new periphery of the molecule is activated for reactions with more monomers; the repletion of this process leads to dendrimers of several generations. The convergent approach is synthesized by starting from the end groups and progressing inward (Oliveira et al., 2012). Commercially available dendrimers polyamidoamine and poly(propyleneimine)s are currently obtained by the divergent method.

In the context of biomimetics, dendrimers have been designed to mimic enzymatic activity (Wei and Wang, 2013), acting as catalysts and displaying flexible folding features as proteins (Wei and Wang, 2013). Dendrimers have as well been used as recognition elements of several types of molecules by incorporating multiple branch ends, which can be readily available for consecutive conjugation reactions and/or host–guest interactions (Yoon et al., 2000; Kesharwani et al., 2014). This includes the detection or delivery of proteins, DNA, or drugs (Gajbhiye et al., 2009; Singh et al., 2009; Malik et al., 2012; Xu et al., 2014; Bhattacharya et al., 2014).

1.2.7 Organosilanes

Organosilanes are building blocks in sol–gel material synthesis (example given in Figure 1.1). Sol–gel materials are colloidal suspensions of silica particles that are polymerized to form a solid gel (Buckley and Greenblatt, 1994). The starting materials (the precursors) used in the preparation of sol are usually inorganic metal salts or metal organic compounds such as metal alkoxides. The hydrolysis of precursor reagents begins when they are mixed with water in the presence of an acid or a base catalyst, but the addition of a mutual solvent (usually alcohol) is not necessarily required. Hydrolysis of precursors leads to the formation of silanol groups (Si–OH), followed by progressive condensation reactions producing siloxane bonds (Si–O–Si), alcohol, and water as by-products. During the sol–gel phase transition, the viscosity of the solution gradually increases as colloidal sol becomes interconnected to form a rigid, porous gel.

Overall, sol–gel process provides a simple way to incorporate numerous organic, organometallic, and biological molecules into a microporous matrix of sol–gel (Hench and West, 1990). In general, sol–gel materials have a combination of advantages over many other polymers when biomolecules are involved. These include: (i) the mild preparation conditions allow entrapped biomolecules to retain much of its physical and chemical properties inside the polymer matrix, (ii) the rigid property of sol–gel cross-linking network favors retaining the shape of the cavities after removal of the templates, and (iii) sol–gel glasses are electro-, photo-, and chemically stable and can be optically transparent. The thickness, porosity, and surface area of the material are easily controlled, while selectivity and diffusion for small template molecules are comparable and even better than acrylic polymer-based imprinted materials (Lahav et al., 2001; Marx and Liron, 2001). There is a wide range of possibilities to obtain well-controlled properties of the materials by varying the chemical composition of the precursors and the ratio of inorganic to organic components (Tripathi et al., 2006). A drawback of the method might be that the fragile polymer network could be less robust than a simple surface or bulk imprinted material.

Sol–gel materials have also been employed with success to produce water-repellent surfaces displaying superhydrophobicity, as plant leafs. Different approaches have been employed for this purpose, including the use of many other nanostructures, most recently reviewed (Latthe et al., 2012).

1.3 Bottom-up arrangement

Scientists have traditionally been designing nanostructured surfaces and supports on a nanometer regimen by *top-down* approaches (Gates et al., 2005). In this approach, macroscopic materials are generated and "carved"/modified to produce nanoscale objects (Figure 1.2a). Several techniques are used in *top-down* approaches, including a series of lithographic methods that are based on traditional photolithography. These methods are generally effective, allowing high nanometer-level precision, accuracy, and registration (Huang et al., 2001), but become very expensive (Perl et al., 2009), while being associated to random geometrical designs.

In biomimetics, *top-down* approaches have also been employed. A typical example is presented in Figure 1.3, concerning the fabrication and construction of three-dimensional scaffolds for tissue engineering. In this, cells are seeded onto a biocompatible and biodegradable scaffold, populating the scaffold and creating their own extracellular matrix (Lu et al., 2013).

In contrast, nature creates structures in nanoscale arrangements, using *bottom-up* processes (Huang et al., 2001; Douglas, 2003; Bazylinski and Frankel, 2004; Veis, 2005; Cheng et al., 2006; Kroeger, 2007). The *bottom-up* approach is where atomic and molecular units are assembled to form molecular structures ranging from atomic

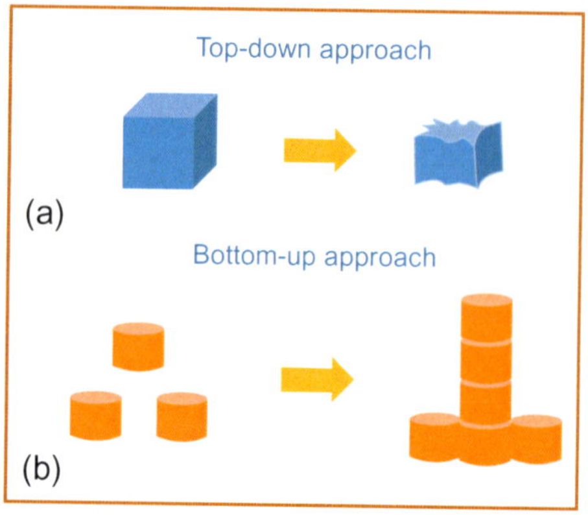

Figure 1.2 Top-down (a) and bottom-up (b) approaches.

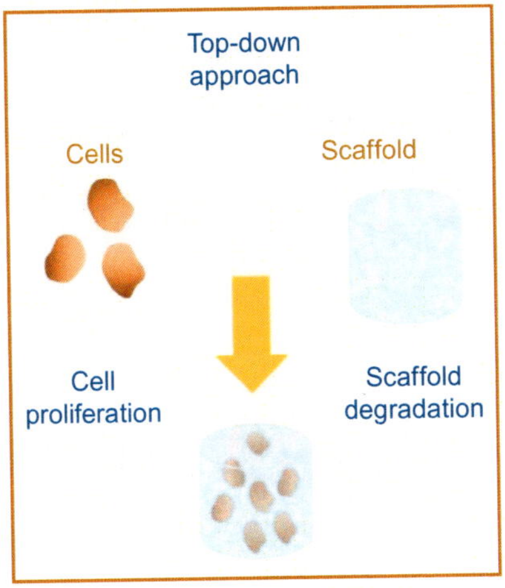

Figure 1.3 Top-down approach.
Based on Lu et al. (2013).

dimension to structures of nanometer size or above, as presented in Figure 1.2b (Ngô and Van de Voorde, 2014). Examples include producing polymers (such as cellulose) from one or several monomers; calcification and silicification found in diatoms; and the formation of magnetite crystals in magnetotactic bacteria. In general, living organisms/cells are capable of organizing nanoscale building blocks into large-scale hierarchical structures that serve different functions, such as mechanical support, filtration, light harvesting, gravity sensing, and locomotion (Calvert, 1992; Aizenberg et al., 2003). Erosion is an exceptional top-down approach of nature, carving macroscopic objects, but this approach does not involve living cells.

In biomimetics, the parallel *bottom-up* approach regarding the construction of three-dimensional scaffolds for tissue engineering would involve the production of microscale tissue building blocks assembled into larger tissue constructs (Lu et al., 2013), as shown in Figure 1.4. Fabrication of tissue building blocks can be achieved via multiple approaches, including fabrication of cell-encapsulating (Yang et al., 2009; Konnova et al., 2013) microscale hydrogels (Sung et al., 2011), self-assembled cell aggregation (Napolitano et al., 2007), generation of cell sheets (Chen et al., 2014), and direct printing of cells (Bose et al., 2013; Zhou et al., 2014a,b). The use of hydrogels in this context is especially relevant and becoming popular. Hydrogels create a similar environment to that of the native extracellular matrix (Geckil et al., 2010) and allow controlling both shape and compositional features of the individual building blocks (Lu et al., 2013).

Many other biomimetic *bottom-up* approaches are currently emerging, putting in practice recent nanotechnology developments (Mann et al., 1993; Zhao et al., 2012). Biomimetics is currently shifting to the molecular level, where the *bottom-up* approach takes advantage of physicochemical interactions for the hierarchical synthesis of ordered nanostructures through the self-assembly of basic building blocks (Hawker and Russell, 2005; Zhao et al., 2012). Self-organizing materials offer simple

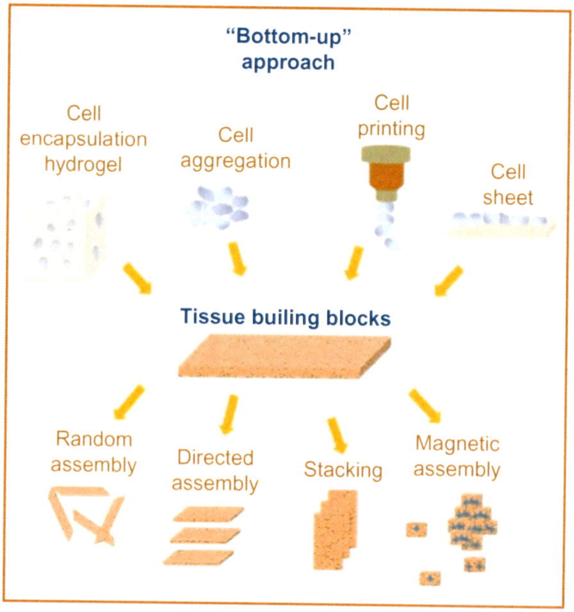

Figure 1.4 Bottom-up approach.
Based on Lu et al. (2013).

and low-cost processes to make huge area of periodic nanostructures (Huang et al., 2001). They contribute in the biological systems form and are sustained as a result of self-organization and can generate ordered three-dimensional (3D) aggregates of components, oscillating in size from the molecular to the macroscopic. This is done mostly by self-assembling, soft lithography, and bulk approaches, among others.

1.3.1 Self-assembled

(a) Self-assembly in living organisms

Self-assembly in living organisms can be generated in different forms. This includes (i) programmed self-assembly (Valery et al., 2003; Chakraborty et al., 2008), (ii) constrained self-assembly (Whitesides and Boncheva, 2002; Tamerler and Sarikaya, 2009), (iii) hierarchical self-assembly (Murnen et al., 2010; Yang et al., 2013; Zhou et al., 2014a,b), and (iv) static and dynamic self-assembly (Zhang et al., 2002; Zhao et al., 2013).

Programmed self-assembly involves the information that is encoded in the living cell, such as nucleic acid sequences that dictate the amino acid residues at the active sites of proteins. In this specific case, the order of the building blocks in such sequences and the surrounding environment determine the "shape" and electrostatic patterns (hydrogen bonds, hydrophobicity, etc.), which in turn determine the function of the material. Overall, both the encoded instructions and the features of the environment determine the outcome of self-organization in living organism. Another example of coded self-assembly concerns the embryonic development where the cell differentiation is governed by the cell origin along with several multitude of environmental signals (Liu and Roy, 2005; Vunjak-Novakovic and Scadden

2011). Neural circuits also assemble themselves from individual cells following a combination of internal program and external guidance (Pistol et al., 2010; Ayers et al., 2011).

Constrained self-assembly regards the existence of constraints that determine the order and asymmetry in self-assembled aggregates of biological molecules. One mechanism of introducing such constraints makes use of chains of monomers: the order of these monomers is fixed, restricting the 3D structures that can be formed. Another mechanism involves geometrical restrictions to self-assemblies. Local geometrical factors are similarly significant at the supramolecular level (Aizenberg et al., 2003) for templating crystal growth during biomineralization, regulation of cell growth and viability (Chen et al., 1997; Johnson and Speir, 1997), and for material exchange between cells and the surrounding environment.

Hierarchical self-assembly concerns the integration of small building blocks into gradually more complex structures in hierarchical designs. These blocks associate into larger and more complex secondary structures, which are, in turn, integrated into increasingly more complex structures. One common example of this living approach is the structural organization of tendons: the triple helices of tropocollagen are organized in microfibrils, arranged next in subfibrils, fibrils, fascicles, and tendons, involving six discrete levels of hierarchical organization (Kastelic et al., 1980).

Static and dynamic self-assembly in living systems generate equilibrium structures. Examples of this process include molecular recognition of globular proteins (Whitesides and Grzybowski, 2002). Some living systems are dynamic, existing out-of-equilibrium and maintaining their characteristic order only while dissipating energy (Whitesides and Grzybowski, 2002).

(b) Artificial self-assembling systems designed using biological principles

In analogy to biological self-assembled structures, the shape and functionality of artificial self-assembled aggregates are related to the shapes of their counterparts, the interactions between these, and the surrounding environment. This approach can be performed by many ways, including the (i) recognition by shape complementarity, (ii) hierarchical self-assembly, (iii) templated self-assemblies, and (iv) dynamic self-assembling systems.

Recognition by complementary shape has been used to design components by molecular and mesoscale self-assembled methods (Martin et al., 1998; Choi et al., 1999a,b; Gracias et al., 2002). A typical example includes the setup of a mesoscale system in which polyhedral, micron-sized electronic components self-assembled on a common substrate by shape recognition and shear forces. The three-dimensional surfaces obtained allowed high specificity in recognition, contributing to the structural stability of resulting self-assembled aggregates. Hierarchical self-assembly assay has been used to build nanostructures for application as optical materials (Drain et al., 2002), tunable nanoporous (Boal et al., 2000) and microporous (Jenekhe and Chen, 1999) materials, nanomaterials with anisotropic properties (Ikkala and ten Brinke, 2002), metal nanostructures on block copolymer scaffolds, (Choi et al., 1999a,b) and extended arrays of polymeric objects at a fluid–fluid interface (Lopes and Jaeger, 2001). Unrestricted and templated self-assemblies of spheres have been shown to give access to only a limited range of structures. The use of a hierarchical approach opens the possibility of generating 3D structures with a variety of 3D lattices. In dynamic self-assembling systems, objects organize into a variety of patterns where the individual components can move autonomously and can interact with one another. Overall, self-assembly is a successful approach to organize components from molecular to macroscopic into functional aggregates.

1.3.2 Soft lithography

Soft lithography includes a collection of methods that uses soft polymeric materials to fabricate stamps, channels, or membranes with micro-sized features (Gates et al., 2005).

Several patterning methods based on imprinting, molding, and embossing with an elastomeric stamp are the basis of soft lithography, currently including: micro-contact printing (Kim et al., 2005), micro-molding in capillary (Jeong et al., 2009), replica molding (Sharma and Madou, 2012), solvent-assisted micro-molding (Han et al., 2009), phase-shifting edge lithography (Ye and Qi, 2011), decal transfer lithography (Childs and Nuzzo, 2004; Childs and Nuzzo, 2005; Kim and Kim, 2007), nanotransfer printing (Hocheng and Hsu, 2008; Errachid et al., 2007; Fox et al., 2012), dip-pen lithography (Henry et al., 2008; Lenhert and Fuchs, 2008; Abrishamchian et al., 2013), and nano-skiving (Xu et al., 2008) assays. Soft lithography is especially used to produce structural patterned surfaces and coatings with specific biomolecules.

Soft-material patterns are often generated on elastomeric stamps, such as poly (dimethylsiloxane) (PDMS) (Jackman et al., 1995; Liao et al., 2012). Typically, this includes creating a mold of the donor surface on an elastomer support and transferring it into a new receptor surface (Figure 1.5). This procedure is an easy way to engineer the properties of surfaces (Jackman et al., 1995; Ko et al., 2008). This approach has been tested so far with different inks, substrate materials, transfer procedures, and pattern-induced reactions (Perl et al., 2009), including the introduction of different chemical approaches for patterning polymeric functional materials, such as "double-click" chemistry and surface-initiated atom-transfer radical polymerization (Cai et al., 2013).

Soft lithography is broadly used in bio-imprinting (Vozzi et al., 2010). The typical imprinting stamp is produced by self-assembly of the template biomolecules on top of a smooth support under appropriate conditions and the self-assembled template stamp is then softly pressed over a prepolymer film for a certain period of time (Mujahid et al., 2013). The template biomolecules should be strictly packed in order to attain high imprinting density (Dickert et al., 2004; Mujahid et al., 2013). Overall, this procedure allows the production of geometrical features of a wide range of biomolecules and translates the chemical information involved in noncovalent interactions between the polymeric functional groups and the receptor surface (Mujahid et al., 2013).

Soft lithography also offers several advantages when compared to other nanofabrication approaches, including low cost, simplicity, and applicability to soft materials.

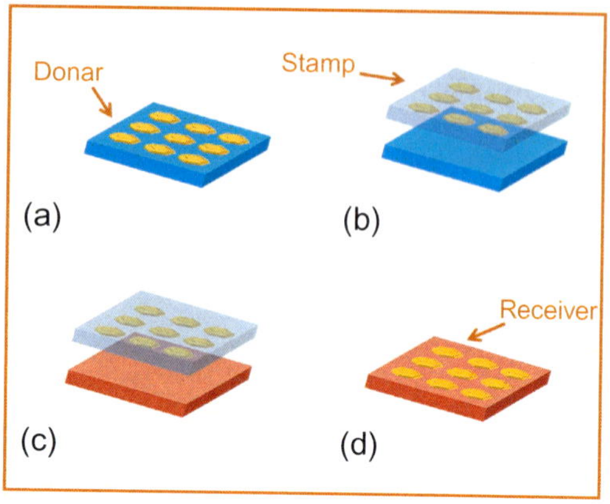

Figure 1.5 Schematic drawing of the process used to transfer microfabricated structures from a donor substrate to PDMS stamp and from PDMS stamp to a receiver substrate. (a) Preparation of the donor substrate by applying a rubber stamp; (b) quickly peel-back stamp grab objects off of donor; (c) apply inked stamp to receiving substrate; and (d) slowly peel-back stamp.

The applications of nanotechnology enabled by soft lithography closest to commercialization will probably be those that reduce the costs of existing devices (Biebuyck et al., 1997; Larsen et al., 1997).

1.3.3 Bulk approaches

In general, bulk approaches are used to entrap biomolecules inside a polymeric matrix. For being a fairly simple procedure, it has been used in many fields, including (i) cell-signaling peptide encapsulation into biomaterials and/or cell encapsulation (Nicodemus and Bryant, 2008; Huang et al., 2013), (ii) incorporation of enzymatically degradable sequences (Schense and Hubbell, 1999; West and Hubbell, 1999; Shin et al., 2003), and (iii) biosensing technology (Moreira et al., 2010; Moreira and Sales, 2011). The cells encapsulated within biomimetic materials can modulate cell proliferation and migration, regulating the amount of secreted matrix from the encapsulated cells (Shin et al., 2004; Stabenfeldt et al., 2010). Cell-signaling peptides are also incorporated into biomaterials, to generate recognition signaling sites on the surface and in the bulk of such materials. The integration of enzymatically degradable sequences in biomaterials is a singular feature of the bulk approach. This includes polymeric bulk materials that can be biodegraded by proteases that are specific to peptide sequences covalently linked to the polymer core (Schense and Hubbell, 1999; West and Hubbell, 1999).

Another promising field of the bulk approach regards its application in biosensing technology (Figure 1.6), where 3D binding sites are formed for the template at a suitable receptor surface. A multitude of facile procedures are shown in the literature for this purpose (Kryscio and Peppas, 2012), including bulk imprinting strategies employing acrylates, hydrogels/sol–gel, and hybrid approaches.

Acrylate imprinting of biomolecules is, so far, the most popular technology for biomolecule imprinting. The overall process is quite simple, and inexpensive, being particularly suited for small biomolecules (Guerreiro et al., 2011a,b; Moreira et al., 2011a, b; Moreira and Sales, 2011; Oliveira et al., 2011; Rebelo et al., 2011). A major limitation of this approach exists when biomolecules to be imprinted are largely insoluble in the solvents where the reaction takes place. In addition, when the biomolecule is present in nonaqueous media, significant conformational changes are expected, which leads to a miss-imprinting process. Imprinting in aqueous environment is therefore an essential

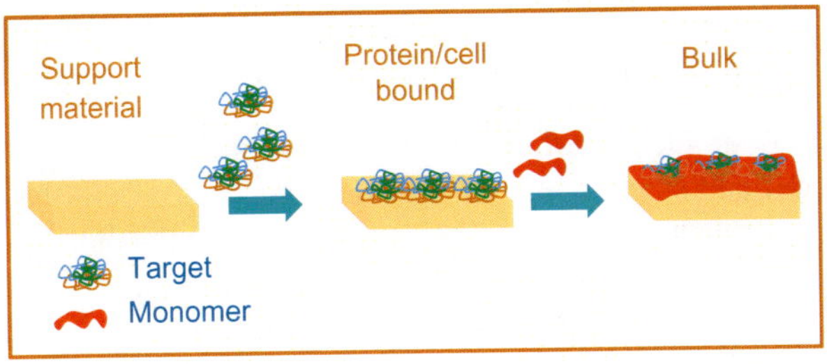

Figure 1.6 Biomimetic sensory approach.

condition to ensure that a correct correlation between imprinted sites and the conformational arrangement of the biomolecule at its native environment are granted.

Hydrogels are another kind of polymeric structure assembled in conventional bulk processes and often used in biomimetics. A hydrogel is a porous polymeric network that may react to external stimulus, such as pH or temperature, by altering its structure. This structural change can be employed to control template releasing, promoting subsequent effects on the polymeric network that memorizes the imprinting shape (Hjerten et al., 1997). Also in this regard, many studies have been performed to mimic the locomotion of organisms by applying external stimulus, such as temperature, pH, and voltage, to polymer gels. Although limitations exist, electrosensitive hydrogels may be triggered by an electrical signal from electro-osmosis and/or electro-kinetic processes to produce mechanical energy (Zhang et al., 2008).

Overall, the controlled synthesis and assembly of tiny building blocks in a *bottom-up* setup, regardless the method by which it is assembled, may be the course to create excellent and reproducible biomimetic materials of specific supramolecular organization (Morales and Lieber, 1998; Law et al., 2004; Xia et al., 2009).

1.4 Supramolecular organization

Supramolecular organization is the aggregation of molecules or ions that are held together by noncovalent forces forming functional nanoscale objects. The supramolecular chemistry has a strong inspiration in biological systems, leading to the development of a great variety of biomimetic materials. One example is the mimicry of enzymes: the supramolecular macrocyclic hosts (such as crown ethers, calixarenes, and phthalocyanines) closely resemble the pyrrole-containing macrocycles at the active sites of enzymes and the metal-containing porphyrins found in hemoglobin. Another example is the biomimetics of photosynthesis with metal terpyridyl complexes that mimics the manganese metal center of the photosystem II, where the manganese ions cycle between Mn(II) and Mn(III) to generate the electrons involved in the conversion of photonic energy into electrical energy. Below are described some synthetic supramolecular organized materials, which resemble analog biomimetic functions.

1.4.1 *Surfactants, micelles, and vesicles*

Nature is full of complex constructions to encapsulate molecules within a confined space. This confined space is particularly relevant considering that the probability and frequency of chemical reactions between atoms and molecules increase with concentration. Actually, cells function well because they encapsulate all the chemicals required for protein synthesis, energy transfer, and their replication. Another example is iron storage proteins (such as ferritin) that are amorphous when the metal ions are absent but form a globular capsule once metals are bound.

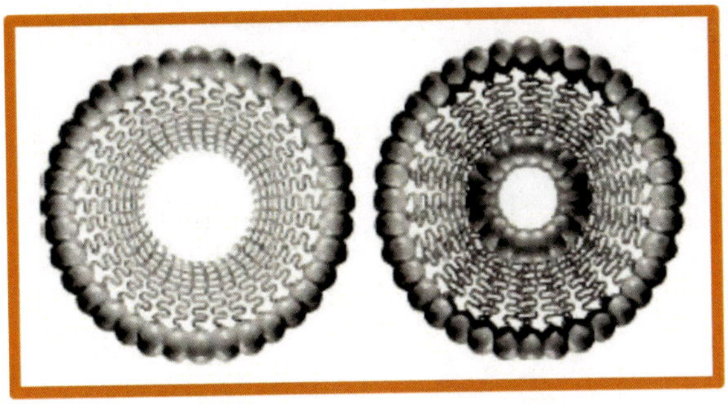

Figure 1.7 Schematics of the amphiphilic aggregates: micelle (left) and liposome (right). Adapted from Steed et al. (2007).

Surfactants are compounds constituted by a hydrophilic (water-soluble) end and a lipophilic (organic-soluble) end that is hydrophobic. Molecules of this type with both hydrophilic and lipophilic characters are named amphiphiles. They form micelles useful to concentrate and compartmentalize hydrophobic compounds from water. Such vesicles have the hydrophilic head groups interacting with water while the other end is oriented to the center forming an insoluble spherical aggregate (Figure 1.7). Another type of capsules is vesicle structures known as liposomes (water-filled spherical structures assembled with phospholipid bilayers in aqueous media) as shown in Figure 1.7. They have the advantage of being formed in water while filled with water with the two media separated by the water-insoluble membrane. The membrane has hydrophilic internal and external surfaces, but a hydrophobic section exists between these. This characteristic makes them ideal vessels to host the chemical constituents of a "living" system. These artificial phospholipid vesicles have been used as transporters to cells or organs of vaccines, enzymes, drugs, and other substances. They are also good models for studying the biologic ion transport across cell membranes because they do not suffer from interfering effects, such as residual ion-channel peptides or ionophores from purified natural cells. For instance, liposomes have been filled with a fluorescent dye to investigate Cl^- transport and study the behavior of artificial anion channel-forming compounds. At high concentrations within the liposome, the dye self-quenches and no fluorescence is observed. When the liposome is treated with a channel-forming compound aimed to transport the hydrated anions, the dye is also released into the external solution and fluoresces (Cragg, 2010).

Additional supramolecular architectures have been designed to encapsulate other species, such as cryptands, sepulchrates, and sarcophagenes (Figure 1.8). These compounds have two bridgehead atoms, often carbon, nitrogen, or boron, connected by three molecular bridges. These molecules are flexible to allow small guests to enter but, once inside, the donor atoms within the bridges surround the guests through weak interactions, thereby establishing a strong complex with the guest ions. A similar encapsulation approach was also proposed, based instead on molecular tetrahedra with bridgehead atoms at the four vertices (Figure 1.8). Molecular capsules composed of covalent bonds with very small internal volumes were also proposed by linking two macrocycles, cavitands and calixarenes, forming carcerands and calixtubes, respectively. In this case, a narrow annulus is formed at both ends of the capsule that is

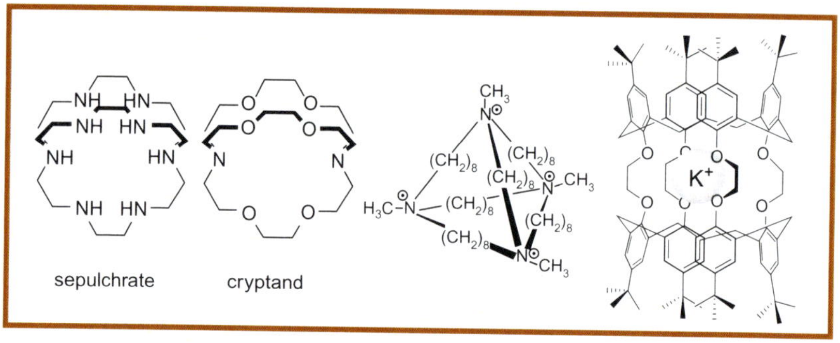

Figure 1.8 Encapsulating molecules.
Adapted from Cragg (2010), Schmidtchen (1977), and Matthews et al. (2002). From left to right: sepulchrate, cryptand, molecular tetrahedral, and calixtube.

too narrow to allow the guests to exit (Figure 1.8). Supramolecular capsules have been made with metal inner cores large enough used to hold molecules and further used as nanoreactors. For example, the co-encapsulation of benzene with cyclohexadiene accelerated the formation of the Diels–Alder cycloaddition product (Kang et al., 1998). Moreover, the shape of the capsule can turn out advantageous in selective reactions, due to the constraints of size and charge imposed by the internal surface. In this regard, these capsules mimic the function of natural compartmentalization: encapsulation of chemical species controls the production of one product over other options.

Supramolecular assembled polymeric capsules have also been developed to mimic proteins, for instance ferritin. The iron concentrations inside ferritin are very toxic, but the protein contains large numbers of sulfur-containing amino acids that isolate the metal ions and hamper their reactivity. In a simple way, this approach is an iron supply of controlled release. One approach used for polymeric capsule synthesis is the self-assembling of complementary polymers forming layer-by-layer vesicular structures by templating the co-assembly of the polymers with a removable core (Wilson et al., 2009). The alternation of polymers with opposite charges allows the composition and thickness of the capsule's walls to be controlled. The porous nature of the polymers used allows the ion species to easily enter and leave the capsule.

1.4.2 Colloids and nanoparticles

Colloids are particles sizing from 5 nm to 0.5 μm that form suspensions showing light diffraction and other optical effects not found in solutions. Many natural macromolecules, such as starch, pectins, latex, nucleic acids, and proteins, fit the definition of colloids. There is no substantial difference between the colloids found in nature and nanoparticles. Common nanoparticles are supramolecular clusters of thousands of atoms with size between 1 and 100 nm usually metallic or semiconducting. They have characteristic electronic optical signatures such as quantum size effects (quantum dots) in semiconductors (fluorescence) and plasma resonance in the metallic nanoparticles.

The phenomenon of quantum size effects in the semiconductor nanoparticles allows their optical features to strongly depend on their size. Actually, the absorption band moves to higher energy (or is blue-shifted) as the particle size decreases. These unique optical properties of quantum dots allow them to be used as sensors for the detection of diseases, such as tumors, mimicking natural processes. Indeed, many biological molecules have intrinsic optical features (such as fluorescence) that change when the molecule is in a specific environment, allowing the distribution or binding of the molecule to be measured. For instance, bilirubin becomes highly fluorescent when bonded to a specific site on serum albumin. In its turn, the zinc protoporphyrin is fluorescent and can be used to detect problems in red blood cells development, when iron is unavailable or lead is present.

Metallic nanoparticles have been largely used in heterogeneous catalysis in the chemistry industry but they have also been used in molecular sensors. For example, an anion sensor that incorporates a zinc metalloporphyrin receptor supported on gold nanoparticles has been developed (Beer et al., 2004; Cormode et al., 2008). Upon anion binding, the electromagnetic coupling perturbed the motion of the free electrons in the nanoparticle, what shifted the plasmon band, allowing an optical detection.

Nanoparticles also have been used in other applications besides exploring their optical properties. One classical success in biomimetics uses the lotus effect, where the surface microstructure and the secretion of wax-like compounds of the lotus leaves produce super-hydrophobic and self-cleaning properties. This is done by introducing hydrophobic silica nanoparticles in a binder material forming paint with self-cleaning properties (Shimomura, 2010).

1.4.3 Surfaces and membranes

A biological surface functions as the interface between a living organism or organelle and its environment, such as the membrane cell. Among its different functions, such as delimiting dimensions and shape, providing mechanical stability, and acting as barriers and chemical reservoirs, the essential aspect of a membrane in Nature is to transport material from the exterior and across it so that the biochemical processes happening inside can occur. Natural membranes have the particular capacity to selectively recognize and transport targets, while excluding others. Thus, supramolecular chemistry with biological inspiration in natural membranes has mainly attempted to mimic simple transporters for ions and small molecules by using artificial methods that employ either a carrier or a channel mechanism.

The artificial carrier transporters usually mimic the naturally occurring siderophores and ionophores. In particular, the macrocyclic crown ethers (Figure 1.9) have been proposed to work by an ionophore-facilitated ion transport. Crown ethers have a high affinity for alkali metals and can transport cations from aqueous solution to nonpolar solvents. This particular attribute has led to their use in phase transfer catalysis (Cragg, 2010).

Regarding channel-forming systems, several approaches have been considered for the design of those supramolecular artificial biomimetics. A bio-inspired method consisted in preparing extended helical molecules to reproduce the channels within the

Figure 1.9 Crown ethers main structure.

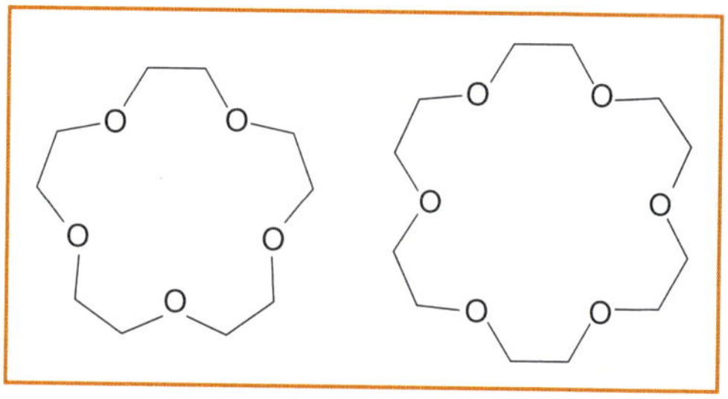

helix. The resulting systems generated membrane-spanning molecules that formed channels, but lacked ion specificity (Cragg, 2010). On the other hand, a size-based selectivity approach has also been considered by designing artificial ion channel mimetic compounds using macrocycles. Macrocycles are selective ion filters that can be attached to amphiphilic membrane-spanning molecules guiding the ions across the membrane. In such approach, chemical links are formed between the membrane-spanning and the size-selective components combining a rigid ion-filtering molecule (the macrocycle) with lengthy substituents that allow the entire molecular assembly to be inserted in the membrane (Cragg, 2010).

Examples of artificial channel-forming systems using helical molecules consider peptides for preparing membrane oligopeptides from serine and leucine (Lear et al., 1988). Heptapeptides of varying 21-residue sequences were linked to form dimers and trimers with 3–4 nm that were capable of spanning a phospholipid membrane (Figure 1.10). The combination of serine and leucine gave the α-helicates a polar yet hydrophobic exterior, making their internal cavity too small (0.8 nm) to act as channels, but permeable to a range of alkali metals although with poor selectivity. The schematic representation of an artificial ion-channel is also shown in Figure 1.10, where a 'closed' position switches to 'open' after ligand binding.

Examples of the size-selectivity approach to construct artificial ion channels comprise supramolecular macrocyclic building blocks such as crown ethers, calixarenes, and phthalocyanines. For instance, each member of the crown family has a particular preference for an alkali metal that can be included in transmembrane channels as selective filters. Crown ether-based ion channels have been developed with a

Figure 1.10 Schematic representation of an artificial pentameric ligand-gated ion channel, in closed (left) and open (right) forms.

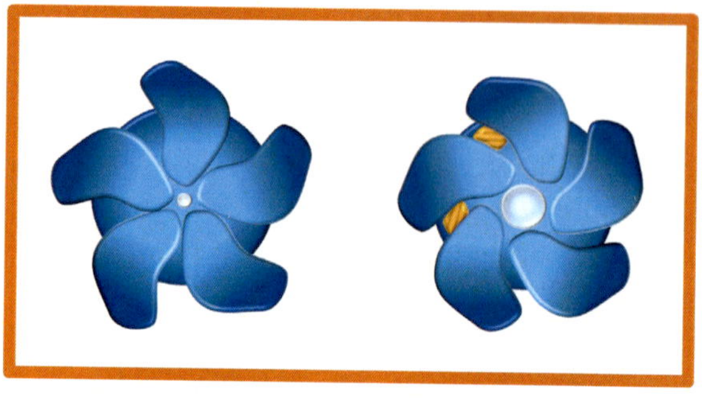

potassium salt of tetracarboamido[18]crown-6 where the macrocycles formed a one-dimensional stack with the hydrated cations allocated in the channels formed by the crowns (Jullien and Lehn, 1988); however, the crown ether substituents were not long enough to span a lipid bilayer. Other approach considered the crown acting as the selectivity filter while cyclic tetraesters provided the membrane-spanning function, showing low transport rates for Li^+ but favoring Na^+ and K^+ (Fyles et al., 1993). Crown ethers were also used as relays within a membrane-spanning structure (Gokel, 2000) with a selectivity of 18 for K^+ instead of Na^+.

The approaches using crown ethers however suffer from lack of rigidity. Cyclic compounds with well-defined central cavities such as CDs and calixarenes have been also employed in ion channel mimetic compounds with the hope that they would be more robust and selective. The crown ethers, usually anchoring in the lipophilic region of the membrane, were replaced by the rigid macrocycles that could anchor at the polar surface of the membrane while their hydrophobic substituents could descend through the lipophilic region. Following such approach, a selectivity for Na^+ in aqueous solution with a factor of 68 over K^+ was observed (Arduini et al., 1988). Although the span of the phospholipid membrane was poor, such approach produced the level of selectivity required for an artificial ion channel.

1.4.4 Polymers

Supramolecular assembled polymers have mainly been used in drug release and in coordination with metals. Regarding drug release, dendrimers, branch-like polymers, were mainly used. Their interest lies in a host–guest chemistry where the dendritic core region, highly porous, exhibits specific host behavior, while the densely packed outer layer protects the interior from the surrounding medium. Related applications are mainly mimicking the hydrophobic pocket regions in enzymes for medicinal purposes. For instance, the outer dendrimer surface could comprise multiple identical binding sites as specific enzymes with a strong pharmacological potential in amplifying substrate binding. Supramolecular dendrimers are prepared by reacting an *n*-directional core with linear or branched building blocks to yield first-generation dendrimers. The peripheral sites then react with more building blocks to form a second-generation dendrimer and further on (Figure 1.11). Each generation is assembled by metal ligand complexes, hydrogen-bonding moieties, or ionic interactions. The main advantage is the ease of tuning the properties of each generation to complement those of a particular guest molecule. Also, it is easier to regulate the dissociation rate to control guest release. This "controlled release" property is the great advantage of dendrimers for being used as drug delivers (Aulenta et al., 2003). Reports have confirmed the advantages of dendrimers in the controlled release of the anticancer drugs cisplatin (Malik et al., 1999) and doxorubicin (Padilla De Jesus et al., 2002). Besides drug release, dendrimers have also been used as molecular antenna in light harvesting and as a blood substitute. To mimic the process that occurs in pigments of some types of algae, bacteria, and green plants, dendrimers were used as a synthetic antenna. The dendrimer was organized in a highly branched macromolecule comprised of rod-like

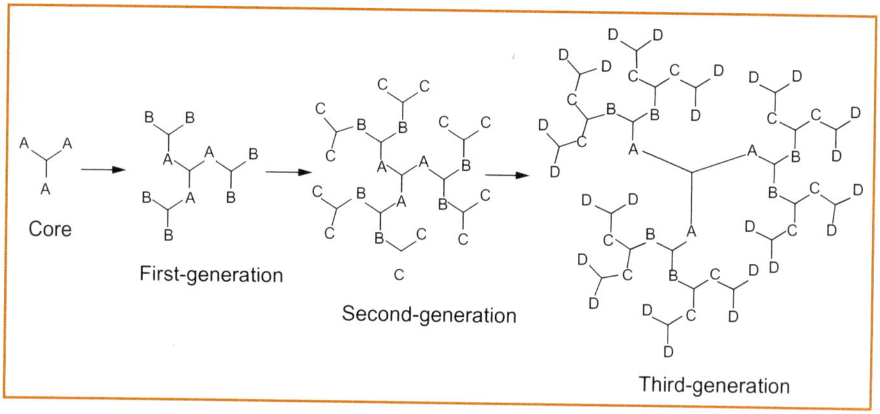

Figure 1.11 Schematic representation of the preparation of a dendrimer.
Adapted from Steed et al. (2007).

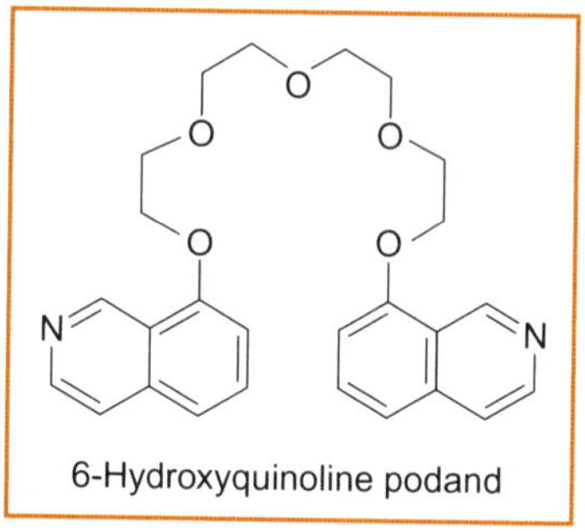

Figure 1.12 Example of a podand.

conjugated groups that were capable of absorbing photons (Steed et al., 2007). As blood substitutes, the steric effect of a dendrimer surrounding a heme center significantly slowed its cytotoxicity when compared to free heme (Twyman et al., 2012).

Coordination with metals has been achieved by using podands. They are functionalized polyethers with variations in the ligand donor groups usually prepared by tosylation of the hydroxyl groups and further reaction with nucleophiles such as benzoic acid and quinoline (Figure 1.12). Originally, podands were applied to alkali metal cation-binding ligands with two or more pendant low-molecular-mass polyether arms capable to bind a number of metal ions. The earliest compounds could coordinate to mainly oxophilic metals, while further developments allowed connection to metals with softer characteristics as pyridine and sulfur donors. Currently, the term podand encompasses a wide range of cation- and anion-binding receptors, as well as hosts for molecular guests based on a multibinding site and is applied to any flexible acyclic host capable of wrapping around a guest. The multi-armed podands lead into the concept of multivalency and they were the precursors of dendrimers.

Coordination polymers are infinite arrays of ligands that bridge metal ions. Transition metals are the common nodes between the organic ligands due to their predictable geometries while the ligands link these precise coordination geometries in a well-defined way. Metals such as Ag(I) that adopt linear coordination geometries are used to form one-dimensional polymers with linear ligands. Similarly, square-planar metal ions usually form two-dimensional sheets when combined with two connecting ligands. The nodes used to form three-dimensional networks are tetrahedral or octahedral metals, which have potential to bind to ligands in the three dimensions.

Coordination polymers are of particular interest due to the mimicking of the structure and host–guest behavior of natural, porous networks such as zeolites. Such networks are able to incorporate a large variety of guests, from simple solvent molecules to molecular hydrogen. Coordination polymers may also display other physical properties, such as nonlinear optical behavior, long-range magnetic ordering, or electrical conduction. The synthesis of large voids can also lead to the phenomenon of interpenetration, when one polymeric network is entangled with other(s), leading to solid state host–guest structures.

1.5 Conclusions and perspectives

The controlled synthesis and assembly of tiny building blocks in a *bottom-up* setup, regardless the method by which it is assembled, has been the course to create excellent and reproducible biomimetic materials of specific supramolecular organization. Biomimetic materials are today promising and powerful tools in the development of synthetic composites, ceramics, and electronics, with successful application in many areas of science and technology. This includes mainly the health domain, with tissue engineering and biomineralization advances, orthopedic implants, biomedical devices, immunoassays, catalysis, nanomedicine, etc., but food safety and environment areas are also interesting fields of application in biomimetics.

Overall, there have been tremendous progresses in the biomimetics and bioinspired materials, leading to the production of amazing materials never expected in the past. The transfer of the nanoscale constructions up to real and practical applications remains however a challenge (Morales and Lieber, 1998; Law et al., 2004; Xia et al., 2009). This is most especially true when biomimetic materials need to be integrated in living systems. There are problems related to material interfacing and compatibility, as well as biological subjects, including viability and stability. Scaling-up effects and dynamic interactions between the different components are also important issues that remain mostly unsolved.

Further developments in the synthesis biomimetics and biomimetic materials will most certainly encompass the parallel developments within biology, biochemistry, physics, chemistry, physiology, and material sciences, all major sources of knowledge of this transversal discipline.

References

Abrishamchian, A., Hooshmand, T., Mohammadi, M., Najafi, F., 2013. Preparation and characterization of multi-walled carbon nanotube/hydroxyapatite nanocomposite film dip coated on Ti-6Al-4 V by sol-gel method for biomedical applications: an in vitro study. Mater. Sci. Eng., C 33 (4), 2002–2010.

Aizenberg, J., Muller, D.A., Grazul, J.L., Hamann, D.R., 2003. Direct fabrication of large micropatterned single crystals. Science 299 (5610), 1205–1208.

Ajayan, P.M., 1999. Nanotubes from carbon. Chem. Rev. 99 (7), 1787–1799.

Almeida, S.A.A., Truta, L.A.A.N.A., Queiros, R.B., Montenegro, M.C.B.S.M., Cunha, A.L., Sales, M.G.F., 2012. Optimizing potentiometric ionophore and electrode design for environmental on-site control of antibiotic drugs: application to sulfamethoxazole. Biosens. Bioelectron. 35 (1), 319–326.

Arduini, A., Ghidini, E., Pochini, A., Ungaro, R., Andreetti, G.D., Calestani, G., Ugozzoli, F., 1988. Molecular inclusion in functionalized macromolecules. 15. Para-tert-butylcalix 4 arene tetra-acetamide—a new strong receptor for alkali cations. J. Incl. Phenom. 6 (2), 119–134.

Aulenta, F., Hayes, W., Rannard, S., 2003. Dendrimers: a new class of nanoscopic containers and delivery devices. Eur. Polym. J. 39 (9), 1741–1771.

Ayers, J., Westphal, A., Blustein, D., 2011. A conserved neural circuit-based architecture for ambulatory and undulatory biomimetic robots. Mar. Technol. Soc. J. 45 (4), 147–152.

Bacsa, R.R., Flahaut, E., Laurent, C., Peigney, A., Aloni, S., Puech, P., Bacsa, W.S., 2003. Narrow diameter double-wall carbon nanotubes: synthesis, electron microscopy and inelastic light scattering. New J. Phys. 5, 131.1–131.9.

Bar-Cohen, Y., 2006. Biomimetics—using nature to inspire human innovation. Bioinspir. Biomim. 1, P1–P12.

Bazylinski, D.A., Frankel, R.B., 2004. Magnetosome formation in prokaryotes. Nat. Rev. Microbiol. 2 (3), 217–230.

Beer, P.D., Cormode, D.P., Davis, J.J., 2004. Zinc metalloporphyrin-functionalised nanoparticle anion sensors. Chem. Commun. 4, 414–415.

Bhattacharya, P., Du, D., Lin, Y., 2014. Bioinspired nanoscale materials for biomedical and energy applications. J. R. Soc. Interface 11 (95), 20131067.

Bhushan, B., 2009. Biomimetics: lessons from nature-an overview. Phil. Trans. R. Soc. A 367, 1445–1486.

Biebuyck, H.A., Larsen, N.B., Delamarche, E., Michel, B., 1997. Lithography beyond light: microcontact printing with monolayer resists. IBM J. Res. Dev. 41 (1–2), 159–170.

Boal, A.K., Ilhan, F., DeRouchey, J.E., Thurn-Albrecht, T., Russell, T.P., Rotello, V.M., 2000. Self-assembly of nanoparticles into structured spherical and network aggregates. Nature 404 (6779), 746–748.

Bose, S., Vahabzadeh, S., Bandyopadhyay, A., 2013. Bone tissue engineering using 3D printing. Mater. Today 16 (12), 496–504.

Buckley, A.M., Greenblatt, M., 1994. The sol-gel preparation of silica-gels. J. Chem. Educ. 71 (7), 599–602.

Cai, X., Wang, Y., Wang, X., Ji, J., Hong, J., Pan, F., Chen, J., Xue, M., 2013. Fabrication of ultrafine soft-matter arrays by selective contact thermochemical reaction. Sci. Rep. 3, 1780, 1–5.

Calvert, P., 1992. Polymer science—tender morsels for microbes. Nature 360 (6404), 535.

Caminade, A.M., Laurent, R., Majoral, J.P., 2005. Characterization of dendrimers. Adv. Drug Deliv. Rev. 57 (15), 2130–2146.

Chakraborty, J., Sarkar, S.D., Chatterjee, S., Sinha, M.K., Basu, D., 2008. Self-assembled structures of hydroxyapatite in the biomimetic coating on a bioinert ceramic substrate. Colloids Surf. B 66 (2), 295–298.
Chen, C.S., Mrksich, M., Huang, S., Whitesides, G.M., Ingber, D.E., 1997. Geometric control of cell life and death. Science 276 (5317), 1425–1428.
Chen, A., Lee, E., Tu, R., Santiago, K., Grosberg, A., Fowlkes, C., Khine, M., 2014. Integrated platform for functional monitoring of biomimetic heart sheets derived from human pluripotent stem cells. Biomaterials 35 (2), 675–683.
Cheng, J.Y., Ross, C.A., Smith, H.I., Thomas, E.L., 2006. Templated self-assembly of block copolymers: top-down helps bottom-up. Adv. Mater. 18 (19), 2505–2521.
Childs, W.R., Nuzzo, R.G., 2004. Patterning of thin-film microstructures on non-planar substrate surfaces using decal transfer lithography. Adv. Mater. 16 (15), 1323–1327.
Childs, W.R., Nuzzo, R.G., 2005. Large-area patterning of coinage-metal thin films using decal transfer lithography. Langmuir 21 (1), 195–202.
Choi, I.S., Bowden, N., Whitesides, G.M., 1999a. Macroscopic, hierarchical, two-dimensional self-assembly. Angew. Chem. Int. Ed. 38 (20), 3078–3081.
Choi, I.S., Bowden, N., Whitesides, G.M., 1999b. Shape-selective recognition and self-assembly of mm-scale components. J. Am. Chem. Soc. 121 (8), 1754–1755.
Collett, J.R., Cho, E.J., Ellington, A.D., 2005. Production and processing of aptamer microarrays. Methods 37 (1), 4–15.
Cormode, D.P., Davis, J.J., Beer, P.D., 2008. Anion sensing porphyrin functionalized nanoparticles. J. Inorg. Organomet. Polym. Mater. 18 (1), 32–40.
Cragg, P.J., 2010. Supramolecular Chemistry: From Biological Inspiration to Biomedical Applications. Springer, Netherlands.
Demchenko, A.P., 2001. Recognition between flexible protein molecules: induced and assisted folding. J. Mol. Recognit. 14 (1), 42–61.
Dickert, F.L., Lieberzeit, P., Gazda-Miarecka, S., Halikias, K., Mann, K.J., 2004. Modifying polymers by self-organisation for the mass-sensitive detection of environmental and biogeneous analytes. Sensors Actuators B Chem 100 (1–2), 112–116.
Douglas, T., 2003. A bright bio-inspired future. Science 299 (5610), 1192–1193.
Drain, C.M., Batteas, J.D., Flynn, G.W., Milic, T., Chi, N., Yablon, D.G., Sommers, H., 2002. Designing supramolecular porphyrin arrays that self-organize into nanoscale optical and magnetic materials. Proc. Natl. Acad. Sci. U. S. A. 99, 6498–6502.
Errachid, A., Caballero, D., Crespo, E., Bessueille, F., Pla-Roca, M., Mills, C.A., Teixidor, F., Samitier, J., 2007. Electropolymerization of nano-dimensioned polypyrrole micro-ring arrays on gold substrates prepared using submerged micro-contact printing. Nanotechnology 18, 485301, 8pp.
Fox, A., Hines, D.R., Li, T., 2012. Probing the adhesion of submicron thin films fabricated on a polymer substrate via nano-transfer printing. J. Micromech. Microeng. 22 (9), 095002, 6pp.
Fyles, T.M., James, T.D., Kaye, K.C., 1993. Activities and modes of action of artificial ion-channel mimics. J. Am. Chem. Soc. 115 (26), 12315–12321.
Gajbhiye, V., Palanirajan, V.K., Tekade, R.K., Jain, N.K., 2009. Dendrimers as therapeutic agents: a systematic review. J. Pharm. Pharmacol. 61 (8), 989–1003.
Gates, B.D., Xu, Q.B., Stewart, M., Ryan, D., Willson, C.G., Whitesides, G.M., 2005. New approaches to nanofabrication: molding, printing, and other techniques. Chem. Rev. 105 (4), 1171–1196.
Geckil, H., Xu, F., Zhang, X., Moon, S., Demirci, U., 2010. Engineering hydrogels as extracellular matrix mimics. Nanomedicine 5 (3), 469–484.

Gokel, G.W., 2000. Hydraphiles: design, synthesis and analysis of a family of synthetic, cation-conducting channels. Chem. Commun. 1, 1–9.

Gracias, D.H., Boncheva, M., Omoregie, O., Whitesides, G.M., 2002. Biomimetic self-assembly of helical electrical circuits using orthogonal capillary interactions. Appl. Phys. Lett. 80 (15), 2802–2804.

Guerreiro, J.R.L., Freitas, V., Sales, M.G.F., 2011a. New sensing materials of molecularly-imprinted polymers for the selective recognition of Chlortetracycline. Microchem. J. 97 (2), 173–181.

Guerreiro, J.R.L., Sales, M.G.F., Moreira, F.T.C., Rebelo, T.S.R., 2011b. Selective recognition in potentiometric transduction of amoxicillin by molecularly imprinted materials. Eur. Food Res. Technol. 232 (1), 39–50.

Guo, T.Y., Xia, Y.Q., Wang, J., Song, M.D., Zhang, B.H., 2005. Chitosan beads as molecularly imprinted polymer matrix for selective separation of proteins. Biomaterials 26 (28), 5737–5745.

Han, L., Zhou, J., Gong, X., Gao, C., 2009. Solvent-assisted polymer micro-molding. Chin. Sci. Bull. 54 (13), 2193–2204.

Hawker, C.J., Russell, T.P., 2005. Block copolymer lithography: merging "bottom-up" with "top-down" processes. MRS Bull. 30 (12), 952–966.

Hench, L.L., West, J.K., 1990. The sol-gel process. Chem. Rev. 90 (1), 33–72.

Henry, O.Y.F., Piletsky, S.A., Cullen, D.C., 2008. Fabrication of molecularly imprinted polymer microarray on a chip by mid-infrared laser pulse initiated polymerisation. Biosens. Bioelectron. 23 (12), 1769–1775.

Hirsch, A., 1994. The Chemistry of the Fullerenes. Georg Thieme Verlag Stuttgart, New York.

Hjerten, S., Liao, J.L., Nakazato, K., Wang, Y., Zamaratskaia, G., Zhang, H.X., 1997. Gels mimicking antibodies in their selective recognition of proteins. Chromatographia 44 (5–6), 227–234.

Hocheng, H., Hsu, W.H., 2008. An Innovative Method for Uniform Pattern Transfer in Nanoimprint. J. Nanosci. Nanotechnol. 8, 1–6.

Hu, W., Li, C.M., 2011. Nanomaterial-based advanced immunoassays. Wiley Interdiscip. Rev. Nanomed. Nanobiotechnol. 3 (2), 119–133.

Huang, Y., Duan, X.F., Wei, Q.Q., Lieber, C.M., 2001. Directed assembly of one-dimensional nanostructures into functional networks. Science 291 (5504), 630–633.

Huang, H., Ding, Y., Sun, X.S., Nguyen, T.A., 2013. Peptide hydrogelation and cell encapsulation for 3D culture of MCF-7 breast cancer cells. PLoS One 8 (3), e59482, 15pp.

Ikkala, O., ten Brinke, G., 2002. Functional materials based on self-assembly of polymeric supramolecules. Science 295 (5564), 2407–2409.

Jackman, R.J., Wilbur, J.L., Whitesides, G.M., 1995. Fabrication of submicrometer features on curved substrates by microcontact printing. Science 269 (5224), 664–666.

Jackman, J.A., Knoll, W., Cho, N.-J., 2012. Biotechnology applications of tethered lipid bilayer membranes. Materials 5 (12), 2637–2657.

Jaime, C., Redondo, J., Sanchezferrando, F., Virgili, A., 1991. Beta-cyclodextrin inclusion complex with adamantane intermolecular H-1(H-1) NOE determinations and molecular mechanics calculations. J. Mol. Struct. 248 (3–4), 317–329.

Jayasena, S.D., 1999. Aptamers: an emerging class of molecules that rival antibodies in diagnostics. Clin. Chem. 45 (9), 1628–1650.

Jenekhe, S.A., Chen, X.L., 1999. Self-assembly of ordered microporous materials from rod-coil block copolymers. Science 283 (5400), 372–375.

Jeong, H.E., Kwak, R., Khademhosseini, A., Suh, K.Y., 2009. UV-assisted capillary force lithography for engineering biomimetic multiscale hierarchical structures: from lotus leaf to gecko foot hairs. Nanoscale 1 (3), 331–338.
Johnson, J.E., Speir, J.A., 1997. Quasi-equivalent viruses: a paradigm for protein assemblies. J. Mol. Biol. 269 (5), 665–675.
Jullien, L., Lehn, J.M., 1988. The chundle approach to molecular channels synthesis of a macrocycle based molecular bundle. Tetrahedron Lett. 29 (31), 3803–3806.
Kang, J.M., Santamaria, J., Hilmersson, G., Rebek, J., 1998. Self-assembled molecular capsule catalyzes a Diels-Alder reaction. J. Am. Chem. Soc. 120 (29), 7389–7390.
Kastelic, J., Palley, I., Baer, E., 1980. A structural mechanical model for tendon crimping. J. Biomech. 13 (10), 887–893.
Kesharwani, P., Jain, K., Jain, N.K., 2014. Dendrimer as nanocarrier for drug delivery. Prog. Polym. Sci. 39 (2), 268–307.
Kim, M., Kim, Y.S., 2007. Advancing decal-transfer lithography with a reusable PDMS-coated nanoscale stamp. J. Am. Chem. Soc. 129 (37), 11304–11305.
Kim, D.J., Lee, K.B., Lee, T.G., Shon, H.K., Kim, W.J., Paik, H.J., Choi, I.S., 2005. Biomimetic micropatterning of silica by surface-initiated polymerization and microcontact printing. Small 1 (10), 992–996.
Knoll, W., 2012. Handbook of Biofunctional Surfaces. CRC Press, Boca Raton.
Ko, H.C., Stoykovich, M.P., Song, J., Malyarchuk, V., Choi, W.M., Yu, C.-J., Geddes III, J.B., Xiao, J., Wang, S., Huang, Y., Rogers, J.A., 2008. A hemispherical electronic eye camera based on compressible silicon optoelectronics. Nature 454 (7205), 748–753.
Konnova, S.A., Sharipova, I.R., Demina, T.A., Osin, Y.N., Yarullina, D.R., Ilinskaya, O.N., Lvov, Y.M., Fakhrullin, R.F., 2013. Biomimetic cell-mediated three-dimensional assembly of halloysite nanotubes. Chem. Commun. 49 (39), 4208–4210.
Kroeger, N., 2007. Prescribing diatom morphology: toward genetic engineering of biological nanomaterials. Curr. Opin. Chem. Biol. 11 (6), 662–669.
Kryscio, D.R., Peppas, N.A., 2012. Critical review and perspective of macromolecularly imprinted polymers. Acta Biomater. 8 (2), 461–473.
Lahav, M., Kharitonov, A.B., Katz, O., Kunitake, T., Willner, I., 2001. Tailored chemosensors for chloroaromatic acids using molecular imprinted TiO2 thin films on ion-sensitive field-effect transistors. Anal. Chem. 73 (3), 720–723.
Larsen, N.B., Biebuyck, H., Delamarche, E., Michel, B., 1997. Order in microcontact printed self-assembled monolayers. J. Am. Chem. Soc. 119 (13), 3017–3026.
Latthe, S.S., Gurav, A.B., Maruti, C.S., Vhatkar, R.S., 2012. Recent progress in preparation of superhydrophobic surfaces: a review. J. Surf. Eng. Mater. Adv. Technol. 2, 76–94.
Law, M., Goldberger, J., Yang, P.D., 2004. Semiconductor nanowires and nanotubes. Annu. Rev. Mater. Res. 34, 83–122.
Lear, J.D., Wasserman, Z.R., Degrado, W.F., 1988. Synthetic amphiphilic peptide models for protein ion channels. Science 240 (4856), 1177–1181.
Lee, C.C., MacKay, J.A., Frechet, J.M.J., Szoka, F.C., 2005. Designing dendrimers for biological applications. Nat. Biotechnol. 23 (12), 1517–1526.
Lenhert, S., Fuchs, H., 2008. Lipid dip-pen nanolithography for functional biomimetic membrane systems. NSTI Nanotech. Tech. Proc. 1, 513–516.
Liao, W.-S., Cheunkar, S., Cao, H.H., Bednar, H.R., Weiss, P.S., Andrews, A.M., 2012. Subtractive patterning via chemical lift-off lithography. Science 337 (6101), 1517–1521.
Liu, H., Roy, K., 2005. Biomimetic three-dimensional cultures significantly increase hematopoietic differentiation efficacy of embryonic stem cells. Tissue Eng. 11 (1–2), 319–330.

Lopes, W.A., Jaeger, H.M., 2001. Hierarchical self-assembly of metal nanostructures on diblock copolymer scaffolds. Nature 414 (6865), 735–738.
Lu, T., Li, Y., Chen, T., 2013. Techniques for fabrication and construction of three-dimensional scaffolds for tissue engineering. Int. J. Nanomedicine 8, 337–350.
Malik, N., Evagorou, E.G., Duncan, R., 1999. Dendrimer-platinate: a novel approach to cancer chemotherapy. Anti-Cancer Drugs 10 (8), 767–776.
Malik, A., Chaudhary, S., Garg, G., Tomar, A., 2012. Dendrimers: a tool for drug delivery. Adv. Biol. Res. 6 (4), 165–169.
Mann, S., Archibald, D.D., Didymus, J.M., Douglas, T., Heywood, B.R., Meldrum, F.C., Reeves, N.J., 1993. Crystallization at inorganic-organic interfaces—biominerals and biomimetic synthesis. Science 261 (5126), 1286–1292.
Martin, T., Obst, U., Rebek, J., 1998. Molecular assembly and encapsulation directed by hydrogen-bonding preferences and the filling of space. Science 281 (5384), 1842–1845.
Marx, S., Liron, Z., 2001. Molecular imprinting in thin films of organic-inorganic hybrid sol-gel and acrylic polymers. Chem. Mater. 13 (10), 3624–3630.
McMahon, K.M., Mutharasan, R.K., Tripathy, S., Veliceasa, D., Bobeica, M., Shumaker, D.K., Luthi, A.J., Helfand, B.T., Ardehali, H., Mirkin, C.A., Volpert, O., Thaxton, C.S., 2011. Biomimetic high density lipoprotein nanoparticles for nucleic acid delivery. Nano Lett. 11 (3), 1208–1214.
Merkoci, A., Pumera, M., Llopis, X., Perez, B., del Valle, M., Alegret, S., 2005. New materials for electrochemical sensing VI: carbon nanotubes. TrAC, Trends Anal. Chem. 24 (9), 826–838.
Molino, N.M., Anderson, A.K.L., Nelson, E.L., Wang, S.-W., 2013. Biomimetic protein nanoparticles facilitate enhanced dendritic cell activation and cross-presentation. ACS Nano 7 (11), 9743–9752.
Morales, A.M., Lieber, C.M., 1998. A laser ablation method for the synthesis of crystalline semiconductor nanowires. Science 279 (5348), 208–211.
Moreira, F.T.C., Sales, M.G.F., 2011. Biomimetic sensors of molecularly-imprinted polymers for chlorpromazine determination. Mater. Sci. Eng, C 31 (5), 1121–1128.
Moreira, F.T.C., Kamel, A.H., Guerreiro, J.R.L., Sales, M.G.F., 2010. Man-tailored biomimetic sensor of molecularly imprinted materials for the potentiometric measurement of oxytetracycline. Biosens. Bioelectron. 26 (2), 566–574.
Moreira, F.T.C., Dutra, R.A.F., Noronha, J.P.C., Cunha, A.L., Sales, M.G.F., 2011a. Artificial antibodies for troponin T by its imprinting on the surface of multiwalled carbon nanotubes: its use as sensory surfaces. Biosens. Bioelectron. 28 (1), 243–250.
Moreira, F.T.C., Freitas, V.A.P., Sales, M.G.F., 2011b. Biomimetic norfloxacin sensors made of molecularly-imprinted materials for potentiometric transduction. Microchim. Acta 172 (1–2), 15–23.
Moreira, F., Sharma, S., Dutra, R., Noronha, J., Cass, A., Sales, M., 2013. Smart plastic antibody material (SPAM) tailored on disposable screen printed electrodes for protein recognition: application to myoglobin detection. Biosens. Bioelectron. 45, 237–244.
Mujahid, A., Iqbal, N., Afzal, A., 2013. Bioimprinting strategies: from soft lithography to biomimetic sensors and beyond. Biotechnol. Adv. 31 (8), 1435–1447.
Murnen, H.K., Rosales, A.M., Jaworsk, J.N., Segalman, R.A., Zuckermann, R.N., 2010. Hierarchical self-assembly of a biomimetic diblock copolypeptoid into homochiral superhelices. J. Am. Chem. Soc. 132 (45), 16112–16119.
Napolitano, A.P., Chai, P., Dean, D.M., Morgan, J.R., 2007. Dynamics of the self-assembly of complex cellular aggregates on micromolded nonadhesive hydrogels. Tissue Eng. 13 (8), 2087–2094.

Nelson, D.L., Cox, M.M. Lehninger Principles of Biochemistry. 5th Edition, Freeman, W. H. & Company, ISBN 071677108X.
Ngô, C., Van de Voorde, M., 2014. Nanotechnology in a Nutshell from Simple to Complex Systems. Atlantis Press.
Nicodemus, G.D., Bryant, S.J., 2008. Cell encapsulation in biodegradable hydrogels for tissue engineering applications. Tissue Eng. Part B 14 (2), 149–165.
Oliveira, H.M.V., Moreira, F.T.C., Sales, M.G.F., 2011. Ciprofloxacin-imprinted polymeric receptors as ionophores for potentiometric transduction. Electrochim. Acta 56 (5), 2017–2023.
Oliveira, J.M., Mano, J.F., Reis, R.L. 2012. Progress in dendrimer-based nanocarriers. Biomimetic approaches for biomaterials development. Wiley-VCH Verlag GmbH & Co. KGaA, Weinheim.
Padilla De Jesus, O.L., Ihre, H.R., Gagne, L., Frechet, J.M.J., Szoka Jr., F.C., 2002. Polyester dendritic systems for drug delivery applications: in vitro and in vivo evaluation. Bioconjug. Chem. 13 (3), 453–461.
Paltauf, F., 1994. Ether lipids in biomembranes. Chem. Phys. Lipids 74 (2), 101–139.
Pan, W., Xin, P., Patrick, S., Dean, S., Keating, C., Clawson, G., 2010. Primer-free aptamer selection using a random DNA library. J. Vis. Exp. 41, pii: 2039.
Perl, A., Reinhoudt, D.N., Huskens, J., 2009. Microcontact printing: limitations and achievements. Adv. Mater. 21 (22), 2257–2268.
Pistol, C., Chongchitmate, W., Dwyer, C., Lebeck, A.R., 2010. Architectural implications of nanoscale-integrated sensing and computing. IEEE Micro 30 (1), 110–120.
Pompe, W., Rödel, G., Weiss, H., Mertig, M., 2013. Bio-Nanomaterials: Designing Materials Inspired by Nature. Wiley-VCH, Weinheim.
Queiros, R.B., Noronha, J.P., Marques, P.V.S., Fernandes, J.S., Sales, M.G.F., 2012. Determination of Microcystin-LR in waters in the subnanomolar range by sol-gel imprinted polymers on solid contact electrodes. Analyst 137 (10), 2437–2444.
Rebelo, T.S.C.R., Almeida, S.A.A., Guerreiro, J.R.L., Montenegro, M.C.B.S.M., Sales, M.G.F., 2011. Trimethoprim-selective electrodes with molecularly imprinted polymers acting as ionophores and potentiometric transduction on graphite solid-contact. Microchem. J. 98 (1), 21–28.
Rebelo, T.S.C.R., Santos, C., Costa-Rodrigues, J., Fernandes, M.H., Noronha, J.P., Sales, M.G. F., 2014. Novel prostate specific antigen plastic antibody designed with charged binding sites for an improved protein binding and its application in a biosensor of potentiometric transduction. Electrochim. Acta 132, 142–150.
Rivas, G.A., Rubianes, M.D., Rodriguez, M.C., Ferreyra, N.E., Luque, G.L., Pedano, M.L., Miscoria, S.A., Parrado, C., 2007. Carbon nanotubes for electrochemical biosensing. Talanta 74 (3), 291–307.
Sandermann, H., 1978. Regulation of membrane enzymes by lipids. Biochim. Biophys. Acta 515 (3), 209–237.
Schense, J.C., Hubbell, J.A., 1999. Cross-linking exogenous bifunctional peptides into fibrin gels with factor XIIIa. Bioconjug. Chem. 10 (1), 75–81.
Schuster, B., Sleytr, U.B., 2014. Biomimetic interfaces based on S-layer proteins, lipid membranes and functional biomolecules. J. R. Soc. Interface 11 (96), 20140232.
Seeman, N.C., Belcher, A.M., 2002. Emulating biology: building nanostructures from the bottom up. Proc. Natl. Acad. Sci. U. S. A. 99, 6451–6455.
Sharma, S., Madou, M., 2012. Micro and nano patterning of carbon electrodes for bioMEMS. Bioinspired, Biomimetic Nanobiomater. 1 (4), 252–265.
Shen, Y.-x., Saboe, P.O., Sines, I.T., Erbakan, M., Kumar, M., 2014. Biomimetic membranes: a review. J. Membr. Sci. 454, 359–381.

Shimomura, M., 2010. The new trends in next generation biomimetics material technology: learning from biodiversity. Sci. Technol. Trends, Q. Review 37, 53–75.
Shin, H., Jo, S., Mikos, A.G., 2003. Biomimetic materials for tissue engineering. Biomaterials 24 (24), 4353–4364.
Shin, H., Zygourakis, K., Farach-Carson, M.C., Yaszemski, M.J., Mikos, A.G., 2004. Attachment, proliferation, and migration of marrow stromal osteoblasts cultured on biomimetic hydrogels modified with an osteopontin-derived peptide. Biomaterials 25 (5), 895–906.
Singh, S.B., Singh, A., 2013. The third allotrope of carbon: fullerene an update. Int. J. ChemTech. Res. 5, 167–171.
Singh, P., Onodera, T., Mizuta, Y., Matsumoto, K., Miura, N., Toko, K., 2009. Dendrimer modified biochip for detection of 2,4,6 trinitrotoluene on SPR immunosensor: fabrication and advantages. Sensors Actuators B Chem 137 (2), 403–409.
Sleytr, U.B., Schuster, B., Egelseer, E.-M., Pum, D., 2014. S-layers: principles and applications. FEMS Microbiol. Rev. 38 (5), 823–864.
Spolar, R.S., Record, M.T., 1994. Coupling of local folding to site-specific binding of proteins to DNA. Science 263 (5148), 777–784.
Stabenfeldt, S.E., Munglani, G., Garcia, A.J., LaPlaca, M.C., 2010. Biomimetic microenvironment modulates neural stem cell survival, migration, and differentiation. Tissue Eng. A 16 (12), 3747–3758.
Steed, J.W., Turner, D.R., Wallace, K.J., 2007. Core Concepts in Supramolecular Chemistry and Nanochemistry. John Wiley & Sons, Ltd, England.
Strehlitz, B., Nikolaus, N., Stoltenburg, R., 2008. Protein detection with aptamer biosensors. Sensors 8 (7), 4296–4307.
Sung, J.H., Yu, J., Luo, D., Shuler, M.L., March, J.C., 2011. Microscale 3-D hydrogel scaffold for biomimetic gastrointestinal (GI) tract model. Lab Chip 11 (3), 389–392.
Tamerler, C., Sarikaya, M., 2009. Molecular biomimetics: nanotechnology and bionanotechnology using genetically engineered peptides. Philos. Trans. R. Soc., A 367 (1894), 1705–1726.
Tripathi, V.S., Kandimalla, V.B., Ju, H.X., 2006. Preparation of ormosil and its applications in the immobilizing biomolecules. Sensors Actuators B Chem. 114 (2), 1071–1082.
Truta, L.A.A.N.A., Ferreira, N.S., Sales, M.G.F., 2014. Graphene-based biomimetic materials targeting urine metabolite as potential cancer biomarker: application over different conductive materials for potentiometric transduction. Eletrochim. Acta 150, 99–107.
Twyman, L.J., Ellis, A., Gittins, P.J., 2012. Pyridine encapsulated hyperbranched polymers as mimetic models of haeme containing proteins, that also provide interesting and unusual porphyrin-ligand geometries. Chem. Commun. 48 (1), 154–156.
Valery, C., Paternostre, M., Robert, B., Gulik-Krzywicki, T., Narayanan, T., Dedieu, J.C., Keller, G., Torres, M.L., Cherif-Cheikh, R., Calvo, P., Artzner, F., 2003. Biomimetic organization: octapeptide self-assembly into nanotubes of viral capsid-like dimension. Proc. Natl. Acad. Sci. U. S. A. 100 (18), 10258–10262.
Veis, A., 2005. A window on biomineralization. Science 307 (5714), 1419–1420.
Vozzi, G., Morelli, I., Vozzi, F., Andreoni, C., Salsedo, E., Morachioli, A., Giusti, P., Ciardelli, G., 2010. SOFT-MI: a novel microfabrication technique integrating soft-lithography and molecular imprinting for tissue engineering applications. Biotechnol. Bioeng. 106 (5), 804–817.
Vunjak-Novakovic, G., Scadden, D.T., 2011. Biomimetic platforms for human stem cell research. Cell Stem Cell 8 (3), 252–261.
Wagner, I., Musso, H., 1983. New naturally occurring amino acids. Angew. Chem. Int. Ed. Engl. 22, 816–828.

Wei, H., Wang, E., 2013. Nanomaterials with enzyme-like characteristics (nanozymes): next-generation artificial enzymes. Chem. Soc. Rev. 42 (14), 6060–6093.
West, J.L., Hubbell, J.A., 1999. Polymeric biomaterials with degradation sites for proteases involved in cell migration. Macromolecules 32 (1), 241–244.
Whitesides, G.M., Boncheva, M., 2002. Beyond molecules: self-assembly of mesoscopic and macroscopic components. Proc. Natl. Acad. Sci. U. S. A. 99 (8), 4769–4774.
Whitesides, G.M., Grzybowski, B., 2002. Self-assembly at all scales. Science 295 (5564), 2418–2421.
Wilson, R., Mehrabi, M., Prior, I.A., Beckett, A., Hutchinson, A., 2009. A reliable method for attaching biological molecules to layer-by-layer self-assemblies. Chem. Commun. 18, 2487–2489.
Xia, Y., Xiong, Y., Lim, B., Skrabalak, S.E., 2009. Shape-controlled synthesis of metal nanocrystals: simple chemistry meets complex physics? Angew. Chem. Int. Ed. 48 (1), 60–103.
Xu, Q., Rioux, R.M., Dickey, M.D., Whitesides, G.M., 2008. Nanoskiving: a new method to produce arrays of nanostructures. Acc. Chem. Res. 41 (12), 1566–1577.
Xu, H., Li, Z., Si, J., 2014. Nanocarriers in gene therapy: a review. J. Biomed. Nanotechnol. 10 (12), 3483–3507.
Yang, W., Thordarson, P., Gooding, J.J., Ringer, S.P., Braet, F., 2007. Carbon nanotubes for biological and biomedical applications. Nanotechnology 18 (41), 412001.
Yang, S.H., Lee, K.-B., Kong, B., Kim, J.-H., Kim, H.-S., Choi, I.S., 2009. Biomimetic encapsulation of individual cells with silica. Angew. Chem. Int. Ed. 48 (48), 9160–9163.
Yang, H., Dou, X., Fang, Y., Jiang, P., 2013. Self-assembled biomimetic superhydrophobic hierarchical arrays. J. Colloid Interface Sci. 405, 51–57.
Ye, X., Qi, L., 2011. Two-dimensionally patterned nanostructures based on monolayer colloidal crystals: controllable fabrication, assembly, and applications. Nano Today 6 (6), 608–631.
Yoon, H.C., Hong, M.Y., Kim, H.S., 2000. Affinity biosensor for avidin using a double functionalized dendrimer monolayer on a gold electrode. Anal. Biochem. 282 (1), 121–128.
Zhang, S.G., Marini, D.M., Hwang, W., Santoso, S., 2002. Design of nanostructured biological materials through self-assembly of peptides and proteins. Curr. Opin. Chem. Biol. 6 (6), 865–871.
Zhang, X., Zhao, N., Liang, S., Lu, X., Li, X., Xie, Q., Zhang, X., Xu, J., 2008. Facile creation of biomimetic systems at the interface and in bulk. Adv. Mater. 20 (15), 2938–2946.
Zhao, Y., Xie, Z., Gu, H., Zhu, C., Gu, Z., 2012. Bio-inspired variable structural color materials. Chem. Soc. Rev. 41 (8), 3297–3317.
Zhao, Y., Sakai, F., Su, L., Liu, Y., Wei, K., Chen, G., Jiang, M., 2013. Progressive macromolecular self-assembly: from biomimetic chemistry to bio-inspired materials. Adv. Mater. 25 (37), 5215–5256.
Zhou, C., Ye, X., Fan, Y., Ma, L., Tan, Y., Qing, F., Zhang, X., 2014a. Biomimetic fabrication of a three-level hierarchical calcium phosphate/collagen/hydroxyapatite scaffold for bone tissue engineering. Biofabrication 6 (3), 035013.
Zhou, Z., Buchanan, F., Mitchell, C., Dunne, N., 2014b. Printability of calcium phosphate: calcium sulfate powders for the application of tissue engineered bone scaffolds using the 3D printing technique. Mater. Sci. Eng. C 38, 1–10.

Bio-inspired fiber composites

2

C. Santulli

2.1 Introduction

The use of composites is desirable whenever a lightweight structure is to be obtained, able to effectively distribute load according to the requirements of material service. Most frequently, composites include fibers, acting as the reinforcement to a matrix, therefore providing a sufficiently strong interface, able to provide an effective load transfer. In nature, a fibrous morphology for reinforcement is often employed, with some notable success, in particular to combine brittle minerals and organic molecules into composites with outstanding fracture resistance and structural performance (Munch et al., 2008). However, composite design in engineering does not usually result in properties to the level of what can be achieved from a simple mixture of their components, so the law of mixtures is more often considered as an indicator of maximal ideal properties for engineered composite materials (Riley and Whitney, 1966). The negative deviation from values provided from the law of mixtures is even larger, whenever sustainable materials, such as lignocellulosic fibers, are inserted as the reinforcement to polymer matrices, especially due to their geometrical variability and the difficulty in providing a sound interface (Facca et al., 2006). In contrast, natural materials, such as bone, wood, and nacre, have often complex hierarchical structures, which on one side allow them to largely exceed the properties predicted from the law of mixture evaluation, but on the other side proved not easy to be replicated, especially as regards the hierarchized construction philosophy (Bhushan, 2009).

This is the situation this chapter moves from, with the aim to consider the real possibility to transfer the knowledge about composite design, which is present in nature, to the production of bio-inspired and multifunctional composites of structural interest. The chapter focuses first on the possible sources of bio-inspiration for composites, in Section 2.2, where relevant natural structures are presented as for their composite nature and the functional possibilities this characteristic offers. The different ways in which multifunctionality is obtained will be discussed in Section 2.3, trying to set a possible scheme for the significance of bio-inspiration when applied to the design of composite materials in Section 2.4. This process can bear some difficulties, especially in specific areas, which are of considerable interest nonetheless for the development of more effective composites, especially for the improvement of interface strength: this is the case for superhydrophobicity; different approaches to it are discussed with reference to bio-inspiration in Section 2.5. Conclusions and future perspectives are briefly presented in Section 2.6.

2.2 Biological materials

Biological materials are typically composites that are both hierarchically structured and multifunctional. The former characteristic allows them offering an outstanding mechanical performance, while the latter is essential for their service in the natural system in which they operate (Meyers et al., 2008). When turning to bio-inspiration, the main question becomes mimicking these two properties, or their effects, considering for example that hierarchization results in the development of high strength, toughness, and fracture resistance and has an influence on an easier achievement of multifunctionality. In other words, the creation of multiscale structure allows achieving an integrated performance of different functions (Liu and Jiang, 2011). The main question about bio-inspiration lies in the fact that it is not always appropriate, in terms of manufacturing procedure, making direct use of natural materials; therefore, the selection of an appropriate material-technology pair is required for exploiting the possibilities that are inherent in the adoption of a biological principle. There are a number of organisms that are particularly inspirational when it comes to the fabrication of a material bearing particular functions or characteristics borrowed from nature. These include, for example, gecko (Rizzo et al., 2006), which is particularly suitable when aiming at obtaining a strong bonding force that is able to withstand a number of cycles of adhesion and de-adhesion; abalone (Lin and Meyers, 2005), which is considered particularly useful to inspire the creation of ceramic matrix composites resistant to crack propagation; nacre (Luz and Mano, 2009), which is an interesting attempt to manufacture together structures with different properties via the use of growth bands as effective crack deflectors; bone, which shows considerable self-healing characteristics (Sanchez et al., 2005); lignocellulosic fibers, which optimize the use of a helical development mode for flexibility, via the programmatic succession of strong and weak parts in the structure, leading to typical kink bands (Monteiro et al., 2011; Gibson, 2012).

In practice, it is possible to concentrate, instead that on the specific materials, on the particular properties that make worth investigating in that bio-inspiration allows obtaining special properties, which can be summarized under the general term multifunctionality, though a bare effect of hierarchization, it is well known that multifunctionality can be declined in a number of ways and structures (Meyers et al., 2006). Examples can be bones, which provide structural support and blood cell formation, or chitin exoskeletons in arthropods, which supply protection, attachment for muscles, and water repellence, not very differently from insect cuticles, which represent a real barrier on the other side allowing fast and effective movement (Miessner et al., 2001). All these properties are realized through the use of hierarchical composites, which are arranged so to exploit to the fullest the possibilities offered by the presence of porosities. The reflection over the properties led to an extended interest for self-healing properties, which in turn carried out an increasing awareness over the potential embedded in the possible use of hollow fibers, such as one of the simplest structural arrangement for the purpose (Pang and Bond, 2005a). In another sense, in terms of restoration of the ideal operational conditions for biological materials after being subjected to harsh environments, self-cleaning surfaces have also received interest as yet another consequence of hierarchical structure (Bhushan et al., 2008). Inspiration from superhydrophobic biological structures has also been applied to obtain superoleophobic properties, once again exploiting the possibility of surface patterning offered by hierarchization, particularly as it is applied in fish scales, leading to different degrees of adhesion at the interface (Liu et al., 2009). On a level of design that involves not only the surface but also the bulk materials, self-assembly strategies applied in nature have the potential to encompass all aspects related to the advantages of designing a material according to a fibrous composite structure (Viney, 2004).

2.3 Sources of bio-inspiration

In this section, the biological structures that can serve as an inspiration for the production of composites for different purposes are briefly discussed. The two main features that are characteristically used with this aim are particularly hierarchization and morphology of fibrous components, which involve nanostructuration as a consequence of self-assembly and presence of hollows. A number of biological artifacts are discussed in the next paragraphs. Their potential in being applied in bio-inspired composites has been only partially exploited so far, but appears clear, at least in principle.

2.3.1 *Nacre*

The composite structure of nacre combines hardness, strength, and toughness to a level not normally achieved in man-made materials (Luz and Mano, 2009). This may be ascribed to the so-called brick-and-mortar arrangement of organic and inorganic elements, which combines the elasticity of composite protein (lustrin) + polysaccharide (β chitin) layers and the strength of calcium carbonate tablets, the latter being normally around an order of magnitude thicker than the former (around 1 μm against 100 nm) (Tang et al., 2003). It has been demonstrated that both "bricks" and "mortar" can be reproduced by the sequential deposition of polyelectrolytes and clays (Tang et al., 2003). In practice, this allowed producing inorganic/organic nanocomposites with clay nanoplatelets and polyimide by centrifugal deposition process, which resulted in an ordered nanostructure with alternating organic and inorganic layers, with mechanical properties comparable to that of lamella bones (Chem et al., 2008). In another study, nanostructured nacre proved to offer antimicrobial properties when assembled in a bio-inspired composite by a layer-by-layer structure (Podsiadlo et al., 2005).

2.3.2 *Gecko*

The hierarchical structure of the gecko foot, comprising different levels, more specifically including setae, each of them containing hundreds of spatulae, appears to have been designed to optimize adhesion strength (Rizzo et al., 2006; Gravish et al., 2008).

In particular, it is suggested that the spatulae terminating with curved ends would reduce the sensitivity of adhesion strength to the presence of defects, such as geometrical irregularities, presence of contaminants, surface roughness, and trapped air bubbles (Gao et al., 2005). As a matter of fact, gecko is an example of this structured patterning aimed at this purpose, another being for example present in some beetles, where dry and safe-from-dirt adhesion is achieved by "mushroom-shaped pillars" protruding from the foot surface (Gorb et al., 2007). This has been expressed as a principle of "contact splitting," widely diffused in insects, arthropods, and reptiles, which can be applied for the development of optimized artificial attachment devices: in practice, adhesion force is enhanced by $n^{1/2}$, where n is the number of subdivided contacts ($n=R^2/r^2$), as it is reported in Figure 2.1, redrawn from Arzt (2006). In this regard, the concept of "adhesion design maps" is also introduced, which in practice relates phenomena, such as fiber fracture, ideal contact strength, fiber condensation, and fiber adaptability with the effects of contact tip radius, Young's modulus, and aspect ratio of the hierarchized fibers on contact strength (Spolenak et al., 2005).

This suggests the possibility to create biomimetic fibrillar interfaces, which bears some interest also for the possible production of a defect-resilient fiber-matrix interface in a composite (Gravish et al., 2010). In this sense, gecko-inspired microfiber arrays have been proposed, which have been realized using polypropylene: the study indicated that contact is maintained and shear force is enhanced with sliding, due to the fact that a partial side contact, in place of a tip contact, is adopted (Lee et al., 2008). In particular, at the microscale, the behavior demonstrates an improvement of adhesion with service, in that fibers shearing over time increases both maximum shear and pull-off forces (Schubert et al., 2008).

2.3.3 *Mussel*

The structure of marine adhesives is essentially analogous to composite thermosets, being formed by fiber, filler, and catalyst molecules dispersed in a cross-linked resin resistant to heat and solvents: to this purpose, different fibers are used, such as collagen, fibroin, and chitin (Waite, 1990). This includes also macro-foulants, such as barnacles, which appear to be equally adapted, using a two-phases adhesion concept, to provide effective bonding both on hydrophilic and on hydrophobic polymer

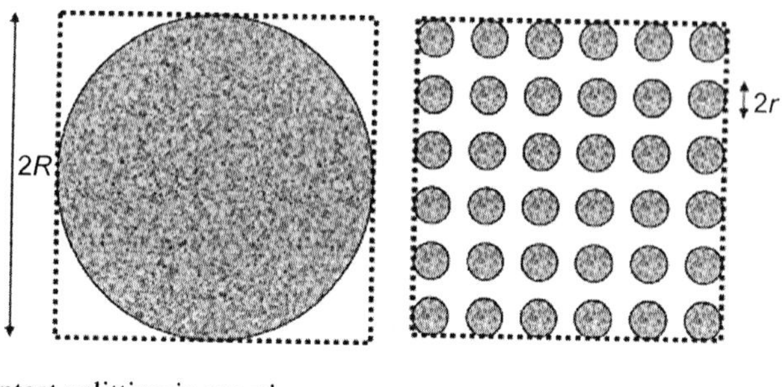

Figure 2.1 Contact splitting in practice.

surfaces, which is promising in terms of prospective composite fabrication (Muthukumar et al., 2011). Dealing with mussel, its adhesive structure, which is referred to as *byssus,* includes a bundle of threads, all of them terminating in an adhesive plaque: the threads are produced using a kind of injection molding process and they are made of proteins not dissimilar from elastin and collagen (Lee et al., 2006).

In addition, while the principal limit of gecko-inspired adhesion is the limited resistance to degree of wetting of the interface, it was indicated that coating gecko-inspired microfibers with a layer of polymer mimicking mussel adhesion process does considerably improve adhesion in wet environments, especially over time (Lee et al., 2007). This property has been also exploited to improve the structural stability of chitosan/polyacrylonitrile composite membranes by the introduction of mussel-adhesive-mimetic carbopol molecule as intermediate layer, with the effect of enhancing the interfacial adhesion strength of the membrane (Ma et al., 2010).

2.3.4 Bone

In general, bone grafting into polymers is a technique that allows effective reparation: some bone replacement products are based on biological structures, such as coral, which, though extremely biocompatible and with optimal pore size, have some difficulties in the manufacture to shape of scaffolds (Olah and Borbas, 2008). Another possibility is the transformation of biological composites, such as *Strombus gigas* (conch) shells and *Tridacna gigas* (Giant clam) into hydroxyapatite (HA), which is supposed to retain some specificity from its biological origin (Vecchio et al., 2007). Biomimetic synthesis of bone scaffold materials included features of natural bone in main composition and hierarchical microstructure, assembling nano-hydroxyapatite and collagen into mineralized fibril, so that the three-dimensional porous scaffold would mimic the microstructure of cancellous bone: this was effective for bio-activity and showed promising properties for clinical repairs of large defects in the bone (Liao et al., 2004). Another possibility of biomimetic synthesis was the preparation of bone-like composites constituted of HA nanocrystals and self-assembled type I collagen fibers; this enabled the growth of HA nanocrystals oriented parallel to the axis of the collagen fiber (Tampieri et al., 2003).

2.3.5 Biological fibers

The use of lignocellulosic fibers in macroscopic form into polymer matrices, giving rise to plant fiber composites, is widely diffused: a number of reviews are available on this subject (Mwaikambo et al., 2001; Kalia et al., 2009; Ku et al., 2011). In contrast, on the nanoscale it is possible to extract cellulose nanocrystals (CNCs) from vegetable biomass, normally by a process of acid hydrolysis (Klemm et al., 2011). Though in general terms both procedures bear considerable interest, these cannot be considered as really exploiting the possibilities offered biomimicking these structures, in particular their hierarchized design and their cellular architecture, including cellular hollows. A few studies oriented to this purpose exist nonetheless, in particular, some work was carried out with low-cost cell wall fragments, obtained from swede root, which was coated with different binders to investigate the possibility of penetration from the polymer matrix into the cell structure (Bruce et al., 2005). The replication of the hierarchical structure allowed also the fabrication of porous metal oxide/polymer hybrid and polymer materials by replication of natural cellulosic substances and subsequent removal of the template cellulose components by treating with a mild sodium hydroxide/urea solution (Gu and Huang, 2009). This latter work is an example of the possibility to apply the hierarchization procedure to the construction of structures not directly linked to the biological origin of the material used.

A work that can be considered as bio-inspired, at least for the application of keratin-based fibrils from wool waste, as a possible reinforcement for polymer matrices, aimed also at elucidating the effect of two possible morphologies, intended as model cases, more in particular plain fibrils and fractal-tree structure fibrils (Yu, 2010). With keratin fibers, other two possible routes have been recently investigated, which more specifically concern the introduction of macrostructures, such as wool felts, as the filler of polymers (Santulli et al., 2013) or the possible extraction of nano-keratin for use as the reinforcement (Aluigi et al., 2014): the latter is also being exposed in slightly more detail in Section 2.4.

2.4 Multifunctional bio-inspired composites

2.4.1 *Auxetic bio-inspired honeycomb cores and matrices for composites*

One of the reasons to use bio-inspired structures in the production of composites, mostly sandwich ones, is the possibility to reduce their weight, for example, via the adoption of adequate cellular structures. These are most likely to be inspired to a honeycomb, therefore involving only cells with planar surfaces with a fixed number of sides, the most common geometry being in practice the centersymmetric hexagonal one with variable internal cell angles. A possibility, which responds in effect to what is achieved in nature, is designing cells with different dimensions and variable aspect ratios, therefore moving away from a regular polygon as for the cell geometry (Seepersad et al., 2005). Moreover, auxetic properties allow obtaining a possible multifunctionality, for example, via the insertion of embedded piezoelectric transducers for sensing or actuation (Miller et al., 2008).

Morphological studies on cellular structures have also been carried out, in particular, to define by geometrical parameters some specific biological tissues, such as, for example, plant cells parenchyma. In the recognition that plant cells have curved edges and undulant faces, possibly with sigmoid curvatures, parenchyma was recognized as being a mixture of tetrakaidecahedral faces with other faces shaped as different polygons (Macior, 1960). Inspiration from nature suggests first that cellular materials, also referred to as honeycomb, do not have by any means to comprise uniquely cells with hexagonal shape. In addition, curvature of the faces leads to the results that a variable amount of cell polygons are in fact concave, which move them away from the possible application for them of concept of Newton's equations for lattice motion; in other words, the concave polygons may partially behave as auxetic structures, i.e., they have negative Poisson's ratios (Evans and Alderson, 2000). Most recently, there has been interest in auxetic structures, which are in practice capable of bending in different directions, instead of showing necking, when undergoing a tensile load, with the additional effect of showing a higher resistance to in-plane indentation, as well as an enhanced shear modulus and compressive strength (Scarpa et al., 2000). In Table 2.1, some types of biological structures that present an auxetic behavior and are conformable as a composite skin or sheath are reported, therefore not including auxetic behavior in minerals, which does not appear relevant as such for application in composites. In Figure 2.2, a number of different auxetic structures, potentially applicable to composite reinforcement and/or to its bulk structure, are presented. Starting from what could be called the pristine auxetic structure in that it is the one that most simply presents a form of repeated concavity, i.e., bow-shaped (also referred to as "reentrant") honeycomb, in the other images different possible geometries are reported, which all have been calculated to have a negative Poisson's ratio.

The interest for auxetic structures, which may lead to significant improvements in honeycomb materials, can easily border with the study of lumens and more generally of the succession of filled and empty area in cell materials, which in turn leads to the observation of different structure arrangements in the fibers. The case for cell fiber structures acting as a possible template for bio-inspired composites has been posed also in the past, based on the study of celery fibers (Santulli, 2008). This has been proposed based on the fact that the distribution of cell geometries has a significant effect on the mode of failure of open cell solids, in particular, relating the position of damage, or notch, to the dimensions of cell struts (Onck et al., 2005). Subsequent

Table 2.1 Some biological structures presenting an auxetic behavior

Biological structure	Characteristics	Reference
Skin of aquatic salamander	Composite made in sheaths with regularly organized collagen fibers in a crossed, fabric-like array	Frolich et al. (1994)
Cow teat skin	Negative Poisson's ratio at low biaxial strains	Lees et al. (1991)
Cat skin	J-shaped stress-deformation curve and out-of-plane auxetic behavior	Veronda and Westmann (1970)
Deployable structures (Dionaea, etc.)	Turgor pressure facilitated by the combined presence of cells with Newtonian and auxetic behavior	Shahinpoor (2011)

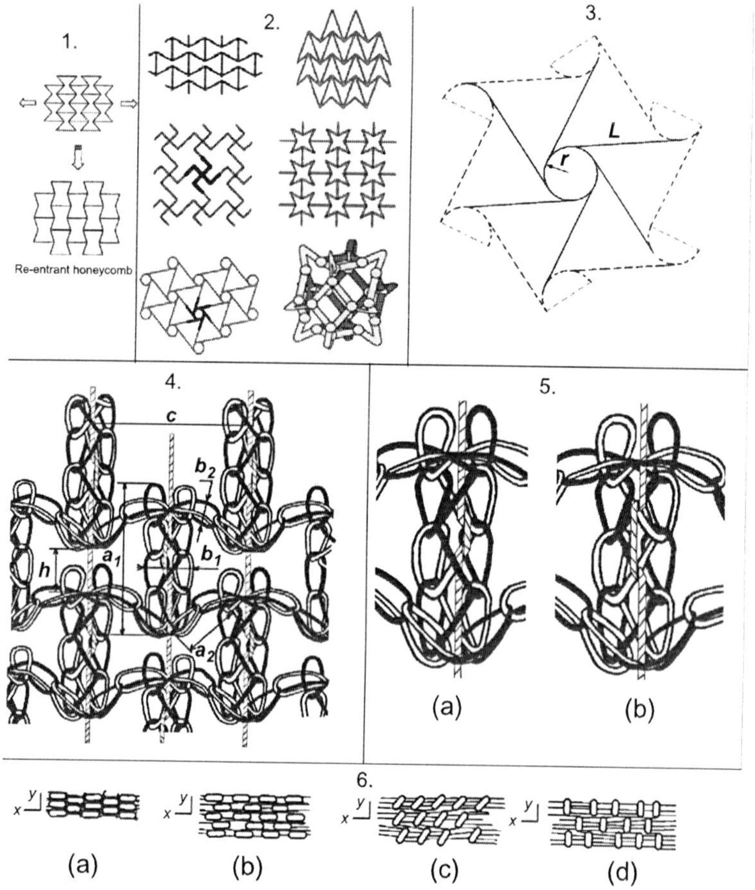

Figure 2.2 Auxetic structures: 1: Re-entrant honeycombs, 2: Different forms of auxetic structures 3: Chiral auxetic honeycombs, 4 and 5: Structure for auxetic textiles, 6: Auxetic behavior of laterally attached rods to polymers (figure redrawn by the author).

morphological analyses have been carried out on other fibers, mainly of herbaceous origin, such as okra bahmia (*Abelmoschus Esculentus*) (De Rosa et al., 2010a) (Figure 2.3) and phormium (De Rosa et al., 2010b). An evolution was represented by another on this aspect, which leads to the consideration of the variety of possible mechanical responses in a fiber, has been carried out by Bouakba et al. on fibers from cactus cladodes, which led to a distinct advantage in fiber extraction. In particular, three different fiber architectures have been discerned based on angles of the pores opening, area pores, and thickness of two hierarchical levels of the fibrils taken in the plane of the sheaths (Bouakba et al., 2013). It is noteworthy though that work on different fiber architectures is still in its infancy and is susceptible of significant developments in the future.

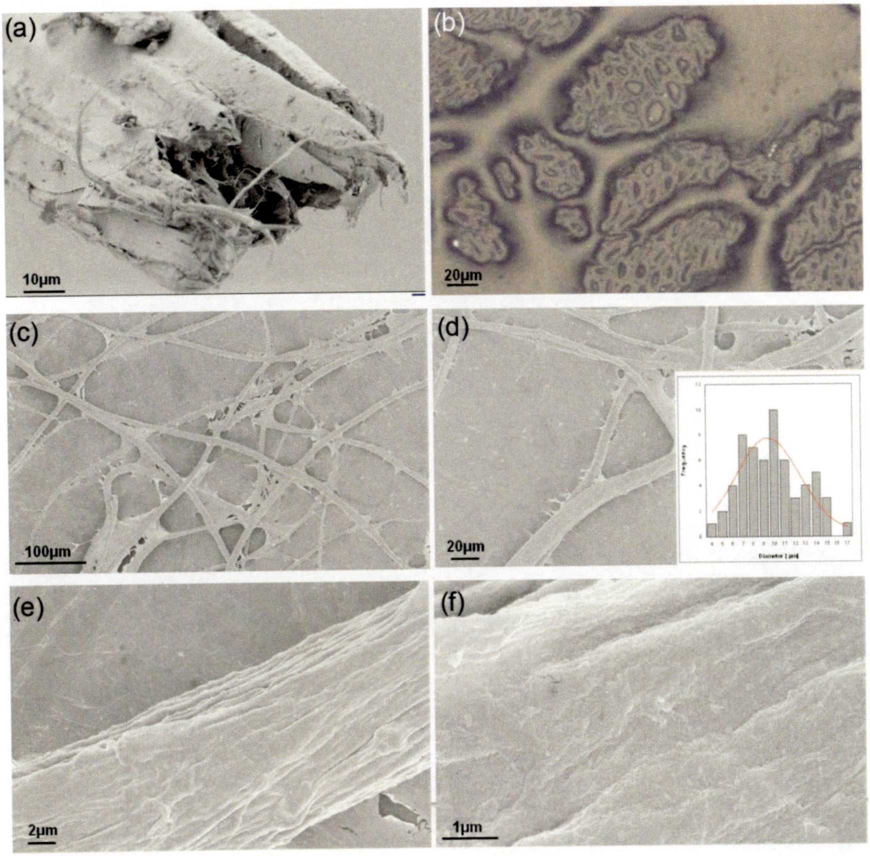

Figure 2.3 Morphological characterization of fractured pristine okra fiber (a–b), and FESEM observation of chemical pretreated okra at different magnifications (c–f). The inset shows the diameter distribution of pretreated okra fibers (Fortunati et al., 2013).

2.4.2 Composites inspired to insect cuticles for stiffness improvement and water retention

The structure of insect cuticle, such as the one of locusts, represented in Figure 2.4, comprises a chitinous and a proteinic phase, joined between them with different degrees of interaction, depending on the species and the function, and usually include also calcium salts, normally carbonates in form of calcite, to increase their stiffness (Vincent and Wegst, 2004). Moreover, the cuticle is multifunctional by representing a sensory barrier in which the deformation of holes tailored on the expected type, level, and direction of strain act as mechanical sensors (Vincent, 2002). Another possibility offered by cuticle is its local hardening by the addition of manganese and zinc (Robertson et al., 1984).

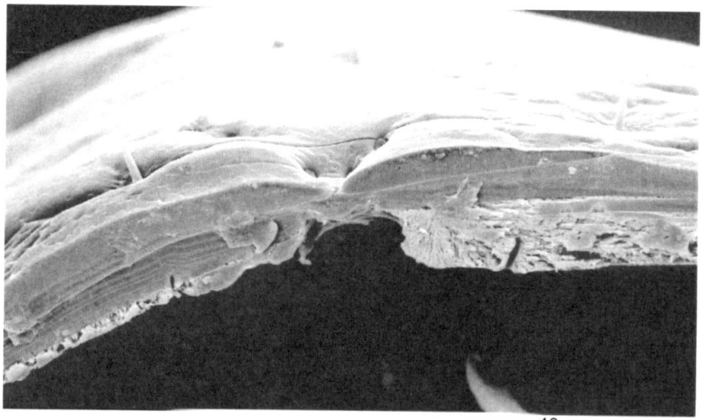

Figure 2.4 Composite structure of a locust cuticle and vibration sensors protruding from it (photograph owned by the author).

A composite mimicking the behavior of insect cuticle was reproduced by replacing chitin with paper cellulose, impregnated with the tripeptide DOPA-Gly-Gly: an alternative route involved treating it with a protein, bovine serum albumin added with catechol, then treated with tyrosinase for catechol oxidization. The resulting material was waterproof and had very high wet strength, decreasing its water retention by repeated wet–dry cycles (Miessner et al., 2001). In practice, interface bonding between chitosan and fibroin suggested that shrilk may be an optimal candidate, which can replace common biopolymers with a biological composite, avoiding its most common defects, first and foremost low toughness and limited resistance to the presence of manufacturing defects (Fernandez and Ingber, 2012).

2.4.3 Function of hollows in composite fibers: self-healing and other properties

Plant stems have been considered as templates for the development of composites, especially for the fact that they are able to control their porosity, due to their tailored presence of hollows: this leads to distinct advantages, including high specific stiffness/tenacity and effective vibration damping. The above properties have suggested concentrating the interest on a few species, in particular giant reed (*Arundo donax*) and horsetail (*Equisetum hyemale*) (Milwich et al., 2007). These properties are obtained by the presence of a stiffness gradient between fibers and cellular parenchyma matrix, obtained by a spiraliform arrangement of layers. This led to the development of a "technical plant stem," which was reproduced by the use of a polyurethane-glass fiber composite to encase microfibrils and fiber, then applying a polyurethane foam matrix between the fiber bundles, which resulted in a very lightweight composite (Masselter and Speck, 2011).

The possibility to successfully exploit hollows and cavities in plant fibers, therefore obtaining other properties, has been proposed also with no need for creation of templates, for example as regards kapok (*Ceiba Pentandra*) fibers, which are particularly suitable for some application, such as oil absorbency and retention capacity, for their low density, large lumens, and waxy surface (Lim and Huang, 2007). However, the literature on inclusion of kapok fibers in composites still remains quite limited. This can be attributed to their low weight and diameter, which is not very suitable for impregnation without misplacement or nonhomogeneous distribution of fiber during conventional composite fabrication: for this reason, only studies on hybrid with other fibers, such as glass or sisal, have been performed (Venkata Reddy et al., 2008).

Another possible application of a simple, yet quite effective, self-healing procedure has been applied in Norris (2011) and Norris et al. (2011) by introducing a vasculature design incorporated into a carbon fiber reinforced polymer via a lost wax process: infusion of a healing resin through the vascule channels resulted in an almost complete recovery of post-impact compression strength.

This leads to the possibility of self-healing for the composite materials, which has been extensively reviewed in Trask et al. (2007), where the different bio-inspired approaches applied for this purpose have been presented. In practice, different bio-inspired approaches did appear suitable for the purpose of self-repair: the inspiration to internal storage mediums for example could be of interest for this task (a large number of these exist in nature, such as cladodes (Bobich and Nobel, 2002) and calla lily (Nechaev and Voituriez, 2001), whose shape has been studied and related to the task of fluid, hence potentially also healing substances, storage. A number of possibilities have been explored, which appeared not only promising but also more easily feasible. This includes hollow fibers aimed at the fabrication of bleeding composites (Pang and Bond, 2005b) and deposition of nanoparticles for remediation of composite matrix (Kolmakov et al., 2010). Further repair strategies would involve remodeling of fractured fibers (Bond et al., 2007) and thermally enhanced cross-links reparation, based on the byssus thread principle (Harrington et al., 2009).

2.4.4 Toward self-assembly of composites

A number of strategies have been developed to explore a route toward self-assembly of engineered composites, as it is the case for biological structures. Such strategies can be considered to be divided in two types, the former being involved in the process of composite structuring, in particular, promoting crystallization according to biological procedures, while the latter is more concerned about the possibility to exploit hierarchization to introduce reinforcements at a different scale in composites, with the aim to improve the interfacial adhesion. It can be observed that the former procedures are bordering on other fields of research, such as bio-inspired crystallization, which are not strictly speaking aimed at the fabrication of composite materials (Yu and Cölfen, 2004). Despite this, in some cases, the principle of using a biological material, such as a polysaccharide, for the growth of a second material with different properties, can be considered pertinent to the development of bio-inspired composites. For example, alginate chains were employed as a template for the growth of the inorganic component and calcium ions present in the HA molecule were exploited to partially cross-link the alginate, giving after lyophilization a macroporous scaffold adapted for the growth of artificial bone (Tampieri et al., 2005).

Recent results on the control of morphology in cryogenic processes of hydrogels and colloid systems, obtained in particular by unidirectional freezing in nitrogen liquid, allow for the fabrication of composites by *in situ* incorporation of biological entities providing hierarchy and functionality to the resulting materials, which are known as "ice-templated" (Gutiérrez et al., 2008). For example, macroporous composite hydrogel, composed of poly(*N*-isopropylacrylamide) clay platelets, was obtained by ice-templated assembly and UV-initiated cryo-polymerization, ensuring a unique hierarchical structure with micrometric aligned pores and nacre-like layered nanostructure (Bai et al., 2013). Ice templating can be possibly applied to the fabrication of nano-reinforcements with tailored via cyclic freezing–thawing of cellulose nanofibril aerogels with ultralow density, superior porosity, and water absorbency, as well as high crystallinity and water-activated shape recovery (Jiang and Hsieh, 2014).

Hierarchization, as it appears in biological structures, has been long suggested to be a common procedure for the production of composites with optimal fiber-matrix adhesion properties (Barthelat, 2007). As a consequence, this method has also been applied in modeling to investigate the behavior of two types of hierarchical materials: "hierarchical tree" (bundles-of-bundles of fibers) and self-similar particle and fiber reinforced composite (in which reinforcements at each hierarchical level represent composites in turn consisting of lower level reinforcements and matrix), which can be mixed as well (Mishnaevsky, 2011). In practice, this procedure has been applied also in dealing with nanocomposites, for example, in producing composites with nanosized bacterial cellulose as a binder for a nonwoven sisal fiber preforms, the whole of them vacuum-assisted infused in hierarchical composites with an acrylated epoxidized soybean oil thermoset resin (Lee et al., 2012). On the other side, a significant contribution to the understanding of the influence of the species, more commonly referred to as *specificity,* on the properties and the morphology of crystalline plant cellulose, can be offered by the extraction of CNC from different plants. In particular, this procedure can confer interest to the use of agro waste from different sources. In practice, nanocellulose has been extracted for example with good yield and considerably high crystallinity from sisal fibers (Morán et al., 2007), from phormium tenax fibers (Fortunati et al., 2012) and from okra bahmia fibers (Fortunati et al., 2013).

However, here bio-inspiration can be considered limited to morphological considerations on hierarchical structure, which for example include the fact that solutions of suspension exhibited strong shear-induced birefringence, highlighting the ability of nanocrystals to form a chiral nematic liquid crystalline (Fortunati et al., 2012). It is significant to stress once again that nanosized cellulose reinforcement is significantly crystalline so that the mechanical performance of the obtained composite is considerably higher than what it is the case for usual plant fiber composites. This principle is by no means limited to the extraction of crystal from cellulose-based materials. Also, the extraction of nanocrystals from keratin obtained from different kind of wool, including Merinos and alpaca, has been realized, which showed similar potential in terms of crystallinity, added to the particular nature of keratin, which involves the presence of cysteine sulfur bonds conferring to the structure at particular rigidity (Aluigi et al., 2014).

2.5 Difficulties in applying bio-inspiration to composites: the case of superhydrophobicity

The above account over the bio-inspiration in composites leads to the consideration that a significant difficulty is still present in reproducing some interesting features of the biological structures, the majority of which requires the fabrication of composite or nanocomposite structures. An example can concern the fabrication of superhydrophobic surfaces, reminding the "lotus effect": in the biological form, this is obtained by the structuration of an epicuticular layer, whose inherent structure is that of a composite of three-dimensional waxes with an underlying wax film (Koch and Barthlott, 2009).

Attempts to obtain the self-cleaning quality in polymer surfaces involved the application of a soft lithography fabrication method, e.g., using polydimethylsiloxane, by replicating prepatterned structures, which were then nanostructured by means of a fluorine carbide plasma treatment (Cortese et al., 2008). The technological limits of this approach are that, rather than curved surfaces for tailoring roughness, square pillars with smoothed edges are obtained: despite this, this may prove quite effective for superhydrophobicity (Jin et al., 2005). Other methods proved more respectful of the natural procedure, therefore being in the end more effective for the purpose: this was for example the case of the transformation of poly(lactic acid) (PLA) film surface in a superhydrophobic one by using a gelation-in-air procedure followed by precipitation in ethanol, which led to the formation of hierarchized flower-like rods or papilla structures on the surface (Shi et al., 2008). Coming even closer to the natural inspiration, UV photografting of silica particles containing vinyl groups over the PLA matrix was also proposed, leading to very effective superhydrophobic properties with water contact angles of up to 150° (Bae et al., 2010). A comparison between the biological artifact, such as first exposed in Barthlott and Neinhuis (1997), and a bio-inspired surface with super-hydrophobic properties is depicted in Figure 2.5 (Ensikat et al., 2011).

2.6 Conclusions and future perspectives

Although representing in general terms a method which can be applied to a number of situations, bio-inspiration has so far produced limited results on composite materials. It is likely that this may change in the near future, given that the bottleneck of this process of exploiting knowledge from nature to address issues in composite materials is given by the necessary material substitution, which leads often to poor reproducibility of the original idea in the engineered structure.

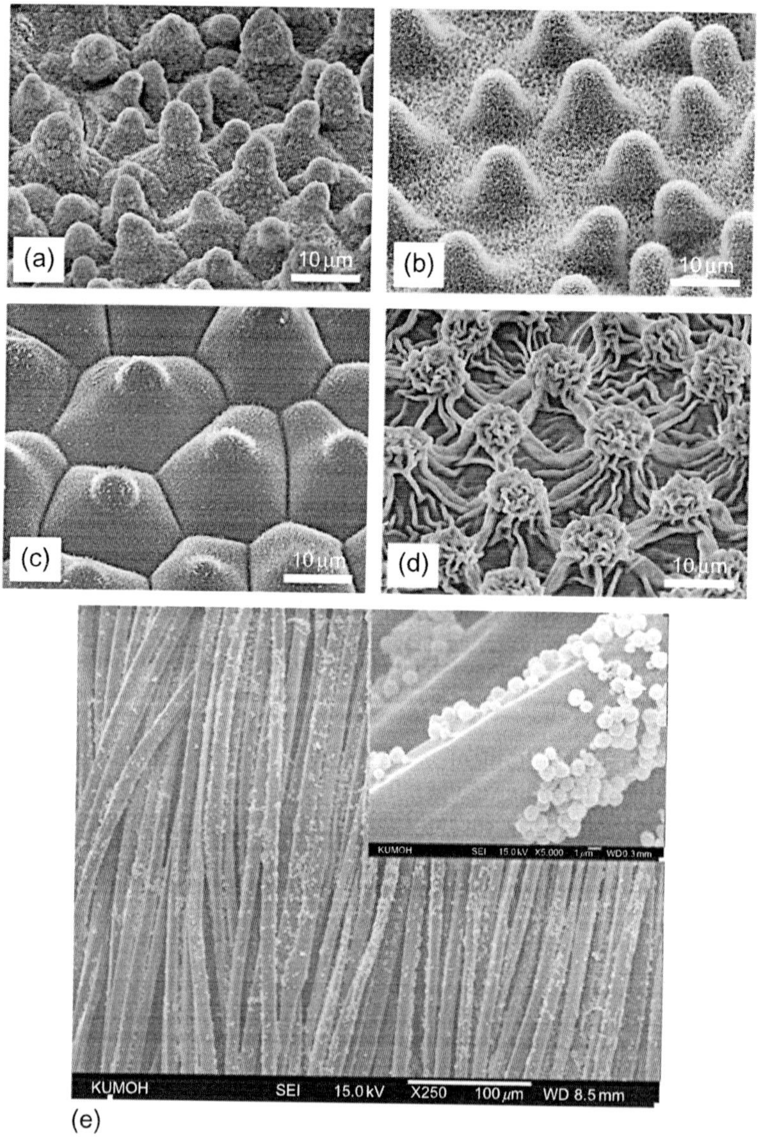

Figure 2.5 SEM images of the papillose leaf surfaces of *Nelumbo nucifera* (Lotus) (a), *Euphorbia myrsinites* (b), *Colocasia esculenta* (c), and *Alocasia macrorrhiza* (d). (e) UV photografting of silica particles containing vinyl groups over the PLA matrix (Bae et al., 2010).

Most promising results have been obtained in the field of the production of hierarchized composites, which may lead to the achievement of multifunctional composites, for which inspirations are multiple, from insect cuticles to plants, such as Venus fly-trap, which have embedded actuating possibilities. Still, difficulties are encountered dealing with practical applications of auxetic materials, potentially adapted especially for use in textile composites to suitably arrange the reinforcement architecture so to offer an improved resistance, especially to flexural loading. Here, the study of the different auxetic morphologies is clearly helpful to expand the range of possible production routes, though it did not lead so far to a significant convergence on optimized manufacturing methods. Other fields are still under development, such as those that are connected with self-healing and self-cleaning properties; here again, it can be suggested that a stricter adherence, though by no means barely formal, to the biological principle may be beneficial for the probability of final success. It is important to conclude that one of the most significant assets for composites would be improvement of fiber-matrix interface, e.g., by acting in adhesion using a contact splitting procedure, as described above, but this appears still not completely realizable when employing engineered materials.

References

Aluigi, A., Tonetti, C., Rombaldoni, F., Puglia, D., Fortunati, E., Armentano, I., et al., 2014. Keratins extracted from Merino wool and Brown Alpaca fibres as potential fillers for PLLA-based biocomposites. J. Mater. Sci. 49, 6257–6269.

Arzt, E., 2006. Biological and artificial attachment devices: lessons for materials scientists from flies and geckos. Mater. Sci. Eng., C 26, 1245–1250.

Bae, G., Jang, J., Jeong, J., Lyoo, W., Min, B., 2010. Superhydrophobic PLA fabrics prepared by UV photo-grafting of hydrophobic silica particles possessing vinyl groups. J. Colloid Interface Sci. 344, 584–587.

Bai, H., Polini, A., Delattre, B., Tomsia, A., 2013. Thermoresponsive composite hydrogels with aligned macroporous structure by ice-templated assembly. Chem. Mater. 25, 4551–4556.

Barthelat, F., 2007. Biomimetics for next generation materials. Philos. Trans. R. Soc. London, Ser. A 365, 2906–2919.

Barthlott, W., Neinhuis, C., 1997. Purity of the sacred lotus, or escape from contamination in biological surfaces. Planta 202, 1–8.

Bhushan, B., 2009. Biomimetics: lessons from nature—an overview. Philos. Transact. A Math. Phys. Eng. Sci. 367, 1445–1486.

Bhushan, B., Koch, K., Jung, Y., 2008. Biomimetic hierarchical structure for self-cleaning. Appl. Phys. Lett. 93, 093101.

Bobich, E., Nobel, P., 2002. Cladode junction regions and their biomechanics for arborescent platyopuntias. Int. J. Plant Sci. 163, 507–517.

Bond, I.P., Trask, R.S., Williams, G.J., 2007. Bioinspired self-healing of advanced composite structures using hollow glass fibres. J. R. Soc. Interface 4, 363–371.

Bouakba, M., Bezazi, A., Boba, K., Scarpa, F., Bellamy, S., 2013. Cactus fibre/polyester biocomposites: manufacturing, quasi-static mechanical and fatigue characterisation. Combust. Sci. Technol. 74, 150–159.

Bruce, D.M., Hobson, R.N., Farrent, J.W., Hepworth, D.G., 2005. High-performance composites from low-cost plant primary cell walls. Compos. A: Appl. Sci. Manuf. 36, 1486–1493.

Chem, R., Wang, C., Huang, Y., Leb, H., 2008. An efficient biomimetic process for fabrication of artificial nacre with ordered-nanostructure. Mater. Sci. Eng., C 28, 218–222.

Cortese, B., D'Amone, S., Manca, M., Viola, I., Cingolani, R., Gigli, G., 2008. Superhydrophobicity due to the hierarchical scale roughness of PDMS surfaces. Langmuir 24, 2712–2718.
De Rosa, I.M., Kenny, J.M., Puglia, D., Santulli, C., Sarasini, F., 2010a. Morphological, thermal and mechanical characterization of okra (*Abelmoschus esculentus*) fibres as potential reinforcement in polymer composites. Combust. Sci. Technol. 70, 116–122.
De Rosa, I.M., Santulli, C., Sarasini, F., 2010b. Mechanical and thermal characterization of epoxy composites reinforced with random and quasi-unidirectional untreated Phormium tenax leaf fibers. Mater. Des. 31, 2397–2405.
Ensikat, H., Ditsche-Kuru, P., Neinhuis, C., Barthlott, W., 2011. Superhydrophobicity in perfection: the outstanding properties of the lotus leaf. Beilstein J. Nanotechnol. 2, 152–161.
Evans, K., Alderson, A., 2000. Auxetic materials: functional materials and structures from lateral thinking! Adv. Mater. 12, 617–628.
Facca, A.G., Kortschot, M.T., Yan, N., 2006. Predicting the elastic modulus of natural fibre reinforced thermoplastics. Compos. A: Appl. Sci. Manuf. 37, 1660–1671.
Fernandez, J., Ingber, D., 2012. Unexpected strength and toughness in chitosan-fibroin laminates inspired by insect cuticle. Adv. Mater. 24, 480–484.
Fortunati, E., Puglia, D., Monti, M., Peponi, L., Santulli, C., Kenny, J.M., et al., 2012. Extraction of cellulose nanocrystals from Phormium tenax fibres. J. Polym. Environ. 21, 319–328.
Fortunati, E., Puglia, D., Monti, M., Santulli, C., Maniruzzaman, M., Kenny, J.M., 2013. Cellulose nanocrystals extracted from okra fibers in PVA nanocomposites. J. Appl. Polym. Sci. 128, 3220–3230.
Frolich, L., La Barbera, M., Stevens, W., 1994. Poisson's ratio of a crossed fibre sheath: the skin of aquatic salamanders. J. Zool. 232, 231–252.
Gao, H., Wang, X., Yao, H., Gorb, S., Arzt, E., 2005. Mechanics of hierarchical adhesion structures of geckos. Mech. Mater. 37, 275–285.
Gibson, L.J., 2012. The hierarchical structure and mechanics of plant materials. J. R. Soc. Interface 9, 2749–2766.
Gorb, A., Varenberg, M., Peressadko, A., Tuma, J., 2007. Biomimetic mushroom-shaped fibrillar adhesive microstructure. J. R. Soc. Interface 4, 271–275.
Gravish, N., Wilkinson, M., Autumn, K., 2008. Frictional and elastic energy in gecko adhesive detachment. J. R. Soc. Interface 5, 339–348.
Gravish, N., Wilkinson, M., Sponberg, S., Parness, A., Esparza, N., Soto, D., et al., 2010. Rate-dependent frictional adhesion in natural and synthetic gecko setae. J. R. Soc. Interface 7, 259–269.
Gu, Y., Huang, J., 2009. Fabrication of natural cellulose substance derived hierarchical polymeric materials. J. Mater. Chem. 19, 3764–3770.
Gutiérrez, M., Ferrer, M., del Monte, F., 2008. Ice-templated materials: sophisticated structures exhibiting enhanced functionalities obtained after unidirectional freezing and ice-segregation-induced self-assembly. Chem. Mater. 20, 634–648.
Harrington, M., Gupta, H., Fratzl, P., Waite, J., 2009. Collagen insulated from tensile damage by domains that unfold reversibly: in situ X-ray investigation of mechanical yield and damage repair in the mussel byssus. J. Struct. Biol. 167, 1115–1123.
Jiang, F., Hsieh, Y.-L., 2014. Super water absorbing and shape memory nanocellulose aerogels from TEMPO-oxidized cellulose nanofibrils via cyclic freezing–thawing. J. Mater. Chem. A 2, 350–359.
Jin, M., Feng, X., Xi, J., Zhai, J., Cho, K., Feng, L., et al., 2005. Super-hydrophobic PDMS surface with ultra-low adhesive force. Macromol. Rapid Commun. 26, 1805–1809.
Kalia, S., Kaith, B., Kaur, I., 2009. Pretreatments of natural fibers and their application as reinforcing material in polymer composites—a review. Polym. Eng. Sci. 49, 1253–1272.

Klemm, D., Kramer, F., Moritz, S., Lindström, T., Ankerfors, M., Gray, D., et al., 2011. Nanocelluloses: a new family of nature-based materials. Angew. Chem. Int. Ed. 50, 5438–5466.

Koch, K., Barthlott, W., 2009. Superhydrophobic and superhydrophilic plant surfaces: an inspiration for biomimetic materials. Philos. Transact. A Math. Phys. Eng. Sci. 367, 1487–1509.

Kolmakov, G., Revanur, R., Tangirala, R., Emrick, T., Russell, T., Crosby, A., et al., 2010. Using nanoparticle-filled microcapsules for site-specific healing of damaged substrates: creating a "repair-and-go" system. ACS Nano 4, 1115–1123.

Ku, H., Wang, H., Pattarachaiyakoop, N., Trada, M., 2011. A review on the tensile properties of natural fiber reinforced polymer composites. Compos. Part B 42, 856–873.

Lee, B., Dalsin, J., Messersmith, P., 2006. Biomimetic adhesive polymers based on mussel adhesive proteins. In: Smith, A., Callow, J. (Eds.), Biological Adhesives. Springer Verlag, Berlin Heidelberg, pp. 257–278.

Lee, H., Lee, B.P., Messersmith, P.B., 2007. A reversible wet/dry adhesive inspired by mussels and geckos. Nature 448, 338–341.

Lee, J., Majidi, C., Schubert, B., Fearing, R.S., 2008. Sliding-induced adhesion of stiff polymer microfibre arrays. I. Macroscale behaviour. J. R. Soc. Interface 5, 835–844.

Lee, K.-Y., Ho, K., Schlufter, K., Bismarck, A., 2012. Hierarchical composites reinforced with robust short sisal fibre preforms utilising bacterial cellulose as binder. Compos. Sci. Technol. 72, 1479–1486.

Lees, C., Vincent, J., Hillerton, J., 1991. Poisson's ratio in skin. Bio-Med. Mater. Eng. 1, 19–23.

Liao, S.S., Cui, F.Z., Zhang, W., Feng, Q.L., 2004. Hierarchically biomimetic bone scaffold materials: nano-HA/collagen/PLA composite. J. Biomed. Mater. Res., Part B 69, 158–165.

Lim, T.-T., Huang, X., 2007. Evaluation of kapok (*Ceiba pentandra* (L.) Gaertn.) as a natural hollow hydrophobic-oleophilic fibrous sorbent for oil spill cleanup. Chemosphere 66, 955–963.

Lin, A., Meyers, M.A., 2005. Growth and structure in abalone shell. Mater. Sci. Eng., A 390, 27–41.

Liu, K., Jiang, L., 2011. Review bio-inspired design of multiscale structures for function integration. Nano Today 6, 155–175.

Liu, M., Wang, S., Wei, Z., Song, Y., Jiang, L., 2009. Bioinspired design of a superoleophobic and low adhesive water/solid interface. Adv. Mater. 21, 665–669.

Luz, G.M., Mano, J.F., 2009. Biomimetic design of materials and biomaterials inspired by the structure of nacre. Philos. Transact. A Math. Phys. Eng. Sci. 367, 1587–1605.

Ma, J., Zhang, M., Wu, H., Yin, X., Chen, J., Jiang, Z., 2010. Mussel-inspired fabrication of structurally stable chitosan/polyacrylonitrile composite membrane for pervaporation dehydration. J. Membr. Sci. 348, 150–159.

Macior, L., 1960. The tetrakaidecahedron and related cell forms in undifferentiated plant tissues. Bull. Torrey Bot. Club 87, 99–138.

Masselter, T., Speck, T., 2011. Biomimetic fiber-reinforced compound materials. In: Cavrak, M. (Ed.), Advances in Biomimetics. InTech, p. 522.

Meyers, M., Lin, A., Seki, Y., Chen, P.-Y., Kad, B., Bodde, S., 2006. Structural biological composites: an overview. JOM 58, 35–41.

Meyers, M.A., Chen, P.-Y., Lin, A.Y.-M., Seki, Y., 2008. Biological materials: structure and mechanical properties. Prog. Mater. Sci. 53, 1–206.

Miessner, M., Peter, M.G., Vincent, J.F., 2001. Preparation of insect-cuticle-like biomimetic materials. Biomacromolecules 2, 369–372.

Miller, W., Smith, C.W., Scarpa, F.L., Abramovich, H., Evans, K.E., 2008. Multifunctional negative poisson's ratio (auxetic) honeycomb cores with embedded piezo-ceramic patches. In: European Conference on Composite Materials 13, Stockholm, Sweden.

Milwich, M., Burgert, I., Seidl, R., Speck, T., Speck, O., Planck, H., 2007. Plant stems as role models for structurally optimized biomimetic composite profiles with gradient structure. Comp. Biochem. Physiol., Part A: Mol. Integr. Physiol. 146, S131–S132.

Mishnaevsky Jr., L., 2011. Hierarchical composites: analysis of damage evolution based on fiber bundle model. Compos. Sci. Technol. 71, 450–460.

Monteiro, S.N., Lopes, F.P.D., Barbosa, A.P., Bevitori, A.B., Da Silva, I.L.A., Da Costa, L.L., 2011. Natural lignocellulosic fibers as engineering materials—an overview. Metall. Mater. Trans. A 42, 2963–2974.

Morán, J.I., Alvarez, V.A., Cyras, V.P., Vázquez, A., 2007. Extraction of cellulose and preparation of nanocellulose from sisal fibers. Cellulose 15, 149–159.

Munch, E., Launey, M., Alsem, D., Saiz, E., Tomsia, A., Ritchie, R., 2008. Tough, bio-inspired hybrid materials. Science 322, 1516–1520.

Muthukumar, T., Aravinthan, A., Lakshmia, K., Venkatesan, R., Vedaprakash, L., Doble, M., 2011. Fouling and stability of polymers and composites in marine environment. Int. Biodeterior. Biodegrad. 65, 276–284.

Mwaikambo, L.Y., Ansell, M.P., Dufresne, A., Hughes, M., Hill, C., Wild, P.M., 2001. Current international research into cellulosic fibres and composites. J. Mater. Sci. 36, 2107–2131.

Nechaev, S., Voituriez, R., 2001. On the plant leaf's boundary, "jupe a godets" and conformal embeddings. J. Phys. A: Math. Gen. 34, 11069–11082.

Norris, C., 2011. Self-healing fibre reinforced composites via a bioinspired vasculature. Adv. Funct. Mater. 21, 3624–3633.

Norris, C.J., Bond, I.P., Trask, R.S., 2011. The role of embedded bioinspired vasculature on damage formation in self-healing carbon fibre reinforced composites. Compos. Part A 42, 639–648.

Olah, L., Borbas, L., 2008. Properties of calcium carbonate-containing composite scaffolds. Acta of Bioengineering and Biomechanics/Wrocław Univ. Technol. 10, 61–66.

Onck, P., Van Merkerk, R., Raaijmakers, A., De Hosson, J., 2005. Fracture of open-and closed-cell metal foams. J. Mater. Sci. 40, 5821–5828.

Pang, J.W.C., Bond, I.P., 2005a. A hollow fibre reinforced polymer composite encompassing self-healing and enhanced damage visibility. Combust. Sci. Technol. 65, 1791–1799.

Pang, J.W.C., Bond, I.P., 2005b. "Bleeding composites"—damage detection and self-repair using a biomimetic approach. Compos. A: Appl. Sci. Manuf. 36, 183–188.

Podsiadlo, P., Paternel, S., Rouillard, J., Zhang, Z., Lee, J., Lee, J., et al., 2005. Layer-by-layer assembly of nacre-like nanostructured composites with antimicrobial properties. Langmuir 21, 11915–11921.

Riley, M., Whitney, J., 1966. Elastic properties of fiber reinforced composite materials. AIAA J. 4, 1537–1542.

Rizzo, N.W., Gardner, K.H., Walls, D.J., Keiper-Hrynko, N.M., Ganzke, T.S., Hallahan, D.L., 2006. Characterization of the structure and composition of gecko adhesive setae. J. R. Soc. Interface/R. Soc. 3, 441–451.

Robertson, B., Hillerton, J., Vincent, J., 1984. The presence of zinc or manganese as the predominant metal in the mandibles of adult stored product beetles. J. Stored Prod. Res. 20, 133–137.

Sanchez, C., Arribart, H., Guille, M.M.G., 2005. Biomimetism and bioinspiration as tools for the design of innovative materials and systems. Nat. Mater. 4, 277–288.

Santulli, C., 2008. A biomimetic approach to the production of sustainable structural composites using plant fibres. In: Ellison, M.S., Abbott, A.G. (Eds.), Biologically inspired textiles. Woodhead Publishing Limited, Rijeka, Croatia.

Santulli, C., Sarasini, F., Tirillò, J., Valente, T., Valente, M., Caruso, A.P., et al., 2013. Mechanical behaviour of jute cloth/wool felts hybrid laminates. Mater. Des. 50, 309–321.
Scarpa, F., Panayiotou, P., Tomlinson, G., 2000. Numerical and experimental uniaxial loading on in-plane auxetic honeycombs. J. Strain Anal. 35, 383–388.
Schubert, B., Lee, J., Majidi, C., Fearing, R.S., 2008. Sliding-induced adhesion of stiff polymer microfibre arrays. II. Microscale behaviour. J. R. Soc. Interface/R. Soc. 5, 845–853.
Seepersad, C.C., Kumar, R.S., Allen, J.K., Mistree, F., Mcdowell, D.L., 2005. Multifunctional design of prismatic cellular materials. J. Comput.-Aided Mater. Des. 11, 163–181.
Shahinpoor, M., 2011. Biomimetic robotic Venus flytrap (Dionaea muscipula Ellis) made with ionic polymer metal composites. Bioinspir. Biomim 6, 046004.
Shi, J., Alves, N.M., Mano, J.F., 2008. Towards bioinspired superhydrophobic poly(L-lactic acid) surfaces using phase inversion-based methods. Bioinspir. Biomim. 3, 034003.
Spolenak, R., Gorb, S., Arzt, E., 2005. Adhesion design maps for bio-inspired attachment systems. Acta Biomater. 1, 5–13.
Tampieri, A., Celotti, G., Landi, E., Sandri, M., Roveri, N., Falini, G., 2003. Biologically inspired synthesis of bone-like composite: self-assembled collagen fibers/hydroxyapatite nanocrystals. J. Biomed. Mater. Res. 67, 618–625.
Tampieri, A., Sandri, M., Landi, E., Celotti, G., Roveri, N., Mattioli-Belmonte, M., et al., 2005. HA/alginate hybrid composites prepared through bio-inspired nucleation. Acta Biomater. 1, 343–351.
Tang, Z., Kotov, N., Magonov, S., Ozturk, B., 2003. Nanostructured artificial nacre. Nat. Mater. 2, 413–418.
Trask, R.S., Williams, H.R., Bond, I.P., 2007. Self-healing polymer composites: mimicking nature to enhance performance. Bioinspir. Biomim. 2, P1–P9.
Vecchio, K.S., Zhang, X., Massie, J.B., Wang, M., Kim, C.W., 2007. Conversion of bulk seashells to biocompatible hydroxyapatite for bone implants. Acta Biomater. 3, 910–918.
Venkata Reddy, G., Venkata Naidu, S., Shobha, Rani T., 2008. Impact properties of kapok based unsaturated polyester hybrid composites. J. Reinf. Plast. Compos. 27, 1789–1804.
Veronda, D.R., Westmann, R.A., 1970. Mechanical characterization of skin—finite deformations. J. Biomech. 3, 111–122.
Vincent, J., 2002. Arthropod cuticle: a natural composite shell system. Compos. A 33, 1311–1315.
Vincent, J., Wegst, U., 2004. Design and mechanical properties of insect cuticle. Arthropod Struct. Dev. 33, 187–199.
Viney, C., 2004. Self-assembly as a route to fibrous materials: concepts, opportunities and challenges. Curr. Opin. Solid State Mater. Sci. 8, 95–101.
Waite, J., 1990. Marine adhesive proteins: natural composite thermosets. Int. J. Biol. Macromol. 12, 139–144.
Yu, W.-D., 2010. The bio-inspired study of homogeneous composite materials. J. Compos. Mater. 45, 113–125.
Yu, S.-H., Cölfen, H., 2004. Bio-inspired crystal morphogenesis by hydrophilic polymers. J. Mater. Chem. 14, 2124–2147.

Solving the bio-machine interface—a synthetic biology approach

3

O. Yarkoni, D.J. Frankel

3.1 Introduction

Interfacing biological cells/tissue with man-made machines has the potential to revolutionize robotics and medical technology. There are a number of biohybrid robots in development with this aim in mind (Ricotti et al., 2012), for example, one device that adheres bacteria to solid substrates to create bacteria-propelled rafts (Kim et al., 2012). However, there are usually insurmountable obstacles to their success. A good illustration to such obstacles is attempts to control a robot with explanted frog muscles. These hybrid devices lack an appropriate mechanism for controlling muscle contraction (Herr and Dennis, 2004), meaning that the robot body could thrash around a water tank but was unable to navigate a path defined by the controller. Similarly, there has been enormous interest in the development of biohybrid machines created from cultured muscle, but again these methods lack any mechanism for controlling contraction (Kim et al., 2008). This chapter has been written to familiarize the reader with the difficulties of cell/electronics communication and introduce some of the many approaches taken to overcome the difficulties. It will be loosely divided into three parts: an introduction to biosensors and the bio-electronic interface, approaches to using cells in devices, and the use of synthetic biology to improve cell/system compatibility. A wide variety of cells and systems designed to facilitate the aforementioned communication will be discussed, including bacterial, mammalian, and functional tissue.

3.2 Definition of the bio-machine interface

Interfacing biological tissue or cells with nonbiological materials does not necessarily produce a bio-machine interface. In the case that no dynamic mechanical or electronic function is to be performed by the device, the interface can be considered as biomaterial. When the interface is between biological systems such as tissue or cells and a functioning device, that is a device that can perform tasks, the interface is bio-machine. This definition can be further expanded to include biosensors that themselves have a bio-machine interface, but one which usually involves individual cells, or groups of cells, rather than tissues. Although these definitions encompass some gray areas, one can generally assume that the bio-machine interface requires overcoming some natural barriers between the biological and nonbiological components. A biosensor is a device that utilizes a mechanism of biological origin to detect a species and subsequently converts the signal into an interpretable reading. It can also include mechanisms that are nonbiological but detect biological species. This can be achieved using enzymes, receptors, or cells as the biological component. The bio-electronic interface is a subset area within biosensors. That is, a biosensor does not necessarily convert biological signal to an electronic output. For example, a much used biosensor is based on the quartz crystal microbalance which can convert specific receptor/ligand interactions into a change in resonant frequency of a quartz crystal (Ogi et al., 2010; Saitakis et al., 2010). The frequency change is subsequently processed via electronics but the signal of interest is the frequency shift. In contrast, the bio-electronic interface involves either a direct conversion of biological signal to electrical current flow or a more indirect route using intermediates but still with the result of trying to measure a difference in electronic signal. We can also open up the bio-electronic interface to include the interfacing of optical devices with biological cells and tissue. The reasoning here is that optical stimuli can be programmed into well-defined patterns, from pulses to continuous emission, thus allowing computer-generated algorithms to be transmitted to biological systems.

3.3 Historical perspective

When discussing the history of the bio-machine interface, it is appropriate to start with biosensors as many of the developments in this technology were later employed in other biohybrid devices. The earliest biosensor was developed in 1962 by Clark and Lyons (1962), an amperometric enzyme reaction-based electrochemical sensor capable of detecting glucose levels from blood samples. This was accomplished using the enzyme glucose oxidase and combining it with an electrode sensitive to dissolved oxygen. In this way, the oxidation of glucose could be monitored via a change in current from the electrode. This allowed the amount of glucose present in the sample to be detected directly. To this day, glucose sensors utilize this principle, a medical application of biosensors which has improved the quality of life for millions of diabetes patients. Although the field has developed significantly since this seminal discovery in the 1960s, the major principles involved remain identical.

A historical perspective on the bio-machine interface would not be complete without a discussion of electrodes/microelectrodes used to stimulate and record from neurons. Microelectrode arrays for *in vitro* interfacing with neural tissue have led to implantable microelectrode arrays for the treatment of blindness caused by macular degeneration. One of the pioneering implantable devices for neural interfacing was the Utah microelectrode array developed in the mid 1980s. These devices are not after single-cell resolution; rather they stimulate many neurons at a time. Consisting of up to 100 spike-like electrodes fabricated from silicon (Figure 3.1), they can be implanted in either the cerebral cortex or the peripheral nerves.

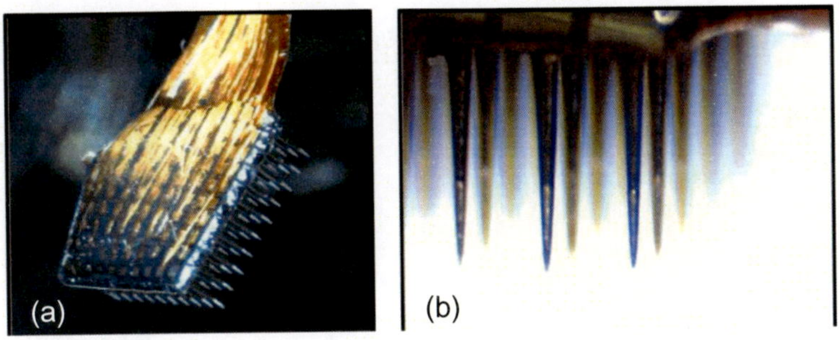

Figure 3.1 Multielectrode arrays used to record and stimulate neuronal activity.
(a) Cyberkinetics silicon-based 100 channel multielectrode array. (b) View of the spike electrodes that interface with the tissue.
Published with permission from Elsevier Ward et al. (2009).

From the early experiments with electrode stimulation of neurons to the fully implantable visual prosthesis, the progress to usable technology has demonstrated the progression from *in vitro* to *in vivo* devices. In much the same vain, new bio-electronic interfacing technology starts *in vitro*. One of the most exciting examples of this is work using novel nanotechnologies to stimulate and take electrical measurements from a single neuron (Patolsky et al., 2006). This was achieved by building arrays of field-effect transistors from silicon nanowires and connecting them to individual neurons. These were then able to record neuronal signals and stimulate the cells at precisely defined locations. For example, the transistors were able to address the neurons at user-defined positions along the cell dendrites (neuronal projections) and along the cell body. The potential of these nanoscale devices lies in the ability to address single cells precisely and also the possibility of integrating these tiny devices into larger electronic systems. A recent breakthrough in fabricating bio-electronic materials was reported in 2012 and involves integrating electronics with tissue (Tian et al., 2012). This "cyborg" tissue uses passivated nanoelectric scaffolds, which demonstrate biocompatibility and the ability to record electrical signals (Figure 3.2). Their fabrication technology offers potential for the wiring of bionic devices within wet and living biological tissue.

3.4 Cells as biosensors

Cell-based biosensors use living cells to monitor the immediate environment and detect changes in physiological conditions. This change in condition could be the introduction of a pathogen, toxins, or a subtle increase in the concentration of an analyte (Stenger et al., 2001). It is also feasible to manipulate the preexisting cellular machinery with the ultimate goal of using cells as sensors in their own right. However, progress is currently limited to subtle manipulation of the cellular machinery transforming the cells into transducers for the conversion of an input into a chemical,

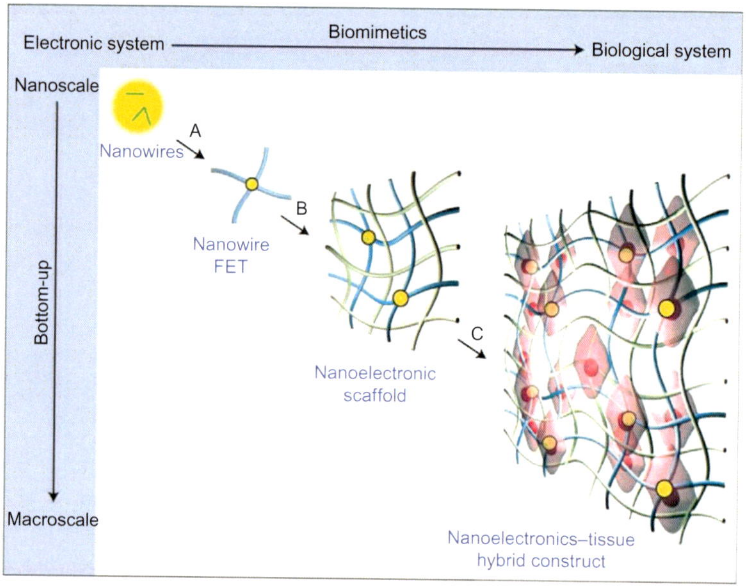

Figure 3.2 General principle of nanoelectric scaffold/tissue hybrid. (a) Fabrication of single nanowire field-effect transistors (FETs). (b) Formation of 3D nanowire FET matrices and hybridization with the extracellular matrix. (c) Integration with cells and tissue through biological processes.
Reprinted by permission from Macmillan Publishers Ltd: [Nature Materials] Tian et al. (2012).

optical, or electrical signal (Aravanis et al., 2001; Feng et al., 2007; Moschopoulou and Kintzios, 2006).

Nature has provided the cell with an extremely specific and subtle detection capability. Combined with the means to process information and parallel pathways, the cell has the potential to be harnessed as the ultimate biosensor. Some sensors use this principle directly, by redirecting the output signal to a stimulus that the cell is already programmed to interpret. It is now also possible, albeit within limits, to adapt preexisting cellular machinery to detect certain changes in extracellular environment. This is achieved using the principles of genetic engineering and the techniques of synthetic biology.

One successful approach to the conversion of cells into sensors utilized cryo-immobilized *Escherichia coli* cells that had been genetically modified to produce organophosphate hydrolase (Owicki et al., 1994). This enzyme is capable of cleaving P–CN, P–F, PO, and P–S bonds, generating two protons per cleavage reaction. Due to the direct relationship between the amount of organophosphate that is hydrolyzed and the increase of protons in solution, the change of pH is proportional to the amount of organophosphate in solution, thus the system could be monitored with a pH sensor. Sensitivities achieved were high at 0.001–1 mM with a response time of 10–20 min. In addition, the cellular component of the sensor was found to be suitably active for over two months when stored appropriately.

A contrasting approach for using cells as transducers can be found in the work of Rider et al. (2014). B cells were genetically modified to produce the luminescent protein Aequorin within their cytosol. This protein is both bioluminescent and sensitive to calcium. The Aequorin is released when the pathogen/antibody-binding event occurs. Detection limits were found to be as low as 20 colony forming units of the chosen pathogen, although higher densities produced more reliable results. However, its potential applications are limited as it requires complex machinery to detect/transduce the cellular signal making the technology only suitable for clinical laboratories. A more direct approach to the conversion of cells into sensor components is seen in the work of Smutok et al. (2007). In this work, *Hansenula polymorpha* yeast was engineered to overproduce Flavocytochrome b_2 and was successfully used to detect L-lactate. The cells were immobilized directly onto a graphite electrode surface, either by use of a dialysis membrane or via electrodeposition of a polymer. Cells were also permeabilized using cetyltrimethylammonium bromide to increase diffusion rates.

3.5 Difficulties in addressing the bio-electronic interface

A major bottleneck to overcome is how to convert a biological input into an electrical output, which is both measurable and accurate. In other words, if a cell senses a molecule by its binding to a receptor, how can this biomolecular event be converted into an electronic signal that is to be read by a computer? What are the obstacles for cells to communicate and/or be stimulated directly with electronics? Some cells present an easily detectable electrical signal, i.e., neurons; however, many events at the cellular level do not present a signal which can be directly communicated to machinery. Cells can function as transducers themselves, transforming a stimulus into a detectable signal such as a photon, a chemical analyte, or a change in cell wall potential.

Neurons are optimal cells for signal transfer and transduction. Their capability of electrical signaling renders their signal directly interpretable by electronics. The ability of neurons to communicate with each other has been widely reported and attempts to harness this trait have already been made. An example can be found in the work of Thewes et al., where neurons were grown into networks on top of a chip (Eickenscheidt et al, 2012). The strategy relies on the precise immobilization of neurons on field-effect transistors. This is accomplished by trapping the neurons within a ring of polyamide pillars so as to ensure contact with the two transistors, a stimulation and an open field-effect transistor. Neuronal connections occur between cells as axons grow and communication signals between cells can be detected and monitored using a CMOS system. Although there is an untold amount of potential in using neurons, their method of operation is still not fully understood and growing them selectively onto electrodes remains a challenge. In addition, this type of cell is highly sensitive to contamination and requires a very specific environment.

There are some additional limitations to interfacing cells with electronics. It has been demonstrated that close proximity to a high potential (such as those generated by electrode surfaces) causes irregular cell growth, hysteresis, and irregular cellular behavior (Oni et al., 2004). This poses a significant problem to the cell-electronic interface as distance between cells and electrodes limits their mode of operation. If cells cannot be in direct contact with the electronic component's surface, then certain methods of signal generation become incompatible, i.e., cell wall potential changes. In their work, the aforementioned group designed a possible solution to this discovered effect. It was proposed that implementing a cellagen© layer separating the cells from the electrode surface would most likely do away with the observed effects of cellular proximity to high potential.

A unique approach to improving the cell-electronics interface was taken by Valderrama et al. (1995). A successful interface between nerve cells and a microelectrode array allowed *in vivo* signal detection and recording. To achieve this difficult feet, the bio-electronic interface was solved using an implantable microelectrode array on silicon-doped chip with *via* holes. It was shown that axons can regenerate through the *via* holes and that communication is resumed in a fashion that becomes measurable. Platinum electrodes were optimal for this task due to their low electrode–electrolyte impedance and good charge delivery. Using *via* holes as an electrode surface greatly increases the interface surface area, which can therefore allow for a greater accuracy of measurement. With this approach, the total exposed surface area is relatively large even though the electrode itself is quite small. Another step to improve the cell-sensor interface was accomplished by including a peptide-functionalized surface to improve cell adhesion and promote neurite growth.

Sensors that are designed to enter the environment of the human body must be non-toxic and not interfere with cell behavior. Achieving the latter can be a complicated task. In the case of electrochemical detection, cells need to remain at a certain distance from the electrode and its operating potential, in order to remain undisturbed (Oni et al., 2004). Conversely as well as the sensor harming the environment, the environment can harm the sensor. *In vivo*, the bodies multiple defense mechanisms can interfere with sensor function. This type of detrimental interaction between the sensor and the host is called biofouling and is one of the major causes of *in vivo* sensor failure. It occurs via the accumulation of cells, compounds, and proteins on the sensor surface and causes a marked decrease in sensor performance and lifetime (Wisniewski and Reichert, 2000).

3.6 Synthetic biology applied to the bio-electronic interface

Over the last decade, the new field of synthetic biology has evolved. It strides to apply engineering principles to biological systems, modifying living cells to perform unnatural functions. By doing this, synthetic biology has the potential to harness the power of biological systems to perform useful tasks. In particular, cells are being engineered to produce high value chemicals, to treat disease, and to produce biologically derived energy sources. It is recent technological advances in DNA sequencing and genetic manipulation that has made this new discipline possible. One of the underlying principles of synthetic biology is the creation of biological "parts" that are interchangeable between organisms, rather like standardized mechanical components in an engineered system. These are built by manipulating the regulation machinery of genetic expression, that is, by controlling the levels of specific genetic products (proteins). In this way, genetic circuits can be built including genetic AND, OR, and NOR gates. These gates can be connected to create cells that can take a specific input and manipulate it to produce the desired output.

Genetic circuits have great potential in their ability to address the bio-electronic and bio-machine interface. A variety of genetic circuits have been implemented a variety of functions, including logic gates (e.g., AND or NOR), switches, oscillators, and time delays (Purnick and Weiss, 2009). The circuits are created by combining genetic parts such as promoters, inducers, repressors, and terminators to control the temporal and spatial expression of the target genes.

There are unique obstacles which must be considered when constructing genetic circuits when applied to the bio/electronic interface. One such obstacle is the potential for toxicity. As many substances (or enzymatic metabolites) can be toxic when present in sufficient quantities, it becomes important to consider about gene expression levels, how active is the protein, and how toxic is the metabolite. Another possible undesirable outcome can arise via the interference of any of the products/elements in the genetic circuit with the endogenous activity of the cell.

3.7 Genetic programs that perform signal processing

An example of a genetic program whose function can be confirmed visually can be found in the work of Tabor and coworkers (Tabor et al., 2009), where *E. coli* bacteria were modified to be capable of photographic edge detection (Figure 3.3). This was

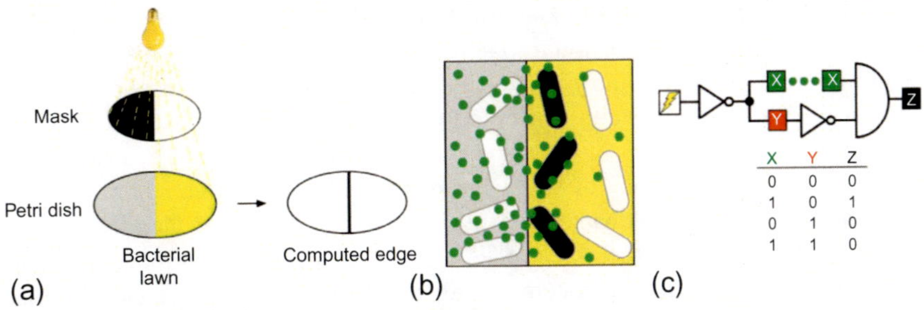

Figure 3.3 Bacterial edge detection via a synthetic biology approach and engineering genetic circuits. (a) Selective illumination of bacteria in a petri dish via use of a mask. (b) Those bacteria in the dark produce signaling molecules (green circles) which diffuse across the dark–light interface. Only bacteria in the light can respond to the signal and are programmed to express a visible reporter gene with the sum of this activity over the two-dimension space corresponding to the edges of the input image. (c) The NOT logic gate represented the lightning bold with the adjacent triangle instigates cell–cell communication, represented by the green X and an inverter represented by the red Y and adjacent triangle. The output of these two circuit elements combine as inputs for an AND gate, the semicircle, which produces the final output Z.
Published with permission from Elsevier Tabor et al. (2009).

accomplished by incorporating a combination of an X AND (NOT Y) logic gates in a genetic circuit. As the terminology implies, the signal is only carried forth when X is present and Y is absent. By having cells produce a pigment as a form of signal, the circuit was made capable of defining edges of light incidence. The engineered cells produce a chemical signal upon light stimulus at the specific wavelength of 650 nm, while having the pigment-producing gene under a restriction that makes it unable to produce in the presence of light. Once switched on, the chemical signal diffuses across the cell population, and over time it activates pigment production in neighboring cells which have not been directly exposed to light.

Quantitative genetic responses are well documented throughout the natural world. This is particularly true in developmental genetics. Gradients of proteins have been found to be at least partially responsible for stem cell division and mother/daughter cell differentiation (Discher et al., 2009). Such processes are part of a complex sequence of expression, transcription, and translation as well as protein migration. Effectively, stem cells are controlling spatiotemporal expression of genes and their products in order to determine which cells will undergo differentiation and which ones will simply undergo self-renewal.

It is important to note, however, that this is mostly thought to be dependent on threshold values rather than specific concentrations. Examining these natural systems has been a key to developing synthetic biology methods of controlling spatiotemporal protein expression. An example of a synthetically engineered quantitative response can be found in the work of Weiss et al. (Basu et al., 2005; Weiss et al., 2003). Cells were engineered to respond to multiple gradients of AHL, with two different responses depending on the concentration of the analyte. Engineering of these mutant cells involved incorporating many of the parts used within the previously described edge detection system, further demonstrating the versatility of the genetic "parts" used.

Synthetic gene circuits have been harnessed to enable cell-based electrochemical detection. A bacterial whole cell sensor was constructed based on cell wall damage reporting for the detection of water toxicity (Neufeld et al., 2006). This was achieved using the *fabA* promoter and *fabR* repressor. The *fabA* gene is responsible for the expression of unsaturated fatty acids (cell wall constituents) and is induced by interruptions in the biosynthesis of fatty acids. This promoter was fused to a promoterless *lacZ* gene so that expression of *lacZ* was controlled by the actions of *fabA* and *fabR*. The resulting recombinant bacteria were then placed into electrochemical cells containing screen-printed carbon electrodes coupled to a Ag/AgCl reference electrode. The resulting bio-electronic system was then tested with varying concentrations of phenol and found to be successful, with a detection time frame of approximately 20 min and sensitivity of up to 1.6 ppm of aminophenol. Aminophenol is the result of the cleavage of *p*-aminophenylgalactoside by *lacZ* and is the agent responsible for electrochemical detection within this system. Due to the system being DNA damage dependant, several other toxic compounds were found to activate the system, including toluene, hydrazine, and ethanol; however, it was unable to detect methanol or the organophosphate DDVP(2,2-dichlorovinyl dimethyl phosphate). This work showed an improvement on a previous system designed to detect cell wall damage using the same promoter/repressor system (Bechor et al., 2002). The new approach also increased lower detection limits as well as decreasing operating time by using electrochemical methods rather than fluorescence.

An additional factor to consider when designing genetic circuits to work with electronics is the time response. Many of the systems based on synthetic biology work over a relatively slow time frame, with response times ranging from tens of minutes to several hours (Tabor et al., 2009; Basu et al., 2005). This is governed by the elements used, as it takes considerably longer to go from an inactive gene to a fully functional protein than to go from an inactive protein to an active one. An example of this would be phosphorylation. Phosphorylation is a post-translational modification common to a host of proteins, and as the process is very fast, a protein can be can activated or inactivated nearly on demand. It is also important to note that there is a major limitation to the use of logic gates for building more complex engineered cells. Only a few can actually be introduced into a host system. In *E. coli*, three gates is the described limit (Weiss et al., 2003).

3.8 Optogenetics for interfacing cells/tissue with machines

Use of light to control biological tissue can allow precisely programmed stimuli to be applied, anything from ultrafast pulses, to slow delay exposure. Thus, by using light in the form of inexpensive light-emitting diodes and optical fibers, it is possible to put biological systems under computer control. Moreover, there is a major advantage of using light to interface with biological tissue as opposed to direct electrical connection. This is that light stimulation allows "action at a distance." That is there doesn't need to be a direct contact between the machine and the biological component, thereby removing the inherent difficulties in terms of resistive losses, and electrical field-induced cell damage.

The emerging field of optogenetics has been particularly successful in coupling light activation to neuronal activity via the expression of light-sensitive ion channels. These light-activated channels called Channelrhodopsins originate from algae. Using genetic engineering, it is possible to express these proteins into the cells of choice, a task made relatively simple by the fact that the single gene coding for Channelrhodopsin is less that 1 kb in size. When exposed to blue light, these transmembrane proteins undergo a conformational change, opening the channel pore, and allowing an influx of cationic ions. The influx of ion will initiate an action potential in the excitable cell (Figure 3.4). As well as Channelrhodopsin, there are a variety of light-sensitive ion channels, excitable by different wavelengths of light, and with different switching characteristics. Moreover, commonly used genetic engineering techniques can be used to vary the expression levels, thus altering the light-sensitive properties of the transfected cells. Stimulation can be via a variety of sources including light emitting diode, laser, or lamp.

A variety of light-sensitive ion channels and advanced genetic engineering strategies have been utilized to photostimulate neurons (Zhang et al., 2006).

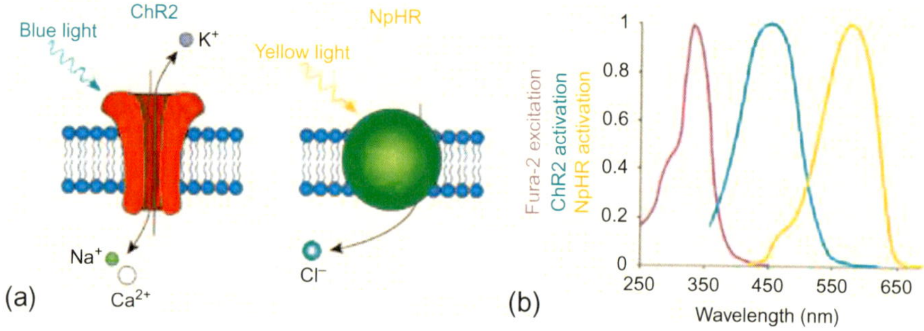

Figure 3.4 (a) Light-sensitive channelrhodopsin-2 (ChR2) and the halorhodopsin (NpHR) pump. Upon illumination with blue light, the light-sensitive ion channel allows the entry of cations into the cell. NphR is activated by yellow light. (b) Adsorption spectra for the two light-activated proteins have sufficient separation so that they can both be excited without interference.

Reprinted by permission from Macmillan Publishers Ltd: [Nature] Hausser and Smith (2007).

Furthermore, mutant Channelrhodopsins have been engineered which are 70 times more light-sensitive than the wild-type variety, and particularly conductive to Ca^{2+}, thus presenting a range of synthetic biology building blocks for the interfacing of electrically excitable cells with light (Kleinlogel et al., 2011). Although the field of optogenetics has been built around applications in neuroscience, more recent work has explored the possibility of using optogenetics to control muscle contraction. Success in this area would allow the interfacing of muscle tissue actuators to control robots, via the programmed flashing of light-emitting diodes. Furthermore, it could even be possible to engineer organs *in vivo* to respond to light impulses.

A major breakthrough in this field has been made whereby cardiac function could be controlled by light impulses inside a living zebrafish (Arrenberg et al., 2010). Light-sensitive ion channels, including channelrhodopsin, were expressed in cardiomyocytes. These genetically engineered pacemaker cells were located within the zebrafish heart and illuminated with light. In this way, the heart could be controllably sped up and slowed down. It was even possible to initiate cardiac arrest. It is with this approach one could envisage the development of biohybrid implantable organs, capable of being controlled using flashing light-emitting diodes, and ultimately controlled by a microprocessor.

Engineered light-activated cells have been taken one step further to create an implantable device capable of aiding blood glucose levels in mice (Ye et al., 2010). Implants containing genetically engineered cells were able to produce a peptide resulting in the attenuation of glycemic excursions in diabetic mice. The novelty of this technique lies in the manipulation and optical control of a complete signaling pathway using transgenic techniques. This could be a starting point for the optically controlled release of drugs via a patient's own cells. In terms of the bio-machine interface, the light source itself can be programmed to maximize genetic expression of the proteins/peptides by either pulsing the light or using continuous exposure.

An optogenetic strategy has been successfully applied to the light-activated control of muscle contraction (Sakar et al., 2012). Muscle cells were genetically engineered to express light-activated ion channels, which upon incidence of blue light would allow an influx of ions, initiating an action potential. The individual cells were encouraged to form muscle tissue and their contraction could be measured by force sensors (Figure 3.5). Response to optical stimulation in terms of dynamic tension in the muscle construct is on the timescale of seconds (Figure 3.6), and the constructs were able to achieve multiple degree of freedom movement. With such a quick response, this technique offers the possibility of biological actuation of mechanical devices, in particular, robots.

A more direct approach to navigating the cell-machine interface has been taken by exploiting biological transduction of an optical input to produce a machine-readable output (Yarkoni et al., 2012). A synthetic biology approach was applied, resulting in cells that can quickly respond to light with a machine-readable signal. Upon light incidence, the mutant mammalian cells release gaseous nitric oxide resulting in a sizeable current increase recorded by the electrode. Furthermore, the cells were able to exhibit switching behavior, which is a current response due to switching on and off

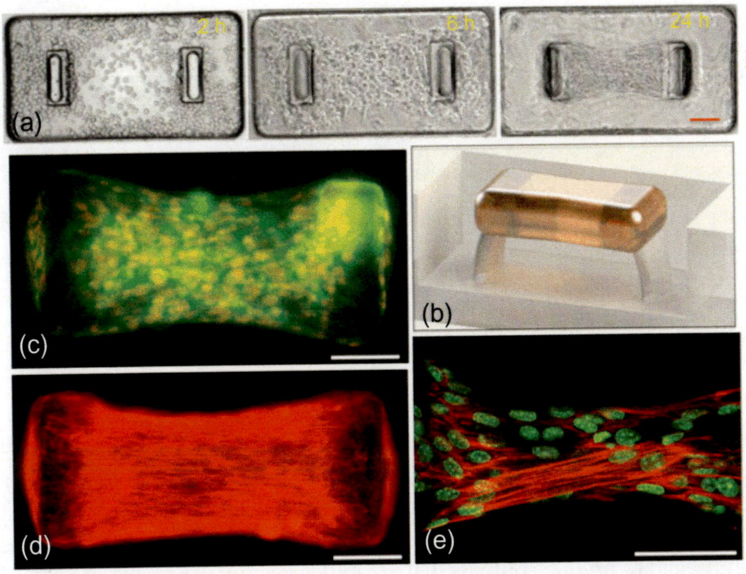

Figure 3.5 Muscle tissue constructs tethered to force sensors. (a) Images representing time course of a tissue construct. (b) CAD model of a single construct. (c) Fluorescence image of construct with nuclei stained red and membrane bound GFP. (d) Fluorescence image of F-actin (red) demonstrating alignment of myoblasts in the direction of stress gradients. (e) Remodeling of actin (red) with multinucleated myotubes.
Reproduced from Sakar et al (2012) with permission of the Royal Society of Chemistry.

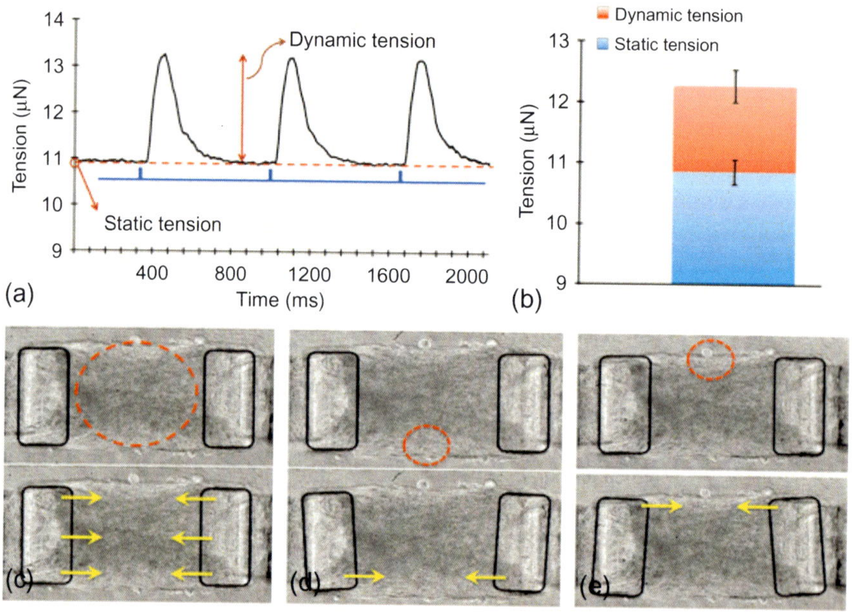

Figure 3.6 Properties of muscle constructs with local stimulation. (a) Recording of the static and dynamic tension of a construct. The tissue is stimulated with a blue light pulse series (indicated by the blue bars). (b) Dynamic and static tension, average of 50 constructs with the error bars being SEM. (c–e) Multidegree of freedom actuation.
Reproduced from Sakar et al (2012) with permission of the Royal Society of Chemistry.

the light source. Mutants were created with two different fusion sites of the LOV (light-capturing domain) with the nitric oxide synthase enzyme. Both mutants show the same magnitude of photosensitivity.

3.9 Conclusions

With the emergence of synthetic biology techniques, cells have a new role in biohyrbid devices that are no longer passive and reliant on natural biological pathways. Cells and biological tissue can be manipulated in order to put biological systems under optical control and to produce outputs that are either machine-readable or useful for driving a device. In particular, genetic circuits allow the "hacking" of biological signaling pathways to allow cells to work in device-like functions. When combined with tissue engineering, synthetic biology can produce muscle constructs capable of device actuation in response to optical stimuli. Development of part biological, part machine devices, which have in the past been out of reach due to the difficulties of traversing the bio-electronic interface, are now a realistic possibility as the limit of electronic probes is no longer the limiting factor.

References

Aravanis, A.M., Debusschere, B.D., Chruscinski, A.J., Gilchrist, K.H., Kobilka, B.K., Kovacs, G.T.A., 2001. A genetically engineered cell-based biosensor for functional classification of agents. Biosens. Bioelectron. 16, 571–577.

Arrenberg, A.B., Stainier, D.Y.R., Baier, H., Huisken, J., 2010. Optogenetic control of cardiac function. Science 330 (2010), 971–974.

Basu, S., Gerchman, Y., Collins, C.H., 2005. A synthetic multicellular system for programmed pattern formation. Nature 434, 1130–1134.

Bechor, O., Smulski, D.R., Dyk, T.K.V., Larossa, R.A., Belkin, S., 2002. Recombinant microorganisms as environmental biosensors: pollutants detection by *Escherichia coli* bearing fabA'::lux fusions. J. Biotechnol. 94, 125–132.

Clark, L.C., Lyons, C., 1962. Electrode systems for continuous monitoring in cardiovascular surgery. Ann. N. Y. Acad. Sci. 102 (1), 29–45.

Discher, D.E., Mooney, D.J., Zandstra, P.W., 2009. Growth factors, matrices, and forces combine and control stem cells. Science 324, 1673.

Eickenscheidt, M., Jenkner, M., Thewes, R., Fromherz, P., Zeck, G., 2012. Electric stimulation of retinal neurons in epiretinal and subretinal configuration using a multicapacitor array. J. Neurophysiol. 107, 2742–2755.

Feng, X., Castracane, J., Tokranova, N., Gracias, A., Lnenicka, G., Szaro, B.G., 2007. A living cell-based biosensor utilizing G-protein coupled receptors: principles and detection methods. Biosens. Bioelectron. 22, 3230–3237.

Hausser, M., Smith, S.L., 2007. Neuroscience: controlling neural circuits with light. Nature 446, 617–618.

Herr, H., Dennis, R.G., 2004. A swimming robot actuated by living muscle tissue. J. Neuroeng. Rehabil. 1 (1), 6.

Kim, J., Park, J., Lee, J., Yoon, E., Park, J., Park, S., 2008. Biohybrid microsystems actuated by cardiomyocytes: microcantilever, microrobot, and micropump. In: Robotics and Automation, IEEE International Conference on, IEEE, pp. 880–885.

Kim, D., Liu, A., Diller, E., Sitti, M., 2012. Chemotactic steering of bacteria propelling microbeads. Biomed. Microdevices 14, 1–9.

Kleinlogel, S., Feldbauer, K., Dempski, R.E., Fotis, H., Wood, P.G., Bamann, C., Bamberg, E., 2011. Ultra light-sensitive and fast neuronal activation with the Ca^{++} permeable channelrhodopsin catch. Nat. Neurosci. 14, 513–518.

Moschopoulou, G., Kintzios, S., 2006. Application of "membrane-engineering" to bioelectric recognition cell sensors for the ultra-sensitive detection of superoxide radical: a novel biosensor principle. Anal. Chim. Acta 574, 90–96.

Neufeld, T., Biran, D., Popovtzer, R., Erez, T., Ron, E.Z., Rishpon, J., 2006. Genetically engineered pfabA pfabR bacteria: an electrochemical whole cell biosensor for detection of water toxicity. Anal. Chem. 78 (14), 4952–4956.

Ogi, H., Nagai, H., Fukunishi, Y., Yanagida, T., Hirao, M., Nishiyama, M., 2010. Multichannel wireless-electrodeless quartz-crystal microbalance immunosensor. Anal. Chem. 82 (9), 3957–3962.

Oni, J., Pailleret, A., Isik, S., Diab, N., Radtke, I., Blöchl, A., Jackson, M., Bedioui, F., Schuhmann, W., 2004. Functionalised electrode array for the detection of nitric oxide released by endothelial cells using different NO-sensing chemistries. Anal. Bioanal. Chem. 378 (6), 1594–1600.

Owicki, J.C., Bousse, L.J., Hafeman, D.G., Kirk, G.L., Olson, J.D., Wada, H.G., Parce, J.W., 1994. The light-addressable potentiometric sensor: principles and biological applications. Annu. Rev. Biophys. Biomol. Struct. 23, 87–113.

Patolsky, F., Timko, B.P., Yu, G., Fang, Y., Greytak, A.B., Zheng, G., Lieber, C.M., 2006. Detection, stimulation, and inhibition of neuronal signals with high-density nanowire transistor arrays. Science 313, 1100–1104.

Purnick, P.E.M., Weiss, R., 2009. The second wave of synthetic biology: from modules to systems. Nat. Rev. Mol. Cell Biol. 10, 410–422. http://dx.doi.org/10.1038/nrm2698.

Ricotti, L., Menciassi, A., Morishima, K., 2012. Guest editorial introduction to the special issue on bio-hybrid systems and living machines. Biomed. Microdevices 14, 965–967.

Rider, T.H., Blanchard, D.J., Bortolin, L.T., Young, A.M., 2014. A B cell-based sensor for rapid identification of pathogens. Science 301 (2003), 213–215. http://dx.doi.org/10.1126/science.1084920.

Saitakis, M., Tsortos, A., Gizeli, E., 2010. Probing the interaction of a membrane receptor with a surface-attached ligand using whole cells on acoustic biosensors. Biosens. Bioelectron. 25 (7), 1688–1693.

Sakar, M.S., Neal, D., Boudou, T., Borochin, M.A., Li, Y., Weiss, R., Kamm, R.D., Chen, C.S., Asada, H.H., 2012. Formation and optogenetic control of engineered 3D skeletal muscle bioactuators. Lab Chip 12, 4976–4985.

Smutok, O., Dmytruk, K., Gonchar, M., 2007. Permeabilized cells of flavocytochrome b 2 over-producing recombinant yeast *Hansenula polymorpha* as biological recognition element in amperometric lactate biosensors. Biosens. Bioelectron. 23, 599–605.

Stenger, D.A., Gross, G.W., Keefer, E.W., Shaffer, K.M., Andreadis, J.D., Ma, W., Pancrazio, J. J., et al., 2001. Detection of physiologically active compounds using cell-based biosensors. Trends Biotechnol. 19 (8), 304–309.

Tabor, J.J., Salis, H., Simpson, Z.B., Chevalier, A.A., Marcotte, E.M., Voigt, C.A., Ellington, A. D., 2009. A synthetic genetic edge detection program. Cell 137 (7), 1272–1281.

Tian, B., Liu, J., Dvir, T., Jin, L., Tsui, J.H., Qing, Q., Suo, Z., Langer, R., Kohane, D.S., Lieber, C.M., 2012. Macroporous nanowire nanoelectronic scaffolds for synthetic tissues. Nat. Mat. 11, 986–994.

Valderrama, E., Garrido, P., Cabruja, E., Heiduschka, P., Harsch, A., Gopel, W., 1995. Microfabrication and characterisation of microelectrode arrays for in vivo nerve signal recording. In: The Ninth International Conference on Solid-State Sensors and Actuators, and Eurosensors IX. Stockholm, Sweden, June 25–29, 1995, pp. 63–66.

Ward, M., Rajdev, P., Ellison., Irazoqui, P., 2009. Toward a comparison of microelectrodes for acute and chronic recordings. Brain Res. 1282, 183–200.

Weiss, R., Basu, S., Hooshangi, S., Kalmbach, A., Karig, D., 2003. Genetic circuit building blocks for cellular computation, communications, and signal processing. Nat. Comput. 2, 1–40.

Wisniewski, N., Reichert, M., 2000. Methods for reducing biosensor membrane biofouling. Colloids Surf., B 18, 197–219.

Yarkoni, O., Donlon, L., Frankel, D., 2012. Creating a bio-hybrid signal transduction pathway: opening a new channel of communication between cells and machines. Bioinspir. Biomim. 7, 046017.

Ye, H., Baber, M.D., Peng, R., Fussenegger, M., 2010. A synthetic optogenetic transcription device enhances blood-glucose homeostasis in mice. Science 332, 1565–1568.

Zhang, F., Wang, L.P., Boyden, E.S., Deisseroth, K., 2006. Channelrhodopsin-2 and optical control of excitable cells. Nat. Methods 3, 785–792.

Part Two

Bio-Inspired Sensors

Biomimetic tactile sensing

4

R. Dahiya, C. Oddo, A. Mazzoni, H. Jörntell

4.1 Introduction

What would happen if we had all sense modalities but the "touch?" A simple experiment of manipulating objects after putting hands on an ice block for a moment can probably provide an answer to this question. In one such experiment, the skin on a volunteer's hand was anesthetized so that tactile information from mechanoreceptors—the specialized nerve endings that respond to mechanical stimulation—was no longer available to the brain (Westling and Johannson, 1984). It was observed that even though volunteers could see what they were doing, they could no longer maintain a stable grasp of the objects. This indicates that the movements become inaccurate and unstable in the absence of "sense of touch." The difficulties that humans could face in the absence of sense of touch also point toward the importance of touch sense modality in robots, especially when they are expected to work in a human environment.

The touch sensing allows us to assess the size, shape, softness, and texture of objects. It helps us understand the interaction behaviors of the real world objects—which depend on their weight; stiffness; on how their surface feels when touched; how they deform on contact; and how they move when pushed. In applications such as robotics, tactile information is useful in a number of ways. In manipulative tasks, the tactile data are used as a control parameter and the tactile information typically includes contact point estimation, surface normal and curvature measurement, and slip detection (Fearing, 1990; Howe, 1994). A measure of the contact forces (both magnitude and direction) allows the grasp force control—needed to maintain stable grasps. In a real world interaction that involves, both, manipulative and exploratory tasks, the tactile information such as hardness/softness (Shikida et al., 2003), temperature, and vibrations are needed to understand diverse properties of the contacted objects.

The need for suitable tactile sensing system in robotics has resulted in a large number of touch sensors and tactile sensing arrays by exploring nearly all modes of transduction, viz., resistive, capacitive, piezoelectric, magnetic, quantum tunneling, etc. (Dahiya et al., 2010b; Lee and Nicholls, 1999; Dahiya and Valle, 2013). Currently, many research groups are also working toward developing skin-like artificial systems for large area tactile sensing. However, the touch sensor technology developed so far is largely insufficient for robotics, even if there is significant success in other areas such as mobile telephony. This could be attributed to a number of factors such as availability of less than satisfactory sensory skins, insufficient methods of processing tactile data, the lack of systems approach, and the lack of mechanical flexibility and robust sensory structures. Often, tactile data are processed with techniques adapted from visual data processing, which may not be a correct approach as the touch sensing is distributed over a much broader area than vision. As a consequence, the dense integration of sensors distributed in large and curved bodies is still lagging behind. This also presents the case for the implementing higher order cognitive functions for tactile action and perception.

Design of a meaningful tactile sensing system must be guided by a broad, but integrated, knowledge of how tactile information is encoded and transmitted at various stages. In this context, evolving biological systems could provide an answer. For centuries, biological systems have inspired engineers and scientists (Crouch, 2003), and for tactile sensing, the human touch sensing could be a good starting point. The human inspiration is also important in the absence of any comprehensive artificial tactile sensing theory as the studies on human touch (e.g., neurophysiology of touch, skin biomechanics, movements for optimum exploration of material properties, object recognition, active and passive perception, and selective attention) could help in specifying important parameters like sensor density, resolution, location, and bandwidth. Starting with a brief discussion on the human touch sensing, this chapter presents the development of artificial tactile sensing arrays that are inspired from touch sensing in humans. System level aspects such as wiring and information processing are discussed with final attention to neuromorphic signaling and the emulation of the neuronal organization and of the human somatosensory system from the periphery to the cortex. As this book focuses on nature-inspired technologies, the discussion on the human sense of touch is brief and limited to the points of inspiration. For deeper understanding on human sense of touch, one may refer to the relevant literature (Wolfe et al., 2006; Purves et al., 2008; Kandel et al., 2000).

4.2 Human sense of touch

The touch sensing in humans comprises two main submodalities, i.e., "cutaneous" and "kinesthetic," or "exteroceptive" and "proprioceptive." The exteroceptive sense is based primarily on receptors with a cutaneous location and provides awareness of the stimulation of the outer surface of body. The proprioceptive or the kinesthetic sense has traditionally been ascribed to sensory receptors located within muscles, tendons, and joints (Loomis and Lederman, 1986) and provides information about the static and dynamic body postures (relative positioning of the head, torso, limbs, and end effectors). However, it is known that the sensors in the skin also play an important role in proprioception or kinesthetic sensation (Edin and Johansson, 1995). The term "tactile sensing," which is discussed in this chapter, is primarily based on the exteroceptive sense of the glabrous skin at the fingertips and the palm.

Our ability to deal with the spatiotemporal perception of external stimuli, to discriminate among surface textures, temperature, and to sense incipient slip and roll of an object between fingers without dropping it, etc., can be attributed to the specialized receptors embedded in the skin (Wolfe et al., 2006; Kandel et al., 2000). The receptors that are sensitive to pressure/vibration stimuli are termed "mechanoreceptors" and those sensitive to pain/damage are called "nociceptors." The response to thermal stimulus is believed to be mediated by separate "warm" and "cold" thermoreceptor population in the skin. The mechanoreceptors are the peripheral ends of neurons (Abraira and Ginty, 2013), which have their cell bodies located just outside the spinal cord, and the events generated at the mechanoreceptors are hence directly transferred into the central nervous system (CNS). The signal is transferred to the CNS via the neuron's axon, which for exteroceptive and proprioceptive sensors are denoted "primary afferent."

The receptors are distributed across the entire body with variable density. As an example, the number of mechanoreceptors, per square centimeter area, is estimated to be about 240 in the fingertips and about 60 in the palm of adult humans (Johannson and Vallbo, 1979). The spatial acuity is highest at fingertips, face, and toes and lowest at thigh, shoulders, and belly. Similarly, the receptors also have different receptive fields—the extent of body area to which a receptor responds—and different rates of adaptation. A fast-adapting (FA) receptor responds with bursts of action potentials when its preferred stimulus is first applied and when it is removed. In contrast, a slow-adapting (SA) receptor remains active throughout the period during which the stimulus is in contact with its receptive field. Thus, spatial-temporal limits and sensitivities of the receptors vary significantly across various body parts. The classification, functions, and location of various mechanoreceptors are given in Figure 4.1.

The moment the skin is stimulated, a variety of mechanical and neural events occur. On contact with an object, the skin conforms to its surface, which may if the object is compressible. The resulting skin deformation elicits mechanical strain patterns in the skin that may differ depending not only on the distance to the actual contact point and the edges of the contact point but also on the local biomechanical properties of the skin and the underlying anatomy of the fingertip, for example. These

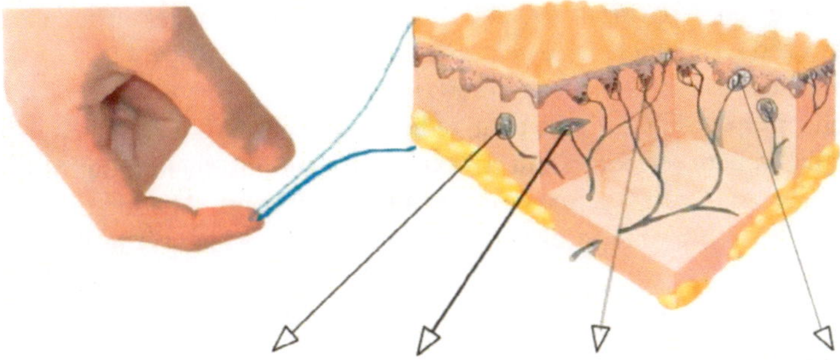

Classification basis		Pacinian corpuscle	Ruffini corpuscle	Merkel cells	Meissner's corpuscle
Type		FA II	SA II	SA I	FA I
Adaptation rate		Fast	Slow	Slow	Fast
Spatial acuity (mm)		10+	7+	0.5	3–4
Vibration/rapid	Best (μm)	0.01	40	8	2
indent threshold	Mean (μm)	0.08	300	30	6
Stimuli frequency (Hz)		40–500+	100–500+	0.4–3	3–40
Conduction velocity (m/s)		35–70	35–70	40–65	35–70
Effective stimuli		Temporal changes in the skin deformation	Sustained downward pressure; lateral skin stretch; skin slip.	Spatial deformation;sustained pressure; curvature, edge, corners.	Temporal changes in skin deformation;
Sensory function		High frequency vibration detection; tool use	Finger position; stable grasp; tangential force; motion direction	Pattern/formdetection;texture perception; tactile flow perception.	low frequenc vibration & motiondetection;grip control tactile flow perception.

Figure 4.1 The classification, functions, and location of various mechanoreceptors present in human glabrous skin (Dahiya et al., 2010b). Recent studies point toward the presence of Ruffini afferents in the hairy skin of human hand and not in the glabrous skin (Pare et al., 2003; Mountcastle, 2005).

varied strain patterns are sensed by the local population of mechanoreceptors, which transforms the local strain pattern into an analogous electrical signal inside the neuron. Each mechanoreceptor thus represents a small portion of the skin-object interaction and encodes the spatiotemporal tactile information as spikes of action potentials—voltage pulses generated when the analogous voltage signal generated in the mechanoreceptor is greater than the threshold of the neuron. The amplitude of the stimulus is then transformed to a train of action potentials, which reflect the intensity and temporal profile of the mechanoreceptor events. Via the primary afferent fiber, the contact event-related information is transmitted to the CNS for higher level processing and interpretation. The first stage in which this occurs is the cuneate nucleus in the lower part of the brainstem. The cuneate nucleus is essentially a mono layer network with local inhibitory interneurons. From the cuneate nucleus, the information is transferred to the thalamus, another monolayer network with local inhibition and recurrent input from the neocortex, and from the thalamus to the primary sensory cortex.

An interesting feature of touch sensing in humans, which is also very useful for artificial tactile sensing, is the processing of tactile information at various stages of data transfer—thus reducing the computational burden of CNS. The processing of tactile data starts right from the peripheral level, i.e., already the local biomechanical properties and the exact forces applied will determine the patterns of skin strain induced by a certain skin-object interaction. As the local strain patterns are effectively transduced in the mechanoreceptors and conducted to the CNS (Hayward et al., 2014), the spikes in the primary afferents already contain information that can be used to distinguish, for example, the curvature and the direction of force in the terminal phalanx (Johannson and Birznieks, 2004). A hypothetical model of human tactile processing, based on coincidence detection of neural events (Figure 4.2), was recently presented in Johansson and Flanagan (2009).

This model proposes that: (i) the relative timing of neural spikes elicited in (neighboring) tactile units of the fingertip conveys significant information during manipulation activities; (ii) the spikes pass through neural afferents showing differentiated delays one to the other (due to dispersion of conduction velocity) in the pathways

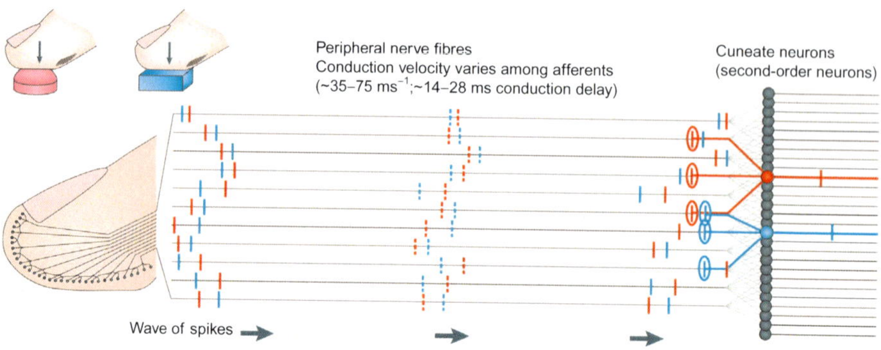

Figure 4.2 Hypothetical model accounted by Johansson and Flanagan (2009), based on coincidence detection of neural events for the fast processing of afferent information.

up to the second-order (cuneate) neurons; (iii) second-order neurons propagate the firing events to the higher stage in case that the differential delay introduced by the afferent pathways compensates the relative spike timing at the level of mechanoreceptors in the fingerpad; (iv) the tactile stimulus is preperceptually represented through the pattern of second-order neurons being activated (i.e., those detecting a coincidence of incoming neural spikes, and thus propagating the firing up to the higher stage) during finger-surface mechanical interaction. Support for a modified version of this hypothesis, where the overall degree of correlation in afferent spike trains were considered rather than the first spike, was recently proposed as an explanation for input feature segregation in the cuneate nucleus (Jörntell et al., 2014).

The implications of the above discussion on the development of artificial tactile sensing systems are (Dahiya and Valle, 2013):

- The presence of varied and distributed receptors with sharp division of functions, which calls for different types of miniaturized sensors, each optimally transducing a particular contact parameter.
- It is desirable to have multifunctional sensors that encode more than one contact parameter, e.g., contact force and hardness detection by a sensor.
- The spatial density of the tactile sensors, distributed or arranged in an array, should be based on the body site or the target application site. For fingertips like sites, it should be about 1 mm—which translates to an approximately 15×10 sensing element grids on a fingertip-sized area.
- The sensors should demonstrate high sensitivity and wide dynamic range. Considering involvement of touch sensors in various exploratory tasks, a contact force sensitivity range of 1–1000 g wt. and a dynamic range of 1000:1 are desirable.
- The touch sensors could encode both magnitude and the direction of contact force. The response of tactile sensors distributed in an area could be used to obtain the direction of contact force as done by population mechanoreceptors in humans.
- Touch sensing elements should detect and encode both static and dynamic contact events. It is desirable to have tactile sensors that can detect vibrations up to 1 kHz.
- In humans, the tactile data are not directly conveyed to the brain. Instead, some processing takes place at various stages of data transfer—perhaps to fit the limited throughput of the nervous system (Johansson and Flanagan, 2009). The tactile arrays or modules, with some level of preprocessing (data selection, local computation, etc.) at the sensory location, can be helpful in reducing the amount of information transfer to the central processing unit. According to this biologically grounded model, computation also occurs along the wires that conduct information from artificial receptors to the central computational units.

4.3 Biomimetic artificial touch

Biorobotics fosters the convergence of technological achievements with new scientific knowledge and helps us understand the underlying natural phenomena and behaviors (Dario et al., 2008). This approach has often been depicted in the light of bioinspiration and biomimetics, and it gives rise to morphological computation, a novel paradigm asserting the role of materials in taking over some of the processes normally attributed to control (Pfeifer et al., 2007; Laschi and Cianchetti, 2014), in conjunction with neuromorphic engineering in case of mimicry of neural mechanisms and architectures (Spigler et al., 2012). The organization of the somatosensory system presented in Section and illustrated in Figure 4.2 represents this understanding with fertile synergies between science and engineering. According to such model, the structure and shape of soft tissues of the skin, the nonregular spatial distribution in array of mechanoreceptors, and the different conduction velocities along the afferent neural pathways up to the second-order cuneate neural stage have been hypothesized to implement computational operations on tactile information at precortical stages (Johansson and Flanagan 2009). This means that the skin, the mechanoreceptors, and the afferent neural pathways are not just a mechanical interface medium, sensors, and wires, respectively, but they implement computation, thanks to their morphological characteristics. Particularly, neural pathways are not the impairment as wires are considered in traditional robotics. Their structure implements processing functions that would have required very complex sequential structures if instantiated centrally at brain level. Artificial touch can therefore show levels of biomimetism with respect to various characteristics, such as:

- the soft artificial skin that mediates the mechanical interaction with the tactile stimuli;
- the mechanotransduction core technology that converts mechanical stimulation to information;
- the neuromorphic representation of tactile information that allows the emulation of and integration with natural neuronal pathways.

These forms of biomimetism are briefly discussed hereafter with respect to current state of the art.

4.3.1 Soft artificial skin

Human tactile transduction is a complex energy conversion mechanism involving populations of mechanosensitive afferent fibers innervating the distal fingerpad and the skin with its different layers including fingerprints (Scheibert et al., 2009; Candelier et al., 2011; Vasarhelyi et al., 2006; Oddo et al., 2011). In the artificial emulation of a tactile sense, soft materials play a crucial role for potential future deployment in domains such as hand prosthetics: indeed, soft materials can increase the size of the contact area, thanks to their higher conformability, increase the contact friction coefficient (and thus the grasp stability), protect distributed embedded sensors, which also provide better contact information, improve cosmetics, the latter being a relevant feature to enhance the final acceptability by the end user (Cabibihan et al., 2006).

Biomimetics in the design of artificial fingers can go beyond the use of soft materials. Indeed, the effectiveness of employing soft materials is enhanced if anatomy and physiology of human fingers are considered (Controzzi et al., 2014). The soft and pulpy tissue that is present between the skeletal bone and the skin addresses several functions, such as dissipating mechanical energy during impacts and protecting the bone tissues from lesions; because of its softness and the elastic nature of the skin, the pulpy tissue can conform to most uneven surfaces of commonly used objects; further, due to its viscoelastic nature, it dissipates strain energy that is induced during manipulation of rigid objects, thus stabilizing the interaction (Montana, 1992; Wettels et al., 2008). Similarly, microstructures such as fingerprints help in stable grasping of the objects, prevent them from slipping and are also reported to help in identifying the roughness or smoothness of various surfaces (Scheibert et al., 2009; Okada et al., 2010; Dahiya and Gori, 2010). Therefore, the fabrication of soft robotic fingers, possibly with microstructures such as fingerprints, is important for a safer, more stable, and reliant interaction with handled objects (Shimoga and Goldenberg, 1992). The packaging used in sensors for synthetic skin is mainly based on polymeric materials, such as silicone elastomers (e.g., polydimethylsiloxane in Dow Corning Sylgard 184® PDMS, polyorganosiloxanes, and silica in Smooth-on DragonSkin™ and Ecoflex©) and polyurethane rubbers (e.g., toluene diisocyanate and polyols in Polytek® Poly-74 Series) (Vasarhelyi et al., 2006; Vasarhelyi et al., 2007). These polymeric materials show compliant nature, resistance to temperature changes, mechanical toughness, and the possibility to be healed. Also, the tensile strength and elongation at break of the elastomer permit to withstand the stretch and abrasion due to forces encountered in object manipulation and exploration (Roy et al., 2012).

4.3.2 Mechanotransduction core technology

Several types of artificial sensitive skin have been proposed and a large number of transduction mechanisms have been reported in the literature. Mechanoelectrotransduction (or mechanoneurotransduction) occurs when an external stimulus transfers energy to the human finger pad, in contact mode (e.g., mechanical probing) or contactless (e.g., heat transfer via radiation), to elicit sequences of electrical discharges that reach the brain via the afferent pathways and code the stimulus in a perceptual form.

Several reviews of tactile sensors have been proposed with respect to synthetic approaches for the design of the skin and transduction mechanisms (Dahiya et al., 2010b; Lee and Nicholls, 1999; Rossi, 1991; Maheshwari and Saraf, 2008; Yousef et al., 2011; Tiwana et al., 2012; Hammock et al., 2013), and novel trends consider the integration of cell-based living structures (Lucarotti et al., 2013; Adamatzky, 2013; Cheneler et al., 2014). Like sense of touch in humans, it is desirable to have tactile arrays, or a coordinated group of distributed tactile sensors, with density and spatial distribution of taxels (tactile elements) depending on the body site where the sensors are installed (Dahiya et al., 2010b). For the sites like fingertips, that are involved in tasks like exploration and fine manipulation, a large number of quick responding (response time of the order of few milliseconds) taxels are needed in a small space (with spatial resolution of about 1 mm). Such spatial constraints can be met by miniaturizing the sensors and placing them over large areas in an array-like fashion. Common synthetic tactile transduction techniques are based on capacitive, piezoelectric, piezoresistive, inductive, optoelectric, and strain gauge methods. The main characteristics associated with these techniques are briefly illustrated hereafter.

Capacitive sensors consist of two conductive plates with a dielectric material sandwiched between them. For parallel plates, the capacitance value is expressed as $C=(A\varepsilon_0\varepsilon_r)/d$, where C is the capacitance, A is the area of the two plates, ε_0 is the permittivity of free space, ε_r is the relative permittivity of the dielectric material, and d is the distance between the plates (Wettels et al., 2008; Cheng et al., 2009; Muhammad et al., 2011a,b; Medler et al., 1996; Moe et al., 2000; Renard et al., 2002). Novel sensor concepts recently being proposed include the capacitive sensors with soft encapsulation materials and textile-based conductive electrodes (Viry et al., 2014).

Piezoelectric sensors are composed of piezoelectric materials, such as poled ceramic lead zirconium titanate (PZT) and polyvinylidene fluoride (PVDF), which respond to the applied force/pressure (Atkinson et al., 2003; Cheng-Hsin et al., 2008; Dahiya et al., 2009b; Krishna and Rajanna, 2004; Li et al., 2008; Hosoda et al., 2006; Caliò et al., 2014). Piezoelectric sensors are often named as *ultrasonic*, when using elements that emit an ultrasonic pulse within a medium (a rubber pad); the pulse is propagated through the medium and reflected. This echo pulse is then received by the emitting source. The transit time of the pulse is proportional to the thickness of the medium; therefore, the strength of the echo pulse depends on acoustic properties of the medium and on the tactile stimulation conditions (Ando, 1995).

Piezoresistive sensors consist of a pressure-sensitive element that changes its resistance upon applied force. The resistance value of a resistor having length l and cross-sectional area A is given by: $R = \rho(l/A)$. According to this relationship, the resistance value is determined by both bulk resistivity ρ and dimensions, with dominant variational effects associated mainly to resistivity changes (Beccai et al., 2005; Wang and Beebe, 2000; Mei et al., 2000; Tibrewala et al., 2009).

Strain gauge sensors consist of a resistive elastic unit, whose change in resistance is a function of the applied strain as shown by the equation $dR/R = G\varepsilon$, where R is the resistance, ε is the strain, and G is the gauge factor. If compared to piezoresistive sensors, the mechanotransduction properties of strain gauge devices are dominated by form factors rather than by variations in resistivity (Lee and Lee, 2010; Hwang et al., 2007; Kwon and Choi, 2010; Tanaka et al., 2007).

Inductive sensors are composed of a primary coil that induces a magnetic field sensed in a secondary sense coil; the mutual inductance between the coils modulates as a consequence of the applied load, thus modulating the amplitude and phase of the voltage measured in the sense coil (Hasegawa et al., 2004; Takenawa, 2009).

Optoelectric sensors employ a light source, a modulatory medium, a transmission medium, and a photodetector, the latter often in the form of camera or photodiode. Transduction occurs when changes in the tactile medium modulate transmission intensity or the spectrum of the source light, as a consequence of variations in the applied force (Begej, 1988; Persichetti et al., 2007; Ahmadi et al., 2012; Maheshwari, 2006; Levi et al., 2013) (Table 4.1).

4.3.3 Neuromorphic representation of tactile information for biomimetic tactile computation

In order to develop biomimetic tactile sensors, the computational characteristics of mechanoreceptors should be reproduced in addition to their physical features, and biomimetic sensors shall convey the same information about external stimuli as the biological sensors. The accuracy of the reproduction of biological information processing

Table 4.1 **Fully synthetic tactile sensing: transduction methods, advantages, and disadvantages**

Transduction method	Modulated parameter	Advantages	Disadvantages
Capacitive	Change in capacitance	– High spatial resolution – Good frequency response – Long-term drift stability – High sensitivity – Low temperature sensitivity – Low power consumption	– Severe hysteresis – Stray capacitance – Complex electronics – Noise susceptible
Piezoelectric	Strain (stress) polarization	– Flexibility – Workability – Chemical stability – Good high-frequency response	– High temperature sensitivity – Poor spatial resolution – Dynamic sensing only – Simple electronics
Piezoresistive	Change in resistance	– Flexibility – High spatial resolution – Good sensitivity – Low noise – Low cost – Simple electronics	– Large hysteresis – Low frequency response – Low repeatability
Strain gauge	Change in resistance	– Sensing range – High sensitivity – Low cost	– High hysteresis – Nonlinear response – Susceptible to temperature changes – Design complexity
Inductive	Change in inductance	– High sensitivity – High dynamic range – No mechanical hysteresis – Linear response – Physical robustness	– Usage limited to nonmagnetic mediums – Low spatial resolution – Low repeatability – Complex electronics
Optoelectric	Light intensity/ spectrum change	– High density – High spatial resolution – Capability to sense both shear and normal contact forces – Immunity from EMI	– Large size – Rigidness – Loss of light by microbending, causing distortion of signal

From Dahiya et al. (2010b), Yousef et al. (2011), Tiwana et al. (2012), Lucarotti et al. (2013), and Dahiya and Valle (2008).

is not straightforward to test, since we can only study a limited set of stimuli, both with natural and artificial sensors. There are two options then. The first is to build *ad hoc* sensors to reproduce some selected aspects of tactile processing, as for instance sharp edge detection or stimulus intensity. The other is to build biomimetic sensors capturing the basic rules of peripheral tactile computation to reproduce the flexibility of natural sensors. As a matter of fact, in humans the long distance signaling between the periphery and the CNS occurs via a temporal sequence of neural spikes flowing in parallel along the afferent pathways, i.e., the communication can be considered as asynchronous digital per each receptor channel (see Section 4.2). Along this direction, an emerging engineering trend is neuromorphic mechanotransduction, i.e., addressing biomimicry in terms of the used tactile code (Spigler et al., 2012). With neuromorphic signaling, no information is therefore associated with the amplitude of the output signals of each taxel, whereas the encoding of tactile experience emerges from the temporal modulation of the (on-off) neural spiking behavior of artificial receptors and from the spatial map of active taxels.

In order to achieve a better information processing performance reproducing the temporal spike modulations of biological neurons, a series of step can be taken, as illustrated in Figure 4.3, and explained in the following. The starting condition, which is not neuromorphic at all but can still be sufficient to convey basic information, is to leave the sensors output unprocessed except for noise filtering and renormalization. The first step to achieve a biomimetic information representation is to convert the continuous output of the sensor arrays into discrete voltage pulses similar to (population) spikes. Besides making the signal closer to real mechanoreceptors output, this operation drastically reduces the size of the signal at the price of small or no information loss. A signal discretization can be achieved with simple signal processing tools, and computing spike times with a biomimetic approach, i.e., by means of a neuronal model reproducing the main features of the neurons biophysics, has a series of advantages. Crucially, such models can nowadays be implemented in hardware (Millner et al., 2010) and ensure high performance even in the case of unexpected stimuli. Moreover, such an approach will be easier to translate into brain-machine interface applications such as upper limb prostheses since it is reasonable to expect that decoding sensors inputs injected into the nervous system will be easier and faster to learn if these inputs are similar to the natural spike trains emitted by mechanoreceptors. Therefore, the neuromorphic approach creates the ground for a natural integration between the artificial sensing system and the natural neural afferent pathways (Kim et al., 2013) and can represent a further advancement of approaches targeting the restoration of a missing sense of touch via neuroprostheses (Raspopovic et al., 2014).

In Section 4.2, we have seen how tactile sensory information is processed by different kinds of mechanoreceptors (Figure 4.2). To take into account, this variety of processing mechanisms, a possible biomimetic approach is to build a parallel layer of computation with different processors reproducing the specific behaviors of the different mechanoreceptors (Bologna et al., 2011, 2013). At a first stage, a single reference neuronal model can be adopted and specific features of the different neuron kinds can be achieved by standard nonbiomimetic signal processing applied to the voltage input. This approach has been, for instance, used by Bensmaia and colleagues

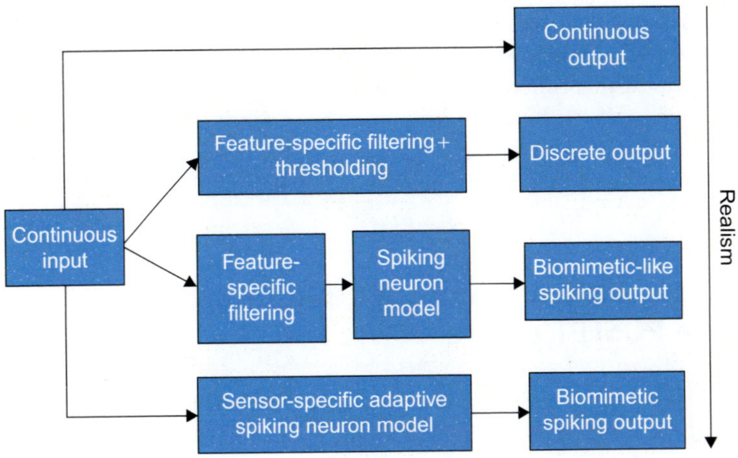

Figure 4.3 Possible approaches for soft-neuromorphic tactile sensing. Middle column shows the processing applied to the continuous output of sensors to obtain the output in the right column. Outputs are arranged from top to bottom in order of increasing realism, i.e., increasing similarity to biological outputs.

(Kim et al., 2010). The final aim, however, should be to achieve the same pattern dynamics with biologically sound neuronal models. In this perspective, simple models like the leaky integrate and fire neuron (Brunel, 2013) should be discarded since they fail to reproduce the adaptation mechanisms that are the very core of the different mechanoreceptors behaviors (Izhikevich, 2004). On the other hand, models such as the Hodgkin and Huxley neuron are computationally expensive since they aim at reproducing the details of the active channels dynamics (Izhikevich, 2004), which does not currently seem to be relevant for this stage of information processing. Appropriate models to reproduce the mechanoreceptors are the Izhikevich neuron model (Izhikevich, 2003) and the Adaptive Exponential Integrate and Fire neuron model (Brette and Gerstner, 2005), both capturing at the same time adaptive mechanisms and the main features of the action potential shape. Which one of the two is more suitable depends on factors such as the hardware implementation or the complexity of the computation.

In Section 4.2, we also highlighted the key role played by the temporal structure of the firing (rather than the total amount of spikes fired) in tactile information processing. It is then crucial to reproduce the main timescales present in mechanoreceptors in the engineered model: as we have seen, the adaptation onset and recovery timescale is probably the most important but also membrane timescale, synaptic opening and closing times, and, as shown in Figure 4.2, the synaptic delays should be taken into account, at least implicitly. Finally, we would like to stress that reproducing the temporal structure of the mechanoreceptors firing does not mean to reproduce the precise time of each spike down to arbitrary high temporal resolution. Every information-processing mechanism has an optimal timescale that can be estimated in different ways (Vázquez et al., 2013; Kayser et al., 2010; Victor and Purpura, 1998).

Timescales faster than the optimal one might then be not discriminated by down-stream layers of information processing because of biophysical constraints. Such a filtering plays also an important functional role since small jitters might be usually due to intrinsic noise. It is then of paramount importance to estimate the optimal time-scale for peripheral tactile processing also to set the indicative temporal resolution at which we must aim to reproduce mechanoreceptors spike patterns.

4.4 Case study of tactile sensing technology: the POSFET device

The POSFET (Piezoelectric Oxide Semiconductor Field Effect Transistor) devices-based tactile sensing arrays presented in this section have been designed for spatio-temporal parameters similar to that of cutaneous sensing at human fingertip. As described later in this section, the POSFET devices on the tactile sensing chips are realized by depositing a piezoelectric polymer, PVDF-TrFE (Polyvinylidene Fluoride—Trifluoroethylene), on the gate area of a MOS transistor (Dahiya et al., 2009a, 2011, 2013, 2014; Adami et al., 2012;). The resulting marriage of transducer and electronics is advantageous in many ways. In addition to minimizing the utilization of space, the marriage of transducer and electronics results in better force resolution, spatial resolution, and signal-to-noise ratio.

4.4.1 Structure and working of a POSFET device

The structure of POSFET touch sensing device, shown in Figure 4.4 (inset), is similar to a metal-ferroelectric-metal-insulator-semiconductor FeRAM (Ferroelectric Random Access Memory). The remanent polarization (P_r), of the piezoelectric polymer film, and the charge neutrality condition result in the appearance of fixed charges $\pm Q$ on the surface of polymer. This results in accumulation of charge carriers at the surface of the semiconductor—according to the polarization direction. When piezoelectric polymer is polarized along thickness and the mechanical stress is also applied along this direction, the mechanical stress T_3, the electric field E_3, and the electric displacement D_3 are related as (Dahiya et al., 2009c,d; Dahiya, 2015):

$$D_3 = d_{33}T_3 + \varepsilon_{33}E_3 \tag{4.1}$$

where d_{33} and ε_{33} are the piezoelectric and dielectric constants, respectively, of piezoelectric polymer. Following Equation (4.1), the electric displacement and hence the polarization can be controlled by the electric field E_3 and the applied force F or stress T_3. While former is used in FeRAM to switch the polarization state, the latter is used in the POSFET touch sensing devices to modulate the charge in induced channel of underlying MOS device (Dahiya et al., 2009a). Thus, the contact force variation is directly reflected into channel current of POSFET devices—which can be amplified by POSFET itself and further processed by the electronic circuitry that may be present

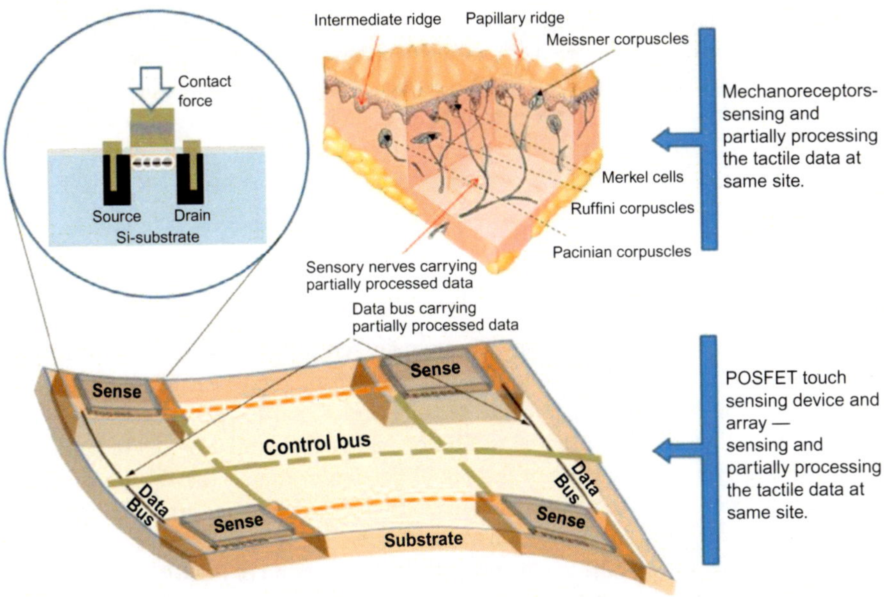

Figure 4.4 The functional comparison of a POSFET touch sensing device with the mechanoreceptors in the skin.

on the same chip. Thus, each touch sensing element or taxel is an integral "sensotronic" unit, comprising transducer and the transistor, which is capable of "sensing and partially processing at same site." In this context, a POSFET touch sensing device can be compared with the mechanoreceptors in human skin—that not only sense the contact parameters but also partially process the tactile data at same site (Johansson and Flanagan 2009). This analogy, between POSFET touch sensing device and the mechanoreceptors in the skin, is shown in Figure 4.4. Another feature of POSFET touch sensing devices is their ability to detect contact temperature variations. With a proper arrangement, this feature can be turned into an advantage and the POSFET device can be made multifunctional—capable of detecting both dynamic contact forces and the contact temperature.

A similar approach, utilizing extended gates, has also been adopted for ultrasonic (Swartz and Plummer, 1979) and force sensing (Graz et al., 2006). The extended gate approach brings the sensor and conditioning electronics closer, and hence, the overall response is better than the conventional approach—where the sensor and conditioning electronics are placed apart. Overall, the sensitivity of POSFET-based tactile sensing devices is higher than that of extended gates-based tactile sensors. The presence of polymer only on the gate area, as in POSFET devices, results in a lesser polymer area (compared to that of an extended gate-based tactile sensor). This means, for same thickness of the polymer, the effective capacitance is lesser and so is the RC time constant. The large interconnects needed for the extended gate are also absent in case of

POSFET—which further reduces the RC time constant. One of the direct fallouts of reduced RC constant is the faster response and improved range of frequencies. Besides this, the absence of extended gates frees some of the real estate on the silicon wafer, which can be used for on-chip electronics as done in the recent version of POSFETs (Dahiya et al., 2013, 2014; Adami et al., 2012). The reliable interconnects between extended gate and MOS transistor is also an issue—more so in case of flexible touch sensing devices.

4.4.2 POSFET tactile arrays—Design, fabrication, and evaluation

As discussed in previous sections, the human sense of touch like spatiotemporal response can be obtained by miniaturizing the sensors and then placing them over large area. The 5 × 5 POSFET tactile sensing arrays, partly shown in Figure 4.5(a), have been designed to have spatial resolution and acuity similar to that of human fingertips. The overall dimension of the initial version of this tactile sensing array was 1.5 cm × 1.5 cm, with each POSFET touch sensing device on the array designed to be 1 mm × 1 mm in size—ensuring human-like spatial acuity. The center-center distance of 1.5 mm between two adjacent taxels in the initial version of POSFET chips ensured human-like spatial resolution. The spatial resolution of about 1 mm possible with POSFET-based devices can be further improved by reducing the spacing between POSFET devices and also by reducing the size of the devices. The most recent version of POSFET chips have reduced number of taxels, i.e., 4 × 4, for optimal use of interconnects when sensors are read in row-column fashion (Dahiya et al., 2013, 2014). The overall size of the chip is 10.1 mm × 8.1 mm, with 1 mm center-to-center pitch of sensor elements. Each POSFET in the most recent version has been designed to have an active area of 0.9 mm × 0.6 mm.

The fabrication steps for POSFET tactile sensing arrays can be divided into two parts: (a) developing MOS device, and (b) depositing the piezoelectric polymer (Dahiya et al., 2009e). The MOS part of the POSFET touch sensing devices is obtained by using the n-MOS technological module of a nonstandard CMOS

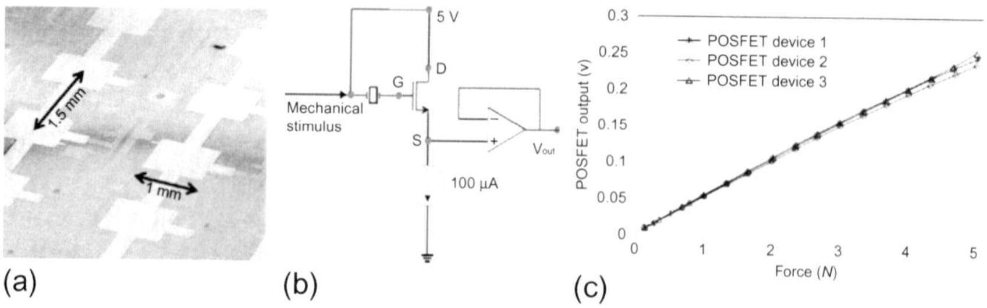

Figure 4.5 (a) The SEM picture of a part of 5 × 5 POSFET tactile sensing array (Dahiya et al., 2010a). The device dimension and distance between two adjacent devices are clearly marked. (b) The source-follower arrangement, with floating gate, used to evaluate the performance of a POSFET touch sensing device. (c) Response of three POSFET touch sensing devices when a 20 Hz sinusoidal force is applied on top in normal direction (Dahiya et al., 2009a).

technology based on 4 μm p-well ion-sensitive FET (ISFET)/CMOS process. A Si_3N_4/SiO_2 double layer is used as a gate dielectric. The piezoelectric polymer-related steps include spin coating of polymer film; annealing; top metallization; and dry etching and poling of polymer films. For a uniform response among various sensors, it is desired to have the polymer film with uniform thickness and hence the deposition method must be carefully chosen. The thickness of polymer film depends on the solution concentration, spinner's speed, and time of spinning. As an example, a 2.5 μm thick PVDF-TrFE polymer film can be deposited by spin coating a 10% solution at 3000 rpm for 30 s (Dahiya et al., 2008). For the same concentration, the thickness of polymer film will decrease with increase in spinner's speed or increase in spinning time. Similarly, a higher concentration solution and higher spinning speed can be used to obtain 2.5 μm thick films. After deposition, the polymer films are annealed at 120 °C for 3 h to enhance the crystallization, to evaporate any left out solvent and to remove any local stress generated during deposition. After this, the piezoelectric film is polarized to introduce the piezoelectric properties. An electric filed strength of 80–100 V/μm is required to polarize the PVDF-TrFE films. The details of fabrication of most recent POSFETs are given in Dahiya et al. (2013, 2014).

To evaluate the performance of a POSFET touch sensing device, a dynamic normal force is applied on the top metal and the change in channel current is observed. The POSFET device is connected in a source-follower circuit arrangement with floating gate, as shown in Figure 4.5(b). The source-follower configuration results in less than unity gain, and hence POSFET devices can be tested for wide range of forces. Alternately, common source configuration can be used to have better force resolution. The response of POSFET touch sensing device is linear, shown in Figure 4.5(c), over tested range of dynamic normal forces (0.15–5 N, sinusoidal 20 Hz). The output of POSFET devices over the tested range is linear with 49 mV/N average slope. The output of the most recent version of POSFET devices is linear with 102 mV/N average slope (Dahiya et al., 2013, 2014). The POSFET devices were tested only up to 2.13 kHz as this frequency is already higher than that perceived by human fingertip. In principle, the POSFETs will have much higher bandwidth due to the higher bandwidth of silicon-based MOS devices and the high pass characteristics of piezoelectric polymers.

The simultaneous excitation of many sensing elements (i.e., application of mechanical stimulus on multiple POSFET elements) is another important test to measure the spatial resolution and the object imaging capability of a tactile sensing array. A snapshot of the response of various POSFET tactile sensors when normal force (670 Hz sinusoidal) is applied on the array with the partial "T" shaped probe is given in Figure 4.6a. The scheme of the probe used for this purpose is also shown in Figure 4.6b. The variation among the responses of the taxels that are pressed is small. A snapshot of the binary images, obtained from the normalized response of various taxels, is also shown in Figure 4.6(c). Similar results are obtained by varying the frequency of applied sinusoidal normal forces. The negligible cross talk confirms that the POSFET tactile sensing arrays have the spatial resolution (1 mm) for which they are designed. The data obtained from these experiments can also be used to detect the edges as shown in Figure 4.6(d). While the dynamic stimulus in above results varies

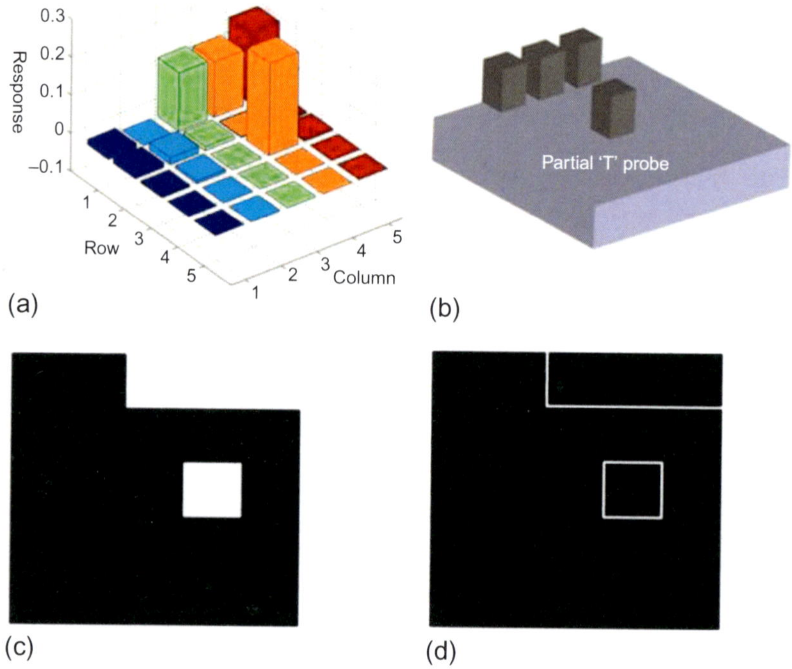

Figure 4.6 (a) Response of various POSFET devices on the array when they are simultaneously pressed with the probe shown in (b); (b) the partial "T" shaped probe; (c) binary image of the response in (a); (d) edge detection using the response data of various POSFET devices on the array.

with time, it is stationary in space. A real-world stimulus may vary both in time and space. When such a stimulus (a ring-shaped probe rolled over the diagonal elements of the array) was applied, the POSFETs yielded good results (Dahiya et al., 2010a)—thus demonstrating their capability to detect stimuli that vary both in time and space. The POSFETS are able to meet many features of human fingertips and they are compared in Table 4.2. Recent development such as flexible or bendable chips (Dahiya et al., 2012a,b; Dahiya and Gennaro, 2013), printing of sensors (Khan et al., 2014a,b; 2015a,b), etc. offer new avenues for cost-effective bio-inspired hardware allowing skin sensor hardware to conform to the 3D curved surfaces.

4.5 Other examples of bio-inspired tactile sensing

There are many studies aiming to realize biologically inspired tactile sensors. These include the neural spike processing-based biologically inspired tactile sensor array reported in Cassidy and Ekanayake (2006). These tactile sensors array integrates

Table 4.2 **The comparison of the tested features of POSFET tactile sensing arrays with the cutaneous/tactile sense of human fingertips**

Feature	Human fingertips	POSFET array
Mechanoreceptor density	241/cm^2	25/cm^2
Multifunctionality	Yes	Yes
Typical range of forces during normal manipulative tasks	0.1–0.9 N	0.15–5 N (tested)
Detectable frequency range of vibration	DC-700 Hz	2–2130 Hz (tested)
Spatial resolution	<1 mm	~1 mm
Receptor level processing of contact data	Yes	Yes

the asynchronous data processing on chip with the sensor array and converts the high-bandwidth raw input data into higher-level information with lower bandwidth requirements. As opposed to traditional rate-based neural spike codes, these tactile sensor arrays use phase-based computation primitives and are able to compute in real time the point of contact, force magnitude, force direction, and the presence or absence of slips, etc. Another example of bio-inspired tactile sensing, reported in Hosoda et al. (2006), embeds many receptors randomly in soft material so as to provide different kinds of sensing modalities. Based on this design principle, an anthropomorphic fingertip is also developed.

Another example of biomimetic tactile sensor array reported in Wettels et al. (2008) mimics the mechanical properties and distributed touch receptors of the human fingertip. Modeled after the human digit, the tactile sensor consists of a rigid central core surrounded by a weakly conductive fluid contained within a silicone elastomeric skin. The sensor uses the deformable properties of the finger pad as part of the transduction process. Multiple electrodes mounted on the surface of the rigid core and connected to impedance-measuring circuitry embedded within the core measure the contacts force. Basically, the external contact forces deform the fluid path around the electrodes, which results in a distributed pattern of impedance changes containing information about those forces and the objects that applied them. As with biological fingertips, the sensor incorporates the low-pass filter effects of cosmetic, protective skin and fluid into the transduction process.

4.6 Conclusion

The ways in which biological systems gather and process information may not always lead to the best engineering solutions. Nevertheless, they provide useful insights into how behaving organisms respond to dynamically changing environments and hence provide a comprehensive multilevel conceptual framework within which to organize the overall task. Thus, rather than imitating, understanding the working of a biological system is more important. Rather than implementing dedicated algorithms to extract specific features, a neuromorphic computational architecture allows to achieve the desired functionality via the implemented structure. Keeping this in view, some of the design cues inspired from human tactile sensing system have been presented in this chapter and used as desiderata for designing the bio-inspired tactile sensing arrays. Some of these cues (structural or functional) have been used in the examples of bio-inspired tactile sensors presented in this chapter.

Acknowledgments

This work was supported in part by the European Commission under grant agreements PITN-GA-2012-317488-CONTEST, EPSRC Fellowship for Growth—PRINTSKIN (EP/M002527/1) and EPSRC First Grant—FLEXELDEMO (EP/M002519/1).

References

Abraira, V.E., Ginty, D.D., 2013. The sensory neurons of touch. Neuron 79, 618–639.

Adamatzky, A., 2013. Slime mould tactile sensor. Sensors Actuators B Chem. 188, 38–44.

Adami, A., Dahiya, R.S., Collini, C., Cattin, D., Lorenzelli, L., 2012. POSFET touch sensor with CMOS integrated signal conditioning electronics. Sensors Actuators A Phys. 98, 502–507.

Ahmadi, R., Packirisamy, M., Dargahi, J., Cecere, R., 2012. Discretely loaded beam-type optical fiber tactile sensor for tissue manipulation and palpation in minimally invasive robotic surgery. IEEE Sensors J. 12, 22–32.

Ando, S., 1995. Ultrasonic emission tactile sensing. IEEE Control Syst. Mag. 15, 61–69.

Atkinson, G.M., Pearson, R.E., Ounaies, Z., Park, C., Harrison, J.S., Midkiff, J.A., 2003. Piezoelectric polyimide tactile sensors. In: 15th Biennial University/Government/Industry Microelectronics Symposium, 2003, pp. 308–311.

Beccai, L., Roccella, S., Arena, A., Valvo, F., Valdastri, P., Menciassi, A., Carrozza, M.C., Dario, P., 2005. Design and fabrication of a hybrid silicon three-axial force sensor for biomechanical applications. Sensors Actuators A 120, 370–382.

Begej, S., 1988. Planar and finger-shaped optical tactile sensors for robotic applications. IEEE Trans. Robot. Autom. 4, 472–484.

Bologna, L.L., Pinoteau, J.R.M., Brasselet, R., Maggiali, M., Arleo, A.A., 2011. Encoding/decoding of first and second order tactile afferents in a neurorobotic application. J. Phys. 105, 25–35.

Bologna, L., Pinoteau, J., Passot, J., Garrido, J., Vogel, J., Vidal, E.R., Arleo, A., 2013. A closed-loop neurobotic system for fine touch sensing. J. Neural Eng. 10, 046019.

Brette, R., Gerstner, W., 2005. Adaptive exponential integrate-and-fire model as an effective description of neuronal activity. J. Neurophysiol. 94, 3637–3642.

Brunel, N., 2013. Dynamics of neural networks. In: Quiroga, R.Q., Panzeri, S. (Eds.), Principles of Neural Coding. CRC Press, Boca Raton.

Cabibihan, J.J., Carrozza, M.C., Dario, P., Pattofatto, S., Jomaa, M., Benallal, A., 2006. The uncanny valley and the search for human skin-like materials for a prosthetic fingertip. In: 6th IEEE-RAS Int. Conf. Humanoid Robots, 2006, pp. 474–477.

Caliò, R., Rongala, U.B., Camboni, D., Milazzo, M., Stefanini, C., De Petris, G., Oddo, C.M., 2014. Piezoelectric energy harvesting solutions. Sensors 14, 4755–4790.

Candelier, R., Prevost, A., Debrégeas, G., 2011. The role of exploratory conditions in bio-Inspired tactile sensing of single topological features. Sensors 11, 7934–7953.

Cassidy, A., Ekanayake, V., 2006. A biologically inspired tactile sensor array utilizing phase-based computation. In: IEEE Biomedical Circuits and Systems Conference (BioCAS) 2006, pp. 45–48.

Cheneler, D., Bowen, J., Kaklamani, G., 2014. Transient bioimpedance monitoring of mechanotransduction in artificial tissue during indentation. J. Electr. Bioimped. 5, 55–73.

Cheng, M.Y., Huang, X.H., Ma, C.W., Yang, Y.J., 2009. A flexible capacitive tactile sensing array with floating electrodes. J. Micromech. Microeng. 19, 115001.

Cheng-Hsin, C., Wen-Bin, D., Wen-Bin, L., 2008. Flexible piezoelectric tactile sensor with structural electrodes array for shape recognition system. In: 3rd Int. Conf. on Sensing Technology, 2008, pp. 504–507.

Controzzi, M., D'Alonzo, M., Peccia, C., Oddo, C.M., Carrozza, M.C., Cipriani, C., 2014. Bioinspired fingertip for anthropomorphic robotic hands. Appl. Bionics Biomech. 11, 25–38.

Crouch, T.D., 2003. Wings: A History of Aviation From Kites to the Space Age. W.W. Norton & Company, Inc., New York.

Dahiya, R.S., 2015. Piezoelectric tactile sensors. In: Webster, J. (Ed.), Wiley Encyclopedia of Electrical and Electronics Engineering. John Wiley & Sons, Inc., New Jersey, pp. 1–15.

Dahiya, R.S., Gennaro, S., 2013. Bendable ultra-thin chips on flexible foils. IEEE Sensors J. 13, 4030–4037.

Dahiya, R.S., Gori, M., 2010. Probing with and into fingerprints. J. Neurophysiol. 104, 1–3.

Dahiya, R.S., Valle, M., 2008. Tactile sensing for robotic applications. In: Rocha, J.G., Lanceros-Mendez, S. (Eds.), Sensors, Focus on Tactile, Force and Stress Sensors. InTech Open Access, Vienna, Austria, pp. 289–304.

Dahiya, R.S., Valle, M., 2013. Robotic Tactile Sensing—Technologies and System. Springer, Dordrecht.

Dahiya, R.S., Valle, M., Lorenzelli, L., Metta, G., Pedrotti, S., 2008. Deposition processing and characterization of PVDF-TrFE thin films for sensing applications. In: IEEE Sensors 2008, Lecce, Italy, 2008, pp. 490–493.

Dahiya, R.S., Metta, G., Valle, M., Lorenzelli, L., Adami, A., 2009a. Piezoelectric oxide semiconductor field effect transistor touch sensing devices. Appl. Phys. Lett. 95, 034105-1–034105-3.

Dahiya, R.S., Metta, G., Valle, M., 2009b. Development of fingertip tactile sensing chips for humanoid robots. In: IEEE Int. Conf. Mechatronics, pp. 1–6.

Dahiya, R.S., Valle, M., Oboe, R., Cattin, D., 2009c. Development and characterization of touch sensing devices for robotic applications. In: IECON '09. 35th Annual Conf. IEEE Industrial Electronics, Porto, Portugal, 2009, pp. 4245–4250.

Dahiya, R.S., Valle, M., Lorenzelli, L., 2009d. SPICE model for lossy piezoelectric polymers. IEEE Trans. Ultrason. Ferroelectr. Freq. Control 56, 387–395.

Dahiya, R.S., Valle, M., Metta, G., Lorenzelli, L., Adami, A., 2009e. Design and fabrication of POSFET devices for tactile sensing. In: 15th IEEE Int. Conf. on Solid-State Sensors, Actuators and Microsystems, Denver, USA, 2009, pp. 1881–1884.

Dahiya, R.S., Lorenzelli, L., Metta, G., Valle, M., 2010a. POSFET devices based tactile sensing arrays. In: IEEE-ISCAS The IEEE Int. Symp. on Circuits and Systems, Paris, France, 2010, pp. 1–4.

Dahiya, R.S., Metta, G., Valle, M., Sandini, G., 2010b. Tactile sensing—from humans to humanoids. IEEE Trans. Rob. 26, 1–20.

Dahiya, R.S., Cattin, D., Adami, A., Collini, C., Barboni, L., Valle, M., Lorenzelli, L., Oboe, R., Metta, G., Brunetti, F., 2011. Towards tactile sensing system on chip for robotic applications. IEEE Sensors J. 11, 3216–3226.

Dahiya, R.S., Adami, A., Collini, C., Lorenzelli, L., 2012a. Bendable ultra-thin silicon chips on foil. In: IEEE Sensors, pp. 1–4.

Dahiya, R.S., Adami, A., Collini, C., Lorenzelli, L., 2012b. Fabrication of single crystal silicon mirco-/nanostructures and transferring them to flexible substrates. Microelectron. Eng. 98, 502–507.

Dahiya, R.S., Adami, A., Collini, C., Lorenzelli, L., 2013. POSFET tactile sensing arrays using CMOS technology. Sensors Actuators A 202, 226–232.

Dahiya, R.S., Adami, A., Pinna, L., Collini, C., Valle, M., Lorenzelli, L., 2014. Tactile sensing chips with POSFET array and integrated interface electronics. IEEE Sensors J. 14, 3448–3457.

Dario, P., Hannaford, B., Takanishi, A., 2008. Guest editorial Sp. issue on biorobotics. IEEE Trans. Rob. 24, 3–4.

Edin, B.B., Johansson, N., 1995. Skin strain patterns provide kinaesthetic information to the human central nervous system. J. Physiol. 487, 243–251.

Fearing, R.S., 1990. Tactile sensing mechanisms. Int. J. Rob. Res. 9, 3–23.

Graz, I., kaltenbrunner, M., Keplinger, C., Schwodiauer, R., Bauer, S., 2006. Flexible ferroelectret field-effect transistor for large-area sensor skins and microphones. Appl. Phys. Lett. 89, 073501-1–073501-3.

Hammock, M.L., Chortos, A., Tee, B.C.Ä., Tok, J.B.Ä., Bao, Z., 2013. 25th anniversary article: the evolution of electronic skin: a brief history, design considerations, and recent progress. Adv. Mater. 25, 5997–6038.

Hasegawa, Y., Sasaki, H., Shikida, M., Sato, K., Itoigawa, K., 2004. Magnetic actuation of a micro-diaphragm structure for an active tactile sensor. In: Int. Symp. Micro-Nanomechatronics and Human Science, pp. 99–104.

Hayward, V., Terekhov, A.V., Wong, S.-C., Geborek, P., Bengtsson, F., Jörntell, H., 2014. Spatio-temporal skin strain distributions evoke low variability spike responses in cuneate neurons. J. R. Soc. Interface 11, 20131015.

Hosoda, K., Tada, Y., Asada, M., 2006. Anthropomorphic robotic soft fingertip with randomly distributed receptors. Robot. Auton. Syst. 54, 104–109.

Howe, R.D., 1994. Tactile sensing and control of robotics manipulation. J. Adv. Rob. 8, 245–261.

Hwang, E.S., Seo, J.H., Kim, Y.J., 2007. A polymer-based flexible tactile sensor for both normal and shear load detections and its application for robotics. J. Microelectromech. Syst. 16, 556–563.

Izhikevich, E.M., 2003. Simple model of spiking neurons. IEEE Trans. Neural Netw. 14, 1569–1572.

Izhikevich, E.M., 2004. Which model to use for cortical spiking neurons? IEEE Trans. Neural Netw. 15, 1063–1070.

Johannson, R.S., Birznieks, I., 2004. First spikes in ensembles of human tactile afferents code complex spatial fingertip events. Nat. Neurosci. 7, 170–177.

Johansson, R.S., Flanagan, J.R., 2009. Coding and use of tactile signals from the fingertips in object manipulation tasks. Nat. Rev. Neurosci. 10, 345–359.

Johansson, R.S., Vallbo, A.B., 1979. Tactile sensibility in the human hand: relative and absolute densities of four types of mechanoreceptive units in glabrous skin. J. Physiol. 286, 283–300.

Jörntell, H., Bengtsson, F., Geborek, P., Spanne, A., Terekhov, A.V., Hayward, V., 2014. Segregation of tactile input features in neurons of the cuneate nucleus. Neuron 83 (6), 1444–1452.

Kandel, E.R., Schwartz, J.H., Jessell, T.M., 2000. Principles of Neural Science, fourth ed. McGraw-Hill Medical, New York.

Kayser, C., Logothetis, N.K., Panzeri, S., 2010. Millisecond encoding precision of auditory cortex neurons. Proc. Natl. Acad. Sci. USA. 107, 16976–16981.

Khan, S., Lorenzelli, L., Dahiya, R.S., 2014a. Bendable piezoresistive sensors by screen printing MWCNT/PDMS composites on flexible substrates. In: 10th Conf. on Ph.D. Research in Microelectronics and Electronics (PRIME), pp. 1–4.

Khan, S., Lorenzelli, L., Dahiya, R.S., 2014b. Screen printed flexible pressure sensors skin. In: 25th Annual SEMI Advanced Semiconductor Manufacturing Conference (ASMC) 2014, pp. 219–224.

Khan, S., Tinku, S., Lorenzelli, L., Dahiya, R., 2015a. Flexible tactile sensors using screen printed P(VDF-TrFE) and MWCNT/PDMS composites, IEEE Sensors J. 15, 3146–3155. http://dx.doi.org/10.1109/JSEN.2014.2368989.

Khan, S., Lorenzelli, L., Dahiya, R., 2015b. Technologies for printing sensors and electronics over large flexible substrates: a review, IEEE Sensors J. 15, 3164–3185. http://dx.doi.org/10.1109/JSEN.2014.2375203.

Kim, S.S., Sripati, A.P., Bensmaia, S.J., 2010. Predicting the timing of spikes evoked by tactile stimulation of the hand. J. Neurophysiol. 104, 1484–1496.

Kim, E., Sugg, K., Langhals, N., Lightbody, S., Baltrusaitis, M., Urbanchek, M., Cederna, P., Gerling, G.J., 2013. An engineered tactile afferent modulation platform to elicit compound sensory nerve action potentials in response to force magnitude. In: World Haptics Conference (WHC), 2013, pp. 241–246.

Krishna, G.M., Rajanna, K., 2004. Tactile sensor based on piezoelectric resonance. IEEE Sensors J. 4, 691–697.

Kwon, H.J., Choi, W.C., 2010. Design and fabrication of a flexible three-axial tactile sensor array based on polyimide micromachining. Microsyst. Technol. 16, 2029–2035.

Laschi, C., Cianchetti, M., 2014. Soft robotics: new perspectives for robot bodyware and control. Bionics Biomim. 2, 3.

Lee, J.C., Lee, D.W., 2010. Flexible and tactile sensor based on a photosensitive polymer. Microelectron. Eng. 87, 1400–1403.

Lee, M.H., Nicholls, H.R., 1999. Tactile sensing for mechatronics—a state of the art survey. Mechatronics 9, 1–31.

Levi, A., Piovanelli, M., Furlan, S., Mazzolai, B., Beccai, L., 2013. Soft, transparent, electronic skin for distributed and multiple pressure sensing. Sensors 13, 6578–6604.

Li, C.Y., Wu, P.M., Lee, S., Gorton, A., Schulz, M.J., Ahn, C.H., 2008. Flexible dome and bump shape piezoelectric tactile sensors using PVDF-TrFE copolymer. J. Microelectromech. Syst. 17, 334–341.

Loomis, J.M., Lederman, S.J., 1986. Tactual perception. In: Cognitive Processes & Performances. John Wiley & Sons, New York.

Lucarotti, C., Oddo, C.M., Vitiello, N., Carrozza, M.C., 2013. Synthetic and bio-artificial tactile sensing: a review. Sensors 13, 1435–1466.

Maheshwari, V., 2006. High-resolution thin-film device to sense texture by touch. Science 312, 1501–1504.

Maheshwari, V., Saraf, R., 2008. Tactile devices to sense touch on a par with a human finger. Angew. Chem. Int. Ed. 47, 7808–7826.

Medler, A., Patel, C., Butcher, J., 1996. A capacitive pressure sensor fabricated by a combination of SIMOX (SOI) substrates and novel etching techniques. J. Commun. 47, 6–8.

Mei, T., Li, W.J., Ge, Y., Chen, Y., Ni, L., Chan, M.H., 2000. An integrated MEMS three-dimensional tactile sensor with large force range. Sensors Actuators A 80, 155–162.

Millner, S., Grübl, A., Meier, K., Schemmel, J., Schwartz, M.-O., 2010. A VLSI implementation of the adaptive exponential integrate-and-fire neuron model. In: Advances in Neural Information Processing Systems, pp. 1642–1650.
Moe, S.T., Schiolberg-Henriksen, K., Wang, D.T., Lund, E., Nysaether, J., Furuberg, L., Visser, M., Fallet, T., Bernstein, R.W., 2000. Capacitive differential pressure sensor for harsh environments. Sensors Actuators A Phys. 83, 30–33.
Montana, D.J., 1992. Contact stability for two-fingered grasps. IEEE Trans. Robot. Autom. 8, 421–430.
Mountcastle, V.B., 2005. The Sensory Hand: Neural Mechanisms of Somatic Sensation. Harvard University Press, Cambridge, Massachusetts and London, England.
Muhammad, H.B., Oddo, C.M., Beccai, L., Recchiuto, C., Anthony, C.J., Adams, M.J., Carrozza, M.C., Hukins, D.W.L., Ward, M.C.L., 2011a. Development of a bioinspired MEMS based capacitive tactile sensor for a robotic finger. Sensors Actuators A Phys. 165, 221–229.
Muhammad, H.B., Recchiuto, C., Oddo, C.M., Beccai, L., Anthony, C.J., Adams, M.J., Carrozza, M.C., Ward, M.C.L., 2011b. A capacitive tactile sensor array for surface texture discrimination. Microelectron. Eng. 88, 1811–1813.
Oddo, C.M., Beccai, L., Wessberg, J., Wasling, H.B., Mattioli, F., Carrozza, M.C., 2011. Roughness encoding in human and biomimetic artificial touch: spatiotemporal frequency modulation and structural anisotropy of fingerprints. Sensors 11, 5596–5615.
Okada, H., Yawata, M., Ishida, M., Sawada, K., Takao, H., 2010. A membrane type Si-MEMS tactile imager with fingerprint structure for realization of slip sensing capability. In: 23rd IEEE Int. Conf. on MicroElectroMechanical Sys., 2010, pp. 608–611.
Pare, M., Behets, C., Cornu, O., 2003. Paucity of presumptive Ruffini corpuscles in the index finger pad of humans. J. Comp. Neurol. 456, 260–266.
Persichetti, A., Vecchi, F., Carrozza, M.C., 2007. Optoelectronic-based flexible contact sensor for prosthetic hand application. In: Int. Conf. Rehab. Robot. pp. 415–420.
Pfeifer, R., Bongard, J., Grand, S., 2007. How the body shapes the way we think: a new view of intelligence. MIT press, Cambridge, Massachusetts.
Purves, D., Augustine, G.J., Fitzpatrick, D., Hall, W.C., LaMantia, A.-S., McNamara, J.O., White, L.E., 2008. Neuroscience, fourth ed. Sinauer Associates Inc., Sunderland, Massachusetts.
Raspopovic, S., Capogrosso, M., Petrini, F.M., Bonizzato, M., Rigosa, J., Di Pino, G., Carpaneto, J., Controzzi, M., Boretius, T., Fernandez, E., 2014. Restoring natural sensory feedback in real-time bidirectional hand prostheses. Sci. Transl. Med. 6, 222ra19.
Renard, S., Pisella, C., Collet, J., Perruchot, F., Kergueris, C., Destrez, P., Rey, P., Delorme, N., Dallard, E., 2002. Miniature pressure acquisition microsystem for wireless in vivo measurements. In: IEEE-EMBS Special Topic Conference on Microtechnologies in Medicine & Biology, pp. 175–179.
Rossi, D.D., 1991. Artificial tactile sensing and haptic perception. Meas. Sci. Technol. 2, 1003.
Roy, D., Wettels, N., Loeb, G.E., 2012. Elastomeric skin selection for a fluid-filled artificial fingertip. J. Appl. Polym. Sci. 127, 4624–4633, pp. 1–10.
Scheibert, J., Leurent, S., Prevost, A., Debregeas, G., 2009. The role of fingerprints in the coding of tactile information probed with a biomimetic sensor. Science 323, 1503–1506.
Shikida, M., Shimizu, T., Sato, K., Itoigawa, K., 2003. Active tactile sensor for detecting contact force and hardness of an object. Sensors Actuators A 103, 213–218.
Shimoga, K.B., Goldenberg, A.A., 1992. Soft materials for robotic fingers. In: IEEE Int. Conf. on Robotics and Automation, pp. 1300–1305.

Spigler, G., Oddo, C.M., Carrozza, M.C., 2012. Soft-neuromorphic artificial touch for applications in neuro-robotics. In: 4th IEEE RAS & EMBS Int. Conf. Biomedical Robotics & Biomechatronics (BioRob), 2012, pp. 1913–1918.
Swartz, R.G., Plummer, J.D., 1979. Integrated silicon-PVF2 acoustic transducer arrays. IEEE Trans. Electron Devices 26, 1920–1932.
Takenawa, S., 2009. A Magnetic type tactile sensor using a two-dimensional array of inductors. In: IEEE Int. Conf. Robot. pp. 1516–1521.
Tanaka, M., Iijima, T., Tanahashi, Y., Chonan, S., 2007. Development of a 3D tactile sensor. J. Mater. Process. Technol. 181, 286–290.
Tibrewala, A., Phataralaoha, A., Buttgenbach, S., 2009. Development, fabrication and characterization of a 3D tactile sensor. J. Micromech. Microeng. 19, 125005.
Tiwana, M.I., Redmond, S.J., Lovell, N.H., 2012. A review of tactile sensing technologies with applications in biomedical engineering. Sensors Actuators A Phys. 179, 17–31.
Vasarhelyi, G., Adam, M., Vazsonyi, E., Barsony, I., Ducso, C., 2006. Effects of the elastic cover on tactile sensor arrays. Sensors Actuators A Phys. 132, 245–251.
Vasarhelyi, G., Fodor, B., Roska, T., 2007. Tactile sensing-processing: interface-cover geometry and the inverse-elastic problem. Sensors Actuators A Phys. 140, 8–18.
Vázquez, Y., Salinas, E., Romo, R., 2013. Transformation of the neural code for tactile detection from thalamus to cortex. Proc. Natl. Acad. Sci. U. S. A. 110, E2635–E2644.
Victor, J.D., Purpura, K.P., 1998. Spatial phase and the temporal structure of the response to gratings in V1. J. Neurophysiol. 80, 554–571.
Viry, L., Levi, A., Totaro, M., Mondini, A., Mattoli, V., Mazzolai, B., Beccai, L., 2014. Flexible three-axial force sensor for soft and highly sensitive artificial touch. Adv. Mater. 26, 2659–2664.
Wang, L., Beebe, D.J., 2000. A silicon-based shear force sensor: development and characterization. Sensors Actuators A 84, 33–44.
Westling, G., Johannson, R.S., 1984. Factors influencing the force control during precision grip. Exp. Brain Res. 53, 277–284.
Wettels, N., Santos, V.J., Johansson, R.S., Loeb, G.E., 2008. Biomimetic tactile sensor array. Adv. Robot. 22, 829–849.
Wolfe, J.M., Kluender, K.R., Levi, D.M., Bartoshuk, L.M., Herz, R.S., Klatzky, R.L., Lederman, S.J., 2006. Sensation and Perception. Sinauer Associates Inc., Sunderland, Massachusetts USA.
Yousef, H., Boukallel, M., Althoefer, K., 2011. Tactile sensing for dexterous in-hand manipulation in robotics—a review. Sensors Actuators A Phys. 167, 171–187.

Bio-inspired hair-based inertial sensors

5

H. Droogendijk, M.J. de Boer, R.G.P. Sanders, G.J.M. Krijnen

5.1 Introduction

In biology, mechano sensors, equipped with differing hair-like structures for signal pick up, are sensitive to a variety of physical quantities like acceleration, flow, rotational rate, balancing, and IR light (Liu, 2007; Schmitz et al., 2012). As an example, crickets have various types of hair-like receptors for measurement of several environmental quantities. For sensing of low-frequency flows (typically <1 kHz) to obtain information about the environment and avoid, e.g., predator attacks, crickets use filiform hairs, which are situated on the dorsal side of two abdominal appendages called cerci, and which are able to sense airflows with velocity amplitudes down to 30 μms^{-1} (Tobias and Murphey, 1979; Shimozawa and Kanou, 1984; Shimozawa et al., 1998; Humphrey et al., 1993) and operate around the energy levels of thermal noise (Shimozawa et al., 2003). Crickets also gather information about their environment by the use of bristle hairs which activate interneurons that respond to tactile stimuli of the cercus and abdomen (Murphey, 1985).

It is these intriguing aspects of biological sensors that inspire engineers on developing artificial counterparts and exploiting the field of biomimetics and bio-inspiration. For example, taking the cricket cercal hair sensors as a source of inspiration, several research groups have worked on the development of bio-inspired hair-based airflow measurements by exploiting microelectromechanical systems (MEMS) technology (Ozaki et al., 2000; Chen et al., 2007; Wang et al., 2007; Sadeghi et al., 2011; Tao and Yu, 2012).

In this chapter, the bio-inspired approach is applied to bio-inspired inertial sensors developed using MEMS technology. Particularly, two types of bio-inspired inertial sensors are discussed: a cricket-inspired accelerometer (Droogendijk et al., 2014b) and a fly-inspired gyroscope (Droogendijk et al., 2014a). The main outline of this chapter is as follows. Section 5.2 deals with two examples of biological sensor systems for measurement of inertial quantities. Subsequently, the design and fabrication of the cricket-inspired accelerometer (Section 5.3) and the fly-inspired gyroscope (Section 5.4) are discussed. Section 5.5 continues with the assessment of the bio-inspired approach within the field of (inertial) hair-based sensors.

5.2 Hair structures for inertial sensing

5.2.1 Cricket's clavate hairs

In addition to flow and tactile perception, crickets have club-shaped sensilla, called clavate hairs, located on their cerci (Figure 5.1), with hair lengths of 20–250 μm (Bischof, 1974). These clavate hairs turn out to be sensitive to (gravitational) acceleration, providing the cricket information on its orientation (Bischof, 1974, 1975; Murphey, 1981; Sakaguchi and Murphey, 1983). For example, a cricket uses its clavate hairs to compensate head movement when it is rotated around its longitudinal axis (Horn and Bischof, 1983), for which such rotations can be measured with a resolution of about 0.1° (Bischof, 1975). Additionally, Bischof (1975) showed that these clavate hairs can respond to harmonic accelerations with frequencies up to 300 Hz.

For measuring (gravitational) acceleration, numerous types of accelerometers have been realized over the past years using MEMS technology, with applications in, e.g., the automotive industry and navigation (Yazdi et al., 1998). Current state-of-the-art commercialized MEMS accelerometers show formidable performance in range, resolution, and noise floor. In contrast to the cricket's clavate system, MEMS accelerometers are usually not hair-based systems and frequently contain feedback electronics. To explore some of the intricacies of the clavate hair system and assess its potential to engineering applications (e.g., automotive industry, robotics, and motion tracking), we aim for the design, fabrication, and characterization of a bio-inspired accelerometer. Bio-inspired hair-based structures have been exploited earlier with applications in both actuation and sensing of physical quantities (Zhou and Liu, 2008; Ginsberg et al., 2013), but

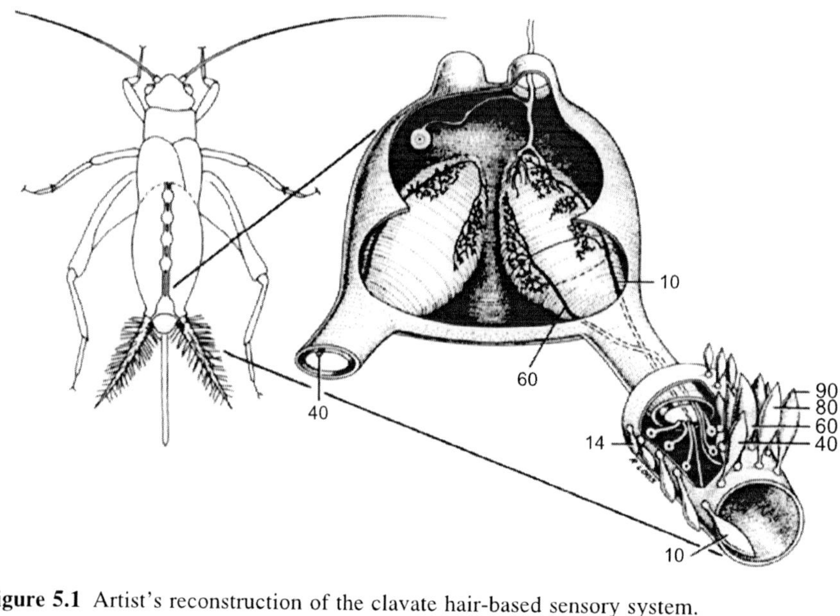

Figure 5.1 Artist's reconstruction of the clavate hair-based sensory system. Adapted from Murphey (1981).

seldom for inertial measurement. Previously, a hair-like accelerometer has been investigated by Tang et al. (2013), but its response to external accelerations was not demonstrated.

5.2.2 Fly's haltere

Another example of a biological hair-based sensory system is the fly's haltere structure. Halteres are tiny club-shaped organs that beat in antiphase to the wings during flight (Fraenkel and Pringle, 1938), and function as gyroscopes[1] by measuring the fly's body rotation using Coriolis forces (Pringle, 1948). The rotation-dependent position of the haltere (Figure 5.2) is measured in sensitive strain fields (Hengstenberg, 1998). It has been demonstrated that this haltere-based system is used for supporting equilibrium reflexes (Sandeman and Markl, 1980; Nalbach and Hengstenberg, 1994; Chan et al., 1998; Ristroph et al., 2010).

For measuring angular rate, numerous types of gyroscopes have been realized over the past years using MEMS technology, where current state-of-the-art MEMS gyroscopes show formidable performance in range, resolution, and noise floor (Yazdi et al., 1998; Xie and Fedder, 2003; Alper and Akin, 2005; Trusov et al., 2011).

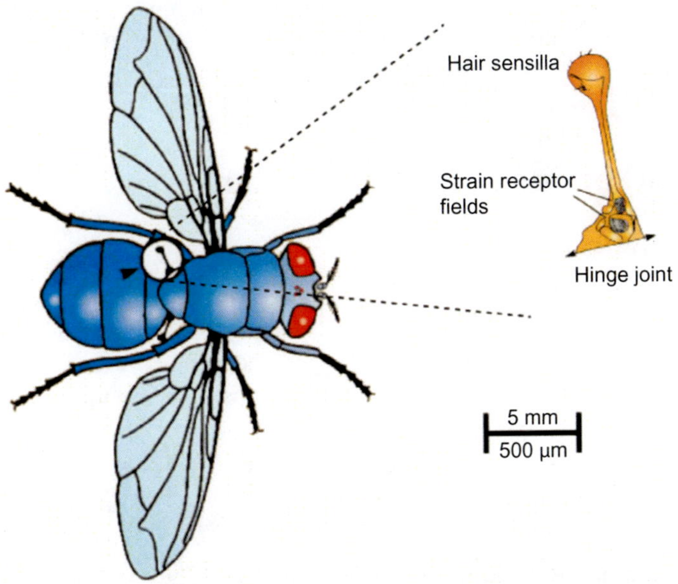

Figure 5.2 Halteres of the blowfly *Calliphora vicina*. During walking and flight, the halteres oscillate in a vertical plane around a proximal hinge.
Adapted from Hengstenberg (1998).

[1] In this work, all gyroscopes are so-called Coriolis vibratory gyroscopes, which are in fact angular rate sensors. By integration of the measured angular rate, information about the angle is obtained.

In contrast to the fly's haltere system, MEMS gyroscopes are typically no hair-based systems, are generally heavily underdamped and operate at rather high frequencies. In contrast, the fly's haltere system is close to critically damped system and operates around the fly's wing beat frequency (130–150 Hz) (Nalbach and Hengstenberg, 1994). Obviously, the fly's haltere system has developed under evolutionary pressure and therefore addresses the sensory needs of the fly. As a result, not only the operation principle is different from those generally employed in MEMS gyroscopes but also the performance may score high on metrics other than normally used for MEMS gyroscopes. For example, bandwidth and response time may be far more essential for flies than (bias-)stability and noise floor, as the halteres have been proven to aid in flight dynamics of flies with fast (10 ms) responses to flight disturbances (Rosner et al., 2009).

Previous research on bio-inspired gyroscopic systems (using foils of stainless steel) shows advantages on using a haltere-based gyroscope by achieving a higher sensitivity and a lower power consumption compared to conventional MEMS gyroscopes (Wu et al., 2002; Wu and Wood, 2006). Also, Tang et al. (1997) and Challoner et al. (2007) fabricated hair-based gyroscopes using MEMS technology, although these devices had still macroscopic dimensions compared to the fly's haltere and were severely underdamped by operating them in vacuum. Wicaksono et al. (2007) discuss the preliminary design and modeling of a bio-inspired MEMS gyroscope with electrostatic driving and piezo-resistive read-out. Smith et al. (2012) report on the design and fabrication of a MEMS haltere to use as a sensor in a micro-autonomous system.

5.3 Cricket-inspired accelerometer

5.3.1 Physics

Mechanically, the hair-based accelerometer can be understood as a so-called inverted pendulum which is subjected to external accelerations (Figure 5.3). It is described as a second-order rotational mechanical system with moment of inertia J, a rotational stiffness S, and a rotational damping R, resulting in a description of the system's response to harmonic accelerations by

$$\theta(\omega) = \frac{T_a}{S - J\omega^2 + J\omega R}, \tag{5.1}$$

where for a cylindrical hair, the moment of inertia can be expressed as

$$J = \frac{\pi\rho d^2}{48}\left(4L^3 + \frac{3}{4}d^2 L\right). \tag{5.2}$$

In these expressions, $\theta(\omega)$ is the rotational angle amplitude of the hair and T_a is the amplitude of the torque acting on the hair. Usually, in the models, the hairs are treated as cylindrical structures (Humphrey et al., 1993), but here the hair is modeled as an

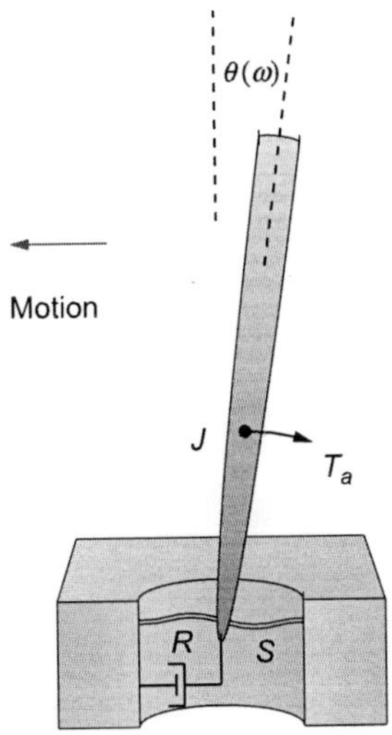

Figure 5.3 Schematic view of inertial measurement by hair-like structures.

inverted conical shape to take the MEMS-hair-shape into account. We will show that this eventually will only lead to a geometry-dependent factor η such that $J \approx \eta \rho d^2 L^3$.

From Equation (5.2), the moment of inertia J depends strongly on the hair diameter d and hair length L. The torque T_a is a consequence of external accelerations, or the projections thereof, in the direction perpendicular to the hair and perpendicular to its rotation axis, denoted here by a_{ext}. Using Newton's second law, T_a is found by integrating the inertial contributions by over the hair:

$$T_a = \int_0^L a_{\text{ext}} \rho \pi \left(\frac{d(z)}{2} \right)^2 z\text{d}z = \Xi \cdot a_{\text{ext}}, \tag{5.3}$$

where Ξ can be expressed as

$$\Xi = \frac{\pi \eta \rho}{8} d^2 L^2. \tag{5.4}$$

In these expressions, ρ is the density of the hair and η is the parameter that depends on the precise geometry of the hair. Further, we assume that the rotational angle amplitudes θ are small, so the torque T_a can be considered directly proportional to the external acceleration a_{ext}.

5.3.2 Design

The hair mechanical system behaves like a classical second-order system, and consequently exhibits the trade-off between responsivity and bandwidth. The responsivity of the hair accelerometer for frequencies well below the system's resonance frequency ($\omega \ll \omega_r$) is defined as

$$\text{Responsivity} = \left.\frac{d\theta\omega}{da_{\text{ext}}}\right|_{\omega=0} = \frac{\pi\eta}{8}\frac{\rho d^2 L^2}{S}. \tag{5.5}$$

The bandwidth of the system is estimated from the system's resonance frequency:

$$\text{Bandwidth} = \omega_r = \sqrt{\frac{S}{J}}. \tag{5.6}$$

By taking the product of responsivity and bandwidth, a figure of merit (FoM) can be defined for the bio-inspired hair accelerometer, similar to the approach described by Krijnen et al. (2007):

$$\text{FoM} = \text{Responsivity} \times \text{Bandwidth}. \tag{5.7}$$

When the hair length is considerably larger than the hair diameter ($L \gg d$), this FoM can be simplified to

$$\text{FoM} \propto \sqrt{\frac{\rho d^2 L}{S}}. \tag{5.8}$$

As a result, to achieve a "good" hair-based accelerometer, the sensor should have a long and thick hair (high d and L), as well as a compliant mechanical suspension (low S).

5.3.3 Fabrication

The fabrication process for the bio-inspired accelerometer is based upon the process for cricket-inspired bio-inspired hair flow sensors, previously developed in our group (Bruinink et al., 2009; Dagamseh et al., 2011). A schematic overview of the bio-inspired accelerometer with the materials indicated is shown in Figure 5.4a.

The sensor is fabricated on a silicon-on-insulator wafer. Trenches are etched in the silicon device layer using deep reactive-ion etching. A layer of 200 nm stoichiometric Si_3N_4 is used for covering and protecting the trenches. The device layer contains two electrodes, which are used for capacitive read-out of the acceleration-induced movement. On top of the Si_3N_4 layer, a sacrificial layer of polysilicon (1.5 μm) is deposited by low-pressure chemical vapor deposition. The sensor membrane and springs are constructed by depositing and patterning a 1-μm SiRN layer on top of the polysilicon. Aluminum (80 nm) is sputtered on top of the membrane to create the electrodes for capacitive read-out. Our artificial clavate hair is created by two layers of SU-8, to release both the center of mass toward the top of the hair structure and a total hair length of about 800 μm with an average diameter of about 80 μm. Finally, to release the membrane, the sacrificial polysilicon layer is removed using XeF_2 etching. The fabrication results are shown by the SEM image in Figure 5.4b.

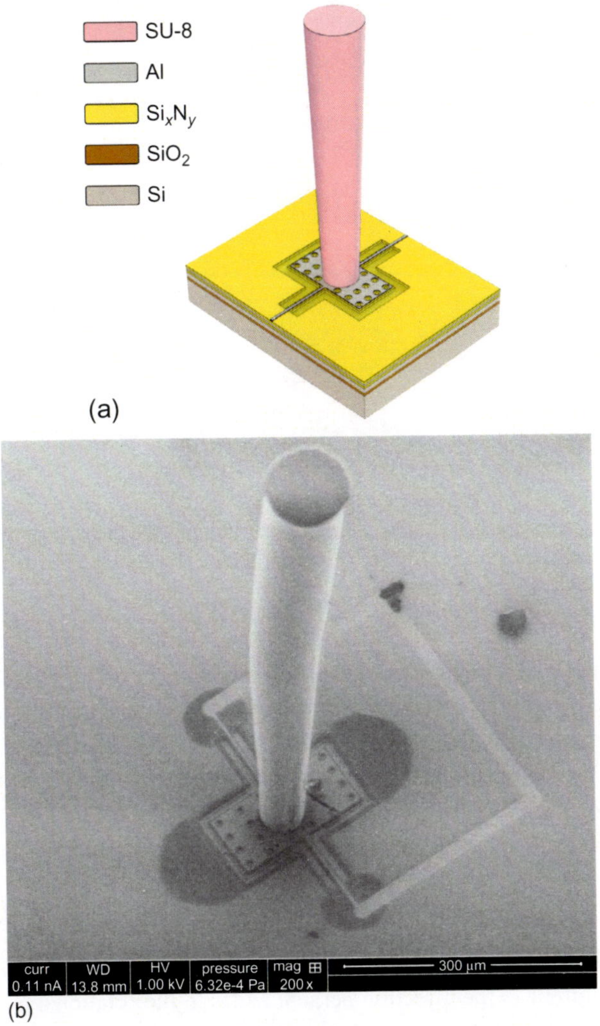

Figure 5.4 Design (a) and fabrication (b) of the MEMS hair-based accelerometer fabricated by surface micromachining and using SU-8 lithography.

5.3.4 Experimental

5.3.4.1 Setup

Experiments to measure the sensor's response are performed using the setup shown in Figure 5.5. A waveform generator (Agilent 33220A-001) is used to produce a sinusoidal signal at a frequency f ($\omega = 2\pi f$) that is supplied to an amplifier. This amplifier drives a voice-coil shaker (MB Electronics PM 50) to generate harmonic acceleration.

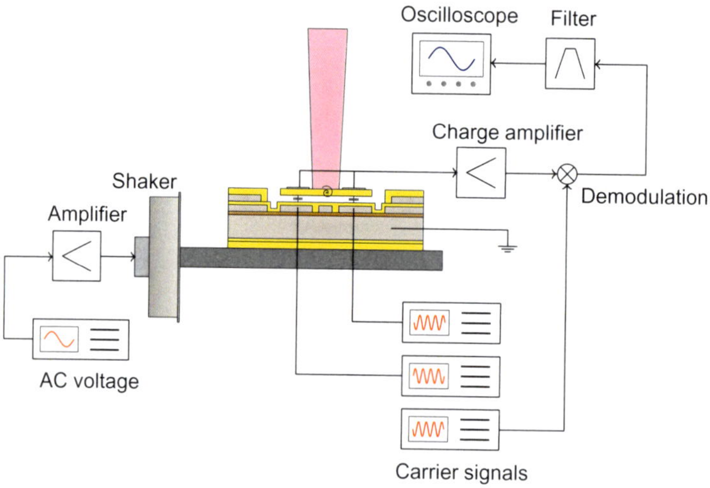

Figure 5.5 Capacitive measurement setup for determining the membrane rotation of the biomimetic accelerometer.

Carrier signals at 1 MHz are supplied to the bottom electrodes of the accelerometer for capacitive read-out. The top electrode is connected to a charge amplifier, and after demodulation and filtering (Stanford SR 650), the sensor's response is monitored on an oscilloscope (Agilent DS1024). For calibration, the applied accelerations were measured by mounting a reference accelerometer (STEVAL-MKI021V1) on the shaker.

5.3.4.2 *Frequency response*

First, the frequency response of the hair-based accelerometer was measured using capacitive read-out in the direction perpendicular to the rotational axis. Frequencies within a range of 50–1000 Hz were applied to the shaker. The reference accelerometer was used to determine the externally applied acceleration amplitude. The resulting measured magnitude response of the bio-inspired accelerometer is shown in red in Figure 5.6. Here, the circles represent the measurements and the dashed line exhibits the analytical model based on Equation (5.1), where the resonance frequency ω_0 and the quality factor Q were fitted. We observe good agreement between model and measurements, where the resonance frequency is found to be about 320 Hz.

5.3.4.3 *Directivity*

The sensor's directivity was measured by rotating it over 360°, with steps of 10°, with respect to the direction of the applied external acceleration, while using capacitive read-out. To this end, a harmonic acceleration with a frequency of 80 Hz was applied

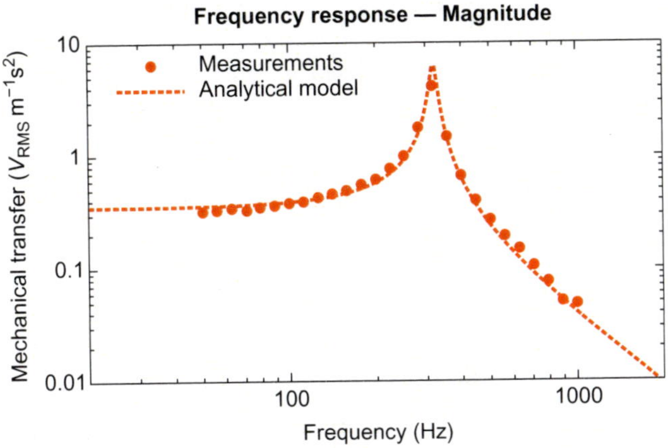

Figure 5.6 Measured mechanical transfer of the hair-based accelerometer using capacitive read-out.

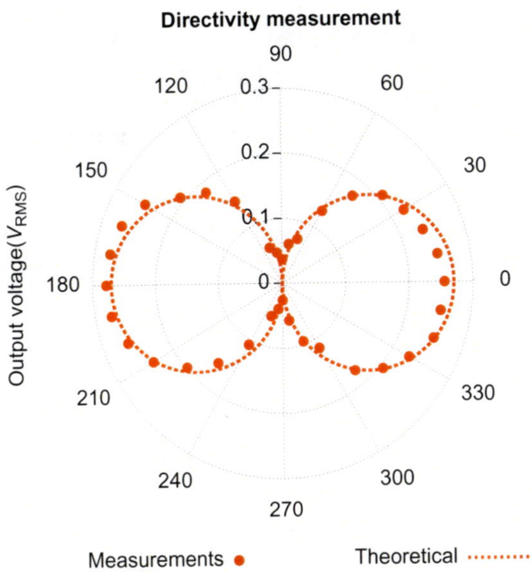

Figure 5.7 Measured directivity of the hair-based accelerometer using capacitive read-out at an acceleration frequency of 80 Hz.

and the output voltage was measured by a multimeter (Keithley, Model 2000). The obtained results are shown in Figure 5.7. We observe that the measurements are in close agreement with the theoretical response for a so-called figure-of-eight. The measurements indicate that the hair-based accelerometer has a maximum responsivity for both 0° and 180°, which coincides with the direction perpendicular to the rotational axis of the hair sensor.

5.3.4.4 Threshold and linearity

To obtain a model which describes the sensor's signal-to-noise ratio (SNR) as a function of acceleration amplitude as well as the sensor's detection threshold, the signal and noise powers are considered. The signal is assumed to have a linear relationship with respect to the acceleration amplitude a_0, given by the coefficient $S_c(\omega)$. This coefficient is directly related to the sensor's rotational angle $\theta(\omega)$ and therefore has a dependency on the acceleration frequency ω. N_c is a constant representing the total noise, giving for the measured output z due to the uncorrelated sources:

$$z(\omega) = \sqrt{(S_c(\omega)a_{\text{ext}})^2 + N_c^2}. \tag{5.9}$$

From this expression, the measured detection threshold $a_{\min}$ can be found by equating the noise and signal powers (or alternatively by calculating the intersection value of the asymptotes) which requires only the values for S_c and N_c:

$$a_{\min}(\omega) = \frac{N_c}{S_c(\omega)}. \tag{5.10}$$

Experiments to determine the sensor's linearity were performed by choosing first a specific acceleration frequency (80 Hz) and then by varying the acceleration amplitude. Subsequently, from the measured output rms voltage, the sensor's detection limit and linearity are derived. The results are shown in Figure 5.8, where the points represent the measurements, the solid line is based on Equation (5.9), and the dashed lines indicate the constant equivalent noise amplitude and ideal linear response asymptotes. We observe that for accelerations with an amplitude of more than 0.1 ms^{-2}, indicated by the intersection of the asymptotes, the hair-based accelerometer exhibits a clear linear relationship with the applied acceleration. Below this amplitude, the sensor's output is dominated by noise (SNR < 1).

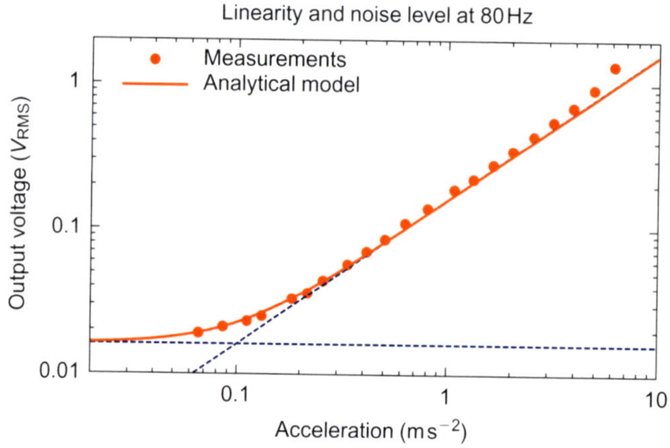

Figure 5.8 Measured response versus acceleration amplitudes at a frequency of 80 Hz using capacitive read-out.

To get some insight into the accelerometer's noise performance and stability, an Allan variance measurement was performed. The zero-acceleration output rms voltage was measured with a time interval of 20 ms for a period of 2 h using a multimeter (Agilent 34401A) connected to Lab VIEW. The results of the subsequently calculated Allan deviation are shown in Figure 5.9, together with asymptotic lines for both the velocity random walk and the bias instability.

From the linearity measurements, the error on full-scale (i.e., the measurement taken at highest acceleration of 6.12 ms^{-2}, see Figure 5.8) was calculated and found to be 3.3%. By considering the detection threshold and the full-scale acceleration amplitude, the dynamic range of the hair-based accelerometer is about 35.6 dB.

The Allan variance results showed a velocity random walk of $1.67 ms^{-1}\sqrt{h^{-1}}$ and a bias instability of 5×10^{-3} ms^{-2}. To summarize, an overview of the sensor performance is shown in Table 5.1.

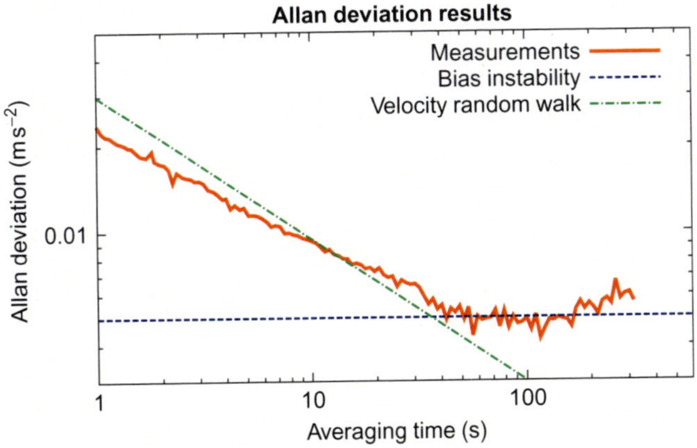

Figure 5.9 Measured Allan deviation using capacitive read-out.

Table 5.1 Experimental values of the bio-inspired hair-based accelerometer

Quantity	Symbol	Value
Mechanical parameters		
Quality factor	Q	12.5
Resonance frequency	f_0	319.6 Hz
Sensor performance (80 Hz)		
Threshold	a_{min}	0.10 ms^{-2}
Dynamic range	DR	≥35.6 dB
Full scale error	ε_{FS}	3.3%
Velocity random walk	VRW	$1.67 ms^{-1}\sqrt{h^{-1}}$
Bias instability	σ_b	5×10^{-3} ms^{-2}
Thermal noise limit	a_{th}	1.1×10^{-3} ms^{-2}

5.3.5 Discussion

The measured threshold of the bio-inspired accelerometer is about 0.10 ms^{-2}, which is about a factor 100 larger than the calculated thermal noise-based value of 1.1×10^{-3} ms^{-2} (Gabrielson, 1993). The relative large detection threshold is due to the presence of comparatively strong noise sources in the read-out electronics (Dagamseh et al., 2013). Improvement of these electronics, by reduction of its noise, will help to bring the detection threshold for the accelerometer toward the thermal noise- limited threshold. Similar differences between measured and (calculated) thermal noise levels have been observed for our previously reported bio-inspired hair flow sensors (Droogendijk et al., 2012b; Dagamseh et al., 2013).

Generally, the susceptibility for (gravitational) acceleration is used by crickets for determination of their position and orientation. The hair-based accelerometer described in this work allows in principle also for determination of orientation using the Earth's gravitational field. That is, by measuring the projection of the Earth's gravitational acceleration, the angle of rotation of the accelerometer with respect to Earth can be determined. However, since the fabricated accelerometer has limits with respect to resolution, an error in this angle will result. Based on the experimental data listed in Table 5.1, this error is calculated to be in the order of 0.7° for accelerations well below resonance ($\omega \rightarrow 0$), which emphasizes the potential use of this accelerometer to determine orientation. Notice that this value approaches the resolution of the cricket's clavate hair system of 0.1° (Bischof, 1975).

As we have shown in Figure 5.7, the hair-based accelerometer has a strong directivity. In our MEMS version, this directivity stems from both the mechanical design, which primarily allows rotation around the torsional axis of the sensor, and the differential capacitive read-out, which causes a strong reduction of signals caused by tilting of the hair. As a consequence, multiple hair-based accelerometers may be used simultaneously to sense acceleration in 3D. In crickets, filiform hairs have been shown to have preferential directions of rotations with ratios in stiffness of "hard" over "easy" directions between 4 and 8 (Kanou et al., 1989). Bischof (1974) demonstrated that such directivity exists in the cricket's clavate hairs. Additionally, Sakaguchi and Murphey (1983) have shown that crickets use many clavate hair sensors on their cerci for determination of their orientation relative to the gravitational field and that they do so both with respect to roll (rotation around longitudinal axis of the animal) and pitch.

5.4 Fly-inspired gyroscope

5.4.1 Physics

The dynamics of the haltere-based gyroscope and common MEMS gyroscopes are similar, since both types consist of vibrating structures governed by two coupled second-order differential equations. The design of these gyroscopes is in general a 2-D isotropic, damped mass-spring system. To describe the haltere mechanics, we first define the force $\vec{F}$ acting on the haltere knob) (Nalbach, 1993):

$$\vec{F} = m\vec{g} - m\ddot{\vec{r}}_\mathrm{i} - m\vec{a}_\mathrm{f} - m\dot{\vec{\Omega}} \times \vec{r}_\mathrm{i} - m\vec{\Omega} \times \left(\vec{\Omega} \times \vec{r}_\mathrm{i}\right) - 2m\vec{\Omega} \times \dot{\vec{r}}_\mathrm{i}, \tag{5.11}$$

where × denotes the vector product, m is the mass of the knob, $\vec{g}$ is the gravitational acceleration, $\vec{r}_\mathrm{i}$ is the position of the knob with respect to the fly, $\vec{a}_\mathrm{f}$ is the linear acceleration of the fly in space, and $\vec{\Omega}$ is the angular rate. Six forces contribute to the total inertial force: gravitational acceleration $\left(m\vec{g}\right)$, primary acceleration $\left(m\ddot{\vec{r}}_\mathrm{i}\right)$, linear acceleration $\left(m\vec{a}\right)$, angular acceleration $\left(m\dot{\vec{\Omega}} \times \vec{r}_\mathrm{i}\right)$, centrifugal acceleration $\left(m\vec{\Omega} \times \left(\vec{\Omega} \times \vec{r}_\mathrm{i}\right)\right)$, and Coriolis acceleration $\left(-2m\vec{\Omega} \times \dot{\vec{r}}_\mathrm{i}\right)$.

Now, we assume that linear accelerations are absent $\left(\vec{a}_\mathrm{f} = 0\right)$, gravitational acceleration $\vec{g}$ is only present in the z-direction (the axial direction of the haltere), angular rates are applied only in the horizontal xy-plane ($\Omega_x = \Omega_y = 0$), the movement of the haltere is harmonic with frequency ω and the angular rate Ω is constant with value Ω_0:

$$\Omega = \Omega_0. \tag{5.12}$$

Consequently, the force amplitude $\vec{F}_0$ for the x and y-directions, since the z-direction is not of interest to us, is given by:

$$\vec{F}_0 = m\begin{bmatrix} \omega^2 + \Omega_0^2 & -j2\omega\Omega_0 \\ j2\omega\Omega_0 & \omega^2 + \Omega_0^2 \end{bmatrix} \begin{bmatrix} x_0 \\ y_0 \end{bmatrix}, \tag{5.13}$$

where, x_0 and y_0 denote the amplitudes in the x and y-directions, respectively. Now, the coordinate system is changed into cylindrical coordinates, as shown in Figure 5.10. The system is continuously driven in a steady-state rotational motion in the drive mode with angle ϑ. Rotation around the haltere induces Coriolis-based motion in the sense mode, with the angle φ proportional to the input angular rate Ω. By using the following relationships, the force acting on the haltere can be written as a torque $\vec{T}$ for small angle amplitudes ϑ_0 and φ_0:

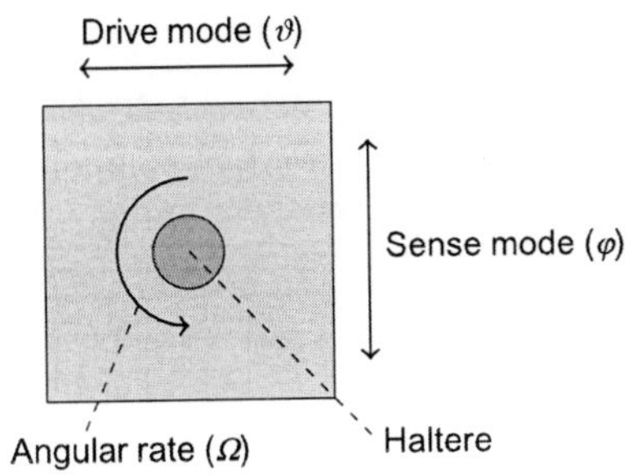

Figure 5.10 Operation principle of the biomimetic gyroscope (top view).

$$J = \eta m L^2, \quad x_0 = L\sin(\vartheta_0) \approx L\vartheta_0, \quad y_0 = L\sin(\varphi_0) \approx L\varphi_0, \tag{5.14}$$

where L is the haltere length, J is the moment of inertia, and η is a parameter depending on the precise geometry. Here, $\eta = 1$ by considering the haltere knob as a point mass. As a result, the torque acting on the haltere for constant angular rates becomes

$$\vec{T} = J\begin{bmatrix} \omega^2 + \Omega_0^2 & -j2\omega\Omega_0 \\ j2\omega\Omega_0 & \omega^2 + \Omega_0^2 \end{bmatrix} \begin{bmatrix} \vartheta_0 \\ \varphi_0 \end{bmatrix}. \tag{5.15}$$

The torque $\vec{T}$ acts on the haltere, which is part of the isotropic gyroscopic mechanical system. The response of this system is described by a coupled second-order differential equation:

$$\begin{bmatrix} G(\omega) & -C(\omega) \\ C(\omega) & G(\omega) \end{bmatrix} \begin{bmatrix} \vartheta_0 \\ \varphi_0 \end{bmatrix} = \begin{bmatrix} \mathcal{T}_{\text{ext}} \\ 0 \end{bmatrix}, \tag{5.16}$$

where $G(\omega)$ is given by:

$$G(\omega) = -\omega^2 + j2\zeta\omega\omega_0 + \omega_0^2 - \Omega_0^2, \tag{5.17}$$

and $C(\omega)$ denotes the coupling between the drive and sense mode due to angular rates:

$$C(\omega) = j2\omega\Omega_0. \tag{5.18}$$

In these expressions, the resonance frequency ω_0, damping ratio ζ, and normalized driving torque $\mathcal{T}_{\text{ext}}$ are defined as

$$\omega_0 = \sqrt{\frac{S}{J}}, \quad \zeta = \frac{R}{2\sqrt{SJ}}, \quad \mathcal{T}_{\text{ext}} = \frac{T_0}{J}, \tag{5.19}$$

where T_0 is the driving torque,[2] S is the torsional stiffness, R is the torsional resistance, and J is the moment of inertia. Further, ϑ_0 and φ_0 are the amplitudes of drive and sense mode, respectively.

From Equation (5.16) follows that the exposure to an angular rate Ω clearly affects the system's behavior; its resonance frequency is reduced by centrifugal forces, and torque contributions by angular Coriolis forces cause coupling between drive and sense mode. Although the reduction in resonance frequency by Ω_0^2 is typically negligible, the principle of a rate-dependent resonance frequency can be used for gyroscopic measurement of large angular rates (Zotov et al., 2011).

[2] This torque is delivered by electrostatic actuation in the case of the MEMS gyroscope and by the muscles in case of the fly.

5.4.2 Design

The governing equation of motion for the drive mode with amplitude has already been stated in Equation (5.16). By driving the gyroscope by a harmonic torque, assuming that the angular rate Ω is small compared to the sensor's resonance frequency ($\Omega_0 \ll \omega_0$), and angular accelerations are small, the drive-mode amplitude ϑ_0 can be approximated well by:

$$\vartheta_0(\omega) = \frac{\mathcal{T}_{\text{ext}}}{\sqrt{\left(\omega_0^2 - \omega^2\right)^2 + \left(2\zeta\omega_0\omega\right)^2}}. \tag{5.20}$$

Generally, MEMS gyroscopes are driven at a frequency ω equal to the gyroscope's resonance frequency ω_0 in the case of underdamped systems. Then, the drive-mode amplitude can be simplified to:

$$\vartheta_0 = \frac{\mathcal{T}_{\text{ext}}}{2\zeta\omega_0^2}. \tag{5.21}$$

Based on the drive mode motion, the normalized Coriolis-induced torque amplitude $\mathcal{T}_{\text{c}}$ of the sense mode is given by:

$$\mathcal{T}_{\text{c}} = 2\omega_0\vartheta_0\Omega_0. \tag{5.22}$$

Using the system of equations (5.16), the corresponding sense-mode amplitude φ_0 can be approximated as:

$$\varphi_0 = \frac{\mathcal{T}_{\text{ext}}}{2}\frac{1}{\omega_0^3\zeta^2}\Omega_0. \tag{5.23}$$

Now, we define the ratio $\mathcal{R}$ between sense- and drive-mode amplitudes, which is a measure for the system's responsivity.[3] Since Coriolis forces in general are small, a large $\mathcal{R}$ is desirable in order to measure correspondingly small angular rates Ω. The ratio $\mathcal{R}$ is defined as:

$$\mathcal{R} = \frac{\text{d}}{\text{d}\Omega_0}\left(\frac{\varphi_0}{\vartheta_0}\right) = \kappa. \tag{5.24}$$

where κ is a design parameter, which is the reciprocal of the product of damping ratio ζ and resonance frequency ω_0:

$$\kappa = \frac{1}{\zeta\omega_0}. \tag{5.25}$$

[3] This ratio is related to the scale factor of MEMS gyroscopes by taking the transfer by capacitive read-out into account (IEEE Aerosp. Electron. Sys. Soc., 2001).

However, in case the gyroscope is critically damped or overdamped, the gyroscope should be operated below its resonance frequency ω_0. A suitable frequency of operation is when the damping term (5.19) becomes equal to the stiffness-related term for small angular rates Ω, and the actuation frequency is chosen half this frequency:

$$2\zeta\omega_0\omega = \omega_0^2, \text{ giving } \omega = \frac{\omega_0}{2\zeta}. \tag{5.26}$$

By operating the device in such a way, in both the drive and the sense mode, the factor 2ζ drops, but the expression for the Coriolis torque given by Equation (5.22) remains unchanged. Therefore, by this analysis, the ratio of the drive- and sense-mode amplitudes of a gyroscope is equal for all classes of damping.

The performance of a gyroscope is also to be determined by its response time; besides a sensitive sensory system, also the ability to quickly respond to changes in angular rate Ω classifies the system. The corresponding response time τ_{95}—a measure for agility—is calculated from the second-order differential equation, describing the mechanical behavior of the system in response to a torque step function. Here, we assume that the gyroscope is driven in steady state with frequency ω, the coupling from sense to drive mode is negligible, and an angular rate Ω is applied stepwise. In that case, the governing equation for analyzing transients in the sense mode becomes

$$\frac{\mathrm{d}^2\varphi(t)}{\mathrm{d}t^2} + 2\zeta\omega_0\frac{\mathrm{d}\varphi(t)}{\mathrm{d}t} + \left(\omega_0^2 - \Omega_0^2\right)\varphi(t) = 2\omega\Omega_0\vartheta_0 \sin(\omega t)H(t), \tag{5.27}$$

where $H(t)$ denotes the Heaviside step function. The general solution of this damped second-order system is:

$$\varphi(t) = \Phi_1 \mathrm{e}^{-r_1 t} + \Phi_2 \mathrm{e}^{-r_2 t}, \tag{5.28}$$

where Φ_1 and Φ_2 need to be derived from initial conditions and r_1 and r_2 are given by:

$$r_{1,2} = \zeta\omega_0 \pm \sqrt{\zeta^2\omega_0^2 - \omega_0^2 + \Omega_0^2}, \tag{5.29}$$

which simplifies under the condition $\Omega_0 \ll \omega_0$ to

$$r_{1,2} \approx \omega_0\left(\zeta \pm \sqrt{\zeta^2 - 1}\right). \tag{5.30}$$

The general solution (5.28) is either real or complex. When the damping ratio ζ is equal or greater than one, the solution is real and the hair moves without oscillations toward the point of torque equilibrium, dominated by the slow-moving mathematical term. When the damping ratio ζ becomes smaller than one, the square root term becomes imaginary and the hair shows overshoot toward its equilibrium, leading to a longer stabilization time. The response time τ_{95}, indicated as the time to get stable within 95% of the end value, is approximated[4] as:

$$\tau_{95} \approx \begin{cases} \dfrac{3}{\zeta\omega_0} & \text{if } \zeta < 0.5, \\ \dfrac{6\zeta}{\omega_0} & \text{if } \zeta > 1. \end{cases} \tag{5.31}$$

The best response time is obtained when $\zeta = 0.707$, corresponding to a close to critically damped system (Shinners, 1998). However, we observe that nearly all described gyroscopic systems shown in Figure 5.11 are clearly underdamped.

The sense/drive ratio and response time are taken as a criterion for designing a gyroscope. However, these quantities exhibit a similar proportionality with respect to the design parameter κ for underdamped gyroscopes:

$$\tau_{95} \propto \kappa, \quad \mathcal{R} \propto \kappa. \tag{5.32}$$

As a consequence, a trade-off exists between the sensitivity parameter $\mathcal{R}$ and the response time τ_{95} (see also Apostolyuk et al., 2002). Namely, to have a good sensitivity $\mathcal{R}$, a large κ-value is required, but to obtain a fast responding system, κ should be small. For design and analysis, we capture this trade-off in a single number by defining a figure of merit:

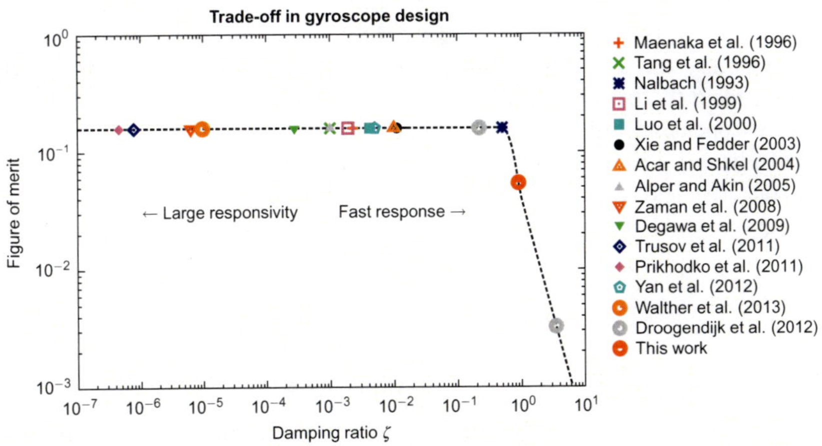

Figure 5.11 Figure of merit for designing a gyroscopic system. The dashed line indicates the figure of merit by Equation (5.33).

4 A precise mathematical solution is rather involved. A spline interpolation is used for connecting the two asymptotes smoothly and obtaining a good approximation, which is not shown here.

$$\text{Figure of merit} = \frac{\text{Sense/drive ratio}}{\text{Response time}} = \frac{\mathcal{R}}{\tau_{95}}. \tag{5.33}$$

An overview of several MEMS gyroscopic systems and the blowfly's haltere-based gyroscope (Nalbach, 1993) is shown in Figure 5.11 by evaluating the figure of merit as function of the damping ratio ζ. We observe that most MEMS gyroscopes are clearly designed with focus on achieving high responsivity at the cost of bandwidth. Especially, the gyroscopes described in Trusov et al. (2011) and Prikhodko et al. (2011) show very low damping factors while having a resonance frequency at 2 kHz, being highly sensitive to angular rate, since the ultimate purpose of these two gyroscopes is angle measurement rather than angular rate measurement. Contrarily, the fly's haltere is clearly geared toward a fast response. Also, MEMS-based gyroscopes typically have operating frequencies which are 1 kHz or more, which is significantly higher than the 150 Hz of the blowfly (Nalbach, 1993). Notice that the figure of merit exhibits a clear decrease when having an overdamped system ($\zeta > 1$), implying that vibratory gyroscopes should preferably be underdamped ($\zeta < 1$).

The eventual design of the bio-inspired gyroscope is based upon the fabrication process for bio-inspired hair flow sensors described by Bruinink et al. (2009) and Dagamseh et al. (2011) to realize a haltere-like structure. Our gyroscope will be actuated in the drive mode with angle ϑ (see Figure 5.10) by exploiting electrostatic actuation. Electrostatic forces induced by judiciously chosen ac voltages bring the artificial haltere in a steady-state resonant rotational motion. Measurement of the Coriolis-induced movement of the artificial haltere in the sense direction with rotational angle φ is achieved by measuring the differential change in capacitance upon tilt of the artificial haltere (Figure 5.12).

Although we reported on the design and fabrication of such a gyroscope earlier (Droogendijk et al., 2012a), we implemented some important design adjustments here. The suspension of the haltere-based gyroscope is changed to a gimbal suspension, like the gyroscope described by Acar and Shkel (2004). Doing so, the effects of residual stress by having a bilayer suspension (i.e., SiRN and Al) can be significantly reduced. Also, the drive and sense modes get mechanically distinguishable, allowing for a separate optimization of both modes. A schematic view of the two modes for our gimbal

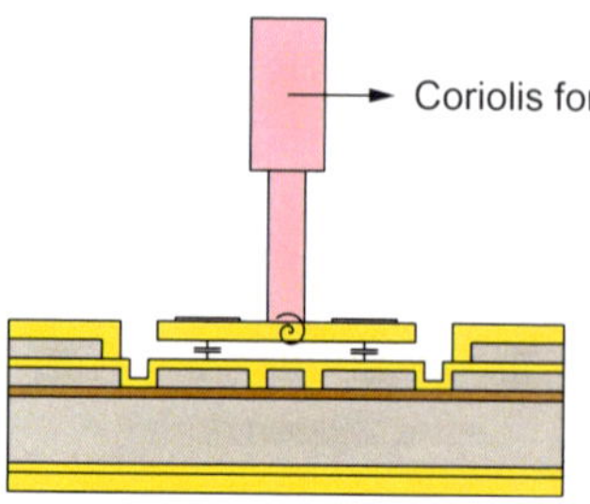

Figure 5.12 Schematic view of the biomimetic gyroscope (side view).

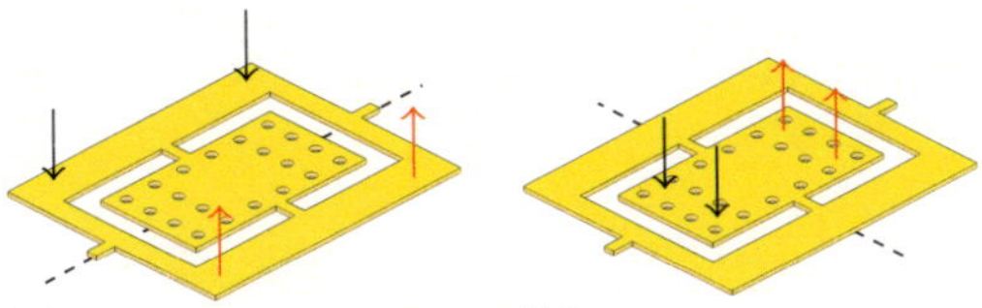

Figure 5.13 Characteristic modes of the gimbal gyroscope: drive (a) and sense (b).

suspension is given in Figure 5.13. A disadvantage of such a gimbal design is the difficulty to achieve mode matching (between drive and sense), which is often aimed for in MEMS gyroscopes to achieve better performance (see e.g., Hu et al., 2011 and Sonmezoglu et al., 2012). However, on following the bio-inspired approach, the quality factor Q of a gyroscope is relatively low, and consequently mode matching plays a less pivotal role for the gyroscope's performance.

5.4.3 Fabrication

An overview of the design and the fabrication process for the bio-inspired gyroscope is shown in Figure 5.14a. The fabrication process is identical to the one shown for the bio-inspired accelerometer described in Section 3.3. The fabrication results for the gyroscope are shown by the SEM image in Figure 5.14b.

5.4.4 Experimental

5.4.4.1 Setup

To characterize the mechanical properties of the gyroscope, an experimental setup based on laser Doppler vibrometry (Polytec, 2005) is used (Figure 5.15). To measure the rotational modes, we differentially applied a sinusoidal signal superposed to a dc offset voltage (Delta Elektronika—Power Supply E 030-1) to a pair of electrodes.

5.4.4.2 Frequency response

The response for the drive mode (Figure 5.13a) was measured by applying a chirp voltage in push-pull configuration. The magnitude and phase response are shown in Figure 5.16, both together with the results of an analytical model based on a classical second-order mechanical system. From both figures, the drive mode turns out to be slightly overdamped ($\zeta = 0.9$) with its resonance frequency found at approximately 550 Hz. Due to the overdamped nature of the system, the bandwidth of the drive mode is calculated by computing the intersection of the stiffness and damping contributing terms in Equation (5.16) and is found to be 305 Hz. Further, we observe that there is a good agreement between the analytical model and the measured response for frequencies up to about 800 Hz.

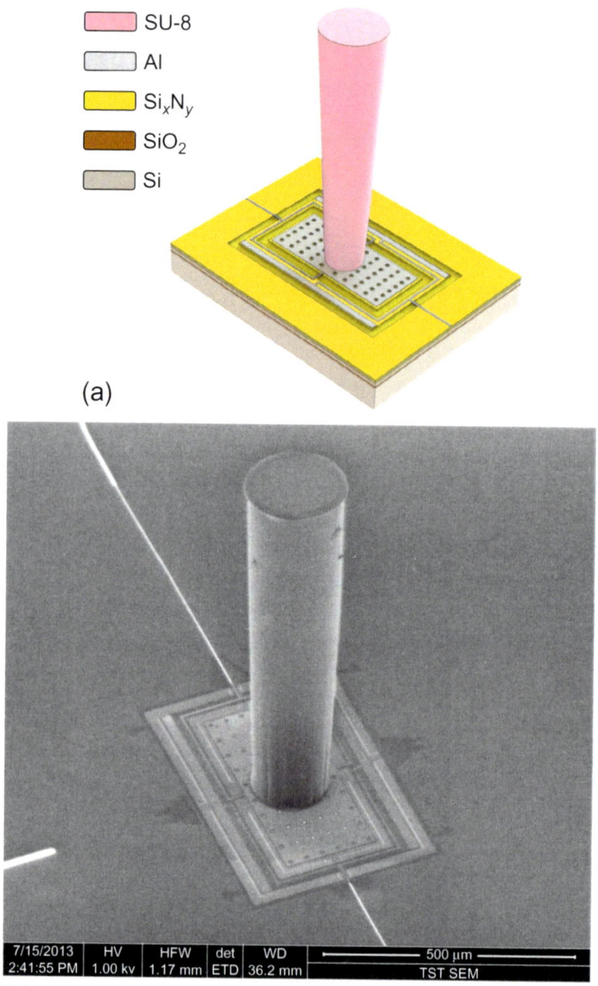

Figure 5.14 Design (a) and fabrication (b) of the MEMS haltere-based gyroscope fabricated by surface micromachining and using SU-8 lithography.

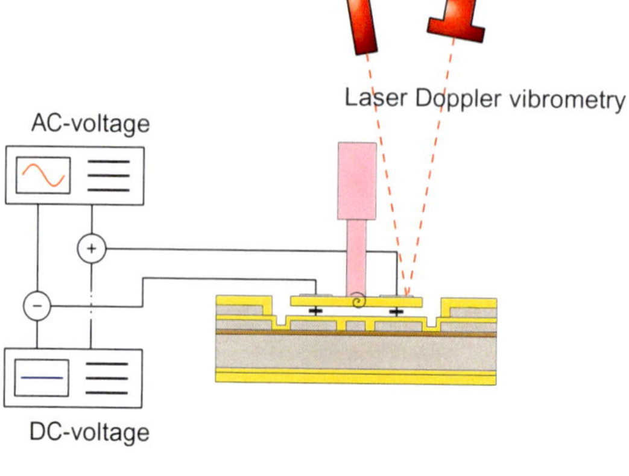

Figure 5.15 Experimental setup for characterization of the biomimetic gyroscope.

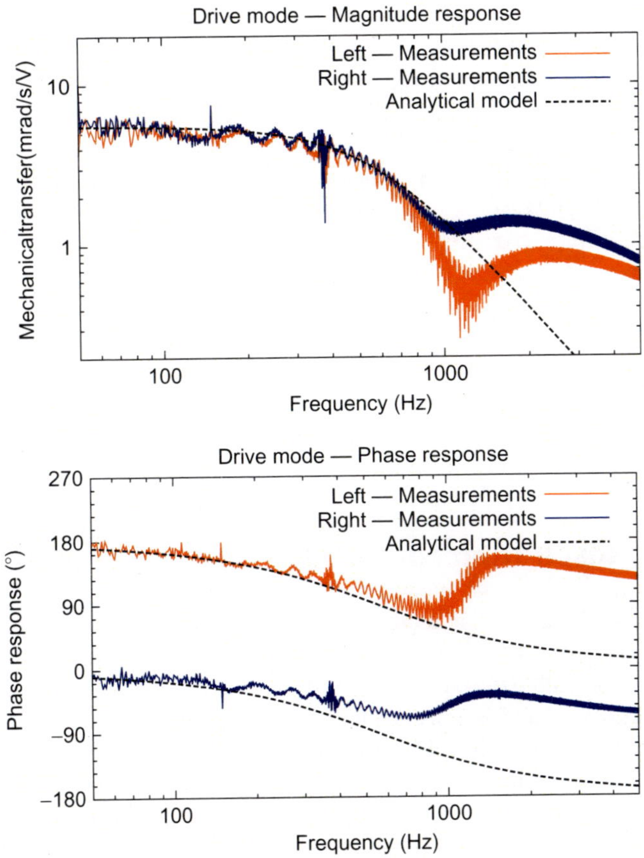

Figure 5.16 Optically measured response of the membrane displacement by electrostatically actuating the drive mode ($f_0 = 550$ Hz and $\zeta = 0.9$).

5.4.5 Discussion

Regarding the fabrication process, the SEM image from the bio-inspired gyroscope (Figure 5.14b) shows that we have successfully fabricated artificial haltere-like structure with increased mass at the top. Optical measurements indicate that the haltere-like structure length is about 800 μm and that the haltere-like structures have a slight negative tapering toward the membrane. This tapering results from the light intensity profile during exposure of the SU-8 as well as the two-step lithography process incorporated in the design. This effectively causes the center of mass to be located in the upper part of the haltere-like structures, similar to the fly's haltere (Figure 5.2).

The measured resonance frequency for the drive mode was measured to be about 510 Hz with a damping ratio of $\zeta = 0.9$. Although this resonance frequency is slightly higher than the wing beat frequency of the fly (130–150 Hz), it remains in the same order of magnitude. Similar results are obtained for the sense mode, wherein the resonance frequency was found to be about 300 Hz with a slightly overdamped system ($\zeta = 1.1$). However, we observed that the measured response is a combination of modes, especially for higher excitation frequencies. Since every mode is expected to be about critically damped, it is difficult to identify each modal resonance frequency due to the absence of clear resonance peaks and phase shifts. Theoretically, using capacitive differential read-out techniques, the contributions of the drive and vertical modes can be commonly rejected for measurement of the sense mode.

A haltere-inspired gyroscope has been designed, fabricated, and partially characterized. However, we were not able to experimentally demonstrate its response to externally applied angular rates using our home-built rate-table, electrostatic actuation of the drive mode, and capacitive read-out of the sense mode. With the current design and the maximum applicable angular rate using our rate table (rate amplitude of about 3000 $°s^{-1}$ at a frequency of 14 Hz), the calculated displacement of the membrane edges for capacitive read-out of the sense mode is in the order of nm, which corresponds to the measurement threshold of our read-out electronics (Dagamseh et al., 2013).

5.5 Bio-inspiration continued

Although a working bio-inspired accelerometer is clearly demonstrated, we believe that a working bio-inspired gyroscope following the "design rules" of a fly and the use of MEMS technology is difficult to achieve, but also possible. However, this will require adaptation of the design and the fabrication process. For our gyroscope, in particular, the value of $\mathcal{R}$ needs to be increased in order to measure the applied angular rates. A possibility is the use of piezo-resistive sensing instead of capacitive read-out, as proposed by Wicaksono et al. (2007). Also, improvement of the mechanical gimbal suspension and the use of more compliant materials will help to increase $\mathcal{R}$. One could also think of exchanging the technology of MEMS for another type of technology (e.g., 3D printing) and investigate its potential for bio-inspired gyroscopes.

The design and fabrication of two hair-based bio-inspired inertial sensors are described in this chapter: an accelerometer to measure external acceleration and a gyroscope to measure angular rates. A next step in the bio-inspired approach is the combination of hair-based sensors to arrive at a multisensor system in which sensor fusion can take place, by adding, e.g., the capability for flow sensing (Bruinink et al., 2009). Also, other types of bio-inspired hair-based sensors offer a potential for integration within such hair-based multisensor systems, like IR light sensing (Schmitz et al., 2012) and tactile sensing (Murphey, 1985).

Over the past years, much research has been done on bio-inspired sensors. Despite all efforts and the many important scientific results on hair-based sensing, it remains a challenge to engineers and scientists to realize the artificial counterpart of the biological sensor system with equal or better performance. Currently, e.g., insects perform still much better on several aspects (e.g., responsivity and detection threshold), provoking the question as to how to "beat nature." To this end, look for improvement of the mechanical design, investigate the use of more compliant materials, and consider the (partial) use of different or new technology.

5.6 Conclusions

In biology, hair-based sensor systems are regularly used for measurement of physical quantities. In this chapter, two types of bio-inspired inertial sensors have been discussed: a cricket-inspired accelerometer and a fly-inspired gyroscope. Both the accelerometer and gyroscope have been developed and fabricated using surface micromachining and SU-8 lithography. We showed that this MEMS hair-based accelerometer has a resonance frequency of 320 Hz, a detection threshold of 0.10 ms^{-2} and a dynamic range of more than 35 dB. Further, the accelerometer has clear directivity and a bias instability of 5×10^{-3} ms^{-2}. For the gyroscope, design rules were investigated and it was shown that haltere-based gyroscopes tend to emphasize a fast response, rather than a high responsivity or low detection threshold, by having a relatively low quality factor. Measurements on our haltere-inspired sensors indicate an excitable gyroscope with a (drive mode) resonance frequency of about 550 Hz and a damping ratio of 0.9. A response to externally applied angular rates was not demonstrated due to the limited applied rotation rates and the very small induced sense-mode amplitude, which is mainly caused by the structures being overdamped and the small achievable drive-mode amplitudes.

Acknowledgments

This work is carried out within the BioEARS-project, funded by STW/NWO.

References

Acar, C., Shkel, A.M., 2004. Structural design and experimental characterization of torsional micromachined gyroscopes with non-resonant drive mode. J. Micromech. Microeng. 14, 15–25. http://dx.doi.org/10.1088/0960-1317/14/1/303.

Alper, S.E., Akin, T., 2005. A single-crystal silicon symmetrical and decoupled MEMS gyroscope on an insulating substrate. J. Microelectromech. Syst. 14 (4), 707–717. http://dx.doi.org/10.1109/JMEMS.2005.845400.

Apostolyuk, V.A., Logeeswaran, V.J., Tay, F.E.H., 2002. Efficient design of micromechanical gyroscopes. J. Micromech. Microeng. 12, 948–954. http://dx.doi.org/10.1088/0960-1317/12/6/327.

Bischof, H.-J., 1974. Verteilung und bewegungsweise der keulenformigen sensillen von gryllus bimaculatus. Biol. Zbl. 93, 449–457.

Bischof, H.-J., 1975. Die keulenförmigen sensillen auf den cerci der grille *Gryllus bimaculatus* als schwererezeptoren. J. Comp. Physiol. A 98, 277–288. http://dx.doi.org/10.1007/BF00656974.

Bruinink, C.M., Jaganatharaja, R.K., de Boer, M.J., Berenschot, J.W., Kolster, M.L., Lammerink, T.S.J., Wiegerink, R.J., Krijnen, G.J.M., 2009. Advancements in technology and design of biomimetic flow-sensor arrays. In: Proc. MEMS 2009, pp. 152–155. http://dx.doi.org/10.1109/MEMSYS.2009.4805341.

Challoner, A.D., Gutierrez, R.C., Tang, T.K., 2007. Cloverleaf microgyroscope with electrostatic alignment and tuning. Patent, US 7159441.

Chan, W.P., Prete, F., Dickinson, M.H., 1998. Visual input to the efferent control system of a fly's "gyroscope" Science 280, 289–292. http://dx.doi.org/10.1126/science.280.5361.289.

Chen, N., Tucker, C., Engel, J., Yang, Y., Pandya, S., Liu, C., 2007. Design and characterization of artificial haircell sensor for flow sensing with ultrahigh velocity and angular sensitivity. J. Microelectromech. Syst. 16, 999–1014. http://dx.doi.org/10.1109/JMEMS.2007. 902436.

Dagamseh, A., Lammerink, T., Sanders, R., Wiegerink, R., Krijnen, G., 2011. Towards high-resolution flow cameras made of artificial hair flow-sensors for flow pattern recognition. In: Proc. MEMS 2011, Cancun, Mexico, Jan. 23–27, pp. 648–651. http://dx.doi.org/10.1109/MEMSYS.2011.5734508.

Dagamseh, A.M.K., Bruinink, C.M., Wiegerink, R.J., Lammerink, T.S.J., Droogendijk, H., Krijnen, G.J.M., 2013. Interfacing of differential-capacitive biomimetic hair flow-sensors for optimal sensitivity. J. Micromech. Microeng. 23, 035010. http://dx.doi.org/10.1088/0960-1317/23/3/035010.

Degawa, M., Jeong, H.W., Sonobe, H., Takubo, C., Yamanaka, K., Goto, Y., 2009. Laterally-driven deformation-robust MEMS gyroscopes with three sets of summetrically arranged folded-beam suspensions. In: Proc. Transducers'09, pp. 664–667, Denver, CO, USA, June 21–25, 2009.

Droogendijk, H., Brookhuis, R.A., de Boer, M.J., Sanders, R.G.P., Krijnen, G.J.M., 2012a. Design and fabrication of a biomimetic gyroscope inspired by the fly's haltere. In: Proc. IEEE Sensors 2012, Taipei, Taiwan, Oct. 28–31 2012, pp. 1400–1403. http://dx.doi.org/10.1109/ICSENS.2012.6411134.

Droogendijk, H., Bruinink, C.M., Sanders, R.G.P., Dagamseh, A.M.K., Wiegerink, R.J., Krijnen, G.J.M., 2012b. Improving the performance of biomimetic hair-flow sensors by electrostatic spring softening. J. Micromech. Microeng. 22 (6), 065026. http://dx.doi.org/10.1088/0960-1317/22/6/065026.

Droogendijk, H., Brookhuis, R.A., de Boer, M.J., Sanders, R.G.P., Krijnen, G.J.M., 2014a. Towards a biomimetic gyroscope inspired by the fly's haltere using MEMS technology. J. R. Soc. Interface 11 (99), 20140573. http://dx.doi.org/10.1098/rsif.2014.0573.

Droogendijk, H., de Boer, M.J., Sanders, R.G.P., Krijnen, G.J.M., 2014b. A biomimetic accelerometer inspired by the cricket's clavate hair. J. R. Soc. Interface 11, 20140438. http://dx.doi.org/10.1098/rsif.2014.0438.

Fraenkel, G., Pringle, J.W.S., 1938. Biological sciences: halteres of flies as gyroscopic organs of equilibrium. Nature 141, 919–920. http://dx.doi.org/10.1038/141919a0.

Gabrielson, T.B., 1993. Mechanical thermal noise in micromachined acoustic and vibration sensors. IEEE Trans. Electron Devices 40, 903–909. http://dx.doi.org/10.1109/16.210197.

Ginsberg, M., Schiano, J., Kramer, M., Alleyne, M., 2013. A case study in bio-inspired engineering design: defense applications of exoskeletal sensors. Def. Secur. Anal. 29 (2), 156–169. http://dx.doi.org/10.1080/14751798.2013.787798.

Hengstenberg, R., 1998. Controlling the fly's gyroscopes. Nature 392, 757–758. http://dx.doi.org/10.1038/33796.

Horn, E., Bischof, H.-J., 1983. Gravity reception in crickets: The influence of cereal and antennal afferences on the head position. J. Comp. Physiol. A 150, 93–98. http://dx.doi.org/10.1007/BF00605292.

Hu, Z.X., Gallacher, B., Burdess, J.S., Fell, C.P., Townsend, K., 2011. Precision mode matching of MEMS gyroscopes by feedback control. In: Proc. IEEE Sensors 2011, Limerick, Ireland, Oct. 28–31, 2011, pp. 16–19. http://dx.doi.org/10.1109/ICSENS.2011.6126998.

Humphrey, J., Devarakonda, R., Iglesias, I., Barth, F., 1993. Dynamics of arthropod filiform hairs. I. Mathematical modeling of the hair and air motions. Philos. Trans.: Biol. Sci. 340, 423–444. http://dx.doi.org/10.1098/rstb.1993.0083.

IEEE, 2001. 528-2001—IEEE standard for inertial sensor terminology. IEEE Std., IEEE Aerospace and Electronic Systems Society.

Kanou, M., Osawa, T., Shimozawa, T., 1989. Mechanical polarization in the air-current sensory hair of a cricket. Experientia 45, 1082–1083. http://dx.doi.org/10.1007/BF01950163.

Krijnen, G., Floris, A., Dijkstra, M., Lammerink, T., Wiegerink, R., 2007. Biomimetic micromechanical adaptive flow-sensor arrays. Proc. SPIE 6592, 65920F. http://dx.doi.org/10.1117/12.721807.

Li, X., Bao, M., Yang, H., Shen, S., Lu, D., 1999. A micromachined piezoresistive angular rate sensor with a composite beam structure. Sens. Act. A: Phys. 72, 217–223. http://dx.doi.org/10.1016/S0924-4247(98)00220-9.

Liu, C., 2007. Micromachined biomimetic artificial haircell sensors. Bioinspir. Biomim. 2, 162–169. http://dx.doi.org/10.1088/1748-3182/2/4/S05.

Luo, H., Fedder, G.K., Carley, L.R., 2000. An elastically gimbaled z-axis CMOS-MEMS gyroscope. In Proc. IS3M, pp 1–6, Hong Kong, October 19–21, 2000.

Maenaka, K., Fujita, T., Konishi, Y., Maeda, M., 1996. Analysis of a highly sensitive silicon gyroscope with cantilever beam as vibrating mass. Sens. Act. A: Phys. 54, 568–573. http://dx.doi.org/10.1016/S0924-4247(97)80016-7.

Murphey, R.K., 1981. The structure and development of a somatotopic map in crickets: the cereal afferent projection. Dev. Biol. 88, 236–246. http://dx.doi.org/10.1016/0012-1606(81)90167-6.

Murphey, R.K., 1985. A second cricket cercal sensory system: bristle hairs and the interneurons they activate. J. Comp. Physiol. A 156, 357–367. http://dx.doi.org/10.1007/BF00610728.

Nalbach, G., 1993. The halteres of the blowfly *Calliphora*—I. Kinematics and dynamics. J. Comp. Physiol. A 173, 293–300. http://dx.doi.org/10.1007/BF00212693.

Nalbach, G., Hengstenberg, R., 1994. The halteres of the blowfly *Calliphora*—II. Three-dimensional organization of compensatory reactions to real and simulated rotations. J. Comp. Physiol. A 175, 695–708. http://dx.doi.org/10.1007/BF00191842.

Ozaki, Y., Ohyama, T., Yasuda, T., Shimoyama, I., 2000. An air flow sensor modeled on wind receptor hairs of insects. In: Proc. MEMS 2000, Miyazaki, Japan, pp. 531–536. http://dx.doi.org/10.1109/MEMSYS.2000.838573.

Polytec, 2005. MSA-400 Micro System Analyzer. Polytec, Waldbronn, Germany.

Prikhodko, I.P., Zotov, S.A., Trusov, A.A., Shkel, A.M., 2011. Sub-degree-per-hour silicon MEMS rate sensor with 1 million Q-factor. In: Proc. Transducers'11, Beijing, China, Jun. 5–9 2011pp. 2809–2812. http://dx.doi.org/10.1109/TRANSDUCERS.2011.5969216.

Pringle, J.W.S., 1948. The gyroscopic mechanism of the halteres of *Diptera*. Philos. Trans. R. Soc. Lond. B 233 (602), 347–384. http://dx.doi.org/10.1098/rstb. 1948.0007.

Ristroph, L., Bergou, A.J., Ristroph, G., Coumes, K., Berman, G.J., Gucken-heimer, J., Wang, Z.J., Cohen, I., 2010. Discovering the flight autostabilizer of fruit flies by inducing aerial stumbles. Proc. Natl. Acad. Sci. U. S. A. 107 (11), 4820–4824. http://dx.doi.org/10.1073/pnas.1000615107.

Rosner, R., Egelhaaf, M., Grewe, J., Warzecha, A.K., 2009. Variability of blowfly head optomotor responses. J. Exp. Biol. 212, 1170–1184. http://dx.doi.org/10.1242/jeb.027060.

Sadeghi, M., Peterson, R., Najafi, K., 2011. Micro-hydraulic structure for high performance biomimetic air flow sensor arrays. In: Tech. Digest – IEDM, 6131638, 2011, pp. 29.4.1–29.4.4. http://dx.doi.org/10.1109/IEDM.2011.6131638.

Sakaguchi, D.S., Murphey, R.K., 1983. The equilibrium detecting system of the cricket: physiology and morphology of an identified interneuron. J. Comp. Physiol. A 150, 141–152. http://dx.doi.org/10.1007/BF00606364.

Sandeman, D.C., Markl, H., 1980. Head movements in flies (*Calliphora*) produced by deflexion of the halteres. J. Exp. Biol. 85, 43–60.

Schmitz, H., Soltner, H., Bousack, H., 2012. Biomimetic infrared sensors based on photomechanic infrared receptors in pyrophilous ("fire-loving") insects. IEEE Sens. J. 12 (2), 281–288. http://dx.doi.org/10.1109/JSEN.2010.2076324.

Shimozawa, T., Kanou, M., 1984. Varieties of filiform hairs: range fractionation by sensory afferents and cercal interneurons of a cricket. J. Comp. Physiol. A 155, 485–493. http://dx.doi.org/10.1007/BF00611913.

Shimozawa, T., Kumagai, T., Baba, Y., 1998. Structural scaling and functional design of the cercal wind-receptor hairs of cricket. J. Comp. Physiol. A 183, 171–186. http://dx.doi.org/10.1007/s003590050245.

Shimozawa, T., Murakami, J., Kumagai, T., 2003. Cricket wind receptors: thermal noise for the highest sensitivity known. In: Sensors and Sensing in Biology and Engineering. Springer, Berlin, pp. 145–159. http://dx.doi.org/10.1007/978-3-7091-6025-1_10.

Shinners, S.M., 1998. Modern control system theory and design, second ed. John Wiley & Sons, Inc.

Smith, G.L., Bedair, S.S., Schuster, B.E., Nothwang, W.D., Pulskamp, J.S., Meyer, C.D., Polcawich, R.G., 2012. Biologically-inspired, haltere, angular-rate sensors for micro-autonomous systems. Proc. SPIE 8373, 83731K. http://dx.doi.org/10.1117/12.918678.

Sonmezoglu, S., Alper, S.E., Akin, T., 2012. An automatically mode-matched MEMS gyroscope with 50 Hz bandwidth. In: Proc. MEMS 2012, Paris, France, Jan. 29 – Feb. 2 2012, pp. 523–526. http://dx.doi.org/10.1109/MEMSYS.2012.6170231.

Tang, T.K., Gutierrez, R.C., Wilcox, J.Z., Stell, C., Vorperian, V., Calvet, R., Li, W.J., Chakraborty, I., Bartman, R., 1996. Silicon micromachined vibratory gyroscope. In: Proc. Solid-State Sensor and Actuator Workshop. Hilton Head Island, SC, USA, pp. 288–293.

Tang, T.K., Gutierrez, R.C., Stell, C.B., Vorperian, V., Arakaki, G.A., Rice, J.T., Li, W.J., Chakraborty, I., Shcheglov, K., Wilcox, J.Z., 1997. A packaged silicon MEMS vibratory gyroscope for microspacecraft. In: Proc. MEMS 1997, Nagoya, Japan, Jan. 26–30 1997, pp. 500–505. http://dx.doi.org/10.1109/MEMSYS. 1997.581911.

Tang, Y., Peterson, R.L., Najafi, K., 2013. Technology for fabricating dense 3-D microstructure arrays for biomimetic hair-like sensors. In: Proc. MEMS 2013, Taipei, Taiwan, Jan. 20–24 2013, pp. 355–358. http://dx.doi.org/10.1109/MEMSYS. 2013.6474251.

Tao, J., Yu, X., 2012. Hair flow sensors: from bio-inspiration to bio-mimicking—a review. Smart Mater. Struct. 21, 113001. http://dx.doi.org/10.1088/0964-1726/21/ 11/113001.

Tobias, M., Murphey, R.K., 1979. The response of cercal receptors and identified interneurons in the cricket (*Acheta domesticus*) to airstreams. J. Comp. Physiol. A 129, 51–59. http://dx.doi.org/10.1007/BF00679911.

Trusov, A.A., Prikhodko, I.P., Zotov, S.A., Shkel, A.M., 2011. Low-dissipation silicon tuning fork gyroscopes for rate and whole angle measurements. IEEE Sens. J. 11 (11), 2763–2770. http://dx.doi.org/10.1109/JSEN.2011.2160338.

Walther, A., Desloges, B., Lejuste, C., Coster, B., Audebert, P., Willemin, J., 2013. Development of a 3D capacitive gyroscope with reduced parasitic capacitance. J. Micromech. Microeng. 23, 025013. http://dx.doi.org/10.1088/0960-1317/23/2/025013.

Wang, Y.-H., Lee, C.-Y., Chiang, C.-M., 2007. A MEMS-based air flow sensor with a free-standing microcantilever structure. Sensors 7, 2389–2401. http://dx.doi.org/10.3390/s7102389.

Wicaksono, D.H.B., Chen, Y., French, P.J., 2007. Design and modelling of a bioinspired MEMS gyroscope. In: Proc. ICEEI, Bandung, Indonesia, Jun. 17–19, 2007, pp. A–05.

Wu, W.-C., Wood, R., 2006. Angular rate sensor using electromechanical haltere. Patent, US 7107842.

Wu, W.-C., Wood, R.J., Fearing, R.S., 2002. Halteres for the micromechanical flying insect. In: Proc. ICRA 2002, Washington, DC, United States, May 2002, pp. 60–65. http://dx.doi.org/10.1109/ROBOT.2002.1013339.

Xie, H., Fedder, G.K., 2003. Fabrication, characterization, and analysis of a DRIE CMOS-MEMS gyroscope. IEEE Sens. J. 3 (5), 622–631. http://dx.doi.org/10.1109/JSEN.2003.817901.

Yan, L., Shangchun, F., Zhanshe, G., Jing, L., Le, C., 2012. Study of dynamic characteristics of resonators for MEMS resonant vibratory gyroscopes. Microsyst. Technol. 18, 639–647, 2012. http://dx.doi.org/10.1007/s00542-012-1492-2.

Yazdi, N., Ayazi, F., Najafi, K., 1998. Micromachined inertial sensors. Proc. IEEE 86 (8), 1640–1659. http://dx.doi.org/10.1109/5.704269.

Zaman, M.F., Sharma, A., Hao, Z., Ayazi, F., 2008. A mode-matched silicon-yaw tuning-fork gyroscope with subdegree-per-hour allan deviation bias instability. J. Microelectromech. Syst. 17 (6), 1526–1536. http://dx.doi.org/10.1109/JMEMS.2008.2004794.

Zhou, Z.-G., Liu, Z.-W., 2008. Biomimetic cilia based on MEMS technology. J. Bion. Eng. 5, 358–365. http://dx.doi.org/10.1016/S1672-6529(08)60181-X.

Zotov, S.A., Trusov, A.A., Shkel, A.M., 2011. Demonstration of a wide dynamic range angular rate sensor based on frequency modulation. In: Proc. IEEE Sensors 2011, Limerick, Ireland, Oct. 28–31, 2011, pp. 149–152. http://dx.doi.org/10.1109/ICSENS.2011.6127269.

Artificial olfactory sense and recognition system

6

H. Araki, S. Omatu

6.1 Introduction

The olfactory sense is one of the five human senses: sight, hearing, touch, taste, and smell (olfactory sense). Research relating to sight and hearing is a popular area of engineering. However, research about taste or smell is less popular.

One of the reasons why these senses are studied less is the difficulty of evaluating taste and smell, as these evaluations are decided by each individual's subjective impressions, and these senses cannot be measured objectively. For example, consider the difficult case of how to decide on a smell for a new perfume. This decision requires that the perfume designers have common perceptions about the perfume. Next, the designers decide the smell of the perfume to fit the design concept for the perfume. If the designers have only a unique smell to consider, it is difficult for them to discuss the feel of the perfume. Therefore, these designers will discuss a well-known smell before discussing the new scent in order to create a common perception. By having this pre-discussion, the designers can create a common smell perception and can use this common perception as a base for the development of the new perfume's scent.

In this case, an artificial olfactory system (often called an electronic nose or e-nose) can potentially provide an easy way to develop a perfume. A comparison model between the human olfactory sense and an artificial olfactory system is shown in Figure 6.1. The e-nose system provides objective data and records them. However, an instrumental system for these data is not yet available for use with a personal computer.

To understand an artificial olfactory system, the human olfactory sense and parts of the artificial olfactory system are explained in this chapter. This chapter is organized as follows:

First, the human olfactory sense and methods to discuss smells are described.

Second, artificial olfactory sensing devices are described. In this section, the metal oxide semiconductor (MOS) sensor and the quartz crystal microbalance (QCM) sensor applied systems are introduced.

Third, classification and recognition methods are described.

Finally, conclusions and future works are described.

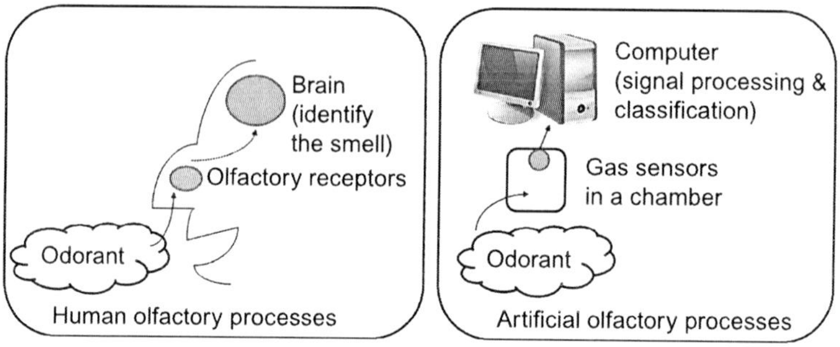

Figure 6.1 Comparison between the human olfactory sense and an artificial olfactory system.

6.2 The human olfactory sense and creating common perceptions of odors

When thinking about an artificial olfactory system, it is useful to study the human sense of smell. The human olfactory sense is created by olfactory receptor cells, the olfactory bulb, and the olfactory cortex. There are many kinds of olfactory receptors; humans have about 300 receptors, while mice have about 1000 (Niimura et al., 2014). Each receptor reacts not only for one fragrance but also for several fragrances. The olfactory receptors react only to evaporated chemicals; they cannot detect nonvolatile chemicals. The human brain is connected to the olfactory receptors through the olfactory bulb, and the olfactory cortex of the brain recognizes scents by combinations of these reactions. As explained, the human olfactory sense is based on sensing and recognition. Figure 6.2 shows how the human sense of smell works.

In animals, the olfactory sense is used to scent danger and to communicate. However, the human olfactory sense is used for several applications, for example,

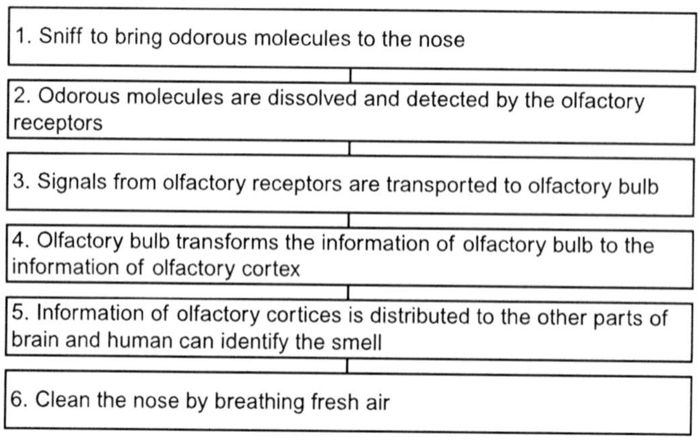

Figure 6.2 How a human's sense of smell works.

searching out chemicals, cooking, and tasting foods and drinks. The human olfactory sense is therefore used for many objectives, but, if a person's sense of smell is contaminated by the same odor for long time or by a strong odor, the sense will be paralyzed. Thus, a person's sense of smell can depend on his or her lifestyle and daily eating habits. Accordingly, the sense of smell is different among different individuals. However, we need common perceptions of smells to discuss fragrances. A standard method for obtaining such a common perception is defined in ISO (4120:1983) or JIS (Z 9080:2004).

A case study of the methodologies used to obtain common perceptions is shown. This case study is constructed by following two steps.

(1) Establish a feeling about and a word describing the smell.
(2) Determine the strength of the smell.

In the first step, members of a group discuss a sample odor. They describe the odor using key words based on their personal feelings, hear other members' words, and talk about the combination of the words and the odor. The discussion creates common perceptions about the odor among the members of the group.

In the next step, the group members discuss the strength of the odor; this feeling about the strength of the smell will differ depending on the members' lifestyles.

After these steps, a discussion based on the common perceptions of a fragrance could be undertaken. However, the common perceptions will be changed by the group members, the environmental conditions, or the air temperature. It is difficult to reconstruct the original discussion with the same conditions.

Subjective assessment has these problems; therefore, objective evaluation by quantity measurement methods of smells are important. However, the results of the quantity method do not always fit with the human olfactory sense. In these cases, the results should be adjusted to match the human sense. Nevertheless, the raw quantity results are very useful to detect trouble such as burning because the results are not influenced by subjective human perceptions.

Due to these features, the quantity result should be used carefully for specific purposes, considering all reasons and motivations.

6.3 The olfactory sensor system for the e-nose

6.3.1 Outline of the sensor system

Olfactory measurements are based on the method used to measure chemicals in air. Humans can smell only volatile chemicals in air; we cannot sense nonvolatile chemicals by smell. Gas sensors and gas-sensing systems have similarly been developed to detect volatile chemicals (Liu et al., 2012). A common volatile chemical detection and measuring system is a gas chromatograph (GC). Gas chromatography can be applied to the e-nose system, but a GC is a large and expensive piece of equipment to use for a personal e-nose system. The GC has the advantages of accurately measuring substances, separating mixed substances, and detecting small amounts of substances. The GC has a column that contains a liquid or polymer; the column is located in an oven where the temperature of the gas can be controlled. A carrier gas is used to force each sample gas through the machine. As each sample gas comes in contact with the column, it interacts with the column, causing each compound to separate at a different time, thus enabling identification of the different compounds. Selection of the column material, carrier gas, and oven temperature are important to accurately measure the substance.

An experimental system for an e-nose is shown in Figures 6.3 and 6.4. The e-nose system can be separated into two blocks: a detection block and a recognition block. The detection block includes an air supply and a gas sensor unit. The sensor unit uses gas sensors as artificial olfactory receptors. Furthermore, the system needs standard dry air and odor-containing air in which the odor strength is controlled. The recognition block includes a data transfer function and a computer.

A diagram of the experimental system is shown in Figure 6.5. As the first step, the system is cleaned by a flow of dry air through valves 1 and 3 (be sure these two valves

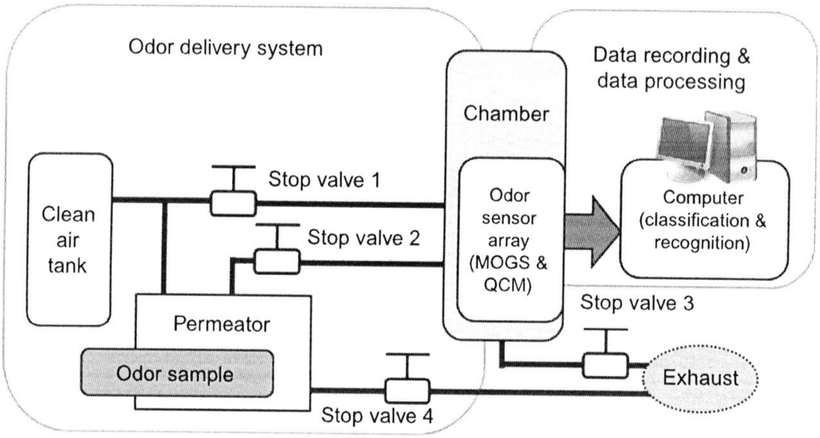

Figure 6.3 An experimental system for an e-nose: diagram.

Figure 6.4 An experimental system for an e-nose: photo.

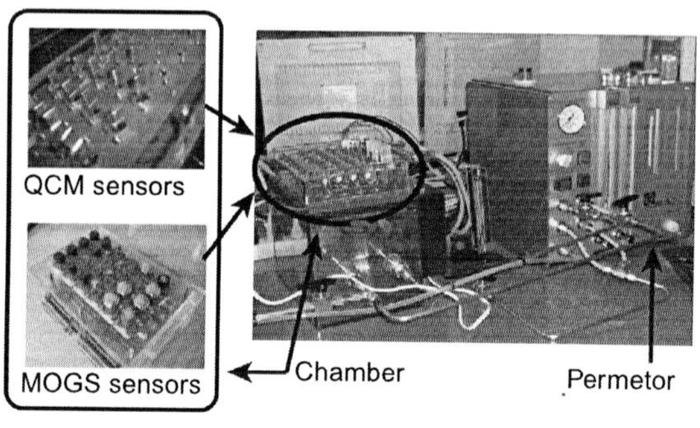

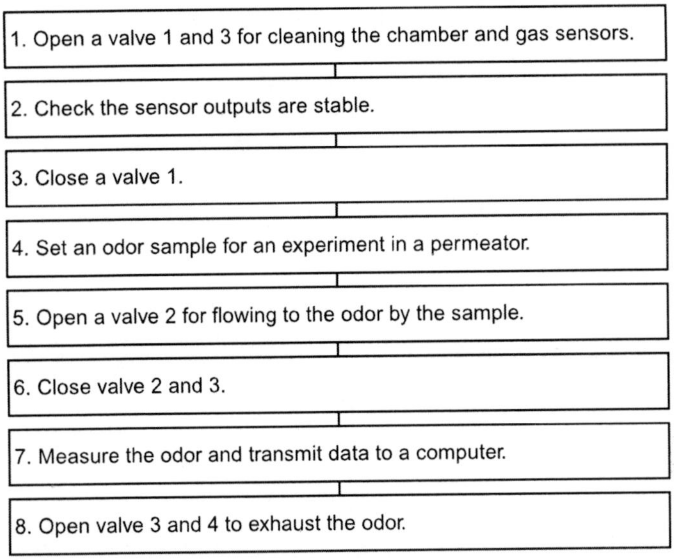

Figure 6.5 A flowchart for the experimental system.

are open). Usually odor sensing is a stable region of the sensor outputs; therefore, the sensor outputs are checked next. Before the odor-containing air flows into the chamber, valve 1 should be closed.

After the chamber and the permeator are ready, an odor sample is placed into the permeator. Then valve 2 is opened, and the odor-containing air flows into the chamber through this valve. However, because the odor-containing air flows out through valve 3, we should be careful about this exhaust to avoid influencing the experiment. After the chamber is filled by the odor-containing air, valves 2 and 3 should be closed.

The start time for measuring, which is created by the recognition system, can be set after the sensors are checked at the beginning of the process and after the data is transmitted to a computer. Finally, the data is selected in the classification and recognition step. After the measurements are completed, valves 3 and 4 are opened to expel the odor-containing air from the system.

The above paragraphs describe the operational process of the e-nose system. However, the e-nose system can use different kinds of gas sensors, and thus two types (the MOS gas sensor and the QCM gas sensor) are shown in this chapter. The differences between these sensors affect the classification and recognition systems. The sensor outputs are connected to controllers because the output data is transmitted from the sensors to a computer. A different controller is used for each kind of sensor.

The chamber of the sensor unit can be improved for each kind of sensor. It is used to stabilize the air that is measured. As the odor is sensed, the condition of the odor-containing air is important. For example, a QCM sensor is very sensitive to physical vibrations of the airflow. Thus, airflow control when using QCM sensors is of greater concern than when using MOS sensors.

If the sensor outputs are different from their design, understanding the sensor's behavior is important. For example, it is important to know that water reacts to MOS sensors because human breath includes a great deal of water.

The data from the sensors is sent to a computer for classification. The classification method is applied via a neural network and other signal-processing technology. In the next sections, the classification systems for MOS and QCM sensors are explained. These systems have different neural network structures because these data each have unique features.

6.3.2 MOS gas sensor system

A MOS gas sensor is a popular gas sensor produced by various manufacturers. This gas sensor works as a variable resister created by the target gas and the oxide surface. The effect is based on the oxidization–deoxidization reaction. Tin oxides or zinc oxides are used in MOS sensors, and the change in resistance occurs by de-oxidization of the material by the target gas. When the sensor is de-oxidized, the resistance becomes low. When the amount of the target gas is low, the surface will oxidize by air, and the resistance becomes high. Therefore, the gas sensor reaction is decided by oxidization via the target gas. To obtain a sensitive reaction, it is important to build a surface of sensors and to control the temperature. Furthermore, sense differences generated by odor are decided by the structure and catalyst of materials.

Tin oxide is an n-type semiconductor, and its carrier is an electron. A sintered block of tin oxide makes up the sensor (see Figure 6.6). If the sintered block is in air which is not contain de-oxidization gas, depletion layers are formed on the surface of the particles of the block. Oxygen molecules are heated with the sensor (400–500°C), and the molecules are adsorbed by the particles. Oxygen on the surface attracts an electron in the conduction band of the particles. The electrical resistance becomes high because the depletion layer is generated on the particle surface.

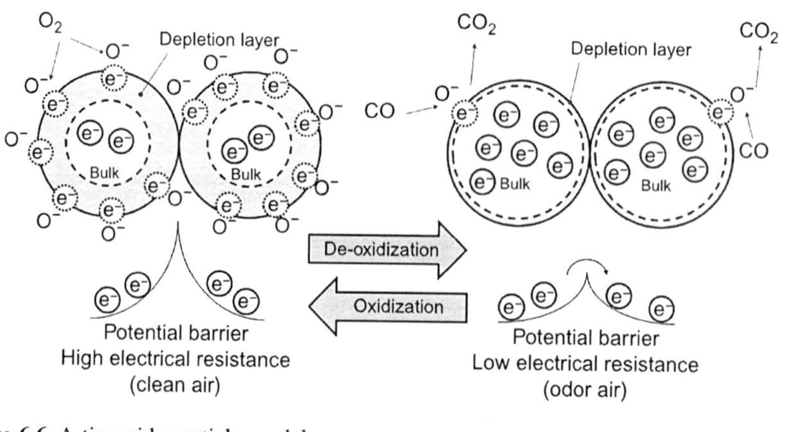

Figure 6.6 A tin oxide particle model.

Next the block is exposed to de-oxidization of the gas (e.g., CO). Oxygen on the surface is removed by the de-oxidization reaction. After oxygen is removed from the surface, the electrons of the carrier become free, and the depletion layer becomes thin. As a result, the electrical resistance becomes low.

Basically, the oxidation or de-oxidation reaction changes the electrical resistance, and the strength of the reaction can be detected with the MOS sensor. However, MOS sensors are produced with individual characteristics for target gases. To acquire these characteristics, the sensors have different materials, structures, and/or catalysts. The produced sensors each have a target gas, and the standard condition and circuit is approved by the suppliers. The usual application is made with the condition and the circuit. A typical circuit for an MOS sensor is shown in Figure 6.7.

The reaction is accomplished at a high temperature (400–500°C) because the MOS sensors have heaters. Before measurement, the sensor should be heated to a stable temperature. If the temperature is not stable, the measurement results might not be accurate. To build an e-nose system, some different kinds of MOS sensors are used. Figure 6.8 shows a multi-MOS sensor unit, and Figure 6.9 shows a typical output waveform of a multi-MOS sensor system for an e-nose. In Figure 6.9, each line is the output from one sensor. These lines can be used to differentiate the sensors' reactions to the gas, which is useful to identify the gas.

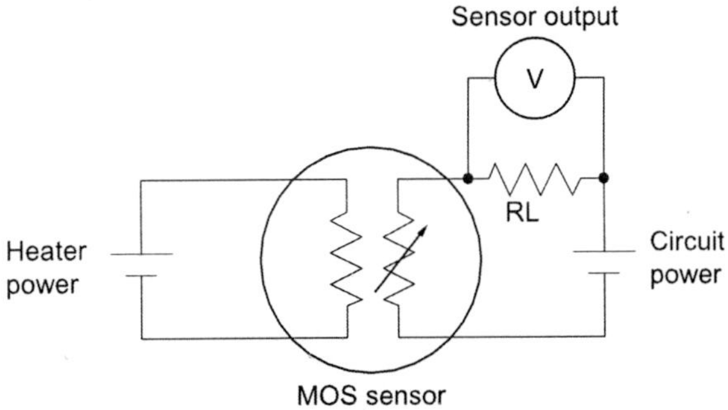

Figure 6.7 A typical circuit for an MOS sensor.

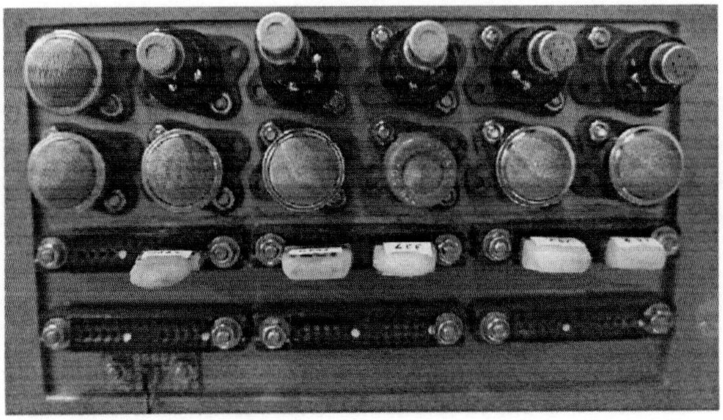

Figure 6.8 A multi-MOS sensor system.

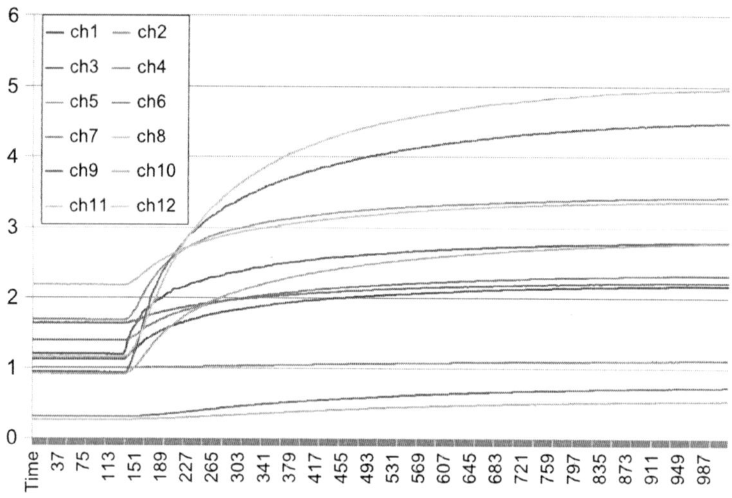

Figure 6.9 Example of multi-MOS sensor system output (instant coffee).

This section demonstrates that the sensor output is affected by the temperature of the sensor. Furthermore, the sensor's character is changed by the temperature. By changing the character of the sensor, researchers can generate more information than is generated when a fixed temperature is studied. To create a sensor system with a heater control, the temperature character of the sensor should be researched for:

- Transition time of the sensor's character
- Voltage value of the heater power
- Heater voltage wave form

The transition time is needed to decide the heater control frequency. However, the frequency differs by the structure or catalyst of the sensor; thus, a control sequence for the heater should be researched to match each sensor. A report of a variable heater control sensor evaluation system with Figaro Engineering gas sensors is described in next paragraph.

Figure 6.10 shows an evaluation circuit with a variable heater control. The gas sensor output signal is sampled at the A/D converter on the microcontroller. The sampling time is decided by the microcontroller program. The sampled data are transmitted to a computer for classification and recognition, and the heater power supply is controlled by the same microcontroller. The gas sensor does not have a temperature sensor; furthermore, the heater is controlled as an open loop by the heater voltage control. These sensors are designed for fixed heater power, and the upper limit of an effective voltage range is determined by the manufacturer's recommendation. However, there is no recommendation about the lower limit. The sensors have various upper and lower limits, and the information about these limits is important if the system has more than one sensor. Furthermore, some sensors need a heater with a PWM controller. In the evaluated system, sensors that need a static heater power are used. Next, consider the

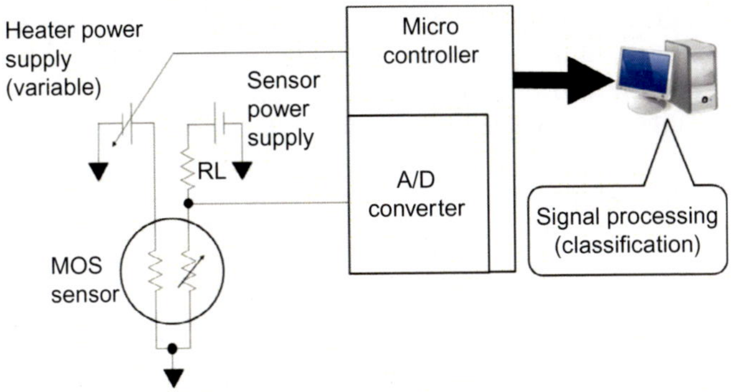

Figure 6.10 Evaluation circuit with a variable heater control.

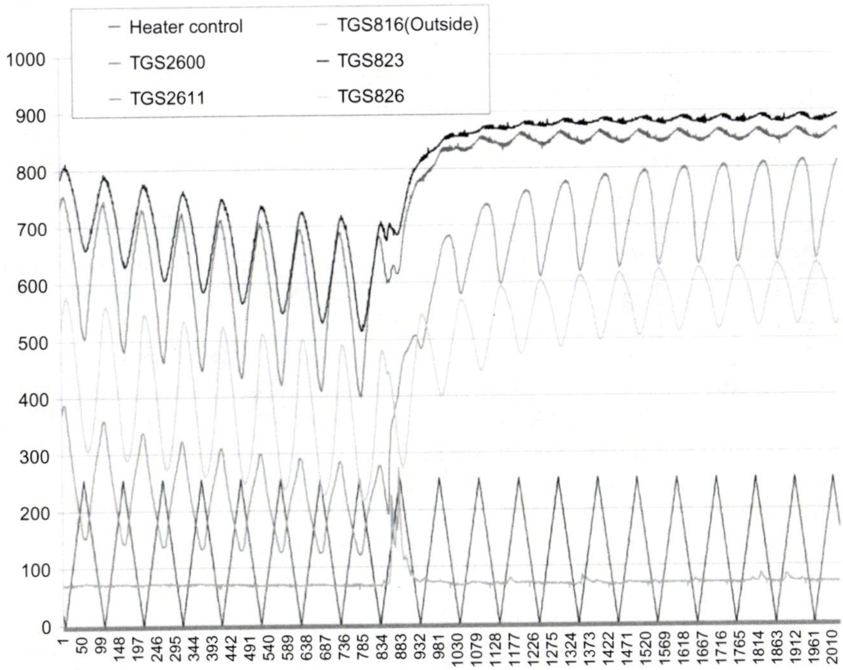

Figure 6.11 A multi-sensor system output with a variable heater control.

voltage wave form of the heater. At first, the system's creators tried a triangle waveform for the control. Next, they tried saw waveforms and reverse-saw waveforms. By the checking the results of these experiments, it was discovered that the triangle waveform generates much more information than any other waveform. Figure 6.11 shows the evaluation system's output. The system has five sensors; four sensors are in the chamber, and they have variable heater power, and the other sensor is placed outside the chamber to monitor the environment, and it has static heater power.

This section explained the fundamentals of MOS sensors and a basic circuit for the sensor. In addition, it explained how to apply the sensor system. Furthermore, an advanced sensor system with a variable heater control was described. More clarification of the classification and recognition process is given in Section 6.4.

6.3.3 QCM gas sensor system

A QCM sensor can measure a small weight of materials on the sensor as a variation in frequency of a quartz crystal resonator. For example, QCM is used to measure proteins in a solution. Crystal is piezoelectric device and has a characteristic vibration, and a crystal device is used for the oscillator circuits (Colpitts oscillator or an unstable multivibrator) with frequency accuracy. The crystal in the QCM sensor has a coating for sensing a gas or vapor. This coating can be adjusted to detect the target gas or vapor (Munoz et al., 2002; Goka et al., 2000).

Figure 6.12 shows QCM sensors that are in a multi-QCM evaluation system. Figure 6.13 shows a diagram for a typical QCM sensor system. For a QCM sensor, a quartz crystal unit is used without a cover; furthermore, the crystal surface is coated with a sensitive membrane. Odor-containing gases touch the surface, and the selected gas or vapor sticks to the membrane.

The QCM oscillation block is based on a multi-vibrator circuit. The multi-vibrator output is connected to the Field Programmable Gate Array (FPGA). The FPGA logic circuit system has two kinds of counters. The first counter is used for each QCM channel oscillation, and the second counter is used for fixed time by the system clock. The first counter is reset by the second counter. The first counter output is sent to a PC at the reset time. Figure 6.14 shows a plot of a QCM counter output. The plot shows that the first counter output is low because the odor or vapor is sticking to the QCM sensor, and, thus, the sensor's characteristic vibration has changed.

This sensor system is created by counting the QCM oscillator output for a fixed time (e.g., 1 s). Counts for each channel are transmitted to a computer for classification and recognition.

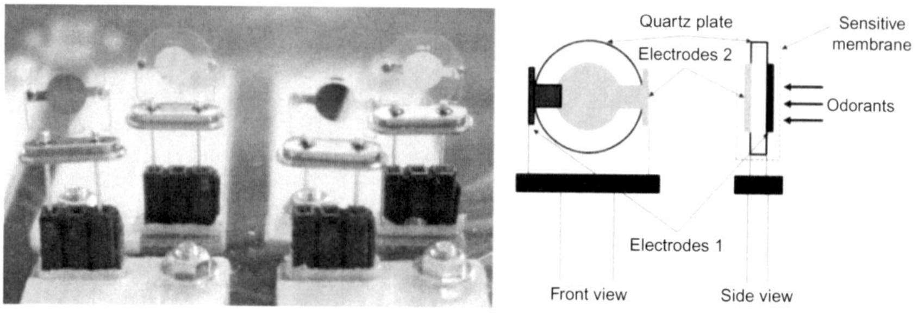

Figure 6.12 QCM sensors.

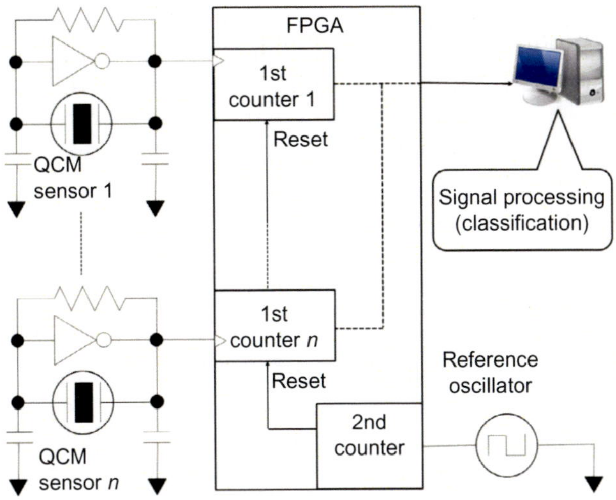

Figure 6.13 A diagram of a QCM system.

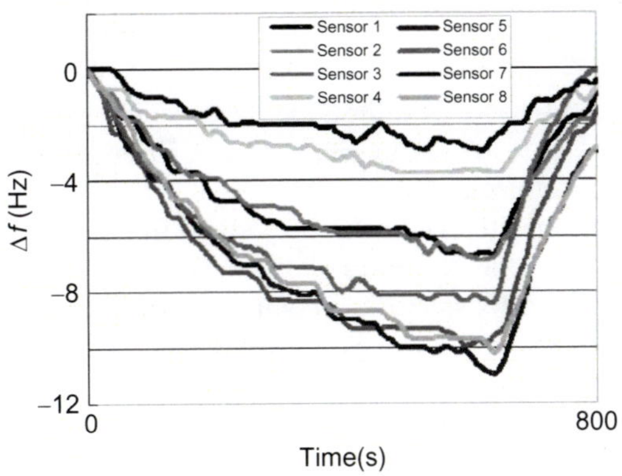

Figure 6.14 Output of the first counter of an FPGA.

To build a QCM sensor system, the following points should be taken into consideration.

- A QCM sensor is fragile.
- QCM sensors are highly sensitive to air flow.
- High-frequency circuits can interfere with each other.

To reiterate the first point, QCM sensors are fragile and easily damaged. Hence, care should be taken when making a QCM sensor system.

To reiterate the second point, QCM systems are highly sensitive to air flow and/or physical vibration. Hence, these systems need a corresponding canceling system for air flows and physical vibrations. For example, the cancellation system can be a plane crystal or a digital filter. A plane crystal can detect air flow and physical vibration, and calculation (subtraction) of the crystal output and QCM sensor output can be used to cancel these vibrations. A digital filter can filter the QCM output using a low-pass filter. A QCM sensor is very sensitive so these sensors' output data should be used cautiously.

To reiterate the third point, a problem occurs with high-frequency electronic circuits: they can interfere with each other. If the system has only one channel, the problem is not serious. However, the problem becomes more serious if the system is a multi-QCM sensor system. The problem is that the interference of each QCM circuit makes it difficult to measure precisely. One way to shield against this interference is to use twisted-pair lines between the QCM oscillator and the FPGA circuit. Figure 6.15 shows a waveform of the QCM oscillator outputs: a single-QCM system output and a multi-QCM system output. The figure shows spurious errors by cross-talking between oscillator circuits and others. Therefore, the multi-QCM sensor system should be considered the best design for an anti-crosstalk and anti-error system.

This section has described the fundamentals of the QCM sensor and its circuit. In addition, the difficulties of creating the single-QCM and multi-QCM sensor unit were described.

6.3.4 Other gas sensor systems

In the previous sections, MOS and QCM sensors were described as the major gas sensors. However, new gas sensors for the e-nose system are being studied. One of the new types of sensors uses receptor cells and biotechnology (Misawa et al., 2010). In one study, researchers created a selective sensor with living cells in a portable fluidic device. The cell in the device had two electrodes, and the electrodes were connected to an amplifier. The analog signal from the sensors was transferred to a computer, changing it to a digital signal. The electrical change occurred by touching odor-containing gases to the receptor cells, and it was observed as an impedance change between the electrodes.

Other types of sensors such as conductivity-changing sensors are also being actively studied (Arshak et al., 2004).

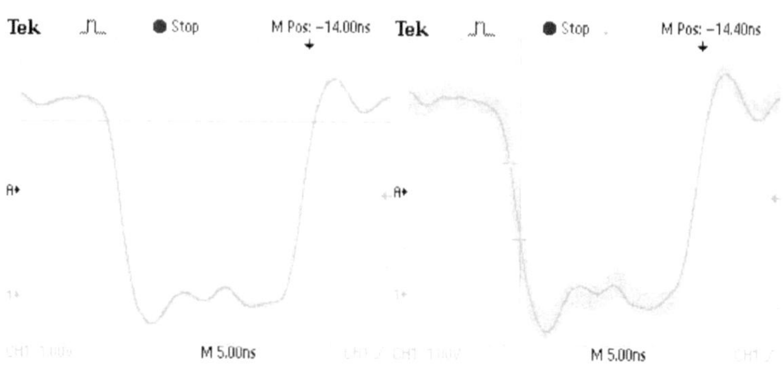

(a) Single QCM oscillator (b) Multi QCM oscillators

Figure 6.15 Comparison of QCM oscillator outputs.

6.4 Olfactory classification—data processing

6.4.1 Outline of olfactory recognition and classification

As already mentioned, olfactory sensor systems use many gas sensors as artificial olfactory receptors; the sensors' output data are recorded in a computer's database. Using the database of odors, we must apply an intelligent signal-processing technique to recognize odors correctly. The odor data are pre-processed, using noise reduction, normalization, and feature extraction techniques. Then neural networks are used to classify odors (Milke, 1995; Bicego, 2005; Gardner and Bartlett, 1998). Basically, we use a layered neural network (Nakamoto, 2013; Omatu and Yano, 2011; Fujinaka et al., 2008) and competitive networks for odor classification because learning ability and robustness are important factors in this classification. The most important process in odor classification is to find features that are robust for different environments (temperature, humidity, and density levels of odors). However, finding these features is very difficult.

Generally, odor sensors are designed to detect some specific odor in an electrical appliance such as an air purifier or a breathylzer. Each of the odor sensors, such as MOS or QCM sensors, has characteristics that respond to different odors. When many odor sensors are combined in one system, their ability to detect an odor is increased. The combination of odor sensors, which is listed in Tables 6.1 and 6.2, is used as the olfactory receptor system in the electronic nose reference system.

Table 6.1 List of MOS sensors from FIS Inc. used in this experiment

Sensor model	Main gas detected	Sensor model	Main gas detected
SP-53	Ammonia, ethanol	SP-31	Hydrocarbons
SP-MW0	Alcohol, hydrogen	SP-19	Hydrogen
SP-32	Alcohol	SP-11	Methane, hydrocarbons
SP-42A	Freon	SP-MW1	Cooking vapors

Table 6.2 Chemical materials used as the membrane

Sensor number	Materials of the membrane
Sensor 1	E(4 ml), DA(0.023 ml)
Sensor 2	W(3.13 ml), E(4 ml), EA(0.043 ml), MTMS
Sensor 3	W(3.13 ml), E(4 ml), EA(0.014 ml), MTMS, PFOE
Sensor 4	W(3.13 ml), E(4 ml), EA(0.015 ml), MTMS, PFOE
Sensor 5	W(0.30 ml), E(4 ml), EA(0.043 ml), MTMS, PFOE
Sensor 6	W(0.05 ml), E(3.0 ml), EA(0.043 ml), MTMS, PFOE
Sensor 7	W(0.30 ml), E(3.2 ml), EA(0.043 ml), MTMS, PFOE
Sensor 8	No membrane

E, ethanol; W, water; DA, dilute nitric acid; EA, ethyl acrylate; MTMS, methyltrimethoxysilane; PFOEA, perfluorooctylethyl acrylate.

In the next section, a classification method and specialized points about the sensors are described. After that, we show experimental results given by the reference system.

6.4.2 Classification method for odor data

To classify odors, we adopt a three-layered neural network based on the error back-propagation method, as shown in Figure 6.16. The neural network consists of three layers: an input layer, i; a hidden layer, j; and an output layer, k. When the input data x_i (i = 1, 2, ..., I) are applied to the input layer, we obtain the output O_k in the output layer. The output O_k is compared to the desired value d_k, which is assigned in advance. The result of the comparison, e_k, is given by $e_k = d_k - O_k$. Then the weighting coefficients w_{ji} and w_{kj} are corrected such that the error becomes smaller based on an error back-propagation algorithm. The algorithm, which is based on a gradient method, is given in the following steps.

Step 1: Set the initial values of w_{ji}, w_{kj}, θ_j, θ_k, and η (>0).
Step 2: Specify the desired values of the output d_k_k, $k = 1, 2, \ldots, K$ corresponding to the input data x_i, $i = 1, 2, \ldots, I$ in the input layer.
Step 3: Calculate the outputs of the neurons in the hidden layer and output layer by

$$\mathrm{net}_j = \sum_{i=1}^{I} w_{ji}x_i - \theta_j, O_j = f\left(\mathrm{net}_j\right), \quad f(x) = \frac{1}{1+\mathrm{e}^{-x}} \tag{6.1}$$

$$\mathrm{net}_k = \sum_{j=1}^{J} w_{ji}O_i - \theta_k, \quad O_k = f(\mathrm{net}_k) \tag{6.2}$$

Step 4: Calculate the error e_k and generalized errors δ_k, δ_j by

$$e_k = d_k - O_k, \delta_k = e_k O_k (1 - O_k) \tag{6.3}$$

$$\delta_k = \sum_{k=1}^{K} \delta_k w_{kj} O_j \left(1 - O_j\right) \tag{6.4}$$

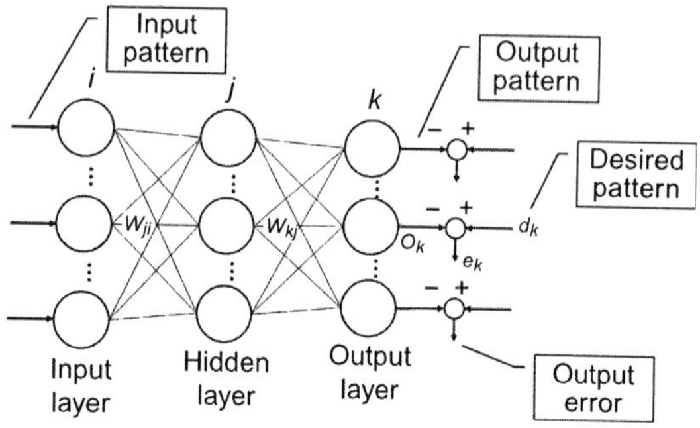

Figure 6.16 A three-layered neural network with error back-propagation.

Step 5: If e_k is sufficiently small for all k, END and otherwise

$$\Delta w_{kj} = \eta O_j \delta_k, \ w_{kj} \Leftarrow w_{kj} + \Delta w_{kj} \tag{6.5}$$

$$\Delta w_{ji} = \eta O_i \delta_j, \ w_{ji} \Leftarrow w_{ji} + \Delta w_{ji} \tag{6.6}$$

Step 6: Go to Step 3.

Using the above recursive procedure, we can train the neural networks to classify odor data.

6.4.3 Classification results using MOS sensors

To evaluate the experimental system using MOS sensors and a classification system, two experiments are examined.

The first experiment (Experiment 1) tried to classify four types of teas using the sensors shown in Table 6.1. The teas are shown in Table 6.3. Note that the chemical properties of these odors are very similar, and it has been difficult to separate them based on the measurement data obtained by using MOS sensors.

The experimental system's neural network contained eight input layers, four hidden layers, and four output layers. The system thus had an 8-4-4 structure.

The odor samples perceived by the MOS sensors consisted of 15 data sets for neural network training and five data sets for classification. The experiment changed the training data set 100 times and checked the classification accuracy for the test samples. Thus, the experiment classified a total of 500 test samples. The classification results are summarized in Table 6.3; the correct classification average was 96.2%.

The second experiment (Experiment 2) tried to classify five kinds of coffees (shown in Table 6.4). The samples labeled A, B, and C are mocha coffees from different companies. The experimental neural network system contained eight input layers, five hidden layers, and five output layers. Thus, the neural network system had an 8-5-5 structure.

The odor samples perceived by the MOS sensors consisted of 20 data sets for neural network training and 15 data sets for evaluation testing. The experiment changed the training data set 100 times and checked the classification accuracy for the test

Table 6.3 Experimental results for classification of teas in Experiment 1

Odor data label	Materials	Samples	Collective answer rate of classification results (average [96.2%])
A	English tea	20	100.0%
B	Green tea	20	98.8%
C	Barley tea	20	85.8%
D	Oolong tea	20	100.0%

Table 6.4 Experimental results for classification of coffees in Experiment 2

Odor data label	Materials	Samples	Collective answer rate of classification results (average [88.8%])
A	Mocha coffee 1	35	79.3%
B	Mocha coffee 2	35	82.5%
C	Mocha coffee 3	35	88.3%
D	Kilimanjaro coffee	35	95.8%
E	Char-grilled coffee	35	98.1%

samples. Thus, the experiment classified a total of 1500 test samples. The classification results are shown in Table 6.4; the correct classification average was 88.8%.

Comparing the results of Experiment 1 and Experiment 2 shows that the results for Experiment 2 are worse by about 7%. In Experiment 2, the classification of mocha coffees 1, 2, and 3 was not good because, although the smells are similar, the coffees are different brands from different companies.

6.4.4 *Classification results using QCM sensors for mixed odor data*

In this section, classification results of evaluation system using QCM sensors and a classification system are shown. This QCM system was evaluated by two experiments.

The first QCM experiment (Experiment 3) tried to measure four types of odors, as shown in Table 6.5. The first counter reset frequency was 1 Hz (see Figure 6.13). The temperatures of the odor-containing gases were 24–26°C, and the humidity of the gases was 6–8%. Diffusion tubes were used to control the density of the gases. Odor data were measured for 600 s. These data may have included impulsive noise due to

Table 6.5 Training data set for Experiment 3

Odor data label	Substance	Output A	Output B	Output C	Output D
A	Ethanol	1	0	0	0
B	Water	0	1	0	0
C	Methyl-salicylate	0	0	1	0
D	Tri-ethyl-amine	0	0	0	1

the extreme sensitivity of QCM sensors. To remove this noise, a median filter, which replaced a value at a specific time by a median value among neighboring data around the specific time, was adopted. Figure 6.14 shows the measurement data for the first substance (ethanol), labeled A, where the horizontal axis is the measurement time, and the vertical axis is the frequency deviation from the standard value (9 MHz) after passing through a five-point median filter.

During Experiment 3, in order to classify the input feature vector, the desired pattern (d_k in Figure 6.16) for the input feature vector, where it was a nine-dimensional vector as shown in Table 6.5, was allocated. The experimental neural network added the coefficient of variation to the usual feature vector to reduce variations in the odors. The training was continued until the total error was less than or equal to 0.5×10^{-2} where $\eta = 0.3$.

After training to classify all the smells (A, B, C, and D) correctly, the system was used to classify mixed data sets. The data sets contained two kinds of odors that were mixed at the same rate and included the following pairs: A and B, B and C, C and D, D and A, A and C, and B and D. The classification results are shown in Table 6.6, where the largest values denote the case where the maximum output values were achieved. The maximum output shows one of the mixed odors.

However, some of the results do not show the correct classification for the remaining odor. Thus, the input is modified as

$$z = x - 0.9y \tag{6.7}$$

where x is the feature, y denotes the top value of each row in Table 6.6, and z is a new feature.

The classification results, obtained using the new feature vector, are shown in Table 6.7. By changing the features according to the above equation, better classification results have been obtained. However, the coefficient 0.9, used above, is not necessarily appropriate. The value might be replaced by the partial correlation coefficient in multivariate analysis.

Table 6.6 Testing the mixed odors in Experiment 3

Odor data label	Output A	Output B	Output C	Output D	Maximum output value and output symbol
A and B	0.673	0.322	0.002	0.001	0.673 (Output A)
B and C	0.083	0.696	0.174	0.001	0.696 (Output B)
C and D	0.001	0.004	0.016	0.992	0.992 (Output D)
D and A	0.003	0.003	0.002	0.995	0.995 (Output D)
A and C	0.992	0.006	0.002	0.000	0.992 (Output A)
B and D	0.003	0.003	0.003	0.995	0.995 (Output D)

Table 6.7 Testing the mixed odors where, except for the largest value, the top was selected as the second odor among the mixed odors in Experiment 3

Odor data label	Output A	Output B	Output C	Output D	The top except for the largest value
A and B	(0.263)	0.290	0.166	0.066	0.290 (Output B)
B and C	0.358	(0.029)	0.631	0.008	0.631 (Output C)
C and D	0.002	0.071	0.644	(0.163)	0.644 (Output C)
D and A	0.214	0.004	0.037	(0.230)	0.214 (Output A)
A and C	(0.031)	0.020	0.527	0.026	0.527 (Output C)
B and D	0.108	0.010	0.039	(0.325)	0.108 (Output A)

6.5 Conclusions

In this chapter, the fundamental technology for an artificial olfactory system was described.

- In Section 6.2, the human olfactory system was described, the difficulty of using the human sense of smell for objective evaluations was explained, and the motivation for studying for an artificial olfactory system was related.
- In Section 6.3, the hardware of an artificial olfactory system was shown, and two types of sensor system, the MOS sensor system and the QCM sensor system, were described.
- In Section 6.4, a classification system using a neural network was described. Experimental classification systems using selective sensor systems (MOS or QCM sensors) were outlined. Furthermore, the experimental results showed that electronic nose systems can be used for many applications.

As explained in the above sections, the three parts (the odor delivery system, the sensor system, and the data processing system) of an artificial olfactory system should be considered and custom-designed for specific purposes, for example, air conditioning control systems or food-processing control systems. These systems often need unique parts for accuracy measurement or stable measurement; furthermore, the systems sometimes need special sensors for various purposes. The human olfactory sense is very sensitive; therefore, studies to create an artificial olfactory system continue in order to obtain the most accurate sensing data and the most objective classification system.

To create a more accurate artificial olfactory system, the following technological improvements will need to be made.

- Develop new gas sensor detectors that are demanded by different applications
- Reduce the number of sensors needed to create a small sensor system
- Stabilize a small gas load system
- Create an accurate and definite classification system

Already, an artificial olfactory system is being used in an air condition management system in a food factory. Furthermore, this system is being studied for applications in the health management field because it can detect human body odors and halitosis, and these odors can be related to disease.

As stated above, the artificial olfactory system has a potential to create these new applications for a computer. For example, the computer is able to know a smell by saving data for a smell by the olfactory system. Furthermore, they will be able to replay the saved data by an odor projection system. These systems make it possible to communicate by the smell between users. When they become popular, computer services with a smell will grow.

The sense of smell is one of fundamental human senses, and there are similar words of smell: odor, scent, fragrance, perfume, aroma and so. These words have each meaning as like a good smell, a bad smell, or a strong smell. An existence of many words for a smell show the smell is important for human life.

When the computer systems utilize sufficiently a smell, they will get along well to people.

References

Arshak, K., Moore, E., Lyons, G.M., Harris, F., Clifford, S., 2004. A review of gas sensors employed in electronic nose applications. Sens. Rev. 24 (2), 181–198.

Bicego, M., 2005. Odor classification using similarity-based representation. Sensors Actuators B 110 (2), 225–230.

Fujinaka, T., Yoshioka, M., Kosaka, T., 2008. Intelligent electronic nose systems for fire detection systems based on neural networks. In: Proceedings of the Second International Conference on Advanced Engineering Computing and Applications in Sciences, ADVCOMP, Sept. 29–Oct. 4, pp. 73–76.

Gardner, J.W., Bartlett, P.N., 1998. Electronic Noses: Principles and Applications. Oxford University Press, Oxford; New York.

Goka, S., Okabe, K., Watanabe, Y., Sekimoto, H., 2000. Multimode quartz crystal microbalance. Jpn. J. Appl. Phys. 39, 3073–3075.

ISO 4120, 2004. Sensory analysis—Methodology—Triangular test.

Japan Industrial Standards Z9080, 2004. Sensory analysis—Methodology.

Liu, X., Cheng, S., Liu, H., Zhang, D., Ning, H., 2012. A survey on gas sensing technology. Sensors 12, 9635–9665.

Milke, J.A., 1995. Application of neural networks for discriminating fire detectors. In: International Conference on Automatic Fire Detection, AUBE, 10th, April 4–6, Duisburg, Germany, pp. 213–222.

Misawa, N., Mitsuno, H., Kanzaki, R., Takeuchi, S., 2010. Highly sensitive and selective odorant sensor using living cells expressing insect olfactory receptors. Proc. Natl. Acad. Sci. 107 (35), 15340–15344.

Munoz, S., Nakamoto, T., Moriizumi, T., 2002. Study of quartz crystal microbalance odor sensing system for apple and banana flavors. IEICE Trans. Elecron. E85-C (6), 1291–1297.

Nakamoto, T. 2013. Human Olfactory Displays and Interfaces: Odor Sensing and Presentation. pp. 105–140. IGI Global, Hershey, PA.

Niimura, Y., Matsui, A., Touhara, K., 2014. Extreme expansion of the olfactory receptor gene repertoire in African elephants and evolutionary dynamics of orthologous gene groups in 13 placental mammals. Genome Res. 24, 1485–1496.

Omatu, S., Yano, M., 2011. Intelligent electronic nose system independent on odor concentration. In: Proceedings of the Second International Workshop on User Modeling.

Bio-inspired engineered sonar systems based on the understanding of bat echolocation

7

S. Kim

7.1 Introduction

Echolocation is an acoustical process which is used to locate and identify a target by sending sound pulses and receiving the echoes reflected back from the target. Echolocation is used by several mammals including dolphins, whales, and bats. The echolocation in bats has attracted large number of scientific researches due to their extraordinary abilities to fly in complete darkness and to use echolocation to capture their prey as well as to communicate between themselves by using self-generated biosonar signals. Since bat echolocation was first observed (Griffin, 1958), their ability has attracted much interest not only from researchers looking at bat's biological and physiological characteristics but also from those in engineering who have been trying to learn from biological echolocating behavior and apply the principles to sonar engineering. Müller and Kuc (2007) have extensively reviewed bio-sonar-inspired technology motivated by echolocating animals. In their review, the importance of insights into various echolocating tasks solved by bats has been stressed as it potentially provides a wide range of methodologies for engineering of any technical sonar system. For example, binaural tracking sensors and rotational sensors have been motivated by the hearing mechanism of two ears and movement of external ears in bats (Barshan and Kuc, 1992; Kuc, 1996, 1997a,b, 2002; Carmena and Hallam, 2001; Carmena et al., 2001).

In this chapter, we will introduce an overview of bat echolocation and explore what is already known from previous research. Then we will investigate further what we can learn from bat bio-sonar to inspire engineers to develop more sophisticated sonar systems.

7.2 Background

This section will provide an overview of bat's echolocation including the species, evolution, and anatomy and major echolocating tasks such as detection, discrimination, and localization of the target will be discussed. Then we will describe the fundamentals of hearing mechanism which is fundamental in designing bio-sonar receivers.

7.2.1 Echolocation in bats

7.2.1.1 Species, evolution, and anatomy

Bats are mammals of the order Chiroptera which has two suborders, *Megachiroptera* (megabats) and *Microchiroptera* (microbats). Microbats live on every continent except Antarctica and all use echolocation for obstacle avoidance and foraging. They are generally smaller than megabats, their ears are often large and complex and many species have nose leaves. These features are known to be associated with their echolocating ability and determine the characteristics of the sound they listen to. Their echolocation sounds are produced in the larynx (vocalizations). All species of the microbats have advanced echolocation capabilities although they often have good vision. Most microbats feed on insects, whereas most megabats eat fruits or suck nectar from flowers. The megabats inhabit tropical Africa and Asia and rely mainly on sophisticated vision and smell for flight and foraging. Except for one genus, *Rousettus aegyptiacus*, megabats are not capable of echolocation. *Rousettus* lives in caves and uses a crude form of echolocation to avoid obstacles when in complete darkness. The echolocation calls that *Rousettus* uses are completely different from microbats in terms of echolocating signal generation. They produce sound by clicking the tongue against the side of the mouth.

An important reason for the evolution of the mammalian auditory system is to localize behaviorally relevant sounds. The shape of the outer ear varies widely across species but all mammals share similar anatomy and physiology in their auditory system. Without exception, the anatomies of bats basically resemble that of other mammals in form and function. However, the outer ear of the bat is highly specialized. The pinnae of bats are relatively large compared to their head size, or even many times bigger, and they have a flap-like shape. Various shapes of pinnae are shown in Figure 7.1. The inside surface of the ear pinna frequently has several transverse ridges or a series of longitudinal ridges, which are presumed to provide structural support from the pinna. The tragus and anti-tragus are also part of the outer ear. The tragus

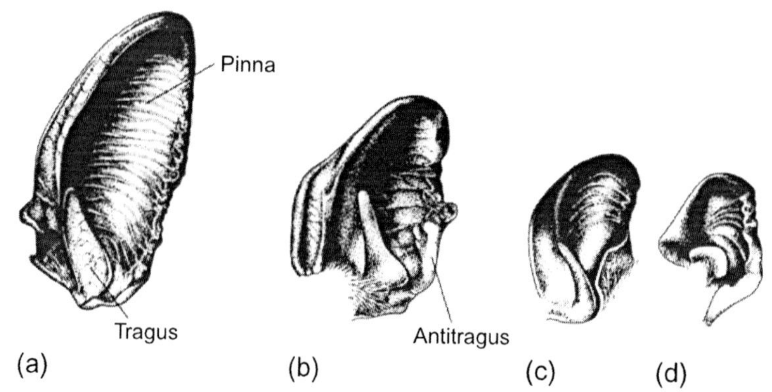

Figure 7.1 Pinnae of several Vespertilionidae (after Hill and Smith, 1984). (a) *Plecotus auritus*. (b) *Barbastella barbastellus*. (c) *Myotis daubentonii*. (d) *Nyctalus noctula*.

is a small "earlet" positioned in front of the ear canal, and it has been known to have a considerable effect on vertical sound localization as well as the pinna (Lawrence and Simmons, 1982). The anti-tragus is a broad flap that is continuous with the outer margin of the pinna (Hill and Smith, 1984). It is noted that the varieties of features in bats' outer ears and their uniqueness have been inspiring researchers in designing an effective sonar device.

7.2.1.2 Echolocation tasks

Sophisticated echolocation systems are found in bats that use echolocating signals for navigation and for foraging in various environments as described in the previous section. During echolocation, target ranging is done by measuring the time delay between the animal's own pulse emission and the echoes. The echoes returning to the two ears arrive at different times and different intensity levels, depending on the position of the target producing echoes. Spectral information in echoes reaching into two ears also varies depending on the target. Information in the returning echoes such as difference in time and intensity levels and the frequency spectrum is used in echolocation including target localization and discrimination.

Echolocating bats depend upon their biological pulse emission to detect, identify, and locate their prey. The echolocation pulses they use consist of short bursts of sound at frequencies ranging from 10 kHz to about 200 kHz (Lawrence and Simmons, 1982). Signal information such as distance, range, angular position, shape, and texture of an object is used in the process.

a. Detection

Although most echolocating bats have a high sensitivity of hearing to their signals, they have to detect these signals against background noise such as wind, self-generated noise during flight, and communication signals produced by other animals. Echolocating sounds used by bats may exceed 100 dB sound pressure level (SPL) at a distance of 10 cm (Griffin, 1958). Because of this intense sound level of vocalization, the middle ear muscle of the bat contracts to protect the inner ear from damage. However, the attenuation effect due to absorption of high frequency sound propagating through the atmosphere and the spreading loss, the returning echolocating signals can be interpreted as relatively "very low level" signals. The schematic diagram of sound level attenuation in this echolocation example is shown in Figure 7.2.

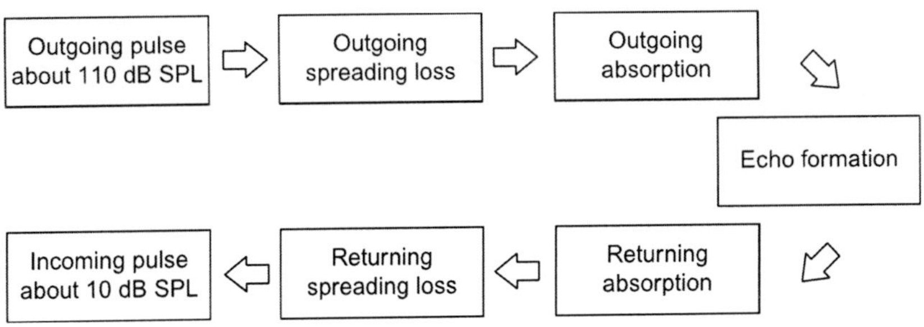

Figure 7.2 Schematic diagram of sound level attenuation in echolocation.

b. Discrimination

There have been a few studies about how bats discriminate objects. The discrimination strategy is known to be different depending on the type of echolocating signal used. Accordingly, the acoustic characteristics of targets also vary depending on the foraging type, habitats, and wing morphology of prey. The bats that use a constant frequency (CF) signal in echolocation utilize the velocity of the flying insect by detecting Doppler shifts. The echoes returning back from the prey when a CF signal is used show the frequency rapidly modulated by the insect's wing beats. Therefore, those bats are able to track the movement of the insect. It has been suggested that frequency modulated (FM) bats also utilize the Doppler-induced changes in echoes to discriminate the fluttering target (Grossetete and Moss, 1998). In addition, a previous study has suggested that FM bats are able to use an "acoustical glint" of the target (Simmons et al., 1990). The acoustic glint is a series of reflections from the complex target in the temporal domain. Simmons et al. examined the acoustic glint from mealworms, spheres, and disks, and the results were shown to provide the profile of them such as the shape information (Simmons et al., 1990). The same study provided the behavioral evidence observed in FM echolocating bats that it showed they can discriminate edible mealworms from the inedible spheres of various sizes. The acoustical properties of those different targets showed the different range profile in terms of temporal spacing of the spectral peaks and notches (Simmons and Chen, 1989). The acoustic glint might not be effectively generated when a CF signal is used because the CF signal consists of a dominant frequency and its harmonics. Hence, it can be expected to carry less information in terms of spectral analysis than the broadband FM signal.

c. Localization

It has been noted that good high frequency hearing is more common among mammals than good low frequency hearing (Heffner and Heffner, 1990). This corresponds to the fact that the "intensity (or level)-difference pathway" in the mammalian ascending auditory system is well established and very similar across almost all mammalian orders. In particular, echolocating bats can be said to have more specialized "intensity-difference pathway" than "time-difference pathway" because they use much higher frequencies than most other mammals. A primary goal of the bats' auditory system is to localize behaviorally relevant sounds in space. It has been generally shown that the interaural level differences (ILDs), caused by a small head (which, for example, is less than 1 cm of diameter for the big brown bat), enable them to localize high frequency sounds. They can resolve the auditory image with high spatial precision because the head acts as an obstacle reflecting sound waves.

In terms of investigation of localization ability in bats, there have been many studies on the big brown bat (*Eptesicus fuscus*). Big brown bats are relatively large in size, from about 10 to 13 cm in length and 14–18 g in weight. Although they are not small among the echolocating bats, their head size is mostly less than 1 cm. Generally, it is known that big brown bats can detect echoes from small objects at a distance of up to 5 m. This species uses broadband FM sweeps, ranging from 100 kHz down to 25 kHz with two or three harmonics. Those FM signals are well suited for spatial localization. Therefore, the big brown bat is considered a good model for the study of echolocating bats. The localization abilities in big brown bats studied from behavioral experiments are summarized in Table 7.1. The result from various angular discrimination experiments in the past suggests that the brown bat can discriminate the angular resolution up to 1.5° of resolution using the echolocation, whereas the smallest angle it is able to discriminate using a passive localization (i.e., without emitted calls and echoes) seems to be 14°. Despite the influence of the differences in methodology, better acuity in echolocation than in passive location in the horizontal plane seems plausible. From those results, it can be argued that binaural hearing works more efficiently in echolocation rather than in passive localization.

Table 7.1 **List of studies of localization ability in big brown bats**

Study	Type	Parameter	Species of bat	Result
Simmons et al. (1983)	Echolocation	Horizontal resolution	*Eptesicus fuscus*	1.5°
Masters et al. (1995)	Echolocation	Horizontal resolution	*Eptesicus fuscus*	1.5°
Lawrence and Simmons (1982)	Echolocation	Vertical resolution	*Eptesicus fuscus*	3°
Wotton and Simmons (2000)	Echolocation	Vertical angle acuity	*Eptesicus fuscus*	2.9–4.1°
Koay et al. (1998)	Passive localization	Horizontal threshold	*Eptesicus fuscus*	14°

7.2.2 Fundamentals of hearing process and modeling

The echolocation phenomenon in bats can be regarded as a mixture of complex problems which is associated with the signal processing of bio-sonar acoustics. More recently, the echolocation in bats has been inspiring engineers and more importance has been given to learning and applying their strategies to sonar systems. In Section 7.2.1, we have reviewed the biological backgrounds of bats (a), echolocation and signals produced (b), and echolocating tasks such as detection, discrimination, and localization (c) as shown in Figure 7.3. Now, we will review how the echolocating task is possibly solved by bats. To reduce the complexity and investigate a single problem one is interested in, a model is useful as it can provide new parameters or limit a given parameter which controls the part of the model. The concept of the echolocation model is that each stage of echolocation, the signal emission, reflection, and reception, is modeled as an individual section and the echolocating process is recreated by combining those different parts in series which is mathematically called "convolution." Convolution is defined as an operation on two functions, producing a third modified version of original function. The convolution can be used to calculate the response of a system to arbitrary inputs by using their impulse responses. Convolving two signals in the time domain equally means that their spectra are multiplied in the frequency domain. The convolution technique is widely used in different areas of signal processing. A similar application of the convolution technique is shown in digital audio processing which recreates virtual sound by convolving the anechoic source with the impulse response of a given room. The advantage of this technique is that it is not necessary to have the source in the room but only the impulse response of the room is required when the source is provided. When it comes to echolocation in bats, it is difficult to measure the echoes from the target when a real bat generates sound during its flight. But using the convolution technique, the same echoes can be recreated theoretically by acquiring the impulse response of the target and the bat's echolocating signal separately. Figure 7.3d and e shows the simplified concept of the model. There are two types of models. One is single receptor and the other is binaural receptors.

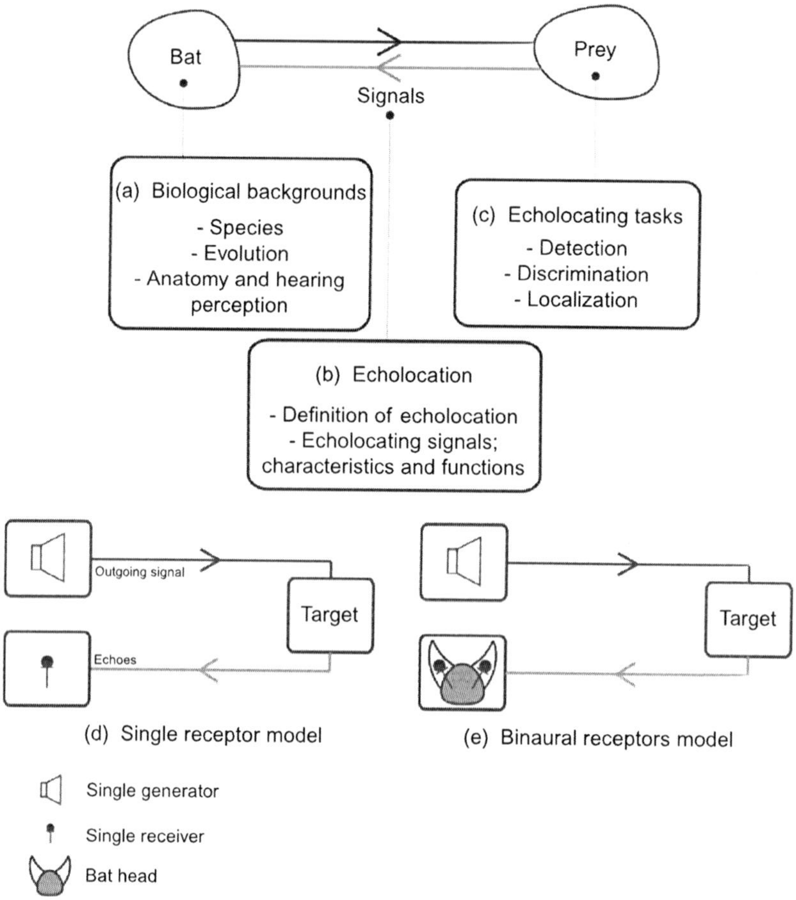

Figure 7.3 Biological backgrounds of bats (a), echolocation and signals produced (b), echolocating tasks (c), single(monaural) receptor model (d), and binaural receptors model (e).

7.2.2.1 Monaural hearing

Figure 7.3d shows the single (monaural) receptor model. This model consists of the echolocating sound source, target reflection, and single receptor. The model would reproduce and predict the signal received in front of the middle of the bat's head in echolocation for a specific target. As the reproduced signal contains the information such as amplitude, temporal characteristics, and spectral characteristics, the target detection and discrimination are considered to be available in this modeling.

7.2.2.2 Binaural hearing

However, as reviewed earlier, the localization task which the bat performs is only available when the binaural hearing is enabled. The function of the external ear and the head is essential to model the localization of the target. Figure 7.3e shows the binaural receptors model. It basically extends from the single receptor model, and it performs binaural processing for the signal received in the single receptor. The information for binaural processing in different locations of the sound source is conventionally known to be completely encoded in the transfer function of the head and external ears. It is commonly referred to as the head-related transfer function (HRTF, H_L, left ear; H_R, right ear), and its time (t)-domain version is the head-related impulse response (HRIR, H_L, left ear; H_R, right ear). Practically, the HRIR is measured at both ears in different azimuth (θ) and elevation (ϕ). It is then transformed into the frequency (f)-domain by the Fourier transform as

$$H_L(f, \theta, \phi) \leftrightarrow h_L(t, \theta, \phi) \tag{7.1}$$

$$H_R(f, \theta, \phi) \leftrightarrow h_R(t, \theta, \phi) \tag{7.2}$$

The amplitude and the phase are described at each ear to provide level and timing information as

$$A_L(f) = 20\log_{10}|H_L(f)| \, \Phi_L = \angle H_L(f) \tag{7.3}$$

$$A_R(f) = 20\log_{10}|H_R(f)| \, \Phi_R = \angle H_R(f) \tag{7.4}$$

The interaural level difference and interaural time difference can be obtained from the interaural transfer function which is represented from the left HRTF and right HRTF as

$$H(f) = \frac{H_R(f)}{H_L(f)} \tag{7.5}$$

Therefore, the ILD is obtained from

$$A(f) = 20\log_{10}|H(f)| = 20\log_{10}\left|\frac{H_R(f)}{H_L(f)}\right| = A_R(f) - A_L(f) \tag{7.6}$$

And the interaural time difference (ITD) is obtained from the group delay (τ_G) information in the interaural transfer function.

$$\tau G = \frac{1}{2\pi}\frac{\partial \Phi(f)}{\partial f} = \frac{1}{2\pi}\frac{\partial(\Phi_R(f) - \Phi_L(f))}{\partial f} \tag{7.7}$$

For humans, since the maximum possible ITD is about 660 μs for a typical radius of human head (approximately 87.5 mm), the ITDs are generally useful only for the frequencies below 1.5 kHz. If the size of the bat is assumed to be 10 times smaller than that of human, the ITD is expected not to be useful below 15 kHz, based on the scaling law. Therefore, one typical method of modeling the auditory system is a series of bandpass filters with a range of center frequencies. For example, octave bandpass filters, which vary the bandwidth depending on the performance of the auditory processing, can be applied and they employ wider bandwidths for higher frequencies. Another alternative method is to compute the envelopes of the signals measured at the two ears, then cross-correlate the envelopes to measure the interaural delay. The envelope of a signal is the outline of the signal and it connects all of the peaks in the signal. Using the envelope delays, one can obtain the interaural delays which increase monotonically with the angle of incidence of the sound relative to the median plane. Extracting an envelope is useful for the analysis of interaural delay in bats as the ITDs are not available for most of the high frequencies in the echolocating signal.

For a symmetrical head, both ILD and ITD are zero in the median plane. Generally, it is accepted that the measured HRTF is a rather complicated joint function of azimuth and elevation. There are also substantial intersubject differences in frequency response. Although the HRTF shows limited systematic variation of frequency response as a function of azimuth and elevation, HRIR measurement and HRTF analysis are required to reproduce and characterize the binaural signals which reach the eardrum in each ear. In conclusion, the HRIRs can be convolved with the signal which is received at the single receptor. This enables simulation of the binaural echolocating signals used in localization.

7.3 Learning from bats

There are a few aspects of echolocation in terms of what we can learn to inspire the development of bio-sonar. To begin with, we will look into the echolocating signal type which varies depending on the species. Each type of signal is regarded to have evolved to serve each species at a given echolocating environment such as type of prey and foliages. Once the emitted echolocating signal is returned and received by the bat, the signal then travels around its head to reach the ears. We will then discuss how the acoustical attributes of returned echoes would be affected by physical dimension and shape of the face features. Next, the echoes received by the outer ears will be processed by the bat's hearing mechanism at the cochlea. We will discuss what is currently known about the auditory processing of bats, and how we can use it for the engineering applications. Finally, there is a lesser known area about the range-dependent characteristics of binaural echolocation and we will review its implications.

7.3.1 Signal types

Microbats fall broadly into two categories depending on the types of echolocating signal they use: those that just use FM signals and those that use a combination of FM and CF signals. The latter category is often referred to as CF bats. Each species of bat emits echolocating signals with different duration, frequency bandwidth, and SPL. The particular type of signal used in each species of bat enables an effective echolocation for its own processing mechanism. Schnitzler and Henson (1980) demonstrated that narrowband, shallow FM components seem to be well suited for the detection of echoes from small insects and target movements, whereas broadband, steep FM components seem to be well suited for accurate target localization by delivering exact time markers. It is generally regarded that broadband echolocating signals carry better spectral information in the target reflection. On the other hand, CF components seem to be suitable for the Doppler shift compensation, in combination with CF bats' specialized hearing system and acoustic fovea. Therefore, the CF echolocating bats can classify fluttering insects by detecting temporal modulation patterns. The observation that each different type of signal has its own advantage and disadvantage corresponds to the fact that the bats live in various conditions. Considering the different foraging environments, such as open or closed spaces, and the types of prey that bats echolocate, the evolution of diverse signal structures seems necessary. In other words, the characteristics of an echolocating call are adapted to the particular environment, hunting behavior, and the type of food source. Although there is a difference between different types of signals, the general characteristics shown in the most of echolocating signals can be described as follows.

a. Sound pressure level (SPL)

The SPL of emitted signal can reach up 100 dB or more with air reference sound pressure 0.02 mPa. It has been recently reported that, at 10 cm distance from the bat, an intensity greater than 125 dB peak level has been shown in the recording from insect-eating bats and 133 dB has been shown in the recording from open space flying bats (Jones and Holderied, 2007).

b. Duty cycle

The duty cycle of a signal is defined as the ratio of the pulse duration (time) and the period between pulses, and is affected by the temporal pattern of signal delivery. In echolocation, the signal duty cycle can be maximized by increasing the signal duration, signal emission rate, or both. The duty cycle in echolocation is important in describing any overlapping pattern between the pulse and the echo.

c. Frequency patterns

In most of the echolocating bats, the FM downward sweep and the CF tones comprise the echolocating signal. The FM sweep is a broadband signal and the CF signal is a narrowband signal. Both of the signals can appear in one frequency range or in multiple harmonics.

d. Harmonics

There exists a dominant harmonic component which has the highest intensity when an echolocating call is composed of multiple harmonics.

e. Duration

A single continuous echolocating signal can last from 0.2 to 100 ms in duration. Typically, these last several milliseconds and are emitted 2–10 times per set of echolocating signal. After the bat detects a target of interest, it increases the repetition rate and decreases the duration of its signals to avoid overlapping between the emitted call and the returning echo.

f. Delay

During the flight while the bat is emitting the signal and searching for the prey, a delay occurs between the call and the returning echoes. This is related to range detection and target separation.

As described above, each echolocating signal carries its own information. The target information from echolocation is encoded by returning echoes and their relationship with the emitted signal. The information obtained by the processing of the signals is as follows.

a. Range

Range is the distance from the target object and it can be calculated from a specific delay between the original call and the echo.

b. Size

Information on size includes length, width, shape, and thickness. It is represented in the waveform characteristics such as amplitude, peaks, and notches in time domain.

c. Velocity

Some echolocating bats, particularly CF-FM bats, can calculate the relative velocity of its target object. This is achieved by analyzing the changes in echo frequency caused by Doppler shift and comparing them to the original echolocating call. The amount of Doppler shift is proportional to the relative velocity.

d. Fine structure

This refers to the spectral characteristics of the returning echo from a specific target. For example, it might be the edibility of various targets from the different echo structures.

e. 3-D location

This is the localization of the horizontal and vertical positions. The basic principle is the same as human localization (Blauert, 1997). The horizontal position is determined by binaural hearing which compares the difference between the signals reaching the two ears. The vertical position is determined by using information varying according to the pinna and tragus in bats. The external ears generate different spectral peaks and notches at different levels of elevation, giving vertical cues.

7.3.2 *Head, nose, and ears*

It is noted that each species of bats show its unique feature in the shape and size of its head, nose, and ears. The characteristics provide evidences as to what we have understood so far in terms of localization in bats and what has been achieved in the bio-inspired application of monaural and binaural receptors until today. The former is mostly investigated in biology and the latter is investigated in engineering such as robotics, electrical engineering, computer science, and acoustics. In biology, a few studies have measured the HRTF in bats, and moreover have shown that binaural cues vary systematically in both azimuth and elevation (Fuzessery, 1996). The pinna of the bat creates systematic changes in the spectral features of transfer functions and performs an important role in localization of targets in different elevations (Jen and Chen, 1988). It is also known that the movements of pinna, which rotate in antiphase, are important for vertical localization (Mogdans et al., 1988). In the engineering field, the application which tracks a fixed or moving object has been developed by using the echo arrival times detected at two receivers (Barshan and Kuc, 1992). Also, two moving receivers with a built-in robot sensor were inspired by pinna movements in the bat and the receivers were able to improve the localization ability using a tone signal (Kuc, 1996). These previous studies have employed narrowband signals and utilized the binaural cues such as ITDs and ILDs. In summary, the bat-specialized features such as types of pinna have been highly motivating the related research. On the other hand, according to the reviewing article about biomimetic sonar system, the effect of binaural hearing has been investigated by employing two receivers in the robotic system (Müller and Kuc, 2007).

7.3.3 Auditory perception and hearing process

The auditory system in bats is structured in the same way as that of other mammals. Once the echolocating signal returning from the target object has reached the two ears, each processes both time and frequency information in the cochlea.

In the inner ear, the cochlea of microbats is specialized for the use of high frequencies. It has been noted that cochleae of microbats are sensitive and sharply tuned at high frequencies up to 160 kHz. Kössl and Vater (1995) have shown that they have narrower and thicker basilar membranes than those of nonecholocating mammals, which explains the adaptation to high frequency selectivity. Also, the hair cells, which play the role of signal receptor, are of shorter length in microbats than those mostly presented in other mammals. This evidence corresponds to the extended high-frequency hearing range of the bats as well.

An interesting and specialized feature of the cochlea is found in the CF/FM bats. Such bats are observed to have an *acoustic fovea* in the cochlea where the neurons are specifically tuned to a narrow frequency range of returning echoes and are seen in Doppler shift-compensating bats such as *Rhinolophus ferrumequinum*, *Pteronotus parnellii*, and *Asellia tridens* (Schnitzler and Henson, 1980). The degree of sharpness in the tuning curve can be characterized by the Q-values (center frequency divided by bandwidth 10 dB from the tip of the bandpass filter). The sharper the tuning, the higher is the Q-value which gives better frequency resolution and accuracy. For example, the mustached bat's cochlear is specialized in response to the first harmonic of the CF component that it is able to measure the target velocity and detect the wing beats of insect prey (Neuweiler, 1990). Its behavior is supported by the evidence that the Q 10 dB values in the tuning curve can reach 600 in that frequency region. The other example shows that the frequencies a few kHz above and below the carrier frequency can reach Q-value up to 400 (Kössl and Russell, 1995). Another piece of biological evidence supporting the notion of the acoustic fovea is that the outer hair cells (OHCs) of the fovea constitute 40% of the total population of the cochlea and OHC responses to the carrier frequency signal dominate the response from the fovea (Russell et al., 2003).

The auditory processing can be simplified based on the bandpass filter banks which model the cochlear function in the previous study by Patterson et al. (1992). According to Patterson's model, each filter bank is modeled using a gammatone characteristic, the impulse response of which is defined in the time domain as Equation (7.8),

$$g(t) = a_g t^{(n-1)} e^{-2bt} \cos(2\pi f_c t + g) \tag{7.8}$$

where n is the filter order, b determines the bandwidth of the filter, and f_c denotes the center frequency of the filter. Also, a_g determines the amplitude coefficient for gammatone impulse response and g determines the phase delay. The equivalent rectangular bandwidth (ERB) is a psychoacoustic measure of the width of the auditory filter at each point along the cochlea and can be defined as Equation (7.9) (Slaney, 1993);

$$\mathrm{ERB} = \frac{f_c}{Q} + \mathrm{minBW} \tag{7.9}$$

where Q is the asymptotic filter quality. When the frequency reaches the high frequency region, minBW can be neglected. In contrast, minBW is the minimum bandwidth possible and occurs when f_c/Q approaches 0. Thus, the minBW term can be neglected as f_c becomes larger. For human auditory modeling, Glasberg and Moore (1990) have recommended data on the ERB of the auditory filter for the Equation (7.9) with $Q = 9.26$ and $\mathrm{minBW} = 24.7$. However, there is no direct evidence of Q-values for bat's auditory modeling. Assuming the auditory processing in bats resembles that of humans in terms of their mammalian cochlea; these values have been adopted and modified for the auditory filter banks of both FM and CF bats. This provides a simple and bio-inspired auditory model based on the more complex bat's system. For example, assuming better performance in resolving frequencies in the cochlear of the FM bats than in those of humans, the Q-value is varied as 10, 20, and above. The higher

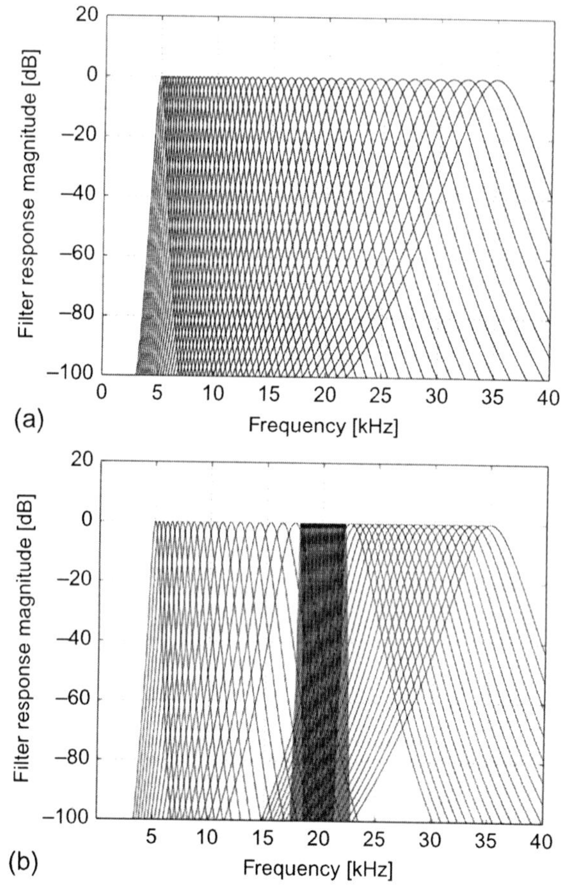

Figure 7.4 (a) Modified gammatone filter banks of auditory processing in FM bats based on Glasberg and Moore parameters (1990). (b) The modified gammatone filter banks of auditory processing in CF bats with acoustic fovea.

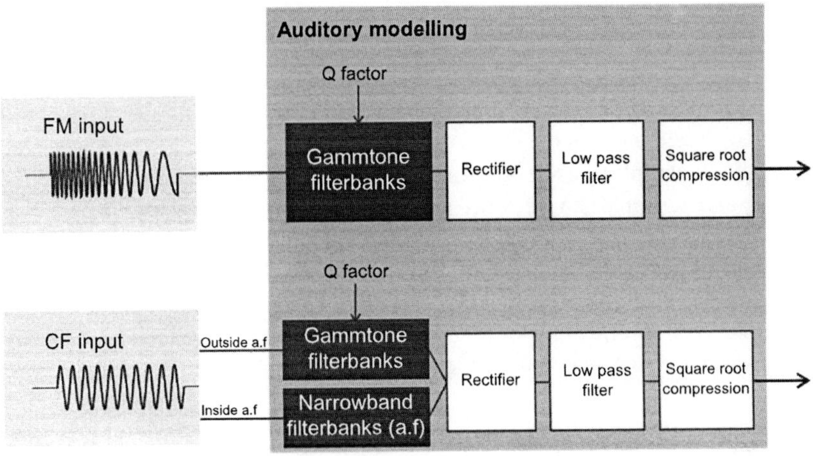

Figure 7.5 Diagram of auditory processing. "a.f" denotes acoustic fovea.

Q-value represents the sharper tuning curve for each frequency in the auditory system. Figure 7.4 shows the example of artificially designed auditory filter banks for FM and CF bats. Note that the CF bat's filter banks show finely tuned collection of filters centered at the frequency where the acoustic fovea is modeled.

Figure 7.5 describes how bat's auditory processing can be modeled. When the gammatone filter banks are modeled, each bandpass filter bank produces the demodulation of the frequency seen through the basilar membrane. The output of a linear filter bank resolves the frequencies to some extent, yet it does not represent the neural activity in the cochlea. After the frequency is resolved by the mechanical motion in the basilar membrane, the inner hair cells convert the motion into neural activity. In the first instance, extraction of the signal envelope from the motion by the inner hair cells can be modeled by half-wave rectification and low pass filtering. As the rectifier generated new frequency components, some of which are unwanted by the specific frequency channel, low pass filters, for example, at 1000 Hz can be chosen to remove these unwanted components. The output is extracted from the envelope of the decomposed signal. The envelope of each channel is applied to the square root compression which reduces the fluctuation of the envelope. The square root compression processing represents the gain control system in the cochlea. As a result, the output signal is fitted within the dynamic range of hearing.

7.3.4 Range-dependent bio-sonar

Echolocation is an active sensing system that is exploited by many species of bats during flight to navigate and locate objects such as prey. The direction and distance-dependent acoustical properties of bats' heads and external ears (pinnae), to which all echoes are subjected before being perceived, are probably crucial to this. Detailed knowledge of these "obligatory" acoustical properties may lead to a better understanding of bat echolocating behavior and the computational processes involved. It may also inspire novel ideas for sonar engineering, as has been the case with other aspects of biological echolocation (Müller and Kuc, 2007). However, the analysis of signals at each ear during the echolocation process is challenging due to active movements, adaptive changes in the signal emitted, and the speed with which bats respond to targets. For example, the bat echolocation process has been categorized into search, approach, and terminal stages (Hill and Smith, 1984), and a typical prey-capture sequence from search to terminal stage takes no longer than 1 s (Ulanovsky and Moss, 2008). During this, a number of acoustically relevant aspects of a bat's behavior also change, including the echolocation calls and the position of the head and pinnae.

The functional implications of these changes have not yet been clearly explained, and may be related to distance-dependent acoustical properties of the head and pinnae. Griffin et al. (1960) observed that many species of bat increase bandwidth and decrease duration of their calls during the approaching stage. Simmons and Stein (1980) have suggested that the bandwidth and average period of echolocation signals can determine the quality of target perception. It has also been reported that bats change their calls not only when they are attacking prey but also when they are approaching obstacles such as tree branches and the ground (Ulanovsky and Moss, 2008). Classic sonar theory explains that increasing bandwidth of the call improves the acoustical image of objects in range resolution, while decreasing the call duration helps bats to avoid overlapping between the emitted call and received echoes. In addition, the other explanation about controlling bandwidth and harmonic frequencies of the call is that adaptive changes in the call structure might compensate for the systematic error of the Doppler-shifted echoes induced during the flight (Hiryu et al., 2005). Increasing bandwidth at high frequency has been found in search calls. Siemers and Schnitzler (2004) have recently demonstrated strong correlation between the ability of prey detection and the respective bandwidth in echolocating calls in the "search" stage. In particular, broadening of the bandwidth was obtained mainly by increasing the starting frequency of a chirp. In addition, Hiryu et al. (2010) have found that increasing the bandwidth by lowering frequencies downward has reduced the pulse-echo ambiguity in clutter. Again, these results emphasize the role of wide bandwidth in better characterization of the prey.

A contribution of the head is observed during the bat's echolocation. Ghose and Moss (2006) have shown that the bat locks its head toward the target when switching from a search to an approach mode and it changes the rate of vocal emission at the same time. It has been shown in several studies that some species of bats move their pinnae in correspondence with echolocating signals (Griffin et al., 1962). Mogdans et al. (1988) have shown that the mobile pinnae contribute to a better performance in target localization. And, Holland and Waters (2005) have suggested that the pinnae might also contribute to controlling the gain of the echoes. They have recently measured the HRTF of *R. aegyptiacus* to demonstrate higher sensitivity in gain when its pinnae are directed forward rather than backward. Kick and Simmons (1984) suggested that the sensitivity in the ear increases with the echo delay due to the fact that the echo level decreases as the distance increases. The intensity compensation, or automatic gain control, during the emission of calls was also studied by Hartley, and the results imply that bats might compensate for the acoustical attenuation during the air transmission of echo signals (Hartley, 1992). Boonman and Jones (2002) have shown that this behavior is not dependent on the target, but it is global and the pattern is stereotyped regardless of the type of target. Surlykke and Kalko (2008) have argued that bats compensate for intensity attenuation of different frequencies in their echolocation call as their findings showed that bats emit the higher intensities for the higher frequencies, which severely attenuate in air. This evidence supports the idea that the echolocating bats might receive stabilized amplitude of the echoes which are independent of the frequencies.

Although the understanding of the relationship between the active echolocating motion and sensing have been made to some extent as described above, there are not many studies about the effect of binaural processing during flight. Recently, Kim et al. have suggested that low-frequency binaural spectral features are strongly distance-dependent such that angular sensitivity can be maintained by lowering the frequency of the echolocation emission at close range. The range-dependent characteristics of bat's echolocation may need further investigation, and sonar engineering application can benefit from its potential implication on designing an active ranging receiver.

7.4 Bio-inspired sonar applications

Many aspects in the design of bio-sonar are challenging. For example, an engineered bio-sonar may demand designing processes from manufacturing right type of transducers to a computational processor involving advanced signal processing techniques. Arguably, one of the most important keys to a successful application is an appropriate and accurate interpretation of the received information.

7.4.1 Development of bio-inspired sonar

The traditional sonar application has been largely based on simple ranging sensors; however, a bat-inspired sonar is potentially capable of extracting much more information from the echoes which will support more intelligent and interactive sonar system (Steckel and Peremans, 2013). As explained in Section 7.3.2, the bat's echolocation recruits its head morphology and facial features, such as nose and outer ears, which process spectral filtering (Reijniers and Peremans, 2007) of the environment on the emitted calls. Understanding the monaural and binaural cues encoded in those filtered calls, i.e., the returning echoes from the specific surroundings, is arguably one of the most critical tasks to be done for the advanced development of more sophisticated bio-sonar.

For example, adaptive changes in ILDs according to the movement of the sonar receiver could be applied to improve its binaural performance. Utilizing both mobility and binaural information can serve to develop sensory system of aids for the blind or for nondestructive testing of manufactured parts, which clearly requires motion of the reception part of the system. However, the performance of moving sonar needs to be tested under controlled conditions where the experimenter is aware of the acoustical characteristics of the receiver, which can be defined by its HRTF. Then, evaluation of the sonar system is required to be accompanied by an investigation of the relationship between its performance and the change of its spatial location and frequency characteristics of the outgoing echolocating signal.

The future work in this field should perhaps also aim to develop an optimized signal and auditory processing tool which can provide better performance in echo detection, discrimination, and localization. It is well known that the signal design changes during a bat's search, approach, and terminal stage. Previous studies have already confirmed that this signal design changes in a predictable manner depending upon the echolocating task required in each stage. Therefore, designing a signal which changes adaptively in a bio-inspired sonar system, and enabling its practical application remain as challenging tasks. It is also noted that signal processing techniques such as the auditory model affect the representation of acoustical images of the echo signals. The performance of the sonar task, such as gain control and spectral representation, can be partly manipulated by those techniques. Therefore, further work is required to develop an effective signal type and its auditory processing which can maximize the performance of practical sonar systems.

7.4.2 Potential applications

The most apparent application of bio-inspired sonar is in advanced sonar systems involving moving sonar capable of decoding the acoustical glints (Kuc, 2004) from random objects to fully interpret the environment, or a device estimating passing ranges while localizing and classifying the objects to avoid a collision (Kuc, 2007a,b). Bat's bio-sonar also provides inspiration to challenge conventional beamforming operation which often uses large number of transducers. Beamforming is a sensor array which uses a signal processing technique to control the direction of sound emission and reception. We have learned that bats are capable of much more sophisticated control over the emitted and received signals and it is partly due to their physical features of face and ears. This lesson might inspire engineers to take a different approach in designing beamforming applications such as radar and acoustic imaging. The bio-sonar is also able to improve the performance of biomedical solutions such as hearing aids. As discussed in Section 7.2, it is already known that the auditory system of bats resembles that of humans. However, how the auditory signals are interpreted in brain processing during echolocation has not yet been revealed. Understanding the bat's exceptional hearing process may provide us with valuable lessons to particularly help blind people who currently depend on hearing aids for their spatial perception of surroundings.

There might be many potential applications engineers can think of, however the methodology to achieve these goals still remain to open question. Müller and Kuc (2007) argue that how bio-sonar-inspired technology could serve as a model system in the search for highly complex technical solution should be approached by a strategy to achieve intermediate goals, such as (a) efficient extraction of exact information from biology, (b) better understanding in technological need, and (c) targeting wider mainstream application area. Also, developing the idea of bio-inspired sonar in the engineering environment is considered necessary because the materials used in engineering are substantially different from those used in nature. Forbes (2006) has expressed an important principle of bio-inspired engineering in this regard:

> *"Scientists try to unravel nature's mechanisms, but technologists use whatever will work. Bio-inspired technical products will almost certainly not mimic the actual materials used by nature."*

Forbes emphasizes the importance of finding global principles which can be adopted to design a system using technical methods. The technical methods may include mechanical/experimental setups, receiver design, and signal processing techniques for example.

7.5 Summary and conclusions

This chapter has reviewed what consists of bat echolocation and discussed what enables bats to perform the echolocation at a highly sophisticated level. Each component of echolocation, such as emitted signals, transmission and filtering of echoes around the bat's head, binaural and auditory processing, still leaves many questions to be answered in order to increase our understanding of how bat's bio-sonar works. The man-made sonar can be developed further from the insights gained about bat's echolocation which invites an attractive possibility to contribute to improving the conventional sonar systems in various applications. However, it is worthwhile for engineers to be reminded that a systematic and strategic approach is necessary to exploit a successfully engineered bio-sonar solution. This is only likely to be achieved by adopting carefully designed technical methods including experimental research and advanced signal processing techniques.

Acknowledgment

The contents of this chapter are largely based on the author's doctoral thesis (Kim, 2010) and her paper published in Bioinspiration and Biomimetics (Kim et al., 2012).

References

Barshan, B., Kuc, R., 1992. A bat-like sonar system for obstacle localization. IEEE Trans. Syst. Man Cybern. 22 (4), 636–646.

Blauert, J., 1997. Spatial Hearing: The Psychophysics of Human Sound Localization. The MIT Press, Cambridge/Massachusetts/London/England.

Boonman, A., Jones, G., 2002. Intensity control during target approach in echolocating bats stereotypical sensorimotor behaviour in Daubenton's bats, *Myotis daubentonii*. J. Exp. Biol. 205, 2865–2874.

Carmena, J.M., Hallam, J.C.T., 2001. Estimating Doppler shift using bat-inspired cochlear filter bank models: a comparison of methods for echoes from single and multiple reflectors. Adapt. Behav. 9 (3–4), 241–261.
Carmena, J.M., Kampchen, N., Kim, D., Hallam, J.C.T., 2001. Artificial ears for a biomimetic sonar head: from multiple reflectors to surfaces. Artif. Life 7 (2), 147–169.
Forbes, P., 2006. The Geckos Foot. Harper Perennial, London.
Fuzessery, Z.M., 1996. Monaural and binaural spectral cues created by the external ears of the pallid bat. Hear. Res. 95 (1–2), 1–17.
Ghose, K., Moss, C.F., 2006. Steering by hearing: a bat's acoustic gaze is linked to its flight motor output by a delayed, adaptive linear law. J. Neurosci. 26 (6), 1704–1710.
Glasberg, B.R., Moore, B.C.J., 1990. Derivation of auditory filter shapes from notched-noise data. Hear. Res. 47 (1–2), 103–138.
Griffin, D.R., 1958. Listening in the Dark. Yale University Press, New Haven, CT.
Griffin, D.R., Webster, F.A., Michael, C.R., 1960. The echolocation of flying insects by bats. Anim. Behav. 8 (3), 141–154.
Griffin, D.R., Dunning, D.C., Cahlander, D.A., Webster, F.A., 1962. Correlated orientation sounds and ear movements of horseshoe bats. Nature 196, 1185–1186.
Grossetete, A., Moss, C.F., 1998. Target flutter rate discrimination by bats using frequency-modulated sonar sounds: behavior and signal processing models. J. Acoust. Soc. Am. 103 (4), 2167–2176.
Hartley, D.J., 1992. Stabilization of perceived echo amplitudes in echolocating bats: II. The acoustic behavior of the big brown bat, *Eptesicus fuscus*, when tracking moving prey. J. Acoust. Soc. Am. 91 (2), 1133–1149.
Heffner, R.S., Heffner, H.E., 1990. Vestigial hearing in a fossorial mammal, the pocket gopher (*Geomys bursarius*). Hear. Res. 46 (3), 239–252.
Hill, J.E., Smith, J.D., 1984. Bats—A Natural History. University of Texas Press, Austin, TX.
Hiryu, S., Katsura, K., Lin, L.K., Riquimaroux, H., Watanabe, Y., 2005. Doppler-shift compensation in the Taiwanese leaf-nosed bat (*Hipposideros terasensis*) recorded with a telemetry microphone system during flight. J. Acoust. Soc. Am. 118 (6), 3927–3933.
Hiryu, S., Bates, M.E., Simmons, J.A., Riquimaroux, H., 2010. FM echolocating bats shift frequencies to avoid broadcast-echo ambiguity in clutter. Proc. Natl. Acad. Sci. U. S. A. 107 (15), 7048–7053.
Holland, R.A., Waters, D.A., 2005. Echolocation signals and pinnae movement in the fruit bat *Rousettus aegyptiacus*. Acta Chiropterol. 7 (1), 83–90.
Jen, P.H.S., Chen, D., 1988. Directionality of sound pressure transformation at the pinna of echolocating bats. Hear. Res. 34 (2), 101–118.
Jones, G., Holderied, M.W., 2007. Bat echolocation calls: adaptation and convergent evolution. Proc. R. Soc. B Biol. Sci. 274 (1612), 905–912.
Kick, S.A., Simmons, J.A., 1984. Automatic gain-control in the bats sonar receiver and the neuroethology of echolocation. J. Neurosci. 4 (11), 2725–2737.
Kim, S.Y., 2010. Development and application of an echolocation model inspired by bats. Doctoral thesis, University of Southampton, Institute of Sound and Vibration Research, Southampton, UK.
Kim, S.Y., Allen, R., Rowan, D., 2012. Range-dependent characteristics in the HRTFs of a bat-head cast: part 2. Binaural characteristics. Bioinspir. Biomim. 7 (4), 046015.
Koay, G., Kearns, D., Heffner, H.E., Heffner, R.S., 1998. Passive sound localization ability of the big brown bat (*Eptesicus fuscus*). Hear. Res. 119 (1–2), 37–48.

Kössl, M., Russell, I.J., 1995. Basilar-membrane resonance in the cochlea of the moustached bat. Proc. Natl. Acad. Sci. U. S. A. 92 (1), 276–279.

Kössl, M., Vater, M., 1995. Cochlea structure and function in bats. In: Popper, A.N., Fay, R.R.R. (Eds.), In: Hearing by Bats, vol. 5. Springer-Verlag, New York.

Kuc, R., 1996. Biologically motivated adaptive sonar system. J. Acoust. Soc. Am. 100 (3), 1849–1854.

Kuc, R., 1997a. Biomimetic sonar locates and recognizes objects. IEEE J. Oceanic Eng. 22 (4), 616–624.

Kuc, R., 1997b. Biomimetic sonar recognizes objects using binaural information. J. Acoust. Soc. Am. 102 (2), 689–696.

Kuc, R., 2002. Binaural sonar electronic travel aid provides vibrotactile cues for landmark, reflector motion and surface texture classification. IEEE Trans. Biomed. Eng. 49 (10), 1173–1180.

Kuc, R., 2004. Neuro-computational processing of moving sonar echoes classifies and localizes foliage. J. Acoust. Soc. Am. 116 (3), 1811–1818.

Kuc, R., 2007a. Biomimetic sonar and neuromorphic processing eliminate reverberation artifacts. IEEE Sens. J. 7 (3–4), 361–369.

Kuc, R., 2007b. Neuromorphic processing of moving sonar data for estimating passing range. IEEE Sens. J. 7 (5), 851–859.

Lawrence, B.D., Simmons, J.A., 1982. Measurements of atmospheric attenuation at ultrasonic frequencies and the significance for echolocation by bats. J. Acoust. Soc. Am. 71 (3), 585–590.

Masters, W.M., Raver, K.A.S., Kazial, K.A., 1995. Sonar signals of big brown bats, *Eptesicus fuscus*, contain information about individual identity, age and family affiliation. Anim. Behav. 50, 1243–1260.

Mogdans, J., Ostwald, J., Schnitzler, H.U., 1988. The role of pinna movement for the localization of vertical and horizontal wire obstacles in the greater horseshoe bat, *Rhinolophus ferrumequinum*. J. Acoust. Soc. Am. 84 (5), 1676–1679.

Müller, R., Kuc, R., 2007. Biosonar-inspired technology: goals, challenges and insights. Bioinspir. Biomim. 2, S146–S161.

Neuweiler, G., 1990. Auditory adaptations for prey capture in echolocating bats. Physiol. Rev. 70 (3), 615–641.

Patterson, R.D., Robinson, K., Holdsworth, J., Mckeown, D., Zhang, C., Allerhand, M.H., 1992. Complex sounds and auditory images. In: Cazals, Y., Demany, L., Horner, K. (Eds.), Auditory Physiology and Perception. Pergamon, Oxford.

Reijniers, J., Peremans, H., 2007. Biomimetic sonar system performing spectrum-based localization. IEEE Trans. Robot. 23 (6), 1151–1159.

Russell, I.J., Drexl, M., Foeller, E., Vater, M., Kossl, M., 2003. Synchronization of a nonlinear oscillator: processing the CF component of the echo-response signal in the cochlea of the mustached bat. J. Neurosci. 23 (29), 9508–9518.

Schnitzler, H.U., Henson Jr., O.W., 1980. Performance of airborne animal sonar system. Microchiroptera in animal sonar systems. In: Busnel, R.G., Fish, J.F. (Eds.), Animal Sonar Systems. Plenum, New York.

Siemers, B.M., Schnitzler, H.U., 2004. Echolocation signals reflect niche differentiation in five sympatric congeneric bat species. Nature, 429 (6992), 657–661.

Simmons, J.A., Chen, L., 1989. The acoustic basis for target discrimination by fm echolocating bats. J. Acoust. Soc. Am. 86 (4), 1333–1350.

Simmons, J.A., Stein, R.A., 1980. Acoustic imaging in bat sonar—echolocation signals and the evolution of echolocation. J. Comp. Physiol. 135 (1), 61–84.

Simmons, J.A., Kick, S.A., Lawrence, B.D., Hale, C., Bard, C., Escudie, B., 1983. Acuity of horizontal angle discrimination by the echolocating bat, *Eptesicus fuscus*. J. Comp. Physiol. 153 (3), 321–330.

Simmons, J.A., Ferragamo, M., Moss, C.F., Stevenson, S.B., Altes, R.A., 1990. Discrimination of jittered sonar echoes by the echolocating bat, *Eptesicus fuscus*—the shape of target images in echolocation. J. Comp. Physiol. A J. Comp. Physiol. A Sens. Neural Behav. Physiol. 167 (5), 589–616.

Slaney, M., 1993. An efficient implementation of the patterson-holdsworth auditory filter bank. Apple Computer Technical Report 35.

Steckel, J., Peremans, H., 2013. BatSLAM: simultaneous localization and mapping using biomimetic sonar. PLoS One 8 (1), e54076. http://dx.doi.org/10.1371/journal.pone.0054076.

Surlykke, A., Kalko, E.K.V., 2008. Echolocating bats cry out loud to detect their prey. PLoS One 3, e2036.

Ulanovsky, N., Moss, C.F., 2008. What the bat's voice tells the bat's brain. Proc. Natl. Acad. Sci. U. S. A. 105 (25), 8491–8498.

Wotton, J.A., Simmons, J.A., 2000. Spectral cues and perception of the vertical position of targets by the big brown bat, Eptesicus fuscus. J. Acoust. Soc. Am. 107, 1034–1041.

Part Three

Biomimetic Actuators

Conducting interpenetrating polymer networks actuators for biomimetic vision system

8

N. Festin, C. Plesse, C. Chevrot, P. Pirim, F. Vidal

8.1 Introduction

Electroactive polymers (EAPs) are a class of polymeric materials that can change dimensions when electrically activated. Those polymers exhibit natural muscle-like behaviors due to their operation principle similar to real muscles and therefore they gained the name of artificial muscles (Bar-Cohen, 2001; Carpi and Smela, 2009; Osada and De Rossi, 1999). As such they are being considered for use to mimic the mechanical performance of biological systems. Their functional modes offer advantages over conventional technologies (thermal engines, hydraulic actuators, electrical motor, etc.) such as lightness, flexibility, and low cost. Therefore, the design of new EAP actuators which can potentially solve inherent limitations of conventional devices becomes a major academic and economic challenge and their favorable properties such as compliance, flexibility, and lightweight now allow many research groups to envision them for soft robotic applications. The EAPs are generally divided into two families operating by fundamentally different principles (Bar-Cohen, 2001): (i) electronic EAPs whose volume changes under application of an electric field and (ii) ionic EAPs whose volume changes with a movement of ions within the material. Electronic conducting polymers (ECPs) belong to the ionic one.

ECPs are chemically reactive polymers. Their oxidation or reduction gives rise to reversible volume variations. Indeed, during redox reactions in electrolytic solution, electrons are extracted from (or injected to) the polymer chains and ions and solvents are exchanged with the electrolyte to keep charge and osmotic balance inside the ECP film (Figure 8.1). These ion expulsion/inclusion motions during redox processes are believed to be the main factors which are responsible for the dimensional changes (Smela, 2003; De Paoli, 1997; Baughman, 1996).

In addition to the previously mentioned advantages, ECP are considered to be biocompatible and can theoretically develop high output forces under low potential (<5 V) without noise. Depending on the device configuration, they can be operated in aqueous/solvent medium or/and in open air. ECP actuators have been proposed among others as caudal paddle or to deflect a camber foil for (under)water vehicles (Alici et al., 2007; McGovern et al., 2009, 2010; Madden, 2004) as well as rat artificial whiskers (Festin and Plesse, 2011; Festin, 2014). Several applications have been also considered in the medical field. For example, guide wires and active catheters based

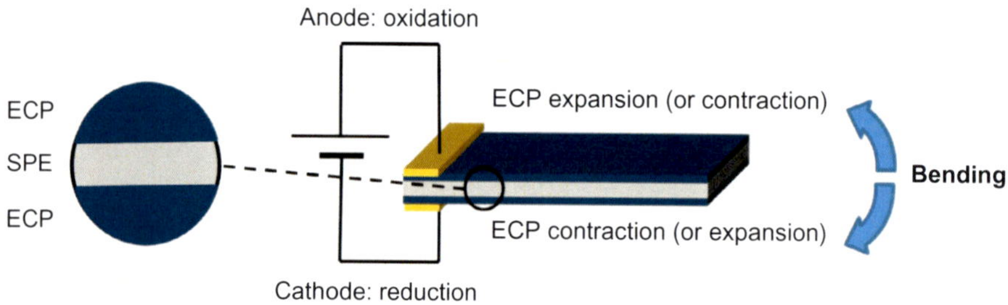

Figure 8.1 Trilayer actuator working principle.

on ECP allowing a tip movement have been proposed by different research groups (Shoa et al., 2010; Krogh et al., 2001; Wilson et al., 2007).

To operate in open air, ECP-based actuators are usually built using a solid polymer electrolyte (SPE) film sandwiched between two ECP layers displaying a trilayer structure: ECP//SPE//ECP (Figure 8.1). The two ECP layers act as the electroactive materials whereas the SPE acting as the ion reservoir providing ions required for the redox reaction (Kaneto et al., 1995).

Even if some interesting prototypes have been already reported (*vide supra*), actuators devices with improved performances (strain, force, speed, etc.) are still needed to expand applications. So far, most efforts have been devoted on ECP synthesis conditions (temperature, electrolyte, solvent, etc.) in order to improve ECP strain, output forces, and response times (Liang et al., 1992; Zhou et al., 2003; Temmer et al., 2012; Madden et al., 2000; Kiefer et al., 2008; Hara et al., 2006). However, performances of open-air actuators are depending not only on the conducting polymer properties but also on the SPE properties. Indeed, the SPE has a strong influence on the electromechanical response. For example, actuation rates can be greatly improved by increasing the SPE ionic conductivity in order to obtain a high ion diffusion rate within the material (Wu et al., 2006; Madden et al., 2000). The SPE also has a major influence on the mechanical properties of actuators since ECPs show usually poor mechanical properties. Thus, open-air actuators have been successfully fabricated, thanks to the presence of PVDF porous films which are usually used as filter membranes. The porous structure is first filled with an electrolyte and the convenient mechanical properties of the PVDF membranes allow the fabrication of actuators (Wu et al., 2006). However, SPE requirements are much greater than for other electrochemical devices such as batteries or supercapacitors and tailoring PVDF membrane properties is rather limited. Thus, custom synthesis of flexible SPEs combining tunable ionic conduction and mechanical properties is a key factor for the elaboration of specific actuators for given applications.

For this purpose, interpenetrating polymer networks (IPNs) represent an interesting class of material as SPE in practical electrochemical devices since they can bring up a certain level of physical and mechanical properties. IPNs are described as an intimate combination of two (or more) cross-linked polymers (Klempner et al., 1994). The tight entanglement of these networks ensures good interpenetration of the two components, and the three-dimensional interpenetration in the networks radically improves dimensional and morphological stability. By choosing two polymer partners for their specific properties, i.e., one for ionic conduction and the other one for mechanical properties, one can design SPE that can meet the specific requirements of ECP-based actuators. When an ECP is incorporated in such an SPE IPN, it can be turned out into conducting IPN. The synthetic pathway used in this study leads to a nonhomogeneous dispersion of the ECP through the thickness of the IPN, i.e., the quantity of poly (3,4-ethylenedioxythiophene) decreases from the outside toward the center of the film mimicking trilayer actuator devices. Thus, the ECP is interpenetrated in the IPN and this complex macromolecular architecture allows overcoming the delamination process (Vidal et al., 2004, 2010; Plesse et al., 2005) which has been reported in laminated trilayer actuators (Bar-Cohen, 2001). Among ECP, PEDOT has received much attention because of its particularly high stability in the doped state and the reversibility of the doping process (Groenendaal et al., 2000, 2003). Therefore, this polymer has been selected for the synthesis of conducting IPN. After the conducting IPNs synthesis, the samples are swollen with an electrolyte to obtain the final electrochemical devices. Ionic liquids have been successfully used as electrolyte (Lu et al., 2002). Among them, 1-ethyl-3-methylimidazolium bis-(trifluoromethylsulfonyl)imide (EMITFSI) is one of the best candidates due to its high ionic conductivity, nonvolatility, and its quite low viscosity (Vidal et al., 2004; Bonhôte et al., 1996; Zhou et al., 2003).

In this chapter, we report the full fabrication of conducting IPN actuator and its first integration in a biomimetic system. First, the SPE matrix synthesis as well as the mechanical and ionic conductivity properties are described. Then the synthesis of the conducting IPN is reported and the resulting actuator performances are characterized. Finally, a specific design of actuators as well as their integration in a first prototype of biomimetic vision system is presented. Each element of the biological vision system (eye ↔ eye muscles ↔ brain) and their relationship will be reproduced by using a combination of microcamera ↔ ECP actuators—electronic board (Figure 8.2).

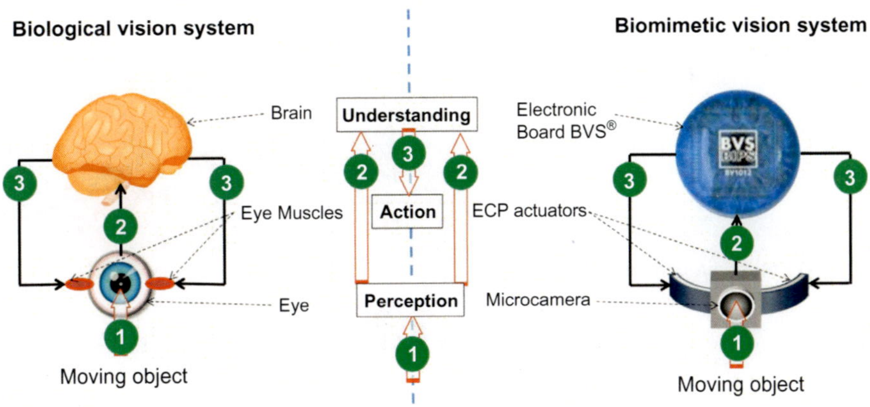

Figure 8.2 Schematic view of the artificial vision system mimicking the biological vision system. (1) Perception of a moving object, (2) analysis and understanding of the visual information, and (3) action on the muscles to track the moving object.

8.2 Interpenetrated polymer network as solid polymer electrolyte

8.2.1 Introduction to SPE and IPNs

As described in the introduction part, SPEs have a major influence on the electro-chemo-mechanical response of actuators. In particular, the redox reaction leading to actuation can only occur if the ionic conductivity within the device is high enough. Therefore, the SPE membrane should be designed in order to obtain high ionic conductivity. On the other hand, and since ECPs have poor mechanical properties, the mechanical resistance of the device is ensured mainly by the SPE. First, a single polyethylene oxide (PEO) network was tested as SPE in actuator device and was synthesized from poly(ethylene glycol) methacrylate derivatives. However, this PEO network was not suitable because of tearing problems leading to the destruction of the electro active material when actuated (Vidal et al., 2003). The PEO network thus has been combined with another polymer into IPN architecture in order to overcome this problem. The presence of nitrile butadiene rubber (NBR) in the PEO network should ensure convenient mechanical properties, i.e., to absorb large deformations during actuations without destruction. Therefore, SPE-based IPNs combining PEO and NBR networks have been prepared (Goujon et al., 2011; Festin et al., 2013). IPNs can be synthesized according to two different ways (Figure 8.3). In the two-step procedure, one network is formed first, and then in a second step, the first network is swollen with the precursors of the second network. Nevertheless, SPE membranes have been prepared according to a second way which is far easier to carry out. Thus, IPNs

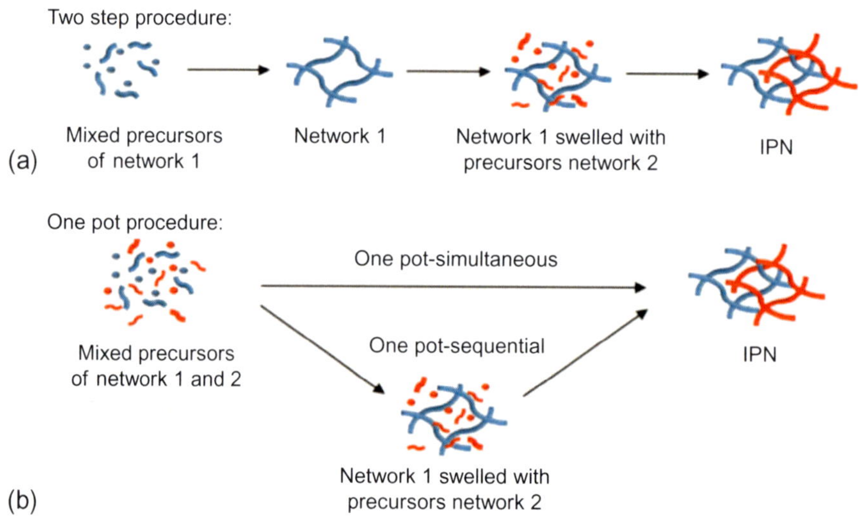

Figure 8.3 Typical pathways of IPN synthesis.

are synthesized in a one-pot procedure in which the PEO network is formed first followed by the NBR cross-linking reaction.

In order to improve the ionic conductivity, dangling chains have been introduced on the PEO network for increasing the proportion of free volume available for the migration of ions (Goujon et al., 2014). As mentioned previously, EMITFSI is one of the best electrolyte candidates due to its high ionic conductivity, nonvolatility, and its quite low viscosity. In addition, EMITFSI has a high affinity to polymer with polar group, which made it compatible not only with PEO but also with NBR which is an asset too to maintain high ionic conductivity within the IPN (Cho et al., 2007; Marwanta et al., 2005). Nevertheless, it should be pointed out here that the combination of properties as ionic conduction and mechanical properties could be obtained only if dual-phase continuity is obtained (Klempner et al., 1994).

8.2.2 IPN SPE synthesis and properties

The synthesis of these materials has been described in detail by Festin et al. (2013). PEO/NBR IPNs are synthesized via a two-step one-pot process where PEO network is composed of 75 wt% polyethylene glycol methacrylate (PEGM) acting as dangling chains and 25 wt% polyethylene glycol dimethacrylate (PEGDM) acting as cross-linkers. The starting medium is a solution of NBR, PEGDM, PEGM, and initiators in trichloroethane containing 70 wt% PEO precursors. The PEO network is shown to proceed within 3 h at 50 °C and a post curing at 100 °C appears necessary to complete the total conversion of methacrylic groups as shown by NIR spectroscopy. In a second step, the NBR network is formed by heating 25 min at 180 °C (Figure 8.4).

Co-continuous morphology is needed to provide a convenient combination of ionic conductivity and mechanical properties in the final SPEs. Thus, the morphology and

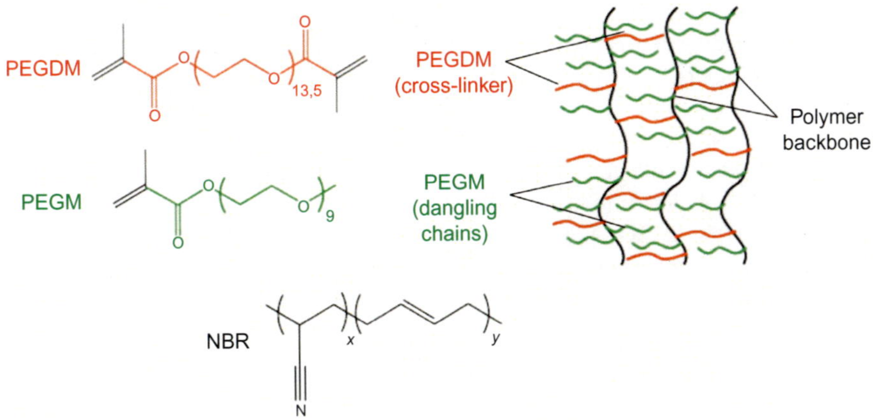

Figure 8.4 Chemical structures of poly(ethylene oxide) methacrylate (PEGM), poly(ethylene oxide) dimethacrylate (PEGDM), and nitrile butadiene rubber (NBR).

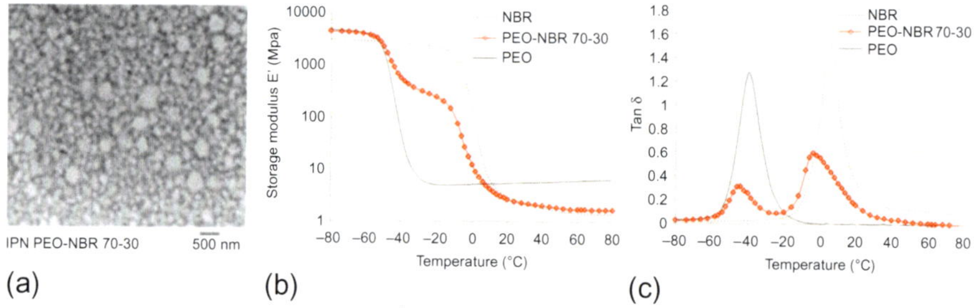

Figure 8.5 (a) TEM picture of a 70/30 PEO/NBR IPN stained by OsO_4. NBR-rich phases appear in black. PEO-rich phases appear in light gray. (b) Storage modulus as a function of temperature of the 70/30 PEO/NBR IPN and corresponding single networks. (c) Loss factor tanδ as a function of temperature of the 70/30 PEO/NBR IPN and corresponding single networks.

phase distribution in IPNs have been studied by transmission electron microscopy (TEM) and by dynamic mechanical analysis (DMA). TEM observations on 70/30 (w/w) PEO/NBR IPN were recorded on OsO_4-loaded stained samples and the picture is shown in Figure 8.5a. Since only NBR partner is marked by OsO_4, the black domains can be interpreted as being NBR-rich phases and thus PEO-rich phases appear as clear-gray domains. On the TEM picture, a macrophase separation takes place giving rise to a PEO-dispersed phase with domain sizes in the range of 500 nm. If the NBR continuity can be stated, additional experiments are required to get insight into the PEO phase continuity. The morphology has been also studied by DMA. The typical viscoelastic behavior of single networks and IPNs was studied. Figure 8.5b depicts the storage modulus and the loss factors (tan δ) for the two single networks and the 70/30 PEO/IPN. Two α relaxations can be clearly observed in the IPN, one about 0 °C corresponding to NBR-rich phases and one about −45 °C corresponding to PEO-rich phases. These results clearly indicate that the IPN presents dual-phase morphology and confirm the results obtained previously by TEM studies.

$LiClO_4$ loading experiments were carried out in order to make a clear assignment of the morphology of the samples. Indeed, we have shown in previous papers that the specific interaction of Li^+ cations within PEO partner can be used to measure the extent of phase separation in the IPN (Gauthier et al., 2007; Plesse et al., 2007). The molar ratio of uptaken Li^+ cations to ethylene oxide units ($r = [Li^+]/[CH_2CH_2O\text{-}]$) is determined by weighing the dried $LiCLO_4$ loaded samples after immersion in the $LiClO_4$ aqueous solution. The molar ratio r in the NBR single network is close to zero. For the PEO network and the IPN, the r values are for both 0.11 meaning that the accessibility of PEO is similar in both networks. In conclusion, these results prove that the PEO domains are continuous or very close to within the IPN material.

The demonstration of the co-continuity allows to consider this material as a good candidate as SPE in electroactive devices. For actuator applications, a critical parameter is the ionic conductivity. The EMITFSI uptake in NBR is 85 wt% and can reach up to 180 wt% in single PEO network (before tearing the network). The synergistic

Table 8.1 EMITFSI saturation swelling and ionic conductivity of networks (25 °C)

Host matrix	NBR	PEO	PEO/NBR 30/70 IPN
σ (S cm^{-1})	3×10^{-5}	$\sim 1.0 \times 10^{-3}$	0.7×10^{-3}

effect of IPNs here is clearly demonstrated since the EMITFSI uptake can reach 230 wt% without any destruction. The ionic conductivity of EMITFSI swollen IPNs (0.7×10^{-3} S cm^{-1}) is just below the conductivity of single PEO network (10^{-3} S cm^{-1}). One can notice that the conductivity value for NBR is too low (3×10^{-5} S cm^{-1}) for open-air actuator applications (Table 8.1). Indeed, from our experience we have noticed that efficient actuators can only be performed if the ionic conductivity is at least higher that 10^{-4} S cm^{-1}.

The second critical parameter is the mechanical properties. Tensile strength experiments have been performed on single networks and IPN. PEO single network has an elongation and a stress at break at 8% and 0.9 MPa, respectively. As already mentioned, these properties make PEO network improper for actuator applications. However, NBR single network breaks at 289% strain for a stress of 1.2 MPa which makes this elastomer interesting for the targeted application. As far as the 70/30 (w/w) PEO/NBR is concerned, the strain at break presents an intermediate behavior between the PEO and the NBR single networks (68%) while the stress at break is around 0.8 MPa (Figure 8.6). The benefit from an IPN macromolecular architecture is demonstrated again here since the poor strain at break of PEO single networks can be overcome by the interpenetration of a NBR network without decreasing significantly the stress at break.

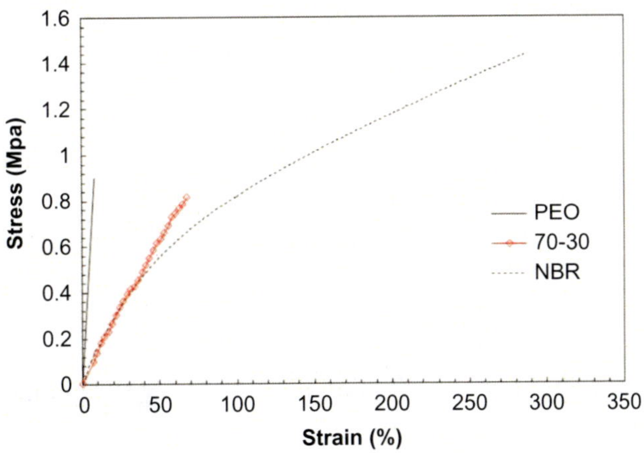

Figure 8.6 Typical stress-strain curves for (a) PEO single network, (b) NBR single network, and (c) 70/30 PEO/NBR IPN.

8.3 Conducting interpenetrating polymer networks actuators

8.3.1 Introduction to actuators based on electronic conducting polymers

ECPs have attracted considerable attention as EAPs because of possible dimensional volume changes during redox processes which can be converted to mechanical work. The expansion/contraction occurring during redox processes are generated by the ion expulsion/inclusion motions. Typically, ions (and solvent molecules) enter or leave the ECP film in order to maintain the electroneutrality during redox reactions as described in Figure 8.7.

Air-working actuators are generally built in a configuration, where the internal layer is an SPE containing ions sandwiched between two ECP layers (ECP//SPE//ECP), and the relative differential expansion between the two ECP layers during redox reaction results in bending (Kaneto et al., 1995; Madden et al., 1999). Thus, IPN-based SPEs are really interesting materials since they can bring up certain level of physical properties such as mechanical strength, elasticity, and ionic conductivity. In others words, IPN strategy allows the design of specific SPE for targeted actuator applications. The principle of the synthesis of conducting IPN implies the chemical synthesis of PEDOT within the IPN-based SPE. This synthesis has been already described by our laboratory (Plesse et al., 2005; Vidal et al., 2010) and summarized in Figure 8.8.

(a)
$$\underset{\text{Neutral chains}}{[(\text{PEDOT}^0)] + n(\text{A}^-)} \underset{\text{reduction}}{\overset{\text{oxidation}}{\rightleftharpoons}} \underset{\text{Oxidized chains}}{[(\text{PEDOT}^{n+}),n(\text{A}^-)] + n(\text{e}^-)}$$

(b)
$$\underset{\text{Neutral chains}}{[(\text{PEDOT}^0),n(\text{MA}^-),n(\text{C}^+)]} \underset{\text{reduction}}{\overset{\text{oxidation}}{\rightleftharpoons}} \underset{\text{Oxidized chains}}{[(\text{PEDOT}^{n+}),n(\text{MA}^-)] + n(\text{C}^+) + n(\text{e}^-)}$$

Figure 8.7 (a) Redox process occurring in the case of mobile anions (A –) and leading to a volume expansion during oxidation. (b) Redox process occurring in the case of immobile anions (MA –) and mobile cation (C+), leading to a volume contraction during oxidation.

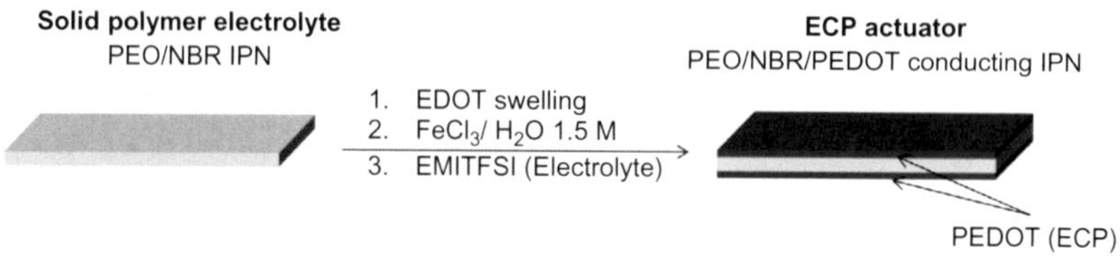

Figure 8.8 Schematic view of the conducting IPN actuator synthesis.

The corresponding monomer EDOT is first introduced in the SPE film by swelling in the pure liquid monomer. Then the polymerization of EDOT is triggered by dipping for controlled lengths of time the swollen film in an aqueous $FeCl_3$ solution. The experimental conditions for the preparation of conducting IPNs have been investigated and now established which allow us the preparation of materials with only a thin layer of PEDOT just under the two opposite faces of the SPE film and with a central part devoid of conducting polymer. The final amount of PEDOT can be controlled from 0.1 to 22 wt% by tuning the duration of immersion in $FeCl_3$. A 250-μm thick actuator with a PEDOT content of 22 wt% displays a PEDOT layer thickness of 40 μm in two symmetrical layers near the surface (Festin et al., 2013). This synthetic route allows the fabrication of actuators which mimics the three-layered device. Furthermore, this process solves *de facto* the problem of delamination which limits the actuator's lifetime (Bar-Cohen, 2001) because the PEDOT is interpenetrated in the PEO/NBR matrix (Vidal et al., 2004).

After EMITFSI uptake, a strip of conducting IPN is subjected to a low voltage, typically ±2 V between the two faces of the actuator film. One conducting layer is connected to the working electrode, whereas the second one to the counter electrode. One layer will be reduced (oxidized), whereas the second PEDOT layer will be oxidized (reduced) leading to an increase of volume on one side and conversely a shrinking of the other side. The net result is a bending movement. Using EMITFSI as electrolyte, the actuation direction corresponds to a decrease in volume at the anode (oxidation) and an increase at the cathode (reduction). The volume increase during reduction indicates the incorporation of EMI^+ in the PEDOT layer in order to balance the negative charge of the nonmobile anion, after that a positive charge on the PEDOT backbone has been removed. Of course after oxidation, the positive charge created on the PEDOT backbone is balanced by TFSI −, after the expulsion of EMI^+. This mechanism is called the "no-mobile anion mechanism" or "cation driven mechanism." More "classical" electrolytes as $LiClO_4$/propylene carbonate (PC) were used. However, the main drawback with those "classical" electrolytes is the solvent evaporation. For instance, conducting IPN actuator can be cycled only few hours before the bending deformation stops due to PC evaporation. Nevertheless, after being immersed again for a few hours in $LiCLO_4$/PC solution, the actuator fully recovers its working capacity indicating that the solvent evaporation is the main issue for long time actuation. In order to prevent the evaporation process, EMITFSI has been used as an electrolyte since it is a nonvolatile compound (Bonhôte et al., 1996). EMITFSI swollen actuators can be cycled (10 Hz) for 3.5×10^6 times without any degradation and/or delamination in open air. Moreover, it could be stored over a period of 6 months without particular precaution and started again thereafter without any sign of weakness (Vidal et al., 2004).

The bending deformation of conducting IPN actuator under ±2 V square wave potential at 0.1 Hz has been quantified by the calculation of the strain difference $\Delta\varepsilon$ (Sugino et al., 2009). A maximum strain difference of 0.35% has been measured in free displacement condition. The measurement of the blocking force (zero displacement) has been performed too and can reach 7.3 mN at 10 mm of the electrical contacts (Figure 8.9a). The corresponding current curve (Figure 8.9a and b) shows the

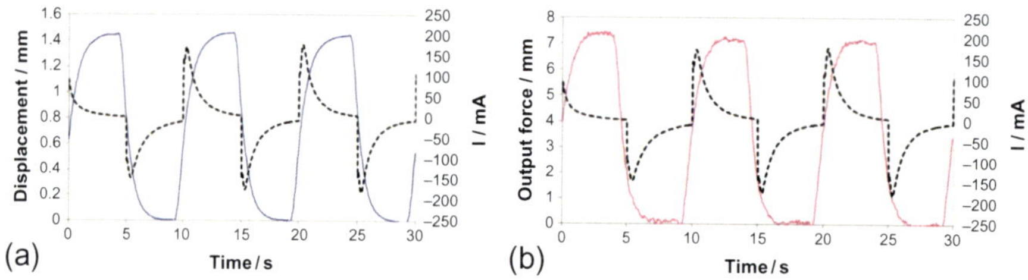

Figure 8.9 Electrical and electromechanical response of the PEO/NBR/PEDOT actuator. Under ±2 V square wave potential stimulation. (a) Free displacement as a function of time at 10 mm from the electrical contacts and corresponding current response. (b) Output force as a function of time at 10 mm from the electrical contacts and corresponding current response. Electrolyte: EMITFSI.

classical electrical charge and discharge profile and the intensity current tends to 0 mA after each potential step. This result indicates that there is no short circuit between the two PEDOT layers and that the desired pseudo-trilayer configuration has been indeed obtained.

8.4 Biomimetic vision systems

8.4.1 Biological vision system: a short introduction

In mammals, the optical system of the eye is mainly composed of the iris, lens, and retina. The iris acts as a diaphragm regulating the amount of light that enters the eye, the lens focuses the image on the retina that acts as light sensor. The retina consists of photosensitive cells and these photoreceptors are connected to the optic nerve. The optical signal is converted to neural signal and transmitted to the brain via the optic nerve (Roorda, 2002). Then the visual cortex of the brain processes the visual information. Neural signal is first transmitted to the primary visual cortex V1 (or striate cortex) in the occipital lobes (Figure 8.10). The area V1 is specialized for processing spatiotemporal information characteristics (orientation, movement, direction, speed). After the area V1, the sensory pathway is split into two new pathways called the dorsal and the ventral streams. The ventral stream deals mainly with information of colors and shapes while the dorsal stream deals with information on locations and motions. The ventral pathway consists mainly of area V4 (temporal cortex) that processes the recognition of information shapes and colors. The dorsal pathway consists mainly of area V5 (parietal cortex) that specializes in locating and movement (Goodale and Milner, 1992; Mishkin et al., 1983; Ungerleider, 1994; Ungerleider and Mishkin, 1982).

Eye movements play also an important role in the mammal vision system (Madelain et al., 2011). These movements are caused by the eye muscles and form part of the visual system. There are several types of eye movements as:

- Saccades: fast movements (50 ms) to explore a particular field.
- Micro-saccades: movements of the same nature as jerks, but at much lower amplitudes that occur during visual fixation.

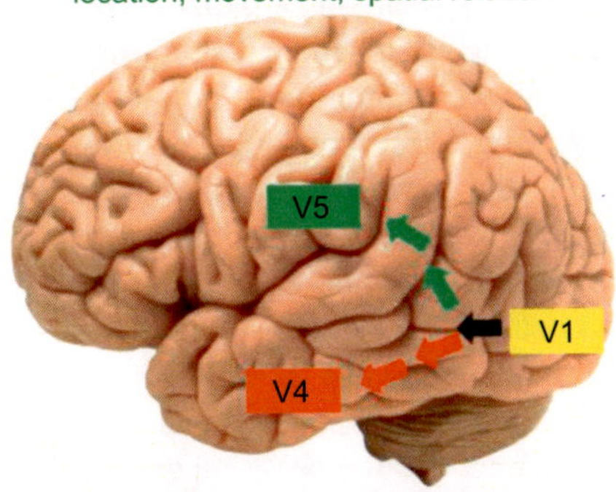

Figure 8.10 The dorsal and ventral cortical pathways.

- Drifts: slow and progressive movements.
- Micro-drifts: motions of the same nature as the drift, but with lower amplitude.
- Micro-tremor: rapid movement and (with) oscillation of small amplitude.

These five types of basic movements combine to allow:

- The smooth pursuit eye movements which allow the eyes tracking a moving object.
- The visual fixation is the maintaining of the visual gaze on a single location. During this step, the eye remains relatively stationary and the visual system extracts detailed information about the fixation point.
- The vestibulo-ocular reflex tends to compensate for the movement of the head to keep the object in the center of the visual field by producing an eye movement in the direction opposite to head movement.
- The optokinetic reflex is a combination of a saccade and smooth pursuit eye movements. For example, when a passenger is watching the landscape through the train window, smooth pursuit is regularly corrected by back motions of eye to the position it was in when it first saw the landscape.

Six extra-ocular muscles control these eye movements and a seventh allows the eyelid elevation.

8.4.2 Conducting interpenetrated polymer network actuator integration in biomimetic vision system

The aim of this present study is to provide an artificial visual system integrating soft actuators as conducting IPNs. This system integrates a microcamera connected to a bio-inspired perception system (BIPS) and conducting IPN actuators. The electronic processor (BIPS) that analyzes sensory information in real time has been developed by the company Brain Vision Systems (BVS; Paris, France). Similar to the brain, the electronic processor from BVS intertwines three aspects of visual perception, related to color vision, to movement detection and to border identification, respectively. The BIPS is designed as a modular system on chip that makes real time multitask perception with learning adaptation. Internally, the BIPS consists of a microcontroller, a flow bank that computes 10 flows (color, motion, structure, etc.) in parallel, and 12 statistical perception cores allowing a biomimetic fast and robust visual perception. Actually, the system performs the same functions as those in area V1 of the brain. Furthermore, the processor visual BIPS is able to command actuators depending on its perception. Using conventional actuators as electric motors, this artificial system based on BIPS board is able to react in real time to colors, movements, and object structures. It can react instantaneously to the speed and direction of a mobile object: it tracks its movement, follows it, and even can anticipate its trajectory. The purpose of this study is to integrate soft conducting IPN actuators in the artificial vision system. Servomotors usually used in the BVS system have been replaced by soft conducting IPN actuators, as described in Figure 8.2. At first, a simple task such as a horizontal visual smooth pursuit and a visual fixation is evaluated.

In this purpose, a rotation system of the microcamera corresponding to the usual eye's rotation angle, i.e., 15–20°, should be designed (Festin et al., 2011). The principle for building up the rotation system is to promote two alternate types of area in the actuator: a first type of area in which there is PEDOT and a second type of area in which the electroactive polymer is not present (Citerin, 2006). In this configuration, the actuating parts can be operated independently since they are not electrically connected, but only mechanically (Figure 8.11). Since those conducting IPN actuators can only bend, the two active parts will therefore operate in the opposite direction in order to obtain the rotation of the microcamera, either in the clockwise direction or in the counterclockwise direction. The presence of a mechanical pivot allows reducing the friction forces during rotation. The actuator parts are 25 mm wide and 50 mm long,

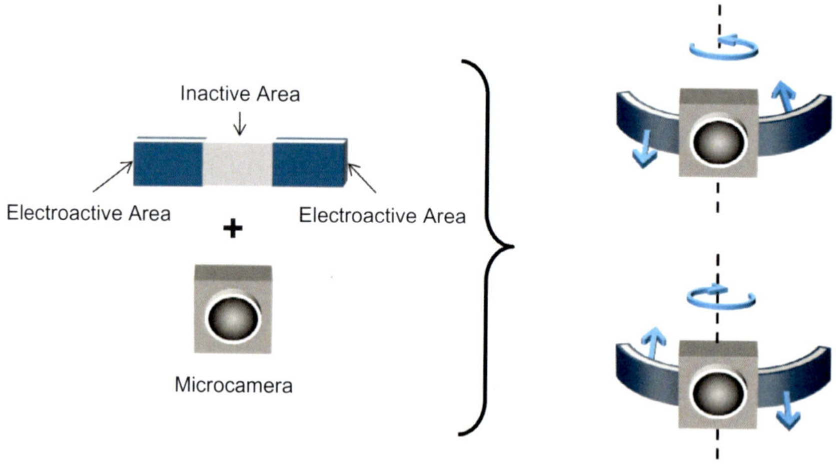

Figure 8.11 Interfacing principle of the ECP actuators and the microcamera and rotation principle of the microcamera.

which is a good compromise between strength and movement. Indeed, as observed previously, the free displacement increases as the actuator length increases and concomitantly a sharp decrease of the output force is observed (Festin, 2014). The microcamera is then fixed on the central part of the film using magnets, and each artificial muscle is connected to the visual processor BIPS which can command them independently. The microcamera position is monitored by a closed loop consisting of two conducting IPNs acting as artificial muscles and a visual perception board BIPS acting as artificial visual cortex.

In this experiment as shown in Figure 8.12, an object is moved in front of the microcamera at a distance of 50 cm. The visual processor analyzes the scene and detects the object by hue, saturation, and motion flow analysis. Consequently, a frame appears on the image on the blue part of the target and as in biological visual systems, the processor tends to place the object in the center of the visual field. Consequently, the processor then commands the two artificial muscles for rotating the microcamera until the target is in the center of the screen. Actuator positions are controlled by the BIPS processor using a Pulse Width Modulation signal (PWM) at a frequency of 100 Hz for an average voltage of ± 2 V. PWM is a very common technique for controlling the power supplied by electrical motors and we have shown that PWM can be successfully used for controlling the position and suppressing the back relaxation of conducting IPN actuators (Festin et al., 2014). In Figure 8.12, the target is moved from position (0) to (-1) or (1) and the visual system is able to track the target in real time and position the object in the center of the screen. The visual system produces a maximum angle

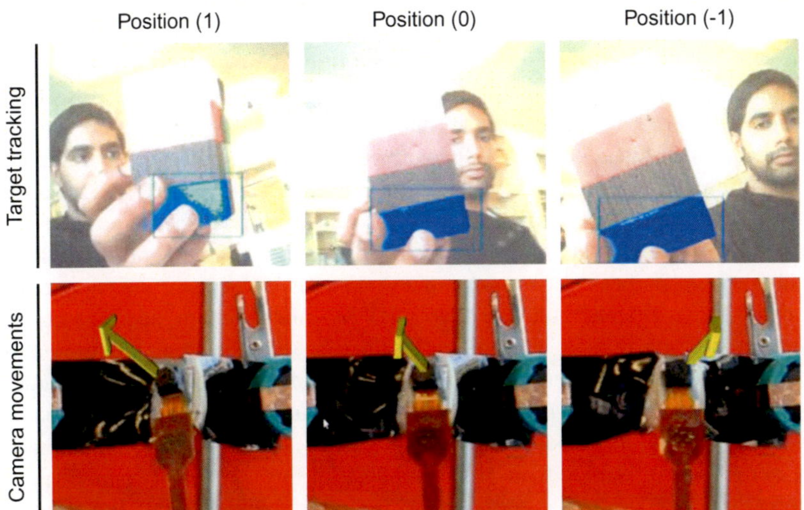

Figure 8.12 (Up) Tracking of the target in real time and closed loop between the microcamera, the ECP actuators, and the electronic perception board. (Down) Rotation of the microcamera controlled by the ECP actuators during the tracking experiment.
(Figure from Festin and Plesse (2011).

movement of 20° during the tracking test with an angular speed of 4°/s. A video of this first visual system prototype can be viewed at: http://www.youtube.com/watch?v=wjJkpKIH8W4&feature=youtu.be

8.5 Conclusion

This chapter presented the synthesis of conducting IPN actuators, from material chemistry to the fabrication of a first biomimetic vision system. The original way used to fabricate those pseudo-trilayer actuators has been thoroughly described. Since these devices are built using an SPE film sandwiched between two ECP film electrodes, each polymer partner has a great influence on the device mechanical properties such as Young modulus and strain at break. First, the synthesis and the characterization of the SPE have been presented. The materials were obtained by *in situ* interpenetration of NBR and PEO networks and we have demonstrated that the presence of 30 wt% NBR improves the mechanical properties of the PEO single network, i.e., the IPN elongation at break is at least seven times higher compared to the PEO single network. Moreover, the presence of the elastomer partner does not decrease significantly the ionic conductivity. The IPN swollen by EMITFSI exhibits ionic conductivity value (0.7×10^{-3} S cm^{-1}) almost comparable to that of PEO. Thus, all these results show that the IPN architecture clearly improves the mechanical properties without decreasing the ionic conductivity and thus they demonstrate the suitability of PEO/NBR IPN for use as base materials in ionic EAPs. In a second step, the synthesis of conducting IPN actuators has been performed with an inhomogeneous distribution of PEDOT across the sample thickness. Indeed, due to a particular synthetic method, the PEDOT is symmetrically interpenetrated in the two outer faces of the SPE IPN. Thus, the delamination process is ruled out by the synthetic pathway and the device is able to work in open air after EMITFSI loading. Under low voltage bias ±2 at 0.1 Hz, the resulting bending actuator exhibits interesting strain and output force. The actuator shows a displacement of 1.4 mm for a 10 mm length sample corresponding to a strain value of 0.35% and a maximum force value of 7.3 mN. The integration of these artificial muscles has been performed. An autonomous biomimetic vision system composed of a visual perception board from BVS, a microcamera, and conducting IPN actuators working in a close loop control have been tested in a smooth pursuit and a visual fixation experiments. The vision system displays angular speed and amplitude of 4 and 20°/s, respectively. It should be pointed out here that the integration of conducting IPN actuators into devices has been possible, thanks to the fabrication of flexible and robust IPN based on NBR and PEO. Thus, the IPN architecture allows tailoring the SPE properties according to the desired applications. For example, by increasing the proportion of NBR, hence the rubber behavior, these active materials have been also used as vibrissae in a biomimetic tactile system. Finally, it should be possible to generalize to other biomimetic system involving artificial muscles. The benefit of the IPN architecture control is thus clearly demonstrated for designing new artificial muscles.

Acknowledgment

This work was supported by ANRT CIFRE number of contract 1201/2008.

References

Alici, G., et al., 2007. Establishment of a biomimetic device based on tri-layer polymer actuators—propulsion fins. Bioinspir. Biomim. 2 (2), S18–S30.

Bar-Cohen, Y., 2001. Electroactive polymer (EAP) actuators as artificial muscles: reality, potential, and challenges. SPIE Press, Bellingham, WA.

Baughman, R.H., 1996. Conducting polymer artificial muscles. Synth. Met. 78 (3), 339–353.

Bonhôte, P., et al., 1996. Hydrophobic, highly conductive ambient-temperature molten salts. Inorg. Chem. 35 (5), 1168–1178.

Carpi, F., Smela, E. (Eds.), 2009. Biomedical Applications of Electroactive Polymer Actuators, John Wiley & Sons, Ltd, Chichester, UK. http://dx.doi.org/10.1002/9780470744697.ins.

Cho, M., et al., 2007. High ionic conductivity and mechanical strength of solid polymer electrolytes based on NBR/ionic liquid and its application to an electrochemical actuator. Sensors Actuators B Chem. 128 (1), 70–74.

Citerin, J., 2006. Fabrication and characterization of linear-moving in air ionic polymer actuators with design and motion simulation tools. In: Bar-Cohen, Y., et al., (Ed.), Proceedings of the society of photo-optical instrumentation engineers (SPIE)p. 616817.

De Paoli, M.A., 1997. Handbook of organic conductive molecules and polymers. In: Nalwa, H.S. (Ed.), In: Conductive Polymers Synthesis and Electrical Properties, 2. Wiley, Chichester.

Festin, N., 2014. Conducting IPN actuator/sensor for biomimetic vibrissa system. In: Bar-Cohen, Y., et al. (Ed.), Proceedings of SPIE Electroactive Polymer Actuators and Devices (EAPAD), p. 90562A.

Festin, N., Plesse, C., 2011. Conducting IPN actuators for biomimetic vision system. In: Bar-Cohen, Y., Carpi, F., et al. (Eds.), The International Society for Optical Engineering, Electroactive Polymer Actuators and Devices, p. 79760K.

Festin, N., Plesse, C., et al., 2011. Actuation and sensing properties of electroactive polymer whiskers. Proc. Comput. Sci. 7, S4–S7.

Festin, N., et al., 2013. Robust solid polymer electrolyte for conducting IPN actuators. Smart Mater. Struct. 22 (10), 104005.

Festin, N., et al., 2014. Electro-active interpenetrating polymer networks actuators and strain sensors: fabrication, position control and sensing properties. Sensors Actuators B Chem. 193, 82–88.

Gauthier, C., et al., 2007. Polybutadiene/poly(ethylene oxide) based IPNs, part II: mechanical modelling and $LiClO_4$ loading as tools for IPN morphology investigation. Polymer 48 (26), 7476–7483.

Goodale, M.A., Milner, A.D., 1992. Separate visual pathways for perception and action. Trends Neurosci. 15 (1), 20–25.

Goujon, L.J., et al., 2011. Flexible solid polymer electrolytes based on nitrile butadiene rubber/poly(ethylene oxide) interpenetrating polymer networks containing either LiTFSI or EMITFSI. Macromolecules 44 (24), 9683–9691.

Goujon, L.J., et al., 2014. Soft and flexible interpenetrating polymer networks hosting electroreflective poly(3,4-ethylenedioxythiophene). Sol. Energy Mater. Sol. Cells 127, 33–42.

Groenendaal, L., et al., 2000. Poly(3,4-ethylenedioxythiophene) and its derivatives: past, present, and future. Adv. Mater. 12 (7), 481–494.

Groenendaal, L., et al., 2003. Electrochemistry of poly(3,4-alkylenedioxythiophene) derivatives. Adv. Mater. 15 (11), 855–879.
Hara, S., et al., 2006. Tris(trifluoromethylsulfonyl)methide-doped polypyrrole as a conducting polymer actuator with large electrochemical strain. Synth. Met. 156 (2–4), 351–355.
Kaneto, K., Kaneko, M., Min, Y., MacDiarmid, A.G., 1995. "Artificial muscle": electromechanical actuators using polyaniline films. Synth. Met. 71 (1–3), 2211–2212.
Kiefer, R., et al., 2008. Cation driven actuation for free standing PEDOT films prepared from propylene carbonate electrolytes containing TBACF3SO3. Electrochim. Acta 53 (5), 2593–2599.
Klempner, D., Sperling, L.H., Utracki, L.A. (Eds.), 1994. Interpenetrating Polymer Networks. American Chemical Society, Washington, DC.
Krogh, M., Inganäs, O., Jager, E., 2001. Fibre-reinforced microactuator. WO03039859.
Liang, W., Lei, J., Martin, C.R., 1992. Effect of synthesis temperature on the structure, doping level and charge-transport properties of polypyrrole. Synth. Met. 52 (2), 227–239.
Lu, W., et al., 2002. Use of ionic liquids for pi-conjugated polymer electrochemical devices. Science (New York, N.Y.) 297 (5583), 983–987.
Madden, J.D., 2004. Actuator selection for variable camber foils. In: Bar-Cohen, Y. (Ed.), Proceedings of the SPIE. In: Smart Structures and Materials 2004: Electroactive Polymer Actuators and Devices (EAPAD), 5385, pp. 442–448.
Madden, J.D., et al., 1999. Encapsulated polypyrrole actuators. Synth. Met. 105 (1), 61–64.
Madden, J.D., et al., 2000. Fast contracting polypyrrole actuators. Synth. Met. 113 (1–2), 185–192.
Madelain, L., Paeye, C., Darcheville, J.-C., 2011. Operant control of human eye movements. Behav. Process. 87 (1), 142–148.
Marwanta, E., et al., 2005. Improved ionic conductivity of nitrile rubber/ionic liquid composites. Polymer 46 (11), 3795–3800.
McGovern, S., et al., 2009. Finding NEMO (novel electromaterial muscle oscillator): a polypyrrole powered robotic fish with real-time wireless speed and directional control. Smart Mater. Struct. 18 (9), 095009.
McGovern, S.T., et al., 2010. Evaluation of thrust force generated for a robotic fish propelled with polypyrrole actuators. Polym. Int. 59 (3), 357–364.
Mishkin, M., Ungerleider, L.G., Macko, K.A., 1983. Object vision and spatial vision: two cortical pathways. Trends Neurosci. 6, 414–417.
Osada, Y., De Rossi, D.E. (Eds.), 1999. Polymer Sensors and Actuators. Springer-Verlag, Berlin.
Plesse, Cédric, et al., 2005. Synthesis and characterization of conducting interpenetrating polymer networks for new actuators. Polymer 46 (18), 7771–7778.
Plesse, C., et al., 2007. Poly(ethylene oxide)/polybutadiene based IPNs synthesis and characterization. Polymer 48 (3), 696–703.
Roorda, A., 2002. Human visual system—image formation. In: Hornak, J.P. (Ed.), Encyclopedia of Imaging Science and Technology. John Wiley & Sons, Inc, Hoboken, NJ, pp. 539–557.
Shoa, T., et al., 2010. Analytical modeling of a conducting polymer-driven catheter. Polym. Int. 59 (3), 343–351.
Smela, E., 2003. Conjugated polymer actuators for biomedical applications. Adv. Mater. 15 (6), 481–494.
Sugino, T., et al., 2009. Actuator properties of the complexes composed by carbon nanotube and ionic liquid: the effects of additives. Sensors Actuators B Chem. 141 (1), 179–186.

Temmer, R., et al., 2012. Combined chemical and electrochemical synthesis methods for metal-free polypyrrole actuators. Sensors Actuators B Chem. 166–167, 411–418.
Ungerleider, L., 1994. "What" and "where" in the human brain. Curr. Opin. Neurobiol. 4 (2), 157–165.
Ungerleider, L.G., Mishkin, M., 1982. Two cortical visual systems. In: Ingle, J., Goodale, M.A., Mansfield, R.J.W. (Eds.), Analysis of Visual Behavior. MIT Press, Cambridge, MA, pp. 549–586.
Vidal, F., et al., 2003. Feasibility of conducting semi-interpenetrating networks based on a poly (ethylene oxide) network and poly(3,4-ethylenedioxythiophene) in actuator design. J. Appl. Polym. Sci. 90 (13), 3569–3577.
Vidal, F., et al., 2004. Long-life air working conducting semi-IPN/ionic liquid based actuator. Synth. Met. 142 (1–3), 287–291.
Vidal, F., et al., 2010. Poly(3,4-ethylenedioxythiophene)-containing semi-interpenetrating polymer networks: a versatile concept for the design of optical or mechanical electroactive devices. Polym. Int. 59 (3), 313–320.
Wilson, S.A., et al., 2007. New materials for micro-scale sensors and actuators. Mater. Sci. Eng. R. Rep. 56 (1–6), 1–129.
Wu, Y., et al., 2006. Fast trilayer polypyrrole bending actuators for high speed applications. Synth. Met. 156 (16–17), 1017–1022.
Zhou, D., et al., 2003. Solid state actuators based on polypyrrole and polymer-in-ionic liquid electrolytes. Electrochim. Acta 48 (14–16), 2355–2359.

Self-oscillating polymer gels as novel biomimetic materials

9

R. Yoshida

9.1 Introduction

In the field of polymer science, polymer gels have made rapid progress since the discovery of "volume phase transition" phenomena by Tanaka in 1978 (Tanaka, 1978, 1981). Many kinds of stimuli-responsive polymer gels that exhibit reversible swelling–deswelling change in response to environmental changes (e.g., solvent composition, temperature, pH change, light, electric field, etc.) have been developed. Especially, from the late 1980s, new functional gels called "intelligent" or "smart" gels have been created, and their applications to bio- or biomimetic materials such as actuator (artificial muscle), drug delivery systems, tissue engineering, purification or separation systems, biosensor, shape memory materials, molecular recognition systems, etc. (Yoshida, 2005; Liu and Urban, 2010; Bauer et al., 2014; Geryak and Tsukruk, 2014; Urban, 2011; Bhattacharyya and Schafer, 2013; Hoffman, 2013; Ottenbrite et al., 2010) has been exploited. In these researches, a concept of "chemo-mechanical gels" to convert chemical energy of chemical/biochemical reaction to mechanical energy of gels has been proposed as a model of artificial muscles to realize soft actuators. Furthermore, with the progress of polymer synthesis technology and supramolecular science, gels with unique network structures have been designed to provide rapid response (Yoshida et al., 1995), toughness (Gong et al., 2003; Okumura and Ito, 2001; Haraguchi and Takehisa, 2002; Sakai et al., 2010), self-healing properties (Urban, 2011; Cordier et al., 2008; Wang et al., 2010; Harada and Takashima, 2013), etc.

In these ways, many stimuli-responsive polymer and gel systems have been inspired by living systems. However, one of the characteristic and important behaviors in living systems is autonomous oscillation, that is, spontaneous changes with temporal periodicity (called "temporal structure") such as the heartbeat, brain waves, pulsatile secretion of hormone, cell cycle, and biorhythm. Nevertheless, there are few studies on polymer and gel systems undergoing self-oscillation under constant condition without any on–off switching of external stimuli. If such autonomous systems can be realized by using completely synthetic polymers, unprecedented biomimetic materials may be created.

From this concept, we have developed polymer gels with autonomous function. In contrast to conventional stimuli-responsive gels, the "self-oscillating" polymer gels autonomously undergo periodic swelling/deswelling oscillation without on–off switching of external stimuli in a closed solution (Figure 9.1). Since the first report in 1996 (Yoshida et al., 1996), we have systematically studied the autonomous

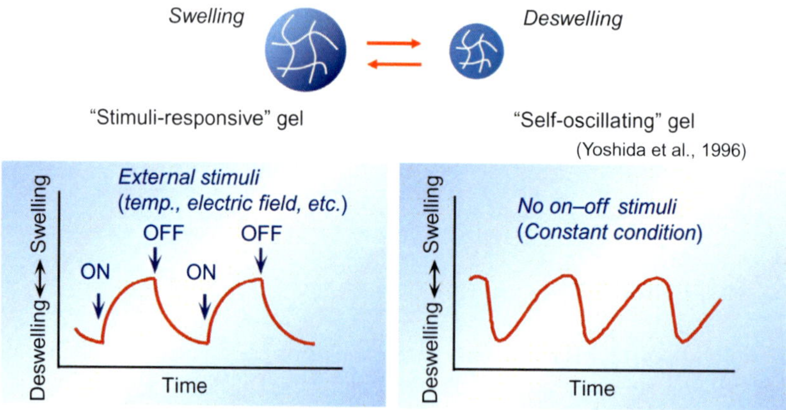

Figure 9.1 Stimuli-responsive and self-oscillating gels.

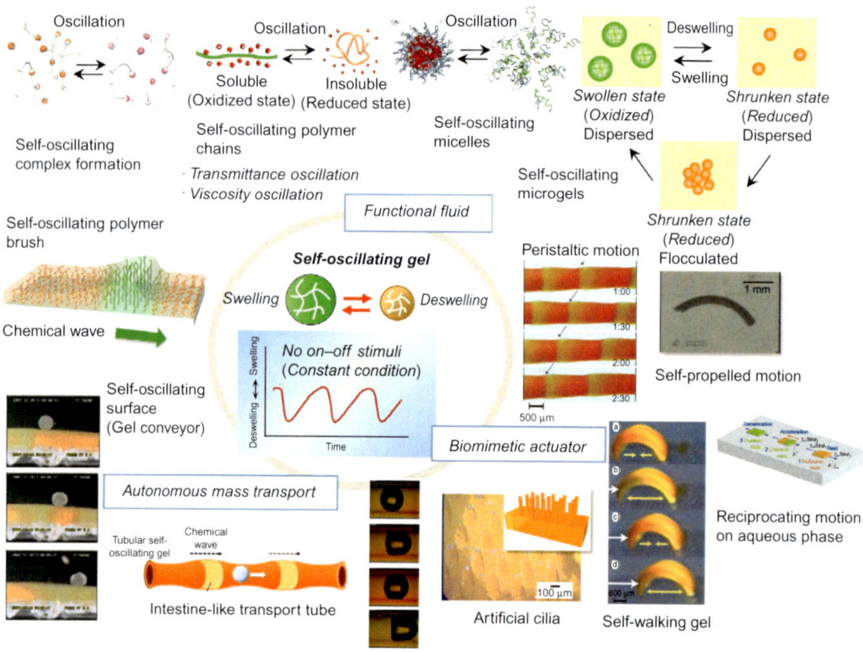

Figure 9.2 Evolution of the self-oscillating polymer gels as functional material systems.

polymer and gel systems on several scales from the order of polymer chains to bulk gels, and have developed many types of biomimetic or smart material systems (Figure 9.2) (Yoshida and Ueki, 2014; Yoshida, 2010; Yoshida et al., 2000, 2003; Maeda et al., 2008a; Takeoka et al., 2003; Sasaki et al., 2003; Ito et al., 2003; Shinohara et al., 2008a,b; Yamamoto and Yoshida, 2013; Murase et al., 2009;

Hara and Yoshida, 2008a,b; Hidaka and Yoshida, 2011; Suzuki et al., 2008, 2009, 2012; Mitsunaga et al., 2013; Tabata et al., 2002, 2003; Maeda et al., 2007, 2008b; Kuksenok et al., 2011; Yashin et al., 2012a; Nakata et al., 2014; Murase et al., 2010, 2011; Yoshida and Murase, 2012; Shiraki and Yoshida, 2012; Masuda et al., 2013; Yoshida et al., 2002; Suzuki and Yoshida, 2008a,b,2010; Taniguchi et al., 2010; Ueno et al., 2010; Ueki et al., 2014; Ueki and Yoshida, 2013, 2014).

9.2 Design of self-oscillating polymer gel

9.2.1 *Oscillating chemical reaction: The Belousov–Zhabotinsky reaction*

For the design of the gel, the Belousov–Zhabotinsky (BZ) reaction (Field et al., 1972; Field and Burger, 1985; Epstein and Pojman, 1998), which is well known as an oscillating reaction which spontaneously exhibits temporal rhythm and spatial pattern, was exploited. The overall process is the oxidation of an organic substrate, such as malonic acid (MA) or citric acid, by an oxidizing agent (bromate ion) in the presence of a metal catalyst under acidic conditions. While the reaction proceeds, the catalyst undergoes spontaneous redox oscillation. Under stirring condition, periodic changes in color of the solution occur. Under stationary condition, concentric or spiral wave patterns propagate in the solution. The wave of oxidized state propagating in the medium is called a "chemical wave." The reaction is often analogically compared with the TCA cycle, a key metabolic process taking place in the living body, and it is recognized as a chemical model for understanding several autonomous phenomena in biological systems.

9.2.2 *Mechanism of self-oscillation for gels*

We attempted to convert the chemical oscillation of the BZ reaction into a mechanical change in gels and generate an autonomous swelling–deswelling oscillation under non oscillatory outer conditions. For this purpose, a gel composed of poly(*N*-isopropylacrylamide) (PNIPAAm) with ruthenium tris(2,2′-bipyridine) ($Ru(bpy)_3$) covalently bonded to the PNIPAAm network was prepared (Figure 9.3) (Yoshida et al., 1996). PNIPAAm is a well-known thermosensitive polymer that exhibits a lower critical solution temperature (LCST) while $Ru(bpy)_3$ acts as a catalyst for the BZ reaction. When the poly(NIPAAm-*co*-$Ru(bpy)_3$) gel is immersed in catalyst-free BZ solution containing the substrates (MA, $NaBrO_3$, and nitric acid), the reaction occurs in the gel. By redox changes in the $Ru(bpy)_3$ moiety, the hydrophilicity as well as the LCST of the poly(NIPAAm-*co*-$Ru(bpy)_3$) changes, resulting in changing swelling ratio of the gel. As a result, the gel undergoes a cyclic swelling–deswelling change in the closed solution under constant condition.

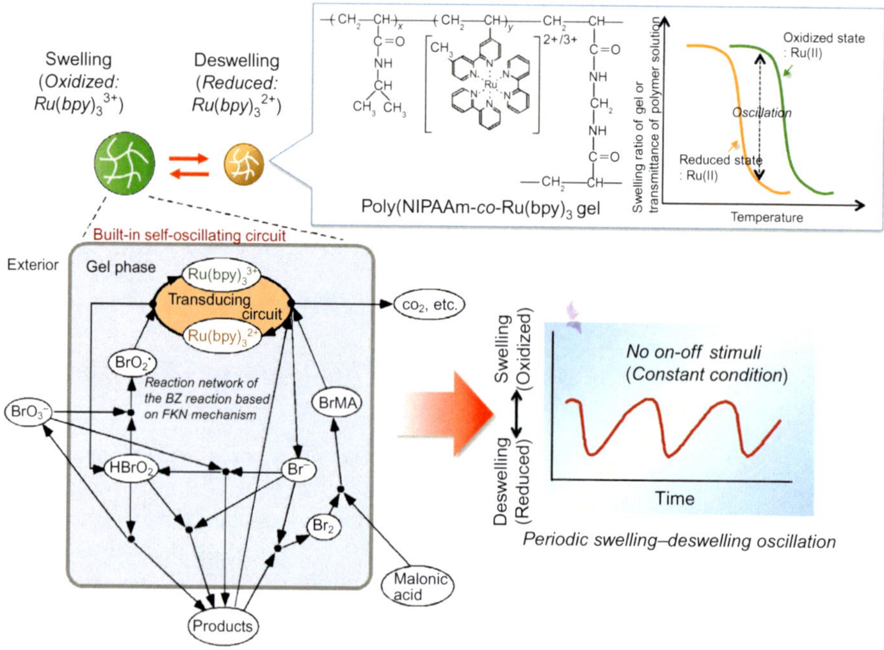

Figure 9.3 Design concept of self-oscillating gel using the BZ reaction.

9.2.3 Self-oscillating behavior on several scales

When the gel is much smaller than the chemical wavelength, redox changes occur homogeneously in the gel without pattern formation (Yoshida et al., 2000). Then the swelling–deswelling change of the gel becomes isotropic. However, when the gel size is larger, chemical waves spontaneously evolve and propagate in the gel. The reduced Ru(II) and oxidized Ru(III) zones represent simply the shrunken and swollen parts, respectively; the locally swollen and shrunken parts move with the chemical wave. As a result, peristaltic motion as living worms or intestines is created (Maeda et al., 2008a; Takeoka et al., 2003; Sasaki et al., 2003) (see Figure 9.2). In the case of the uncross-linked linear polymer, the polymer solution exhibits self-oscillations of optical transmittance and viscosity due to spontaneous cyclic soluble–insoluble changes of the polymer, which will be mentioned later.

9.3 Control of self-oscillating chemomechanical behaviors

9.3.1 Concentration and temperature dependence of oscillation

The oscillating behavior of the BZ reaction changes depending on concentration and temperature as characteristics of chemical reaction. Typically, the oscillation period increases with a decrease in the initial concentration of substrates. Further, in general, the oscillation frequency (the reciprocal of the period) of the BZ reaction tends to increase as the temperature increases, in accordance with the Arrhenius equation. The swelling–deswelling amplitude of the gel increases with an increase in the oscillation period and amplitude of the redox potential changes (Yoshida et al., 2000). Therefore the swelling–deswelling amplitude of the gel is controllable by changing the initial concentration of substrates as well as the temperature.

9.3.2 On–off regulation of self-oscillation by external stimuli

On–off regulation of self-oscillation by external stimuli such as temperature change (Ito et al., 2003), addition, and removal of organic acid (Yoshida et al., 2003), and photo-irradiation is also possible. In particular, $Ru(bpy)_3$ is photosensitive in the reduced state. By utilizing such photochemical characteristics of the BZ reaction, photo-regulation of the self-oscillating motion of the gel was experimentally demonstrated (Shinohara et al., 2008a,b). Further, we have designed photo-regulated self-oscillating systems based on hydration and dehydration changes of the polymer by photo-irradiation. For this purpose, spirobenzopyran (Sp) was introduced into the poly(NIPAAm-*co*-$Ru(bpy)_3$) as a photochromic site (Yamamoto and Yoshida, 2013) (Figure 9.4a). Even under the acidic conditions necessary for the BZ reaction, photochromism of the spirobenzopyran occurs, and the LCST of the polymer solution shifts to a lower temperature with isomerization from McH to Sp by photo-irradiation. As a result, on–off switching of the soluble-insoluble self-oscillation for the polymer solution is possible by photo-irradiation.

9.3.3 Control of self-oscillating behaviors by designing the chemical structure of the gel

The self-oscillating behaviors can also be controlled by designing the chemical and physical structures of the gels. For example, it was found to be effective to copolymerize 2-acrylamido-2′-methylpropanesulfonic acid (AMPS) with a poly (NIPAAm-*co*-$Ru(bpy)_3$) gel network to generate a large amplitude of volume change of the gel because the gel had a microphase-separated structure due to poor solvation during the polymerization process (Figure 9.4b) (Murase et al., 2009). To induce self-oscillation under physiological conditions for biomedical applications, BZ substrates other than organic ones (MA, citric acid, etc.) must be built into the polymer system itself. For this purpose, a quaternary copolymer that includes both pH control and oxidant-supplying sites in the poly(NIPAAm-*co*-$Ru(bpy)_3$) chain was synthesized, and (Hara and Yoshida, 2008a) (Figure 9.4c) self-oscillation was observed by adding only the organic acid (i.e., MA).

To induce self-oscillation while maintaining a larger amplitude at higher temperatures and at physiological body temperatures, a self-oscillating gel composed of a thermosensitive *N,N′*-ethylmethylacrylamide polymer exhibiting a higher LCST than that of PNIPAAm (Hidaka and Yoshida, 2011) was prepared. The design concept of self-oscillation at higher temperatures without a decrease in swelling–deswelling amplitude was demonstrated by utilizing a thermosensitive polymer exhibiting a higher LCST.

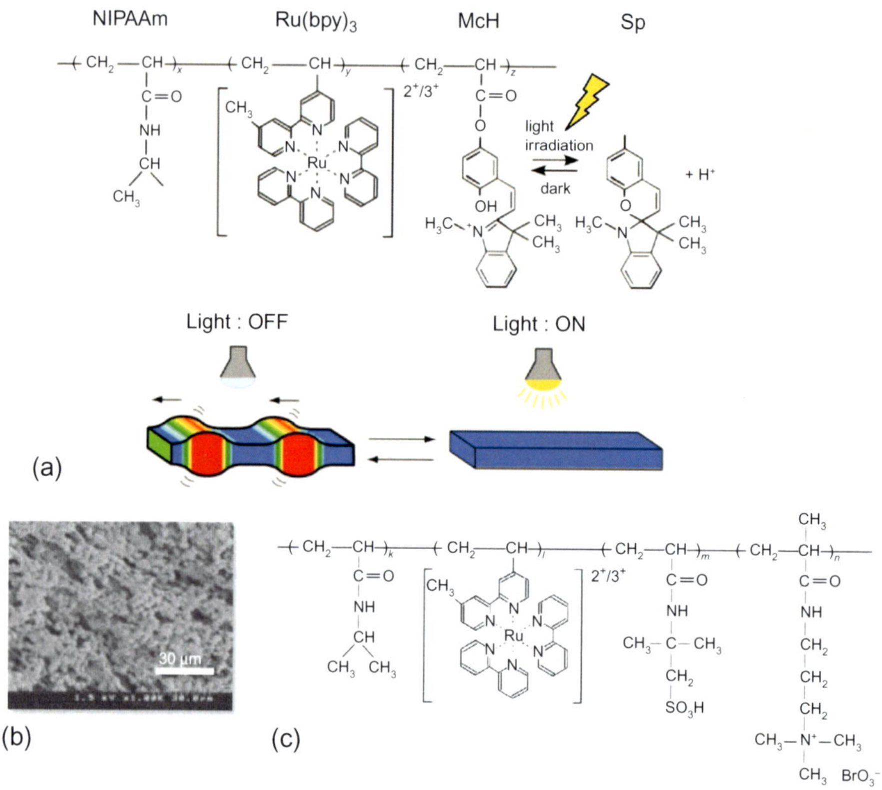

Figure 9.4 (a) Chemical structure of poly(NIPAAm-*co*-Ru(bpy)$_3$-*co*-Sp) (PNRS). (b) SEM micrograph of the poly(NIPAAm-*co*-Ru(bpy)$_3$-*co*-AMPS) gel. (c) Chemical structures of poly (NIPAAm-*co*-Ru(bpy)$_3$-*co*-AMPS-*co*-MAPTAB) gel.

9.3.4 Remarkable swelling–deswelling changes by assembled self-oscillating microgels

Several strategies have been used to improve the response of gels, such as introducing porous microstructures and decreasing the size of the gels. Additionally, in living muscle, a hierarchical structure exists to amplify the microscopic movements of actin–myosin to macroscopic displacements. Such a hierarchical structure was introduced into the self-oscillating gel to obtain a large amplitude of swelling–deswelling oscillation. Soft actuators assembled from self-oscillating submicron-sized particles (microgels) were fabricated (Suzuki et al., 2012) (Figure 9.5a). First, the self-oscillating microgels with amino groups were prepared by aqueous free-radical precipitation polymerization. Then, the microgels were assembled and cross-linked to each other using glutaric dialdehyde. The resulting macrogels have a porous structure

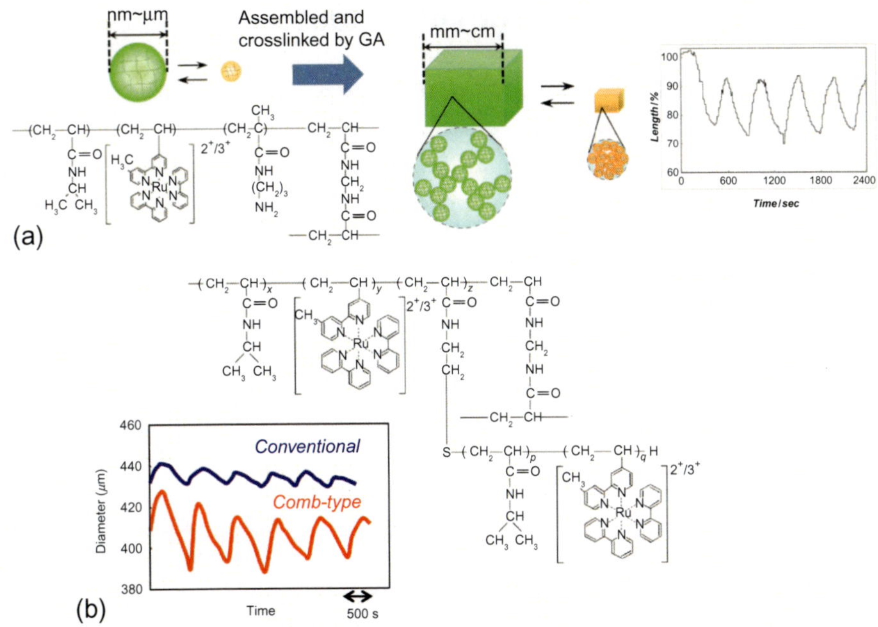

Figure 9.5 (a) Chemical structure of poly(NIPAAm-*co*-Ru(bpy)$_3$-*co*-APMA) microgel and the swelling–deswelling oscillating behavior of the macrogel prepared by assembling and cross-linking the microgels. (b) Chemical structure of comb-type poly(NIPAAm-*co*-Ru(bpy)$_3$)-grafted poly(NIPAAm-*co*-Ru(bpy)$_3$) gel and self-oscillating behaviors for conventional poly(NIPAAm-*co*-Ru(bpy)$_3$) gel and the comb-type gel at 20 °C in the BZ substrate solution containing $NaBrO_3$, MA, and HNO_3.

and exhibited large displacements due to the cooperative dispersing/flocculating motion of the constituent microelements.

9.3.5 Comb-type self-oscillating gel

As an effective method to improve the response of the gels, introduction of grafted side chains with freely mobile ends on the backbone networks of the gels was reported. For example, comb-type grafted PNIPAAm gels were shown to exhibit a fast deswelling response to temperature change by the guiding effect of hydrophobic interaction between side chains that have freely mobile ends (Yoshida et al., 1995). Such designs of physical network structure are expected to be applicable for improving the swelling–deswelling kinetics of the redox change in the self-oscillating gel. We prepared a comb-type self-oscillating gel that has Ru(bpy)$_3$ on both the main chain and grafted side chains (Figure 9.5b) (Mitsunaga et al., 2013). Compared with the conventional self-oscillating gel, faster swelling–deswelling changes were observed because the grafted side chains can respond to the redox change of Ru(bpy)$_3$ more quickly than the main chains. As a result, self-oscillation with a larger swelling–deswelling amplitude was achieved.

9.4 Design of biomimetic soft actuators

9.4.1 Ciliary motion actuator using self-oscillating gel (artificial cilia)

By exploiting such swelling–deswelling oscillation of the gel, novel biomimetic actuators can be created (Figure 9.2). As applications to autonomous biomimetic actuators, ciliary motion actuators (artificial cilia) (Tabata et al., 2002, 2003) were fabricated by microfabrication technique. With propagation of chemical waves, dynamic rhythmic motion of the microprojection arrays on the surface of self-oscillating gel membrane was actually observed.

9.4.2 Self-walking gel

We successfully developed a novel biomimetic walking-gel actuator made of self-oscillating gel (Maeda et al., 2007). To produce directional movement of gel, asymmetrical swelling–deswelling is desired. For these purposes, as a third component, AMPS was copolymerized. During polymerization, the monomer solution faces two different surfaces of plates: a hydrophilic glass surface and a hydrophobic Teflon surface. Since $Ru(bpy)_3^{2+}$ monomer is hydrophobic, it easily migrates to the Teflon surface side. As a result, a nonuniform distribution along the height is formed by the components, and the resulting gel has gradient distribution for the content of each component in the polymer network.

In order to convert the bending and stretching changes to one-directional motion, we employed a ratchet mechanism. A ratchet base with an asymmetrical surface structure was fabricated. On the ratchet base, the gel repeatedly bends and stretches autonomously. In Figure 9.2, successive profiles of the "self-walking" motion of the gel like a looper in the catalyst-free BZ solution under constant temperature is shown. During stretching, the front edge can slide forward on the base, but the rear edge is prevented from sliding backward. Oppositely, during bending, the front edge is prevented from sliding backward while the rear edge can slide forward. This action is repeated, and as a result, the gel walks forward. The walking velocity of the gel actuator was approximately 170 μm/min. Since the oscillating period and the propagating velocity of chemical wave change with concentration of substrates in the outer solution, the walking velocity of the gel can be controlled. By using the gel with gradient structure, other type of actuator which generates a pendulum motion is also realized (Maeda et al., 2008b).

9.4.3 Self-propelled motion

Furthermore, the self-propelled motion of these gels was theoretically and experimentally demonstrated (Kuksenok et al., 2011). A cylindrical self-oscillating gel with a gradient in cross-linking density was prepared by photo-polymerization with UV light irradiated from one direction. The resulting gel has denser cross-linking at the photo-irradiated side and bends toward that direction in the reduced state. In the catalyst-free

BZ solution, the gel repeated the bending and stretching motion, and the position of the center of the gel appeared to shift slowly toward the region with lower cross-linking density.

Control of the motion was attempted also by preparing a composite gel made of self-oscillating and nonactive gels (Yashin et al., 2012a). The disk-shaped self-oscillating gels were arranged around the corners of a polygonal sheet of poly(acrylamide) (PAAm) gel. Wave propagation was controlled by changing the patch size, the catalyst content of the BZ gel, and the spacing between the patches.

Additionally, it was observed that the gel shows periodic reciprocating motion on an aqueous phase synchronized with the BZ reaction (see Figure 9.2) (Nakata et al., 2014). When the Ru catalyst in the gel was rapidly oxidized, the gel was accelerated in a direction opposite to the side of oxidation. The gel then returned to its original position while the Ru catalyst in the gel was slowly reduced. To clarify the mechanism of this periodic reciprocation of the gel, the contact angle between a sessile bubble and the gel and the time variation of the adhesive force of the gel on the aqueous phase were measured. The experimental results suggest that the periodic reciprocation of the gel is driven by the periodic change in the contact angle of the gel induced by the BZ reaction

9.4.4 Theoretical simulation of the self-oscillating gel

To understand these chemomechanical behaviors, Balazs et al. (Yashin and Balazs, 2006; Yashin et al., 2010, 2012b; Kuksenok and Balazs, 2013) developed a mathematical model for simulating the behaviors of the self-oscillating gels. Since their first report in 2006 (Yashin and Balazs, 2006), several aspects of the self-oscillating behavior of the gels have been demonstrated by theoretical simulation. The theoretical studies will provide helpful guidelines for robotic applications, understanding living phenomena, etc.

9.5 Design of autonomous mass transport systems

9.5.1 Self-driven gel conveyer: Autonomous transportation on the self-oscillating gel surface by peristaltic motion

By utilizing the peristaltic motion of the self-oscillating gel, a novel autonomous mass transport system can be constructed. First, we attempted to transport an object on the gel surface to realize a self-driven gel conveyer (Murase et al., 2009, 2010, 2011; Yoshida and Murase, 2012). A model object, such as a cylindrical or spherical PAAm gel, was put on the surface of a self-oscillating gel sheet. It was observed that the object was transported on the gel surface with the propagation of the chemical wave as it rolled (see the photograph in Figure 9.2). The velocity and the inclination angle of the chemical wave were changed by changing the concentration of the outer solution. For analyzing these results, we proposed a model to describe the mass transport phenomena based on the Hertz contact theory, and the relationship between the transportability and the peristaltic motion was investigated. The influence of these surface properties on the transport behaviors has also been investigated (Murase et al., 2011).

9.5.2 Autonomous intestine-like motion of tubular self-oscillating gel

To construct autonomous mechanical pumping systems such as intestines, we fabricated a self-oscillating gel in a tubular shape (Shiraki and Yoshida, 2012) (Figure 9.6) by photopolymerization. In the tubular gel, a CO_2 gas bubble adheres to the inner surface and is autonomously transported showing an intermittent motion caused by the peristaltic pumping of the gel (Figure 9.6c–e). From this result, an autonomous pulsatile flow for a fluid inside the tubular gel is expected. Actually, it was demonstrated that we can cause autonomous pulsatile flow in a tubular gel by utilizing the peristaltic motion of the tubular self-oscillating gel-like intestine. The autonomous flow was proved by using latex beads as tracer particles and analyzing the motion. A new possibility of the self-oscillating gel as an autonomous chemomechanical gel pump was demonstrated.

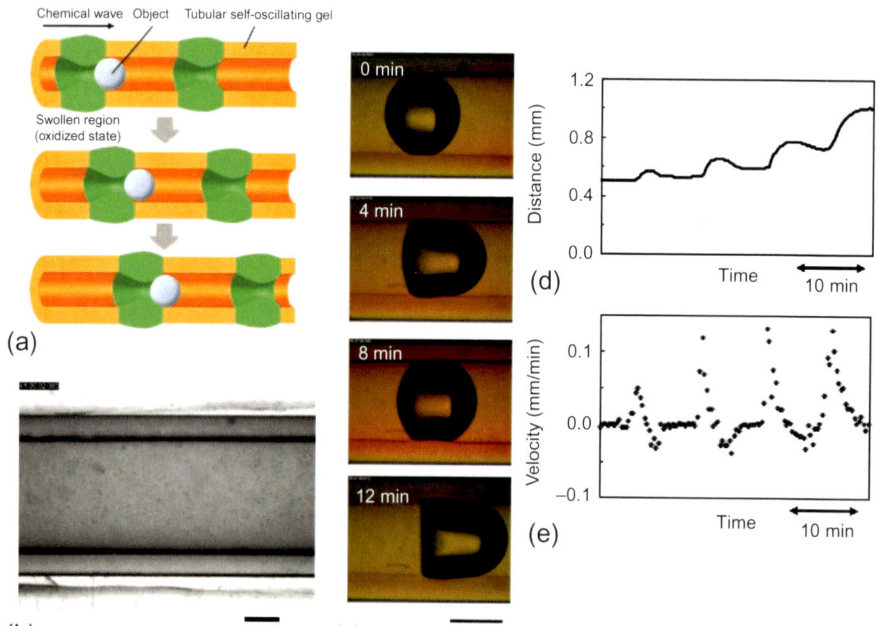

Figure 9.6 (a) Schematic illustration of autonomous mass transport by peristaltic pumping of a tubular self-oscillating gel. (b) Photograph of the tubular poly(NIPAAm-*co*-Ru(bpy)$_3$-*co*-AMPS) gel. (c) Behavior of the autonomous transport of a CO_2 bubble in the gel tube by peristaltic pumping. (d) Change in the position of the bubble. (e) The velocity of the bubble.

9.5.3 Self-oscillating polymer brushes

Recently, surface modification techniques for polymer chains have progressed a great deal with the development of new polymer synthesis methods. In particular, surface-initiated atom transfer radical polymerization (SI-ATRP) is one of the most effective modification methods for preparing a well-defined dense polymer brush structure, or polymer brush, on substrates. Thus, a self-oscillating polymer brush prepared by SI-ATRP can be expected to create a new self-oscillating surface with autonomic function, such as cilia, which will lead to potential applications in transporting systems for nanomaterials or flow control in microfluidics.

We prepared self-oscillating polymer brushes on glass substrates through SI-ATRP (Masuda et al., 2013) (Figure 9.7). The self-oscillating polymer was grafted onto the inner surface of a glass capillary. The BZ reaction occurred on the self-oscillating polymer brush surfaces, and the propagation of the chemical wave was observed in the polymer brush layer on the inner surface of a glass capillary (Figure 9.7b and c). A self-oscillating surface to generate spontaneous periodic changes was

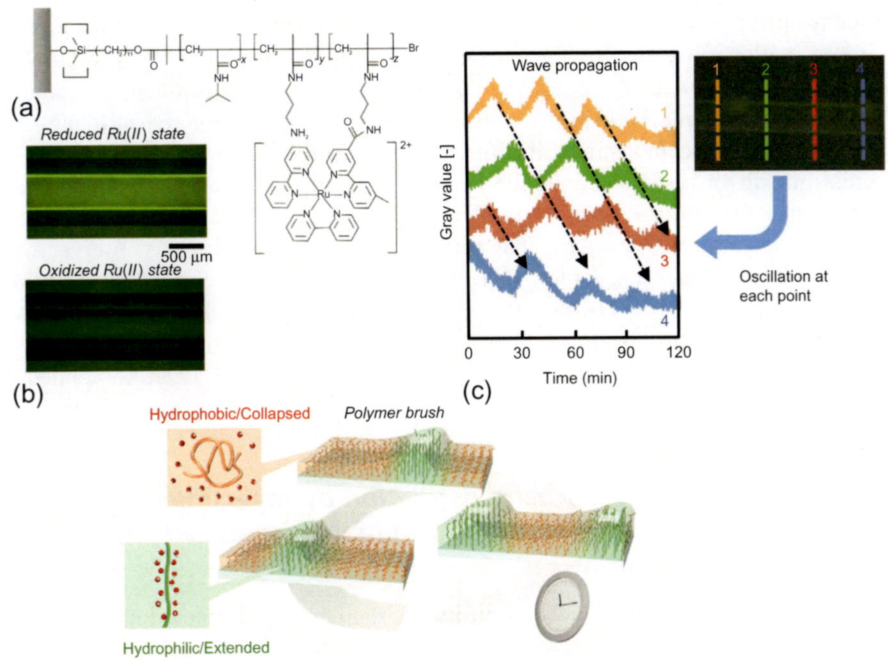

Figure 9.7 Preparation of self-oscillating polymer brush by surface-initiated atom transfer radical polymerization (SI-ATRP). (a) Chemical structure of the self-oscillating polymer brush. (b) Images of glass capillary modified with the self-oscillating polymer observed by fluorescence microscopy. (c) Oscillating profile of fluorescence intensity at each position for the self-oscillating polymer brush on the inner surface of the glass capillary. The solution containing MA, $NaBrO_3$, and HNO_3 is enclosed in the capillary at 25 °C.

demonstrated using synthetic polymers as a novel autonomous functional surface, which has potential applications in systems such as nano-transport systems.

9.6 Self-oscillating fluids

9.6.1 Transmittance and viscosity oscillation of polymer solution and microgel dispersion

As mentioned before, in the case of the uncross-linked linear polymer, the polymer (poly(NIPAAm-*co*-Ru(bpy)$_3$) undergoes spontaneous cyclic soluble–insoluble changes, and the transmittance of the polymer solution oscillates autonomously (Yoshida et al., 2002). Also, in the case of submicron-sized poly(NIPAAm-*co*-Ru(bpy)$_3$) gel beads prepared by surfactant-free aqueous precipitation polymerization (Suzuki et al., 2008; Suzuki and Yoshida, 2008a,b, 2010), the microgel dispersion exhibits transmittance oscillation due to swelling–deswelling changes of the microgels. With increasing temperature, the oscillation period decreased and the amplitude increased slightly. When the temperature increased to near the volume phase transition temperature of the reduced microgel, the microgels showed dispersing/flocculating oscillation as well as swelling–deswelling oscillation (see Figure 9.2) because the reduced and shrunken microgels lost colloidal stability, which resulted in a remarkable increase of amplitude in the optical transmittance oscillation. By utilizing such behaviors, it was demonstrated that the macroscopic self-oscillating gel prepared by cross-linking the assembled microgels exhibits a faster response and leads to a larger amplitude of swelling–deswelling oscillation (Suzuki et al., 2012). In both cases of the polymer solution and the microgel dispersion, viscosity oscillation was observed with optical transmittance oscillation (Hara and Yoshida, 2008b; Suzuki et al., 2009; Taniguchi et al., 2010). The oscillating behavior can be controlled by changing the concentration of microgels, Ru(bpy)$_3$ contents, cross-linking density, etc. It is expected that these polymer solutions and microgel dispersions can be applied as novel functional fluids.

9.6.2 Autonomous viscosity oscillation by reversible complex formation of terpyridine-terminated branched PEG in the BZ reaction

Further, we realized autonomous viscosity oscillations of polymer solutions coupled with metal–ligand association/dissociation between Ru and terpyridine (tpy) (Ueno et al., 2010; Ueki et al., 2014; Ueki and Yoshida, 2014), driven by the BZ reaction. The tpy ligand for the Ru catalyst was attached to the terminals of branched poly(ethylene glycol) (PEG) (linear-, tetra-, and octa-PEG) (Figure 9.8). In supramolecular chemistry, it is well known that mono-tpy coordination is more stable when Ru is oxidized (Ru(tpy)$^{3+}$), whereas bis-tpy coordination is more stable when the Ru is reduced

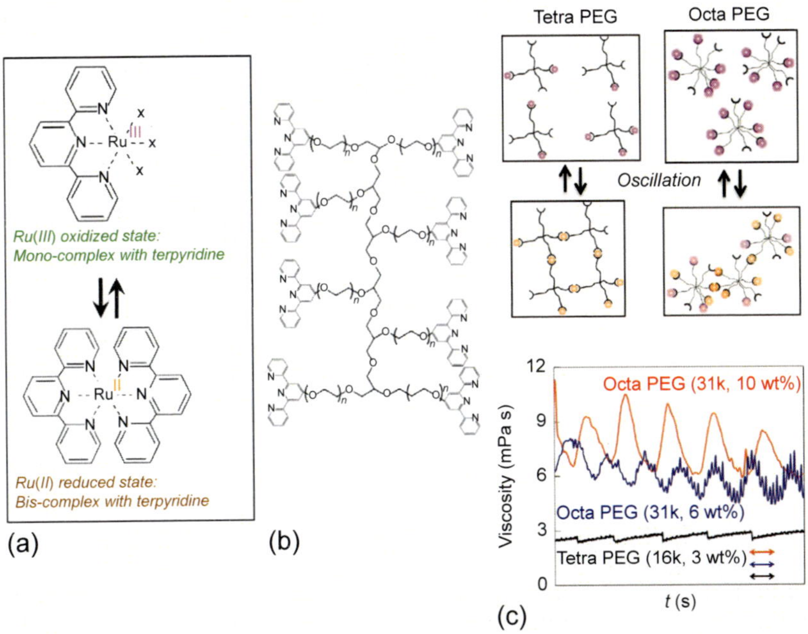

Figure 9.8 (a) Reversible complex formation of terpyridine (tpy) and Ru. (b) Chemical structure of tpy-terminated octa PEG. (c) Oscillating profiles of viscosity of the aqueous solution containing $Ru(tpy)_2$-tetra or $Ru(terpy)_2$-octa PEG, HNO_3, $NaBrO_3$, and MA at 25 °C.

($Ru(tpy)_2^{2+}$) (Figure 9.8a) (Lohmeijer and Schubert, 2002). In the oxidized state, as a result, these polymers existed as solutions. In contrast, when the Ru was reduced, gels were obtained for the tetra- and octa-PEG owing to the formation of a three-dimensional polymer network through Ru–tpy coordination. By increasing the number of PEG branches, the number of cross-linking points necessary for gelation can be decreased, as explained by the tree-like structure theory stating a rate of reaction of cross-linking points for a branched polymer at the gelation point. The polymer solutions of Ru^{2+}-tpy-modified tetra- or octa-PEG exhibited self-oscillation of absorbance and viscosity after adding the BZ substrates. This indicated that the $Ru(tpy)_2^{2+}$ attached to the polymer ends could serve as a catalyst for the BZ reaction. As a result of comparing the viscosity oscillation profiles between the tetra- and octa-PEG systems, it was found that the octa-PEG was much more effective than the tetra-PEG system in providing a large oscillation amplitude as well as a higher baseline viscosity (Figure 9.8c). This is likely because the number of cross-linking points necessary for gelation was decreased by increasing the branch number of PEG, as predicted from the tree-like structure theory. Consequently, the maximum value of cross-linking points in oscillation is closer to that necessary for gelation, and viscosity oscillation occurred in the region of higher viscosity with a larger amplitude.

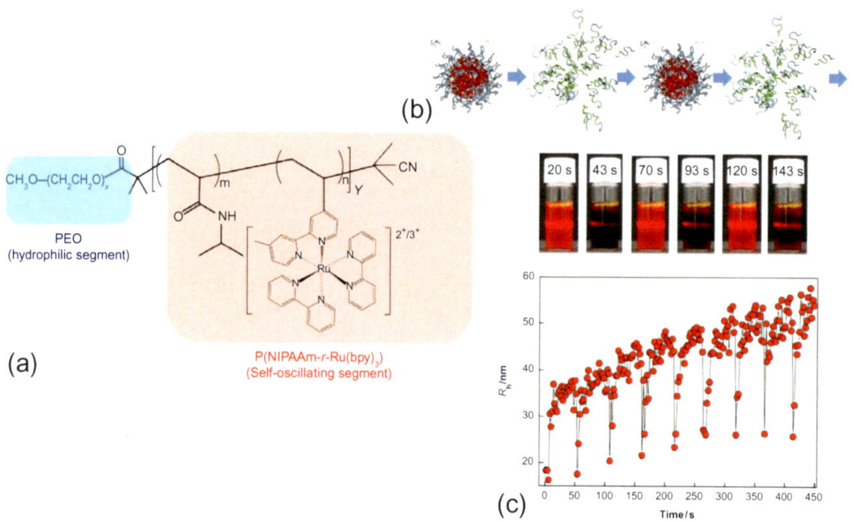

Figure 9.9 (a) Chemical structure of PEO-*b*-P(NIPAAm-*r*-Ru(bpy)$_3$). (b) Schematic illustration of unimer–micelle oscillation and photographs of the block copolymer solution showing periodic changes in the Tyndall effect derived from the self-oscillating micelle synchronized with the BZ reaction. The sample was irradiated with a red laser from the left-hand side. (c) The oscillating profiles of the hydrodynamic radius (R_h) of the diblock copolymer determined by time-resolved DLS measurements.

9.6.3 Self-oscillating micelles

As novel oscillating polymer systems showing structural changes, we prepared a block copolymer that could undergo spontaneous unimer–micelle oscillation under constant conditions (Figure 9.9) (Ueki and Yoshida, 2013). The diblock copolymer (PEO-*b*-P (NIPAAm-*r*-Ru(bpy)$_3$) was successfully prepared by RAFT random copolymerization from poly(ethylene oxide) (PEO)-based macro-CTA. Rhythmical oscillation of the scattering intensity and hydrodynamic radii of the block copolymer solution driven by the BZ reaction was demonstrated without any on–off switching of external stimuli. There have been numerous studies on block copolymers in the area of controlled self-assembly, focused mainly on the formation of static structures under equilibrium conditions. However, this is the first report of a synthetic block copolymer that exhibits "temporal structure," undergoing self-oscillation between unimer and micelle, as an example of a dissipative structure. This result provides a novel concept for self-organization of block copolymers by combining self-assembly with dissipative structures.

9.7 Future prospects

In these ways, as novel biomimetic chemomechanical gels, we developed "self-oscillating" polymer gels that exhibit autonomous swelling–deswelling oscillation similar to those of heart muscle under constant external conditions. Since the first report in

1996 (Yoshida et al., 1996), we have systematically studied these polymer gels. In this chapter, our recent progress on the self-oscillating polymer gels as functional materials has been summarized. Recently, it was found for the first time that hydrated protic ionic liquid (PIL) can act as an acid in the BZ reaction (Ueki et al., 2012), and we attempted to create self-oscillating polymer systems using the PILs. As an innovative study to propose a new concept of functional gels and to expand the potential of these gels, our studies have attracted much attention in many research fields of polymer science, materials science, physical chemistry, robotics, theoretical simulation, biophysics, and others. Actually, there are many studies related to self-oscillating gels inspired by our researches (Zhou et al., 2013). We will continue to advance our research toward more innovations.

References

Bauer, S., Bauer-Gogonea, S., Graz, I., Kaltenbrunner, M., Keplinger, C., Schwödiauer, R., 2014. A soft future: from robots and sensor skin to energy harvesters. Adv. Mater. 26, 149–162.

Bhattacharyya, D., Schafer, T. (Eds.), 2013. Responsive Membranes and Materials. John Wiley & Sons, Ltd, West Sussex, UK.

Cordier, P., Tournilhac, F., Soulié-Ziakovic, C., Leibler, L., 2008. Self-healing and thermoreversible rubber from supramolecular assembly. Nature 451, 977–980.

Epstein, I.R., Pojman, J.A., 1998. An Introduction to Nonlinear Chemical Dynamics: Oscillations, Waves, Patterns, and Chaos. Oxford University Press, New York.

Field, R.J., Burger, M. (Eds.), 1985. Oscillations and Traveling Waves in Chemical Systems. John Wiley & Sons, New York.

Field, R.J., Körös, E., Noyes, R.M., 1972. Oscillations in chemical systems. II. Through analysis of temporal oscillation in the bromate-cerium-malonic acid system. J. Am. Chem. Soc. 94, 8649–8664.

Geryak, R., Tsukruk, V.V., 2014. Reconfigurable and actuating structures from soft materials. Soft Matter 10, 1246–1263.

Gong, J.P., Katsuyama, Y., Kurosawa, T., Osada, Y., 2003. Double-network hydrogels with extremely high mechanical strength. Adv. Mater. 15, 1155–1158.

Hara, Y., Yoshida, R., 2008a. Self-oscillating polymer fueled by organic acid. J. Phys. Chem. B 112, 8427–8429.

Hara, Y., Yoshida, R., 2008b. A viscosity self-oscillation of polymer solution induced by the BZ reaction under acid-free condition. J. Chem. Phys. 128, 224904.

Harada, A., Takashima, Y., 2013. Macromolecular recognition and macroscopic interactions by cyclodextrins. Chem. Rec. 13, 420–431.

Haraguchi, K., Takehisa, T., 2002. Nanocomposite hydrogels: a unique organic–inorganic network structure with extraordinary mechanical, optical, and swelling/de-swelling properties. Adv. Mater. 14, 1120–1124.

Hidaka, M., Yoshida, R., 2011. Self-oscillating gel composed of thermosensitive polymer exhibiting higher LCST. J. Controlled Release 150, 171–176.

Hoffman, A.S., 2013. Stimuli-responsive polymers: biomedical applications and challenges for clinical translation. Adv. Drug Delivery Rev. 65, 10–16.

Ito, Y., Nogawa, N., Yoshida, R., 2003. Temperature control of the Belousov–Zhabotinsky reaction using a thermo-responsive polymer. Langmuir 19, 9577–9579.

Kuksenok, O., Balazs, A.C., 2013. Modeling the photoinduced reconfiguration and directed motion of polymer gels. Adv. Funct. Mater. 23, 4601–4610.

Kuksenok, O., Yashin, V.V., Kinoshita, M., Sakai, T., Yoshida, R., Balazs, A.C., 2011. Exploiting gradients in cross-link density to control the bending and self-propelled motion of active gels. J. Mater. Chem. 21, 8360–8371.

Liu, F., Urban, M.W., 2010. Recent advances and challenges in designing stimuli-responsive polymers. Prog. Polym. Sci. 35, 3–23.

Lohmeijer, B.G.G., Schubert, U.S., 2002. Supramolecular engineering with macromolecules: an alternative concept for block copolymers. Angew. Chem. Int. Ed. 41, 3825–3829.

Maeda, S., Hara, Y., Sakai, T., Yoshida, R., Hashimoto, S., 2007. Self-walking gel. Adv. Mater. 19, 3480–3484.

Maeda, S., Hara, Y., Yoshida, R., Hashimoto, S., 2008a. Peristaltic motion of polymer gels. Angew. Chem. Int. Ed. 47, 6690–6693.

Maeda, S., Hara, Y., Yoshida, R., Hashimoto, S., 2008b. Control of dynamic motion of a gel actuator driven by the Belousov–Zhabotinsky reaction. Macromol. Rapid Commun. 29, 401–405.

Masuda, T., Hidaka, M., Murase, Y., Akimoto, A.M., Nagase, K., Okano, T., Yoshida, R., 2013. Self-oscillating polymer brushes. Angew. Chem. Int. Ed. 52, 7468–7471.

Mitsunaga, R., Okeyoshi, K., Yoshida, R., 2013. Design of comb-type self-oscillating gel. Chem. Commun. 49, 4935–4937.

Murase, Y., Maeda, S., Hashimoto, S., Yoshida, R., 2009. Design of a mass transport surface utilizing peristaltic motion of a self-oscillating gel. Langmuir 25, 483–489.

Murase, Y., Hidaka, M., Yoshida, R., 2010. Self-driven gel conveyer: autonomous transportation by peristaltic motion of self-oscillating gel. Sens. Actuators, B 149, 272–283.

Murase, Y., Takeshima, R., Yoshida, R., 2011. Self-driven gel conveyer: effect of interactions between loaded cargo and self-oscillating gel surface. Macromol. Biosci. 11, 1713–1721.

Nakata, S., Yoshii, M., Suzuki, S., Yoshida, R., 2014. Periodic reciprocating motion of a polymer gel on an aqueous phase synchronized with the Belousov–Zhabotinsky reaction. Langmuir 30, 517–521.

Okumura, Y., Ito, K., 2001. The polyrotaxane gel: a topological gel by figure-of-eight cross-links. Adv. Mater. 13, 485–487.

Ottenbrite, R.M., Park, K., Okano, T., Peppas, N.A. (Eds.), 2010. Biomedical Applications of Hydrogels Handbook. Springer, New York.

Sakai, T., Akagi, Y., Matsunaga, T., Kurakazu, M., Chung, U., Shibayama, M., 2010. Highly elastic and deformable hydrogel formed from tetra-arm polymers. Macromol. Rapid Commun. 31, 1954–1959.

Sasaki, S., Koga, S., Yoshida, R., Yamaguchi, T., 2003. Mechanical oscillation coupled with the Belousov–Zhabotinsky reaction in gel. Langmuir 19, 5595–5600.

Shinohara, S., Seki, T., Sakai, T., Yoshida, R., Takeoka, Y., 2008a. Chemical and optical control of peristaltic actuator based on self-oscillating porous gel. Chem. Commun. 4735–4737.

Shinohara, S., Seki, T., Sakai, T., Yoshida, R., Takeoka, Y., 2008b. Photoregulated wormlike motion of a gel. Angew. Chem. Int. Ed. 47, 9039–9043.

Shiraki, Y., Yoshida, R., 2012. Autonomous intestine-like motion of tubular self-oscillating gel. Angew. Chem. Int. Ed. 51, 6112–6116.

Suzuki, D., Yoshida, R., 2008a. Temporal control of self-oscillation for microgels by cross-linking network structure. Macromolecules 41, 5830–5838.

Suzuki, D., Yoshida, R., 2008b. Effect of initial substrate concentration of the Belousov–Zhabotinsky reaction on self-oscillation for microgel system. J. Phys. Chem. B 112, 12618–12624.

Suzuki, D., Yoshida, R., 2010. Self-oscillating core/shell microgels. Polym. J. 42, 501–508.

Suzuki, D., Sakai, T., Yoshida, R., 2008. Self-flocculating/self-dispersing oscillation of microgels. Angew. Chem. Int. Ed. 47, 917–920.

Suzuki, D., Taniguchi, H., Yoshida, R., 2009. Autonomously oscillating viscosity in microgel dispersions. J. Am. Chem. Soc. 131, 12058–12059.

Suzuki, D., Kobayashi, T., Yoshida, R., Hirai, T., 2012. Soft actuators of organized self-oscillating microgels. Soft Matter 8, 11447–11449.

Tabata, O., Hirasawa, H., Aoki, S., Yoshida, R., Kokufuta, E., 2002. Ciliary motion actuator using self-oscillating gel. Sens. Actuators, A 95, 234–238.

Tabata, O., Kojima, H., Kasatani, T., Isono, Y., Yoshida, R., 2003. Chemo-mechanical actuator using self-oscillating gel for artificial cilia. In: Proceedings of the International Conference on MEMS 2003, pp. 12–15.

Takeoka, Y., Watanabe, M., Yoshida, R., 2003. Self-sustaining peristaltic motion on the surface of a porous gel. J. Am. Chem. Soc. 125, 13320–13321.

Tanaka, T., 1978. Collapse of gels and the critical endpoint. Phys. Rev. Lett. 40, 820–823.

Tanaka, T., 1981. Gels. Sci. Am. 244, 124–136.

Taniguchi, H., Suzuki, D., Yoshida, R., 2010. Characterization of autonomously oscillating viscosity induced by swelling/deswelling oscillation of the microgels. J. Phys. Chem. B 114, 2405–2410.

Ueki, T., Yoshida, R., 2013. Self-oscillating micelles. Chem. Commun. 49, 6947–6949.

Ueki, T., Yoshida, R., 2014. Recent aspects of self-oscillating polymeric materials: designing self-oscillating polymers coupled with supramolecular chemistry and ionic liquid science. Phys. Chem. Chem. Phys. 16, 10388–10397.

Ueki, T., Watanabe, M., Yoshida, R., 2012. Belousov–Zhabotinsky reaction in protic ionic liquids. Angew. Chem. Int. Ed. 51, 11991–11994.

Ueki, T., Takasaki, Y., Bundo, K., Ueno, T., Sakai, T., Akagi, Y., Yoshida, R., 2014. Autonomous viscosity oscillation via metallo-supramolecular terpyridine chemistry of branched poly(ethylene glycol) driven by the Belousov–Zhabotinsky reaction. Soft Matter 10, 1349–1355.

Ueno, T., Bundo, K., Akagi, Y., Sakai, T., Yoshida, R., 2010. Autonomous viscosity oscillation by reversible complex formation of terpyridine-terminated poly(ethylene glycol) in the BZ reaction. Soft Matter 6, 6072–6074.

Urban, M.W. (Ed.), 2011. Handbook of Stimuli-responsive Materials. Wiley-VCH, Weinheim.

Wang, Q., Mynar, J.L., Yoshida, M., Lee, E., Lee, M., Okuro, K., Kinbara, K., Aida, T., 2010. High-water-content mouldable hydrogels by mixing clay and a dendritic molecular binder. Nature 463, 339–343.

Yamamoto, T., Yoshida, R., 2013. Self-oscillation of polymer and photo-regulation by introducing photochromic site to induce LCST changes. React. Funct. Polym. 73, 945–950.

Yashin, V.V., Balazs, A.C., 2006. Pattern formation and shape changes in self-oscillating polymer gels. Science 314, 798–801.

Yashin, V.V., Kuksenok, O., Balazs, A.C., 2010. Modeling autonomously oscillating chemo-responsive gels. Prog. Polym. Sci. 35, 155–173.

Yashin, V.V., Suzuki, S., Yoshida, R., Balazs, A.C., 2012a. Controlling the dynamic behavior of heterogeneous self-oscillating gels. J. Mater. Chem. 22, 13625–13636.

Yashin, V.V., Kuksenok, O., Dayal, P., Balazs, A.C., 2012b. Mechano-chemical oscillations and waves in reactive gels. Rep. Prog. Phys. 75, 066601.

Yoshida, R., 2005. Design of functional polymer gels and their application to biomimetic materials. Curr. Org. Chem. 9, 1617–1641.

Yoshida, R., 2010. Self-oscillating gels driven by the Belousov–Zhabotinsky reaction as novel smart materials. Adv. Mater. 22, 3463–3483.
Yoshida, R., Murase, Y., 2012. Self-oscillating surface of gel for autonomous mass transport. Colloids Surf., B 99, 60–66.
Yoshida, R., Ueki, T., 2014. Evolution of self-oscillating polymer gels as autonomous polymer systems. NPG Asia Mater. 6, e107.
Yoshida, R., Uchida, K., Kaneko, Y., Sakai, K., Kikuchi, A., Sakurai, Y., Okano, T., 1995. Comb-type grafted hydrogels with rapid de-swelling response to temperature changes. Nature 374, 240–242.
Yoshida, R., Takahashi, T., Yamaguchi, T., Ichijo, H., 1996. Self-oscillating gel. J. Am. Chem. Soc. 118, 5134–5135.
Yoshida, R., Tanaka, T., Onodera, S., Yamaguchi, T., Kokufuta, E., 2000. In-phase synchronization of chemical and mechanical oscillations in self-oscillating gels. J. Phys. Chem. A 104, 7549–7555.
Yoshida, R., Sakai, T., Ito, S., Yamaguchi, T., 2002. Self-oscillation of polymer chains with rhythmical soluble-insoluble changes. J. Am. Chem. Soc. 124, 8095–8098.
Yoshida, R., Takei, K., Yamaguchi, T., 2003. Self-beating motion of gels and modulation of oscillation rhythm synchronized with organic acid. Macromolecules 36, 1759–1761.
Zhou, H., Ding, X., Zheng, Z., Peng, Y., 2013. Self-regulated intelligent systems: where adaptive entities meet chemical oscillators. Soft Matter 9, 4956–4968.

Biomimetic muscle—The slipping/ sliding friction mechanism (SFM) for dynamic agile animal robots* 10

F. Nickols

10.1 The need for a biomimetic muscle

The reader is asked to wonder how our very own muscles work. How do animals and humans walk, run, jump, fly, and swim with such accuracy, fluidity, elegance, poise, and ease? Currently, Man is not able to create robots that can run like Usain Bolt, dance like Ginger Rodgers and Fred Astaire, do an overhead scissor kick like Wayne Rooney, swerve and chase like a Cheetah, swim and leap from the water like a dolphin or take off, swoop, soar, hover, perch, and pluck a fish from a lake like an eagle. Instead, what we have at present are stiff, clumsy, jerky robots such as the Asimo robot with bent knees or the less inelegant but power-hungry robots from Boston Dynamics. These robots are very impressive but still there is a problem with their physical performance. Why is this so? What is frustrating this new science of Dynamic Agile Animal Robots? Is it the state of the art in sensors?. . .in computers?. . .in software algorithms?. . .in batteries? No, the answer is none of these.

Instead, the problem lies in the inadequate state of the art of actuators that articulate the limbs. If engineers have a range of actuators from the size of an insect wing muscle up to the size of a race horse's hind leg muscle that emulates biological skeletal muscle, then the exciting new genre of Dynamic Agile Animal robots will be entirely possible, and with it, a fascinating new challenge, previously untapped, of the associated control methodology of managing individual biomimetic muscles and synergistically acting groups of biomimetic muscles. Daniel Wohlpert outlines a fascinating theory (Wolpert) of the brain evolving to primarily control muscles. Creating an effective biomimetic muscle will enable scientists and engineers to mimic the brain's control of muscles and thus give greater understanding of this phenomenon since it is difficult to "read" the algorithms in the brain. Furthermore, the energetics of animals will be much better understood by scientists and engineers if we can recreate dynamic agile animal robots because it is difficult if not near impossible to measure accurately muscle energies and powers during the active behavior of animals.

Dynamic Agile Animal Robots will create a new industry and, with it, new jobs and opportunities. Interestingly, Hollywood films, such as "I-Robot," illustrate how

* F. Nickols, Singapore patent no. 190737 awarded 29 May 2014 entitled; "Apparatus and an assembly for emulating an impulse force exerted by a skeletal muscle." Patent owned by Nanyang Technological University, Singapore.

humanoid robots, being one branch of Dynamic Agile Animal Robots, will be used effectively in society. In the background will be significant job-creating supporting industries concerned with servicing and maintenance together with business opportunities that we can hardly imagine.

10.2 Review of biomimetic artificial muscles

The most exciting recent development in biomimetic muscles has been carried out by a team led by Sangbae Kim who is Director of the MIT Biomimetic Robotics Lab. His work and that of his collaborators can be seen at Kim and Seok which is concerned with the design and construction of a dynamic agile Cheetah robot. It is very interesting to see how this team developed their biomimetic muscles for the robot. They used large diameter, caseless, direct drive brushless DC motors and obtained exceptional results but still not good enough to make the Cheetah gallop more than 22 kph. This speed has only been bettered by Boston Dynamics hydraulically actuated Cheetah robot (Boston Dynamic's Cheetah robot) that has obtained 45 kph, but this speed is still well short of a Cheetah's 100 kph. Boston Dynamics has also developed other impressive robots such as Petman and Big Dog, which all use hydraulically driven actuators. Now, let us analyze why actuators are not performing well enough to articulate dynamic agile animal robots with the grace agility, speed, and precision of their biological counterparts.

Currently existing actuators use a range of physical phenomena to provide force such as (in approximate order of popularity of use) (i) electromagnetic force, i.e., electric motors, (ii) hydraulic cylinder force, and (iii) pneumatic cylinder force. Other, less common actuators acting as artificial robot muscles are (iv) piezoelectric, (v) shape memory alloy, (vi) electric charge force, (vii) electrically activated polymers (EAPs), and (viii) thermal, e.g., bimetallic strip. There are also other methods for providing artificial muscle actuation ranging from twisted string Spanish windlass type to methods based on carbon nanotubes and myogenics (Myogenesis). These less common actuators generally cannot provide sufficient force or performance to match skeletal muscle or are inadequately developed and are thus deemed inadequate (by this author) for use as artificial muscles. So, the only viable contenders are actuators that use electric motors or piston/cylinder combinations actuated by liquid or gas. We will see shortly that even these contenders, i.e., the electric motor, pneumatic and hydraulic actuators, fall short of being able to satisfy the criteria for biomimetic muscles and as a result a new species, the SFM (Figure 10.1) has been evolved to satisfy the criteria.

Aerovironment has pushed the limits of biomimetic muscle design with their highly impressive robot, hummingbird (Keennon et al., 2012). This is notable because an electric motor and ingenious gear system are used to flap the wings and phase the wing attack angles. However, such a system would lack versatility in its application, meaning that it is designed only for controlled hovering flight. Such an electromechanical system is unlikely to serve as a generic biomimetic muscle in other animal robots.

Barrett Technology has invented a very interesting actuating technique for robots (Barrett Technology). A direct drive DC brushless electric motor is used to drive a low

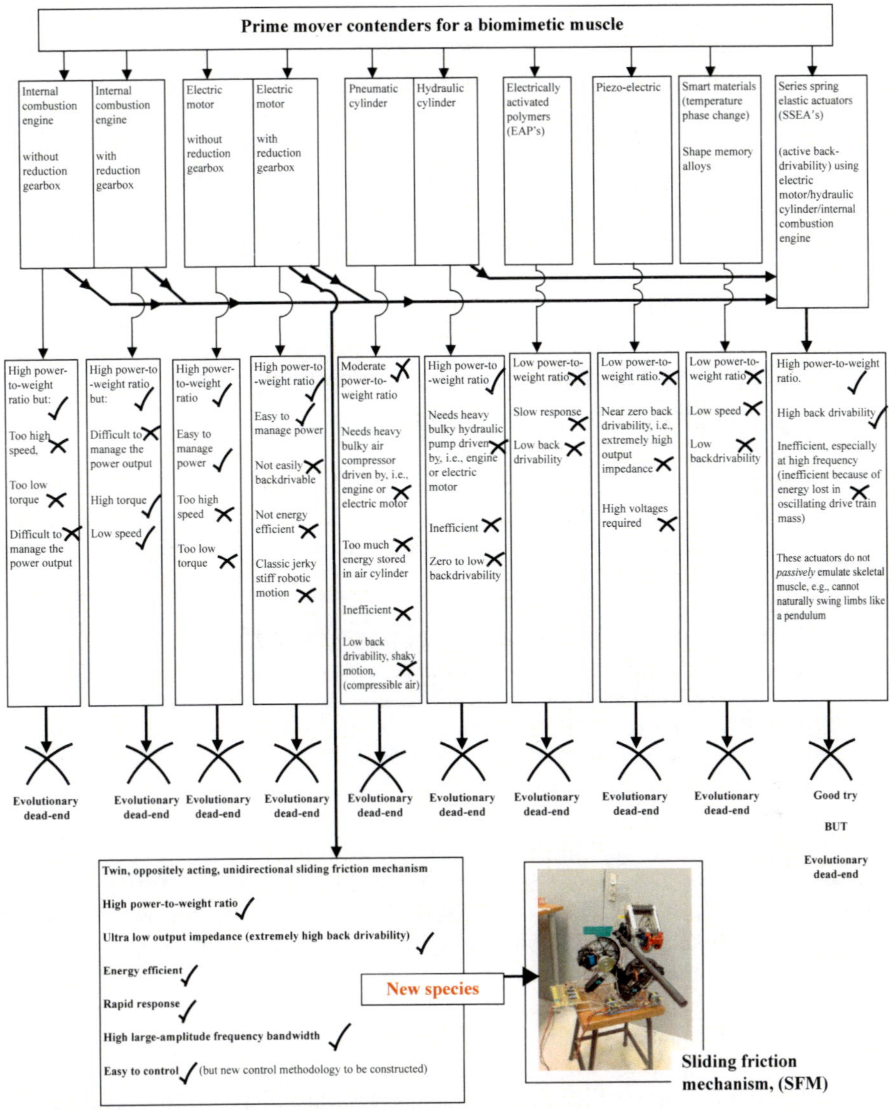

Figure 10.1 Sliding friction mechanism (SFM), evolutionary tree diagram. The SFM accurately emulates the sliding filament model of biological skeletal muscle. The SFM is a new species of artificial muscle.

friction cable pulley system that articulates robot arms. The cable system serves as a reduction gearbox transmission system. Since it is an extremely efficient transmission, coupled with a low-friction electric motor, the back drivability seems low, but this is deceiving since the inertia seen at the end effector will be significant thus rendering the design unsuitable for biomimetic muscles. This reasoning will be explained shortly but is due to low energy efficiency during, for example, running and flapping.

MIT has invented the Series Spring Elastic actuator, MIT SEA (Raibert), which appears to be used in many dynamic agile robots around the world. This biomimetic muscle solves, simply, elegantly and ingeniously, compactly and with low mass, the next most significant requirement of biomimetic muscles which is high back drivability, low output impedance, with an active system. However, the highly significant requirement of high energy efficiency during fast oscillation of robot limbs is not solved since the whole gear train and electric motor armature masses, together with their friction, are dragged along with the oscillating limb. Or in the case of hydraulic servomechanisms, the pumping friction losses in pipes and valves.

10.3 Reasons for the inadequate performance of existing biomimetic muscles

In summary, inadequacies of currently existing actuators concern their inability to mimic accurately biological skeletal muscle. Even Marc Raibert, founder of Boston Dynamics, expresses his concern as quoted below over the state of actuators in his Big Dog robot (Pratt et al., 1997);

> *One notable area that needs improvement is in the actuators. The hydraulic actuators used have very little compliance, unlike real muscles, and their force-length characteristics are such that the robot cannot hold its own weight if it crouches down. Both of these issues are partially compensated for by the control algorithm, using fast feedback to simulate compliance and maintaining the legs in a stretched posture, but the lack of a better artificial muscle is a major obstacle to improving the robustness of this robot.*

Biological skeletal muscle tissue has the following 11 key properties: (i) high force-to-weight ratio, (ii) fast reaction time (less than 0.1 s response time to maximum force) that in alliance with (i) produces high mechanical power-to-weight ratio, (iii) low physical volume, (iv) low strain energy stored in the muscle fibers, implying high stiffness output shaft supplying the force, (v) significant latent energy stored in the muscle for approximately 1 min in order to permit initial explosive output of power such as an Olympic sprinter or a four legged Cheetah, (vi) almost soundless in operation, (vii) self-centering, meaning that the muscle, when relaxed will tend to attain a length half way between fully contracted and fully stretched, (viii) high force resolution, (ix) low reflected inertia seen by the limb, (x) negligible forward and back-drivable force, otherwise known as high back drivability or low output impedance, which will be mathematically defined later, (xi) ease of controllability (which generally favors electric motors and microcomputer systems).

It should be noted that when the power-to-weight ratio of actuators is assessed, then the weight of the whole system including energy production and/or its storage should be taken into account and not just the actuator alone because the actuator should be considered as actuating a stand-alone mobile robot or autonomous machine system, e.g., an animal robot. For example, the weight of a pneumatic or hydraulic actuator should include the petrol/battery plus the internal combustion engine/electric motor plus the compressor/pump and the weight of control components such as pneumatic/hydraulic valves, electric circuits, computers, wires, pipes and in the case of hybrid systems, such components as electric generators.

State-of-the-art actuators for use in robots follow the design methodology of (i) using closed loop position and velocity servomechanisms that give high stiffness and high accuracy and (ii) the trajectory of robot limbs is found using mathematical techniques such as Jacobian matrices. Whereas this can be highly suitable for most engineered systems, e.g., CNC machine tools, it is not considered the way biological systems, i.e., animals, articulate their limbs. Animals use their high back drivability, low output impedance muscles to provide force impulses to their limbs thus resulting in an energy-efficient system. In contrary to state-of-the-art robot servomechanisms, the position and velocity of these limbs may not be fed back into closed loop servomechanisms. Instead, the force impulse applied to the limb is accurately delivered, probably from an open loop, but nonetheless accurate, force-producing muscle. The force-time signature is a relationship that is the result of an in-built program and/or is a learnt process. The open loop position or velocity control of limbs, nonetheless, produces an accurate position-time and or velocity-time signature as can be seen with any animal walking or running. Herein lies the fundamental difference between traditional taught control theory based on closed loop feedback of position, velocity, or acceleration of motion system and that of biological brain-muscle systems that provide a force-time signature (an impulse (N s)) from an actuator possessing high back drivability that is obtained passively.

Negligible forward and backward drivable force relates to, (i) a limb such as a human arm being able to become limp and easily moved when its muscles are not activated and (ii) the limb being able to be moved against the muscle when the muscle is activated. Most of the aforementioned currently existing actuators cannot be easily forward driven or backward driven with the exception of a direct drive, brushless electric motor that is energized by a current-controlled electrical circuit. However such a system, while being forward and backward drivable, will fail the test of possessing low inertia and high force/high mechanical power-to-weight ratio; hence, a direct-drive electric motor is also inadequate as a biomimicking artificial muscle.

The reason for this is that electric motors possess adequate mechanical power-to-weight ratio for artificial muscles but in the wrong format meaning that electric motors produce high power only at high speed with low torque rather than low speed and high torque, the latter being suitable for biomimetic muscles. Hence, electric motors require the speed to be reduced and the torque increased using a high reduction gearbox with a reduction ratio typically in the order of 300:1. A gearbox introduces (i) friction and (ii) added inertia due to the inertia of moving gears and motor armature magnified by the square of the gear ratio. Thus, a gearbox will decrease the forward and backward drivability giving high bidirectional output impedance which is undesirable because it results in large energy losses as a limb is oscillated. An electric motor using Neodymium Boron Iron magnets together with a planetary or harmonic drive gearbox results in a prime mover that possesses both high power-to-weight ratio and high power-to-volume ratio, both ratios of which are highly suitable for biomimetic muscles, but the motor/gearbox combination gives undesirable high output impedance due to increased gearbox friction and extremely high reflected inertia which amounts to almost 100,000 times the inertia of the electric motor rotating armature (300:1 gearbox ratio squared).

So, the conclusion is that currently existing electric motor/gearbox combination actuators directly connected to robot limbs are unsuitable as biomimetic muscles.

Now, we come to examining pneumatic and hydraulic systems. Both types use a piston and cylinder or swash plate motors, but the pneumatic type can also use a bag that as it fills with air becomes fatter and shorter similar to the apparent shape change of a real muscle. (Skeletal muscle does not get fatter but instead becomes more erect as it is energized). Both pneumatic and hydraulic types suffer from lack of forward and backward drivability due to piston friction and valve flow losses. Both types require on-board compressors or pumps and a bank of fluid control valves that are heavy, bulky, and not as easy to control as an electric motor system and neither can they respond with the rapidity of an electric motor system.

So, the conclusion is that pneumatic and hydraulic system actuators are unsuitable as biomimetic muscles.

This is a critical situation. There appears to be no actuation methodology that is suitable for emulating biological skeletal muscle. This seems to be the conclusion arrived at by other inventors such as the MIT SEA inventors and that is why they developed their force feedback system as a way out of the trap which is; we need the gearbox in an electric motor system but it is also our worst enemy. The MIT SEA solves the problem actively with a mechanical spring at the force-providing output shaft. The problem is that it does not solve the problem of energy efficiency. This is solved with the SFM.

However, before the SFM is described, some theory and definitions will be outlined.

10.4 Theory and definitions

The SFM device described here can be considered an impulse servomechanism producing an impulse as follows:

$$\text{Impulse, } I = \int_{t_1}^{t_2} F \cdot \mathrm{d}t (\text{N s}) \tag{10.1}$$

where I is the impulse (N s), F is a fixed or variable force (N) applied to a mass M (kg) from time, t_1 (s) to time t_2 (s).

An impulse, I, applied to a mass, changes its momentum, p, according to Equation (10.2):

$$\text{Momentum change, } \Delta p = I \tag{10.2}$$

Momentum, $p = M \cdot v$, where v (m/s) is the velocity of a mass, M. For simplicity, we can assume that a constant force, F, acts on a constant mass, M, for time Δt. Thus, an impulse is produced that results in a change in velocity, Δv, of the mass where, in this case, the change in velocity is proportional to the impulse, I. Since robots are largely composed of rotary joints and limbs with polar second moments of inertia, J, a similar analysis means that a limb acted on by a torque, T, has its angular velocity, ω, changed by an amount proportional to the rotational impulse, $I_{rot} = \int T \cdot dt$(N ms) applied to it.

This means that, if we know the required change in velocity of the mass, and we have a device that can apply a precise impulse with respect to time, then, we can control the velocity of the mass with respect to time. The SFM does just that without interfering with the free motion of the limb that the mechanism is actuating, thus enabling dynamic robots. In contrast, limbs driven by an electric motor-gearbox combination can never be freed from the friction and mass effects of the electric motor and gearbox; the limb is forever dragging with it the mass and friction of the attached actuator. For example, a running humanoid robot has legs that oscillate forward then backward at 2.5 Hz. This means that a traditional bidirectional electric motor and gearbox will accelerate its moving mass (armature plus gears) to its maximum velocity forward then decelerate to its maximum velocity backwards at 2.5 times every second. This is enormously wasteful of energy and unnecessary if you have a pair of oppositely acting, clutched, unidirectional electric motor gearboxes, which is the working methodology of the SFM.

It needs to be borne in mind that muscles are also required to apply an impulse to a limb or set of limbs even when there is zero velocity change. This case refers to the muscles applying impulses that overcome the force due to gravity acting on the limbs when a body is standing still. The analysis of a multijointed robot is more complicated than expressed above since an impulse applied at the arm applies an equal and opposite impulse to the rest of the body and ultimately to the ground if the robot is standing on the ground. Thus, limb impulses are reflected through the body. Nonetheless, the basic principles remain as above. Almost without exception, state-of-the-art robots are articulated by closed loop angular/linear displacement servomechanisms or angular/linear velocity servomechanisms. Rarely, if at all, are robots articulated by impulse servomechanisms. Probably, the MIT SEA is the exception.

This SFM is based on the premise that skeletal muscles are not to be seen as displacement or velocity servomechanisms but rather seen as impulse servomechanisms that position the limb in the correct displacement or with the correct velocity or acceleration. The implication of an impulse force-producing actuator is that the force produced should be independent of the limb position, velocity, and acceleration. We define this property as high forward and backward drivability. We will call this phenomenon, ultra low, negligible, or near-zero bidirectional output impedance. The meaning of "impedance" is the resistance to an applied quantity. Here, the applied quantities are (i) displacement, (ii) velocity, and (iii) acceleration, and the resistance will be the change of force to each of these applied quantities. The output impedance will be quantified as the ratio of the change in force to these applied quantities. The meaning of "output" is that the applied quantities are applied external to the artificial muscle via the output shaft that is connected to the limb. Low bidirectional output impedance is defined as low values of all of the following three output impedance coefficients, k_{displ}, k_{vel}, k_{accel}, with the actuator programmed to exert a demanded force, F_{dem}. However, F_{muscle} is the actual force produced by the muscle which will be a different value from F_{dem} due to friction and inertial effects. Ideally, for perfect forward and backward drivability, and zero bidirectional output impedance, F_{muscle} is always equal to F_{dem}. In practice, we aim F_{muscle} and F_{dem} to be as near equal as possible with a passive system in contrast to an active system such as the MIT SEA. We now set about quantifying low output impedance as follows:

(1) $F_{muscle} = F_{dem} + k_{displ} x$

where F_{dem} is the force or torque demanded by a muscle controller, F_{muscle} is the actual force or torque produced by the muscle, k_{displ} is displacement output impedance, N/m or N m/rad, and x is displacement (m) or (rad).

Zero or negligible displacement impedance will be produced when, $k_{displ} \approx 0$, which means that force, F_{muscle}, is independent of actuator displacement. Thus, there should be no springiness in the actuator output shaft.

(2) $F_{muscle} = F_{dem} + k_{veln}(\mathrm{d}x/\mathrm{d}t)^n$

where k_{veln} is the velocity output impedance and consists of (i) friction output impedance (N) or (N m) for $n=0$, (ii) viscous output impedance (N/(m/s)) or (N m/(rad/s)) for $n=1$, and (iii) fluid dynamic output impedance (N/(m/s)^2) or (N m/(rad/s)^2) for $n=2$ and $\mathrm{d}x/\mathrm{d}t$ is actuator velocity (m/s) or (rad/s).

Zero or negligible velocity output impedance will be produced when $k_{veln} \approx 0$ which means that force, F_{muscle}, is independent of actuator velocity. Thus, there should be no coulomb, viscous, or fluid dynamic losses in the actuator output shaft.

(3) $F_{muscle} = F_{dem} + k_{accel}\mathrm{d}^2x/\mathrm{d}t^2$

where k_{accel} is acceleration output impedance (N/(m/s^2) = kg) or (N m/(rad/s^2) = kg m^2) and $\mathrm{d}^2x/\mathrm{d}t^2$ is actuator acceleration (m/s^2) or (rad/s^2).

Zero or negligible acceleration output impedance will be produced when $k_{accel} \approx 0$ which means that force, F_{muscle}, is independent of actuator acceleration. Thus, the moving elements of the output shaft should be as lightweight as possible to produce as little inertia force as possible.

To help the reader's intuitive understanding of the meaning of zero bidirectional output impedance, we can imagine getting hold of the actuator and pushing and pulling against it. The result will be that the force felt from the actuator remains constant, equal to $F_{muscle} = F_{dem}$, whatever is the actuator bidirectional displacement, bidirectional velocity, or bidirectional acceleration. In other words, the biomimetic muscle will possess negligible bidirectional output impedance. Another important property of a biomimetic muscle is that of force resolution meaning that the force exerted by the muscle should be resolute to, for example, 0.1% of its maximum force, e.g., 1 N force resolution for a 1000 N maximum force biomimetic muscle.

The SFM is also modeled on biological skeletal muscle in that such muscle tissue cannot exert pushing forces but can only exert pulling forces due to contraction. In other words, skeletal muscles can only contract, they cannot extend. Biological muscles are thus inherently unidirectional. This unidirectionality is not slavishly copied just because Nature has evolved the muscle this way. The fundamental advantage in being unidirectional over that of a bidirectional system is that there is no energy loss in reversing the direction of the muscle system. The cost of a unidirectional system is that a pair of unidirectional systems is required to achieve bidirectionality.

Since skeletal muscles cannot extend themselves, they are in fact extended due to their partner muscle contracting on the opposite side of the limb. Skeletal muscles thus work in pairs and are known as *agonistic* and *antagonistic* muscles. Each skeletal muscle is capable of being agonistic or antagonistic depending on whether the limb is being flexed or extended. The agonistic muscle is the one overcoming the load exerted on the limb and the antagonistic muscle is the one relaxing itself to allow its partner to contract against the external load.

It is highly instructive to examine the working principle of skeletal muscle because it directs the mind toward a biomimetic muscle design solution.

10.5 Working principle of biological skeletal muscle

The following account is based on *The Sliding Filament Theory*, Movie clip2, Huxley and Niedergerke (1954), Huxley and Hanson (1954), and Chen and Zeltzer, and is the author's interpretation of information and events given by these references. In other words, the author has taken some creative license and liberties with the information but at the same time has made effort to remain as accurate and factual as possible.

Muscles are manufactured from five compounds which are:

1. *Myosin*, which forms the very axially stiff *thick filament*
2. *Actin* which is the main constituent of the very axially stiff *thin filament*
3. *Tropomyosin* which is used in the *thin filament*
4. *Troponin* which is also used in the *thin filament*
5. *Titin* also known as *Connectin* which is a rope-like, sometimes elastic (sometimes elastic followed by relatively inextensible behavior at the end of its travel), long chain molecule that connects the thick and thin filaments together at their sarcomere centers.

The muscle-building blocks will now be built up in sequence. We will start with the articulated myosin unit (Figure 10.2). The articulated myosin unit consists of a single myosin filament with a 2 degree-of-freedom (2dof) articulated walking mechanism at each end of the filament. The unit is symmetric about a central axis as shown in Figure 10.2.

Each 2dof articulated walking mechanism "walks" similar to a foot connected to a leg. However, the walking mechanisms walk in opposite directions in a mirror image as if walking away from each other (Figure 10.3).

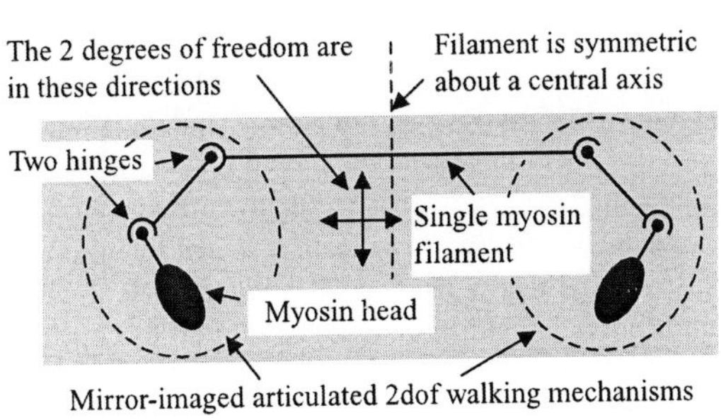

Figure 10.2 Articulated myosin unit with a 2 degree-of-freedom articulated walking mechanism at each end of a myosin filament.

Figure 10.3 Path of the opposing walking 2dof mechanisms at each end of the myosin filament.

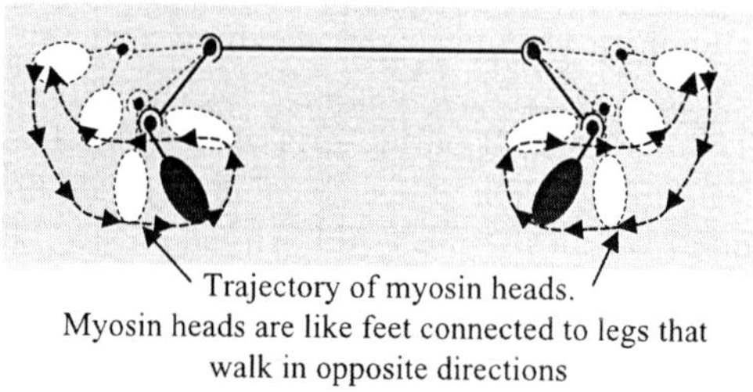

But the walking myosin heads are not allowed to walk anywhere because (i) they are connected together and (ii) they are walking in opposite directions. Instead, they do the only alternative option which is, so as to speak, to make the floor move under their feet meaning that the thin filaments are pulled, or contracted, together. These thin filaments are largely composed of actin but have an amazingly ingenious electrical–chemical–mechanical mechanism that utilizes tropomyosin and troponin to create force. These thin filaments (Figure 10.4) are pulled together as the myosin heads walk and thus form the basis of a contractile mechanism. An important point to realize is that the myosin heads can still walk and produce contractile force even though the thin filaments are inhibited from movement. In other words, the myosin heads apparently slip but still apply force. It will be shown shortly that continuous force is possible despite the myosin heads periodically releasing their grip during their circulatory 2dof motion because there are many walking myosin heads acting at random times.

The walking mechanisms only "walk" when energized by nerves from the brain and they walk at a speed in proportion to the nervous excitation. As already stated, the nervous excitation of muscle tissue is ingenious and involves electro-chemical—physical—mechanical mechanisms. However, it is only necessary to describe the mechanical properties here. When there is no nervous excitation, the myosin heads

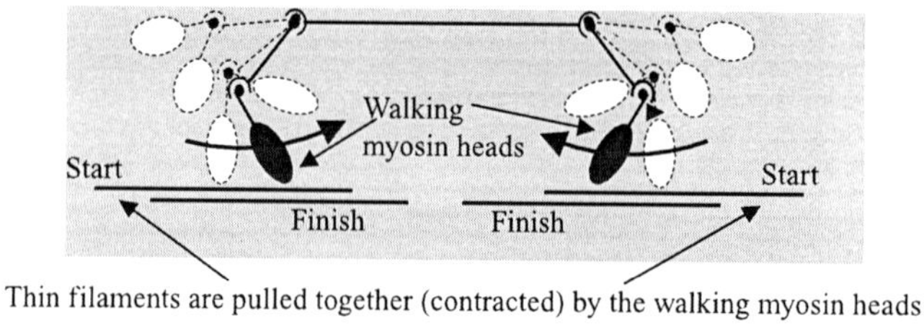

Figure 10.4 The walking myosin heads apply force to pull the two thin filaments closer together thus forming a contractile mechanism. Note that the myosin heads slip on the surface of the filaments.

Figure 10.5 The myosin heads can retract away clear from the thin filaments.

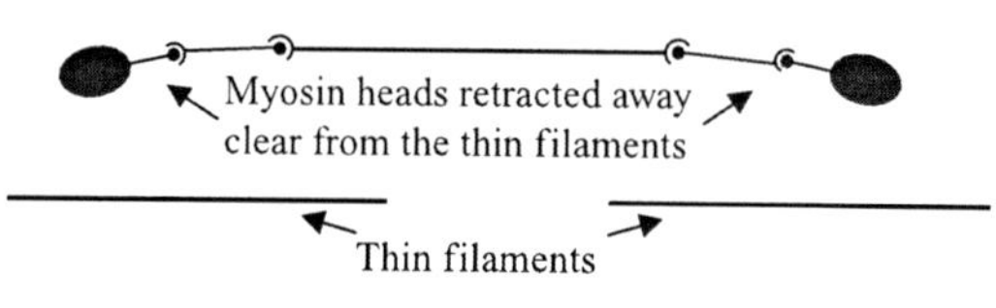

cease to walk and retract, like an aeroplane undercarriage, away clear from the thin filaments (Figure 10.5).

This complete physical disassociation between the myosin heads and the thin filaments is a key feature of muscle tissue. It means that skeletal muscle tissue can allow, if necessary, free unhindered motion of limbs meaning there is no feeling of friction or little feeling of inertial mass connected to the limp limb. This is one of the key features of obtaining low output impedance and high back drivability.

The method by which the myosin heads pull on the thin filaments appears not to be known accurately. The literature uses the phrase, "the myosin heads *bind* with the thin filaments." Precisely what is meant by *bind* is not clear. For example, is it a frictional force or an electric charge force or do the myosin heads slot into grooves in the thin filaments? Whatever is the precise mechanism, the SFM utilizes friction to emulate the *binding* mechanism.

Figures 10.2–10.5 above already show the basic micromechanism of skeletal muscle. The next step is to assemble, en masse, many of these micromechanisms to form a complete muscle. To do this, natural biology stacks together many articulated myosin units of various lengths into a bundle to form what is called a myosin "thick filament" (Figure 10.6).

The author considers that the core (not the heads) axial stiffness of these myosin bundles is very stiff. The right-hand side of Figure 10.6 also shows the thick filament viewed from the end, where it can be seen that the myosin units are arranged into a hexagon format. This is because the thick filaments can form a three-dimensional

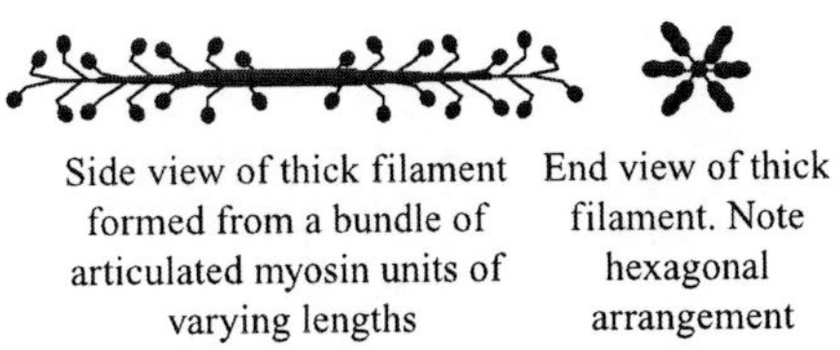

Figure 10.6 Side view and end view of thick filament consisting of a bundle of numerous 2dof articulated myosin units of various lengths.

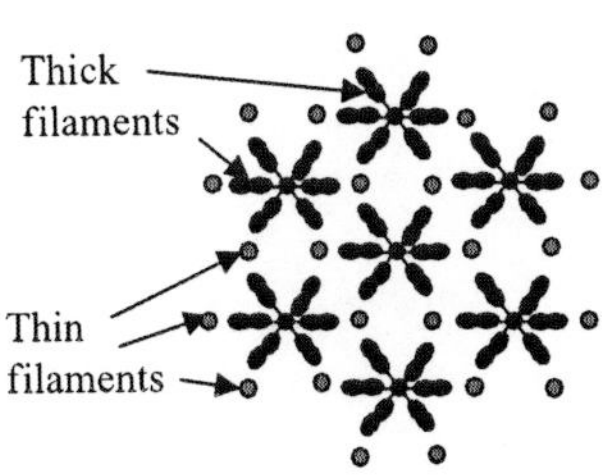

Figure 10.7 Cross-sectional view muscle showing thick and thin filaments packed in a hexagonal arrangement.

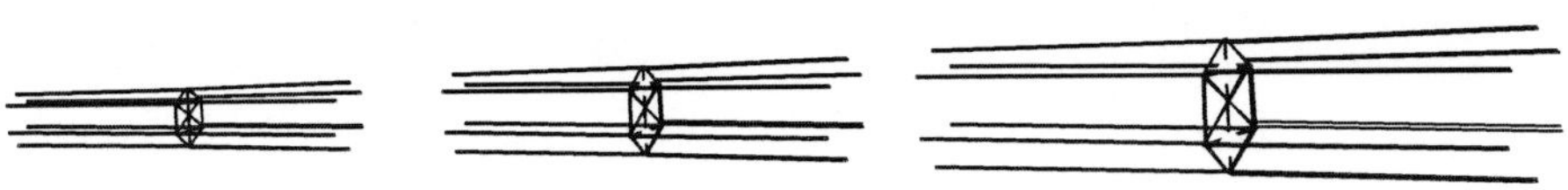

Figure 10.8 The thin filament opposing "wire cups" shown in perspective (not tapered).

nested hexagonal honeycomb arrangement that matches with the thin filaments that are arranged also in a hexagonal arrangement (Figure 10.7). Figure 10.8 shows three sets of thin filament "wire cups" with their myosin bundles and titin ropes removed. Likewise, as with the high axial stiffness of the thick filament myosin bundle, the author also considers that the axial stiffness of the thin filament actin wires is also highly stiff.

One thick filament bundle and a pair of opposing thin filament wire cups form the basis of a single muscle contractile unit called a *sarcomere* (Figures 10.9 and 10.10). Figure 10.9 also shows a short length of sarcomeres joined together. Sarcomere size varies according to muscle application but for humans, they are approximately 2 μm in length; so, a bicep muscle of 200 mm in length will consist of approximately 100,000 sarcomeres strung together in a continuous line. There will, of course, be many more strings of sarcomeres all mutually connected in parallel.

It is easier to explain further action of skeletal muscle by reverting back to a two-dimensional arrangement in order to simplify explanation of the muscle contractile principle (Figure 10.10).

In Figure 10.10, the basic muscle contractile unit, known as a *sarcomere*, is of the-order of 2 μm in length. The sarcomere is composed of three items which are (i) the already described, thick filament with numerous walking myosin heads, (ii) the already mentioned thin filaments but this time shown as a pair of opposing "wire cups" (see Figure 10.8), and (iii) a further component in the muscle system which is a pair of centralizing tensile ropes made from titin. These two ropes are mounted at each end of the thick myosin filament.

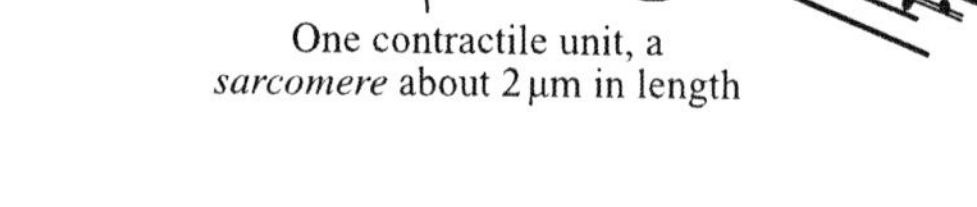

Figure 10.9 Sarcomeres are single contractile units. Here they are joined together. Note the constituent parts: the actin thin filament wire cups, the myosin thick filament articulated units, and the titin elastic ropes.

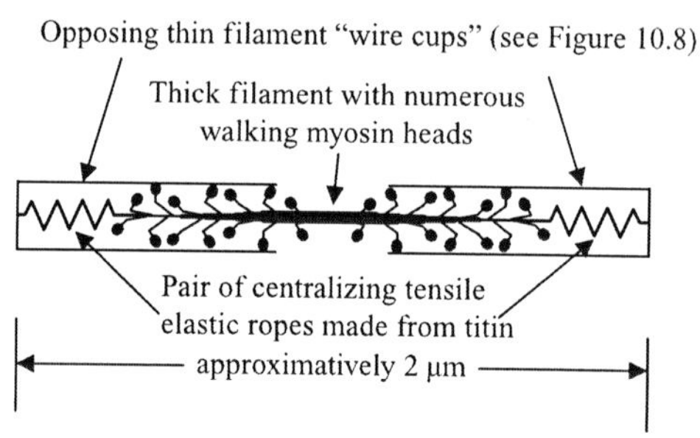

Figure 10.10 Basic muscle contractile unit, the *sarcomere*.

Mechanically speaking, the probable purpose of these ropes is twofold; one is to keep the thick filament centralized with respect to the thin filament cups and the second is to stop the muscle being pulled apart. The titin also appears to possess springiness that is nonlinear in the respect that its restoring force is low except until it reaches the end of its travel. Thus, it can be that it acts more like an *uncoiling tethered rope*. No doubt, Nature has evolved the titin to be a linear spring in some muscles such as bird wing flapping muscles. Since the thick filament can be considered stiff, it can be understood that the titin spring acts in parallel, thus forming an external resonant system as shown later in Figures 10.21 and 10.24. External resonant system means that the mass-spring system exists separately and is disconnected from the force excitation system.

We are now in the position of explaining the contractile action. We start with the sarcomere in its fully extended state (Figure 10.11), which occurs, for example, in the bicep arm muscle when the arm is straightened by contracting the opposing triceps muscle. It is to be remembered that the articulated myosin heads can only walk one way which is to drag the thin filaments together, not apart. The sarcomere in its fully extended state results in a large gap between the thin filament wire cups. The gap is known as the *H-zone*.

If, now, the articulated myosin heads are activated, then the thin filament wire cups are pulled together (Figure 10.12) and the H-zone now decreases to a small size. The sarcomere can extend and contract +/− 15% from its mid-range length of 2 μm.

The sarcomere muscle unit has a very special property which is that it can apply a contractile force, F, which is largely independent of the position, x, velocity of contraction, dx/dt, and due to its low mass is largely unaffected by the acceleration of contraction, d^2x/dt^2 (Figure 10.13).

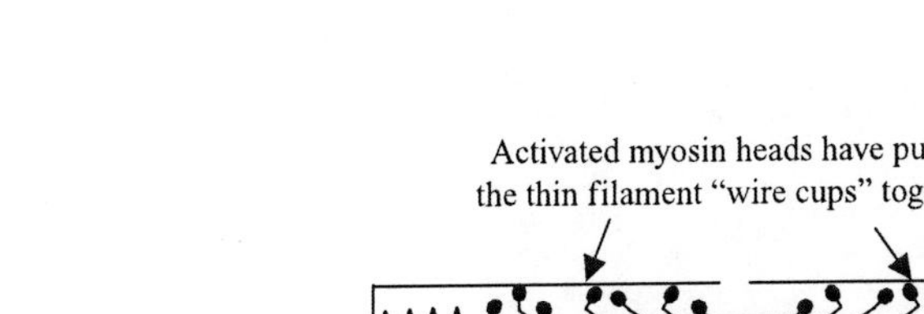

Figure 10.11 Sarcomere shown fully extended showing large gap between the thin filament wire cups.

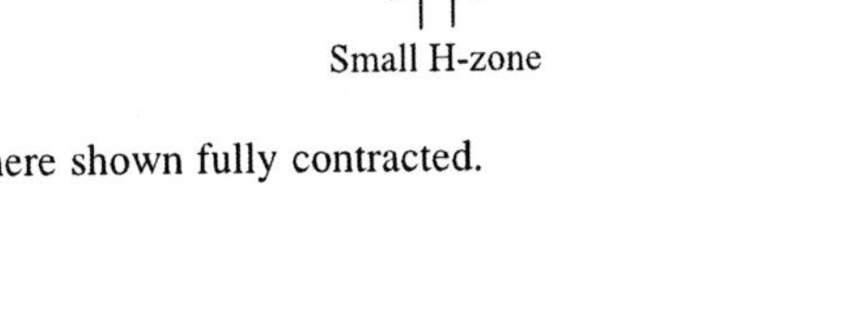

Figure 10.12 Sarcomere shown fully contracted.

Figure 10.13 Contractile force, F, is largely independent of x, dx/dt, and d^2x/dt^2.

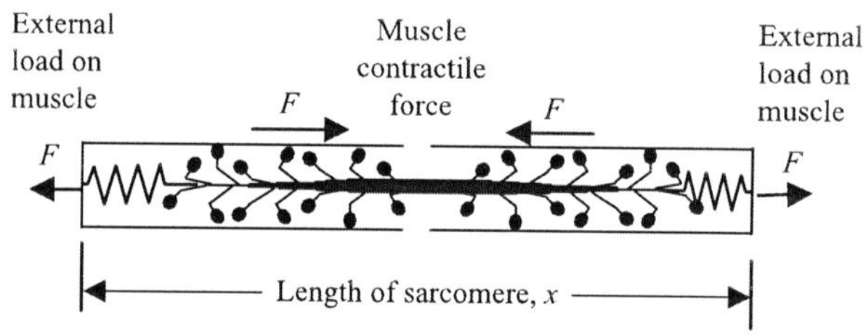

Figure 10.13 shows the sarcomere resisting an external tensile load, F, by exerting an equal and opposite contractile force, F. The special property means that the sarcomere will allow the relative free sliding, in both left and right directions, of the wire cup thin filaments over the thick filament myosin heads while still exerting a constant force, F. This means that skeletal muscle tissue is forward and backward drivable and thus is essentially a force-producing device. The implication is that the myosin heads "slip" over the thin filaments while still applying a contractile force.

It can be seen that the workings of biological muscles are very interesting and a fundamental departure from engineered systems that are position and/or velocity and/or acceleration producing actuators. Yes, engineered systems do apply a force to achieve a position and/or velocity and/or acceleration and yes paradoxically, biological muscles do control the position and/or velocity of limbs, but the difference between the two actuating methods is manifested by the forward and backward drivability of skeletal muscle tissue.

There are relatively high forward and backward drivable actuators on the market at present such as those by Barrett Technology. The drawback of these actuators is either too much reflected mass seen at the end effector. Skeletal muscle tissue in contrast is low in mass so engineers still largely have not solved the problem of creating an artificial muscle that closely mimics skeletal muscle. The two exceptions seem to be (i) the MIT SEA and (ii) the SFM.

We will now wind up the discussion on the workings of biological skeletal muscle at the sarcomere level by just saying that a complete muscle is orderly assembled from many sarcomeres placed in parallel and series (Figure 10.14). Adding sarcomeres in

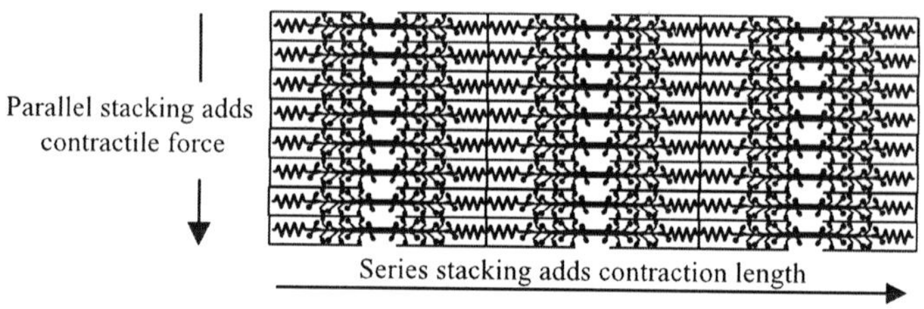

Figure 10.14 Sarcomeres are stacked in series and parallel. Playing with the parallel and series stacking causes effective impulse matching of different length limbs and different length moment arms. This is an interesting area to research.

parallel will increase contractile force while adding in series will increase the change in length. Thus, the work capability of a muscle is proportional to its volume.

The next step in developing our discussion of the effectiveness of the SFM is to explain how force-producing contractile muscles work in pairs to articulate limbs. We first make a simplification in the representation of the contractile muscle by showing it as a sliding telescopic system with a force-producing contractile element which applies a variable and controllable force that is exerted to contract the telescopic system (Figure 10.15).

Figures 10.15 and 10.16 above show the muscle in its fully extended position and in its fully contracted position, respectively.

It is interesting to note that the simplified representation of the muscle (Figure 10.15) can be realized as a linear electromagnetic telescopic device. It can be designed to be accurately forward and backward drivable, so why it is not being used? The answer is that the mechanical power-to-weight ratio is too low. As already stated, achieving high mechanical power output from an electromagnetic device requires a small electric motor running at high speed delivering mechanical power through a reduction gearbox.

As already stated, muscles cannot apply an extending force; they can only apply a contractile force. Thus, the only way for a muscle to extend is by the muscle contracting on the other side of the limb. The following figures make this clearer. Figure 10.17

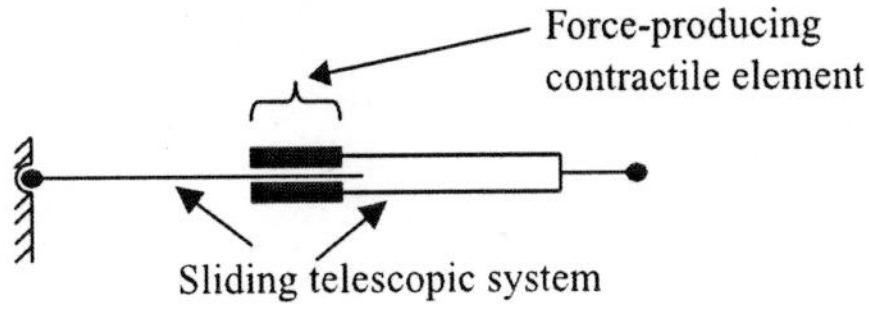

Figure 10.15 Simplified muscle in fully extended position.

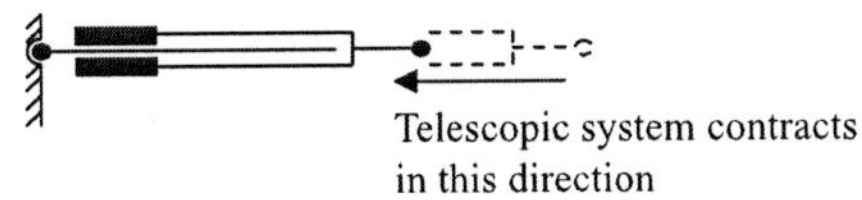

Figure 10.16 Artificial muscle in fully contracted position.

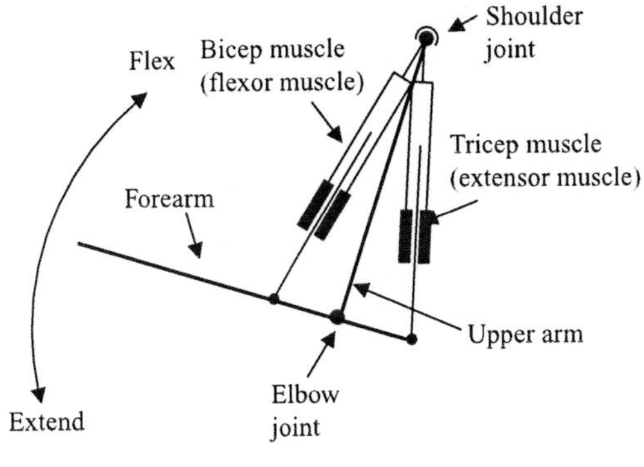

Figure 10.17 Human forearm and upper arm shown in mid-range position with bicep and triceps muscles that flex and extend the forearm.

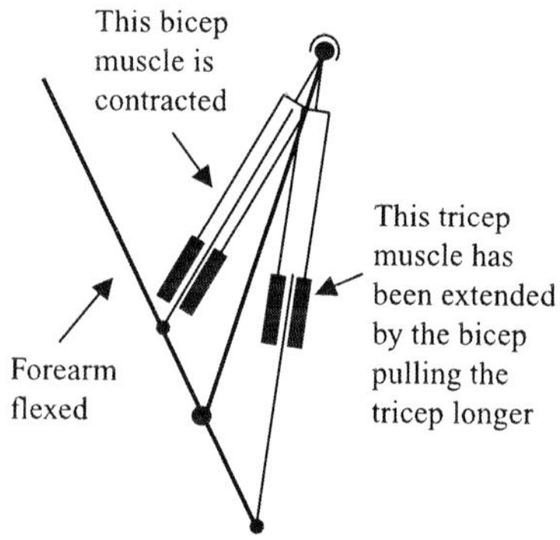

Figure 10.18 Forearm shown in a flexed position due to the bicep muscle contraction.

shows a human forearm and upper arm in its mid-range position. If the forearm is brought closer to the upper arm, then the joint is said to be "flexed" (Figure 10.18).

Since skeletal muscles can only apply a contractile force, the only muscle that can flex the forearm is the bicep muscle which is also known as the flexor muscle. The triceps muscle, on the other hand, relaxes its contractile element which allows the forearm to flex and, in turn, the triceps muscle becomes extended.

If the arm is straightened, then the joint is said to be "extended" (Figure 10.19). This time the bicep muscle relaxes and the triceps muscle (the extensor muscle) is contracted to extend the forearm. Thus, this time the bicep muscle extends. The arm is typical of most skeletal muscles in the body and typifies skeletal muscles existing in pairs, i.e., one muscle is used to flex a limb and the other is used to extend the limb thus exhibiting bidirectional motion.

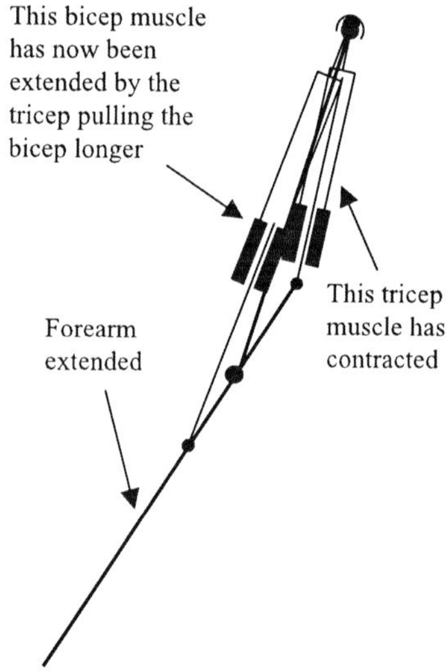

Figure 10.19 Forearm shown in an extended position due to the triceps muscle contraction.

Three more terms will now introduced; they are "reciprocal inhibition," "agonistic muscle" and "antagonistic muscle," all three of which will now be explained via an example in the next few paragraphs.

You would expect that when the forearm flexes, only the bicep will contract, but this is not true. First of all when the brain commands the forearm to flex, both biceps and triceps muscles are activated, but of course there can be no movement until the triceps relaxes and allows the bicep to overpower the bicep. What happens is that the flexing bicep muscle sends a signal to its opposing mate to allow flexing to occur by reducing the contractile force in the triceps muscle. The process is known as "reciprocal inhibition." The inhibition of the triceps muscle is greatest at the start of flexing and the least at the end of motion. In other words, the contractile force of the triceps is lowest at the beginning of flexing and greatest at the end of motion. The bicep works inversely by being the most strongly activated at the beginning of motion and decreasing at the end of motion. The effect can be considered analogous to velocity feedback that is used in engineered control systems.

The bicep, which is overpowering the triceps muscle to create flexing, is called the "agonistic" muscle because it is the muscle undergoing the greater stress or agony (Greek, agon = struggle). On the other hand, the triceps muscle, which is moderating the forearm motion to ensure it does not slam into the upper arm and cause damage, is called the "antagonistic" muscle (="the one that fights against").

If now the forearm is extended, the roles of the bicep and triceps muscles are reversed. In this case, the more highly activated triceps muscle becomes the agonistic muscle because it has to overpower, using reciprocal inhibition, the bicep muscle which now becomes the antagonistic muscle.

We now conclude the description of biological skeletal muscle and turn our attention to engineering a man-made solution to a biomimicking skeletal muscle which is the main subject of this chapter. First, we formulate a mechanical model of skeletal muscle.

10.6 Modeling skeletal muscle

Researchers have created a mechanical model of skeletal muscle (Shadmehr & Wise). The model, known as the Hill/Huxley model, is shown in Figure 10.20.

The author considers that the model can be better represented if the series spring and the damper are not present. The reasons relate to (i) the difficulty in controlling a

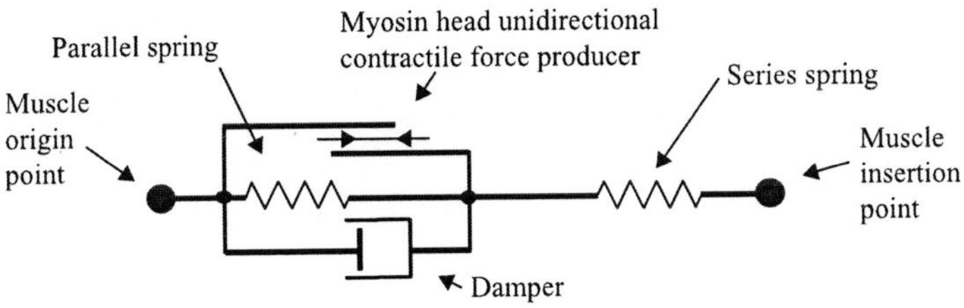

Figure 10.20 Hill/Huxley model of skeletal muscle. Note that all thick black lines are considered infinitely stiff.

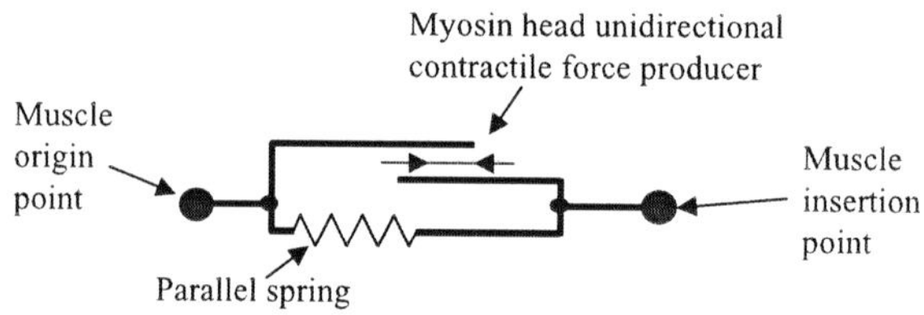

Figure 10.21 Simplified model of skeletal muscle.

muscle system if the series spring is present and (ii) the low energy efficiency if the damper is present. The author considers that the antagonistic muscle is used to damp motion via reciprocal inhibition which is a well-known physiological phenomenon. Hence, the author proposes the simplified model of Figure 10.21.

It can be considered that Nature plays with the parallel spring stiffness rate depending on its application. For example, the rate is low in humans allowing freedom of movement but would be a high rate in an avian breast muscle resulting in a high efficiency oscillating tuned mass-spring system for its flapping wings. We now move on to implement the model (Figure 10.21) in a mechatronic system, the SFM.

10.7 Description of the SFM

The SFM biomimetic muscle has evolved by choosing to mimic biological skeletal muscle tissue by creating a force via clamping a pair of friction pads onto a unidirectional continuously running surface such as a brake disk (Figure 10.22). This brake disk can be seen in a picture of the SFM (Figure 10.23), which is a proof-of-concept apparatus. Note that the friction pads are clamped on opposite sides of the rotating surface and in opposing directions, by a pair of Futaba integrated-servos.

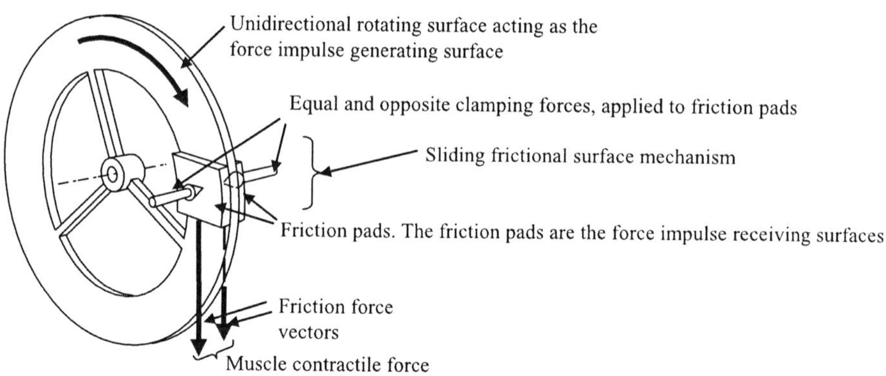

Figure 10.22 Principle of muscle contractile force generation from clamped friction pads that mimic the myosin heads interacting with actin thin filaments.

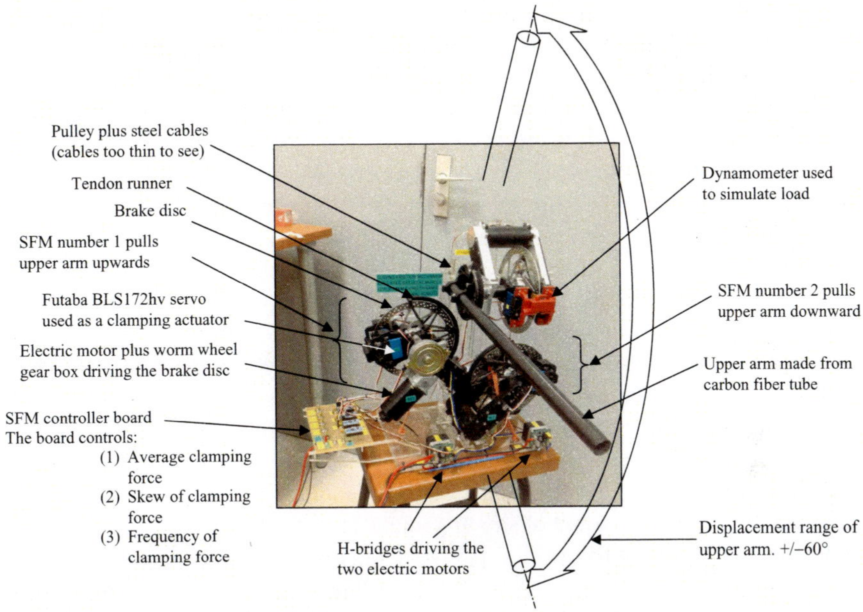

Figure 10.23 Sliding friction mechanism of proof-of-concept apparatus.

The force produced is from sliding frictional force between the continuously rotating surface and the friction pads. The millions and maybe billions of minutely sized protuberant sliding friction areas that are in sliding contact with the running surface and the friction pads can be considered to mimic the millions and maybe billions of sliding filament myosin walking heads that exist in skeletal muscle. Both the minutely sized friction areas and the minutely sized myosin heads produce nano Newton-second randomly applied force impulses that when summed together produce a smooth, low noise, high value force for each second that they are in operation.

Friction pads such as automotive or bicycle disk brake pads are chosen because they (i) are capable of exerting very large braking forces, (ii) are small and lightweight, (iii) are low cost, and (iv) are capable of long life being designed for this application. We will assume a constant friction coefficient, independent of the slip speed, between the rotating surface and friction pads equal to the coefficient of kinetic friction. We use the kinetic friction coefficient by arranging the unidirectional running surface to always run faster than the pad speed. The heating energy loss is minimized by ensuring the slip speed is kept as low as possible. The rotating surface runs in one direction only, i.e., it is unidirectional; it does not change direction. However, it can change its surface speed. The force, which represents the muscle contractile force, is extracted from lightweight friction pads that are freely allowed to rotate independently about the rotating disk axis, thus providing a force independent of position, velocity, and acceleration of the friction pads. The continuously rotating surface provides the source from which is tapped the force. The force from the friction pads is continuously variable from zero up to the maximum force available from the continuously rotating surface. The force is varied by varying the pad clamping force. Since the rotating surface is unidirectional, the friction pad force will also be unidirectional and thus will mimic skeletal muscle. The clamping force can be reduced to zero such that there is no contact between the friction pads and rotating surface, thus mimicking the myosin heads being completely retracted (Figure 10.5).

The speed of the continuously rotating surface is arranged to be greater, or marginally greater, than the maximum speed of the friction pads which are connected to a telescopic slider. Thus, there will always be a slip occurring between the friction pads and the rotating surface. If there is always a slip, then the contractile friction force provided by the friction pads is dependent on a constant friction coefficient which is the coefficient of kinetic friction. Hence, the contractile friction pad force will be directly proportional to the clamping force. Thus, the contractile friction pad force which represents the muscle contractile force can be accurately controlled by accurately controlling the friction pad clamping force. Slip, occurring between the friction pads and the rotating surface, means there will be energy wasted that is manifested as heat dissipated between the friction pads and the rotating surface. A control system is to be used to limit the amount of slip to a minimum in order to minimize energy loss. Biological muscles also have this slipping energy loss that manifests itself as muscles getting hot even if the limb is not moving but supporting a weight; anyone practicing Yoga or Pilates will know this well. This energy loss appears to be a natural law of inevitable payment in return for obtaining the property of ultra-low output impedance that is created passively.

The SFM solves the problem associated with energy wastage caused by reversing the rotation direction of the electric motor/gearbox together with solving the problem of achieving low oscillating mass. First of all, the electric motor/gearbox is kept rotating in one direction only, and second, the high inertia of the motor/gearbox is not seen by the moving limb or the moving parts of the muscle. In fact, the relatively high kinetic energy of the motor/gearbox is an advantage because it reduces the fluctuations in the speed of the rotating surface as the friction pads extract periodic impulses from it. The moving mass, which is connected to the limb, is low because it is equal to the mass of the friction pad clamping system which can be made a low value.

It is also to be noted with the SFM that it is capable of absorbing shock loads without damaging the motor. This is due to the maximum clamping force applied to the friction pads being purposefully limited such that the maximum contractile force remains safely less than the force that will do damage to the motor gearbox teeth or the rotating surface.

The SFM, albeit, does not suffer from the need of the motor/gearbox having to reverse direction, but it does bear the disadvantage of requiring a pair of artificial muscles to actuate one limb. In fact, herein lays the dualism which is either two separate unidirectional muscles to actuate one limb or one bidirectional muscle to actuate one limb. The disadvantage of requiring two unidirectional artificial muscles is that the weight and cost will be higher than one bidirectional muscle. This disadvantage has to be overcome by future research and development.

As regards cost, the SFM will spur the development of a manufacturing process that should make a pair of unidirectional actuators that is no more expensive than one bidirectional actuator. Anyway, if a device solves a difficult problem, then cost is not of immediate importance. It should also be made clear that the unidirectional muscles of the SFM operate interdependently which means that both muscles can be activated at the same time such that one reciprocally inhibits the force of the other. It is important to note the high reaction speed of the SFM. The rapid speed of the unidirectional and bidirectional force response of this device together with the large amplitude bandwidth is two of its key advantageous features. The reason is due to the lightweight tendon runners together with the speed of response of the Futaba BLS172hv friction pad clamping servos. Furthermore, when a pair of muscles is used to cause oscillation and/or reversal in a robot limb, then this device has the potential to excel over the state of the art.

10.8 Model of the SFM

Figure 10.24 shows a rectilinear mechanical model of the SFM shown in Figure 10.23. The model is equipped with a parallel spring, stiffness K(N/m) and the system is responsible for giving rectilinear motion to a mass, M along the x-axis.

The parallel spring system represents the potential of the SFM to actuate high efficiency oscillations to a tuned mass-spring system of a sprinting or flapping limb. The system is not dissimilar to that of inputting sufficient energy to the pendulum of a grandfather clock via a Geneva wheel escapement mechanism.

The rotating surface is already rotating at speed and does not have to speed up or slow down and reverse; it runs in one direction at a certain speed which can be set to a low speed for leisurely operations or at high speed for highly active behavior patterns. The friction pads are placed very close to the rotating surface such that with zero force when the pads are not in contact at all, the combined gap on each side of the rotating surface will be of the order of 0.1 mm. This gap can be closed very quickly, especially since the pads are small and lightweight, in the order of 1 ms with a model aircraft

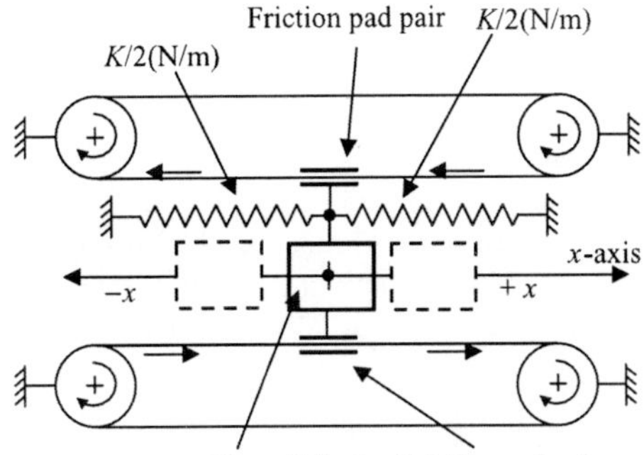

Figure 10.24 Rectilinear mechanical model of the SFM that is shown in Figure 10.23. Dual, unidirectional, opposite-acting impulsive force excitation using two, single acting, sliding friction mechanisms.

servomechanism, e.g., Futaba BLS172hv which has a maximum torque rating 3 N m. The time to reach a torque of 1 N m is approximately 5 ms. If the Futaba servo exerts a clamping force on the friction pads through a 2-mm radius arm, then a clamping force of 500 N on either side of the rotating surface can be applied in approximately 5 ms. The friction pads, e.g., automotive brake pads, are very stiff in a direction perpendicular to the clamping direction. Furthermore, so also is the stiffness very high of the rotating surface, e.g., a steel brake disk, in the direction of clamping. Hence, the clamping force is increased rapidly as the friction pads are clamped through a small distance and this clamping force of 500 N, as already calculated, is exerted in 5 ms. The kinetic friction coefficient of brake pads is approximately 0.25 and thus a muscle contractile force of 250 N is possible from an opposing pair of friction pads with a rise time of 5 ms.

To show the SFM more clearly, we show an agonistic–antagonistic arrangement (Figure 10.25). Two mirror-imaged SFMs running in opposite directions flex and extend the limb. Herein, we can see a disadvantage of just one artificial muscle acting alone, that of gyroscopic precession of the unidirectional rotating surface plus the motor and gearbox combination as the mobile platform, to which the muscle is attached. However, placing two SFMs back to back with the rotating surfaces rotating in opposite directions but at the same speed means that gyroscopic precession moments will be canceled out. Figures 10.26 and 10.27 show how the arrangement extends and flexes a limb.

10.9 SFM basic control methodology

The control methodology is in its early stages since only a proof-of-concept SFM has been constructed. In the pipeline is a much improved SFM that uses a 2.8-kW (mechanical output power) brushless D.C. motor together with a harmonic drive gearbox. This device will have a mass of 3.5 kg and produce a pulling force of 2000 N and large angle (+/−60°) full power response at 3 Hz.

Currently, the proof-of-concept bidirectional SFM system has a specification as follows:

(i) A twin unidirectional SFM system mounted in an agonistic–antagonistic arrangement similar to Figures 10.25–10.27 produces bidirectional motion of a carbon-fiber arm via a steel cable and pulley arrangement. The arrangement mimics the pectoralis/supracoracoideus breast muscle set that actuates, down and up, respectively, the upper arm of a bird wing.

(ii) Each SFM is driven by a brushed DC motor and worm-wheel gearbox that drives a 160 mm diameter bicycle brake disk (150 mm mean diameter). The motor gearbox has a maximum mechanical power output of 60 W at 120 rpm ($\approx$ 13 rad/s), thus producing a torque of 4.8 N m at this angular velocity. The torque constant of motor gearbox seen at the gearbox output is 1 N m/A.

(iii) The force is extracted from each SFM via a clamping system that provides clamping force from a pair of oppositely acting Futaba BLS172hv integrated servos. Each servo produces a maximum torque of 3 N m at a torque constant of 1 N m/A. The clamping force acts via a 20 mm long radius arm on a friction pad that is a commercially available component that

(Continued on page 222)

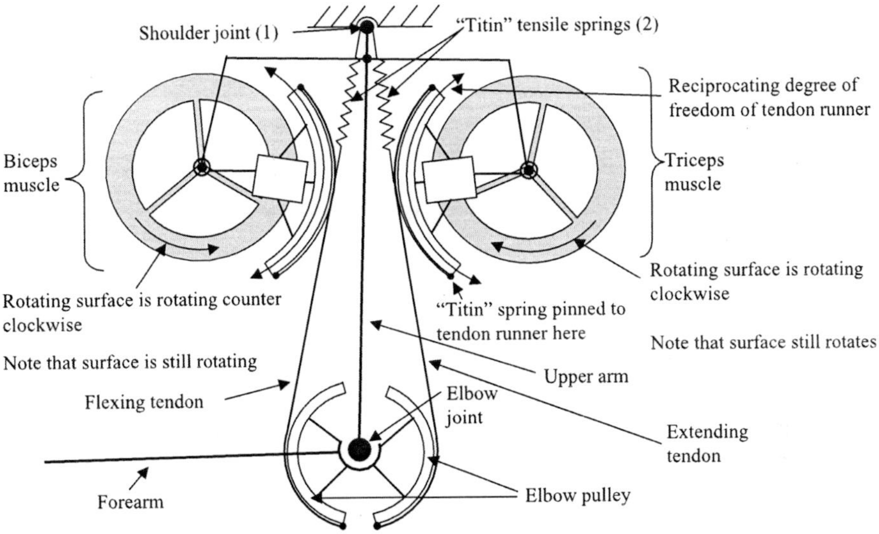

Figure 10.25 Arrangement using rotary to rectilinear unidirectional sliding friction mechanisms in an agonistic/antagonistic pair arrangement to produce bidirectional motion of a robot limb, e.g., humanoid robot forearm. The muscles are shown oversize for clarity. In practice, the muscles will be more compact and resemble the shape of human biceps and triceps muscles. Note that the line of action of each contractile force vector passes through the shoulder joint thus applying no moment of force at the shoulder joint when the muscles are in action. (1) The two muscles have an "origin" (medical term) at the shoulder joint such that the contractile force line of action passes through the joint. This design in synergy with the elbow tendon runner applies no moments to the upper arm to sustain throughout the range of movement of the forearm. In other words, a pure couple is applied at the elbow joint, and no other torques or moments are applied to the upper arm. If this were not the case, then the muscles actuating the upper arm would require additional corrective energy to correct the undesirable and superfluous moments acting on the upper arm thus resulting in an inefficient muscle system. Of course, there will be an unavoidable moment applied to the upper arm brought about by any acceleration of the forearm that creates inertial forces that have to be resisted by the upper arm muscles. (2) The "titin" springs have low stiffness spring rate if it is not required to create a resonant spring-mass system. Low rate springs do not serve the purpose of centralizing the forearm although in practice there will be a small centralizing force. In fact, low rate springs serve the purpose of keeping the flexing and extending tendons taut without any significant energy required to flex and extend the forearm limb. High rate springs not only have a similar effect of keeping the tendons taut but also provide a resonant spring-mass dynamic oscillating system; however, they have the disadvantage of requiring significant energy to displace the forearm limb when the muscles are used to statically position the limb or to velocity profile the limb. Thus, adjustable variable rate "titin" springs will permit the muscle system to operate in static, dynamic, and velocity profiling modes.

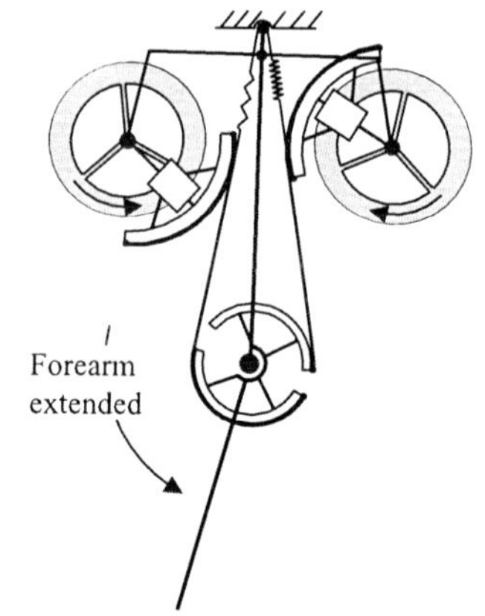

Figure 10.26 Muscle pair arrangement displacing the forearm into the extended position.

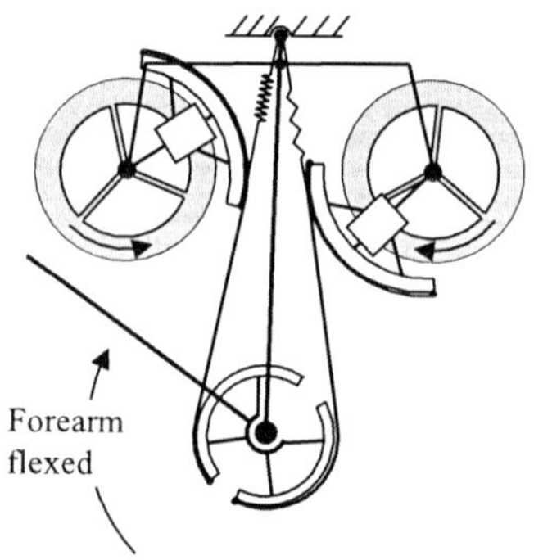

Figure 10.27 Muscle pair arrangement displacing the forearm into the flexed position.

matches the bicycle brake disk. A clamping force of 150 N is achieved with a 3A per servo current (6A total servo current because there are 2 servos per SFM). Such a clamping force produces a friction force of 75 N with a 3A per servo current.

(iv) The SFM force is applied via a tendon runner of 86 mm radius that actuates a pulley of radius 43 mm via a steel cable. Thus, a maximum torque of 43 mm × 75 N = 3.2 N m can be applied to the carbon fiber upper arm. A current of 3A per servo is not advisable since it will significantly decrease servo life. Hence, the proof-of-concept SFM system is driven with a maximum servo current of 2.1A per servo, thus producing a maximum upper arm torque of 2 N m. The maximum angular velocity of the upper arm is thus 13 rad/s × 86 mm/43 mm ≈ 25 rad/s. Thus, the maximum possible angular velocity of the upper arm is 25 rad/s. It is advisable that the upper arm maximum angular velocity is less than 25 rad/s since that is one basic premise of the SFM that there should always be some slip, albeit minimum, between the brake disk and the tendon runner. Assuming an amplitude of 1 rad and assuming that the upper arm is oscillated sinusoidally at ω_{arm}, then:

(a) the upper arm angular position, θ_{arm} can be represented as, $\theta_{\text{arm}} = 1 \sin \omega_{\text{arm}} t$

(b) the upper arm angular velocity, $\omega_{arm} = \omega_{arm} \cos 20t$
(c) the upper arm angular acceleration, $\alpha = -\omega_{arm}^2 \sin \omega_{arm} t$

The polar second moment of inertia, J_{arm} of the upper arm, including pulley, tendon runner, two Futaba servos, and steel cables was calculated as 0.005 kg m^2. The maximum torque available to drive the upper arm is 2 N m. Hence, the upper arm angular velocity of oscillation is given by:

$$Jx\omega_{arm}{}^2 = 2\,\text{N m}$$

Thus,

$$\omega_{arm} = \text{sqrt}\left(2\,\text{N m}/0.005\ \text{kg m}^2\right) = 20\ \text{rad/s}\ (3.2\ \text{Hz})$$

An experiment was carried out to oscillate the upper arm at 3.2 Hz and amplitude of 1 rad. The result was that 3 Hz was possible which is encouragingly close to the calculated value of 3.2 Hz.

(v) A controller board manually controls the following quantities for oscillating motion: (a method not devised yet to control displacement)
   (1) Average clamping force of the two SFMs
   (2) Skew of clamping forces, meaning, that the average force stays the same but one increases and the other decreases and vice versa, in order to counterbalance an offset load
   (3) Frequency of clamping force
   (4) Duration of clamping force
   (5) Rotation speed of brake disk

   This controller board was used to obtain the results in (iv) above.

10.10 Conclusions and future work

The SFM through reasoning and experiment shows potential and promise as a good candidate for a high performance biomimetic muscle for dynamic agile animal robots. The SFM is aimed to replace traditional biomimetic muscles but only after it has been further developed. Hurdles to overcome concern:

(i) Proving its performance by actuating the leg of an animal robot or the wing of an eagle bird robot.
(ii) Reducing its weight and volume.
(iii) Modeling its performance to inspect its scalability from an insect muscle up to a horse's leg muscle.
(iv) Designing a heat, sound, and wear management system.

References

Barrett Technology WAM robot arm USA patents, 4903536, 5046375, 5388480.
Boston Dynamic's Cheetah robot. https://www.youtube.com/watch?v=chPanW0QWhA.

Chen D.T., Zeltzer, D., Computer graphics and animation group. The Media Laboratory Massachusetts Institute of Technology. http://www.chrisevans3d.com/files/reference/pump_it_up.pdf.

Huxley, A.F., Niedergerke, R., 1954. Structural changes in muscle during contraction. Nature 173, 971–973.

Huxley, H., Hanson, J., 1954. Changes in the cross striations of muscle during contraction and stretch and their structural interpretation. Nature 173, 973–976.

Keennon, M., Klingebiel, K., Won, H., Andriukov, A., 2012. Development of the nano hummingbird: a tailless flapping wing micro air vehicle. In: Presented at 50th AIAA Aerospace Sciences Meeting including the New Horizons Forum and Aerospace Exposition, 09–12 January, Nashville, Tennessee.

Movie clip2: http://www.youtube.com/watch?v=Vlchs4omFDM.

Myogenesis. http://darbelofflab.mit.edu/?q=node/7.

Pratt et al., 1997. Elastic actuator for precise force control, US Patent No. 5650704.

Prof. Daniel Wolpert of Cambridge University Engineering Department explaining why the brain primarily evolved to control muscles. http://www.ted.com/talks/daniel_wolpert_the_real_reason_for_brains.html.

Quote by Boston Dynamics founder, Mark Raibert concerning inadequacies of actuators. http://spectrum.ieee.org/automaton/robotics/robotics-software/meeting_on_biologically-inspired_robots.

Sangbae Kim's Cheetah robot gait transition from trot to gallop. https://www.youtube.com/watch?v=UBHJqnM8RTU.

Sangok Seok et al. Actuator design for high force proprioceptive control in fast legged locomotion. http://ieeexplore.ieee.org/xpl/login.jsp?tp=&arnumber=6386252&url=http%3A%2F%2Fieeexplore.ieee.org%2Fxpls%2Fabs_all.jsp%3Farnumber%3D6386252.

Shadmehr, R., Wise, S.P., A simple muscle model. http://www.shadmehrlab.org/book/musclemodel.pdf.

The sliding filament theory. Movie clip 1: http://www.youtube.com/watch?v=EdHzKYDxrKc.

Part Four

Applications of Biomimetic Technologies

Artificial intelligence through symbolic connectionism—A biomimetic rapprochement

11

A. Ellery

11.1 Introduction

It would be impossible to review the whole field of artificial intelligence (AI) in a few short pages—from its beginnings, the field *in toto* may be regarded as bio-inspired in attempting to emulate human reasoning, said humans being biological animals albeit with enhanced cognitive faculties. The AI program has evolved and has been peppered with paradigms and paradigm shifts, faster than any other academic field I can think of. Furthermore, these paradigm shifts have not yielded any single dominant paradigm, merely a multiplicity of paradigms embattled with each other. Every decade or so, a new paradigm joins the flock to declare its divine right as the foundation of cognition. Yet, a multiplicity of cognitive processes is probably likely—human cognition has evolved piecemeal involving many interlocking faculties in conflict with the illusion of the unity of consciousness. Marvin Minsky's 1988 book *Society of Mind* was an early statement of this notion. His *K*-lines theory was essentially connectionist with linked nodes, each node represented by a simple frame. Cognitive dichotomies abound: inaccessible, unconscious, and procedural processes versus accessible, conscious, and declarative processes that are suited to connectionist and symbolic approaches, respectively (Holyoak and Spellman, 1993). Further complications occur such as in language acquisition involving an innate universal grammar combined with learning of the parameters of that grammar associated with specific languages. More generally, humans and other animals are limited to learning knowledge that conforms to specific structural regularities based on some naive physics—innate knowledge has been acquired through evolutionary processes and it shapes learned knowledge acquired through experience.

I shall focus on two dominant paradigms—symbolic processing and connectionism—that emerged early in the field and have been engaged in a spirited conflict as to which represents the key to human cognition, and ergo, the importation of intelligence into the machine. Connectionist models are adept at pattern matching, while symbolic systems encapsulate logic. Connectionist links serve to transmit activation signals between simple units rather than implementing structured relationships between symbols. Hence, the neurons of a typical neural network obviously cannot readily transmit structured symbolic information (Feldman and Ballard, 1982). Yet, symbols occur throughout biological systems—the genetic code is symbolic (Cariani, 2001). A symbol is an arbitrary designation that refers to an object, event, or relation in the outside world. It is a unitary concept but can be formed into composite symbol structures such as linguistic expressions. However, the early neural networks of McCulloch–Pitts neurons comprising binary maximum-of-sum threshold units implemented logic gates of AND, OR, and NOT with the appropriate weights and thresholds, indicating an early synergy between connectionism and symbolicism. A more recent variation on this theme is the adaptive connectionist expert system (ACES) built on a neural logic network that performs both pattern recognition and logical inferencing using past examples within a unified network architecture (Low et al., 1991). The neural logical network is a finite directed graph in which input nodes feed into output nodes with three logical values (TRUE, FALSE, and UNKNOWN). Each link is characterized by a number pair (x,y) representing both excitatory and inhibitory excitations rather than a single weight value with (1,0) for TRUE, (0,1) for FALSE, and (0,0) for UNKNOWN. The net excitatory and inhibitory weights for each link are summed independently. Logic gates may be implemented readily; for example, $A \rightarrow B$ may be implemented by two input nodes A and B feeding into a single output node with weights $(-1/2, -2)$ and (2, ½). Initially, input nodes are assigned known values, while output nodes are assigned UNKNOWN values. The weights then implement logical inferencing to determine the values of the output nodes. Another approach is the neural tree network that comprises neuronal nodes connected in a decision tree architecture similar to ID3 (Sankar and Mammone, 1993). It thus combined neural networks with decision trees in a hybrid format. These constitute what might be regarded as integrated approaches to symbolic connectionism.

The physics of the outside world is determined by causal relations between objects and events (Hatfield, 1990). The connection between the representation and the referents is arbitrary—hence, the multitude of possible representations and their processes. The only constraint is that the representation and its evolution over time should match the represented real-world processes. In good old-fashioned AI (GOFAI), it is first-order logic that is employed to model the real-world states. In connectionism, it is learning from past correlations. The attraction of symbolic rule-based systems rooted in first-order logic is transparency of reasoning. Symbols are discrete, categorical representations of the external world. Symbols are defined in terms of their syntax and the operations on those symbols. Furthermore, symbols are specific representations that permit binding to a value (filler) that may be variable or constant. Furthermore, the same variable may occur in several places in a formula or sequence of formulae. In language, it is represented by the problem of assigning pronouns to their referred objects. Most importantly, symbolic reasoning based on logic offers the prospect of provability by virtue of its transparency.

In a connectionist system, different segments of a formula are represented independently within a network. Connectionism is based on neural networks that can be modeled by differential equations—they are based on finer grained microfeatures than symbols; that is, they are subsymbolic, intermediate between neural foundations and cognitive systems (Smolensky, 1988). Neural networks learn from example by generalizing from input–output pairings of the training data. Knowledge is represented as numerical weights. The neural network is commonly treated as a black box in which its internal mechanism is hidden from analysis. Such neural networks do not offer transparency in that knowledge and inferencing are distributed within a network as a set of microfeatures that by themselves are not readily analyzable—it is the interrelationships between these entities that are important. Subsymbolicism implies that connectionist processing involves microfeatures that are elements distributed through the network—they are not semantically interpretable into properties of the world unless constituted with other microfeatures into symbols through patterns of activation. Higher level cognition involves symbolic processing whereby cognition emerges from lower (subsymbolic) level of neurons and neural assemblies (Fodor and Pylyshyn, 1988). The neural network's set of weights cooperate in a shared subsymbolic representation. The symbol then emerges as a collective cooperation between the distributed set of neurons. This form of representation is analogous to a hologram. Neural networks process truth values of instances to variables from which they learn a model theory (Komendantskaya, 2009). They offer the ability to learn from training examples through adaptation of their connection weights. Connectionism can determine the effect of an input on the output by tracking the error terms in each step of learning. The relative contributions of each input on output errors can thus be determined over time. The chief advantage of neural networks lies in their learning ability.

Rather than adding fuel to the fires of conflict that have been kept plenty-stoked for decades, I shall explore the narrow area of the peace-makers—symbolic connectionism (Wermter and Sun, 2000). Symbolic connectionism offers the prospect of combining the expressiveness of symbolic processing with the adaptability of connectionism. The key factor is in matching two different forms of representation of objects and events (referents) in the world. I believe that it is through these attempts to hybridize symbolic processing and neural networks that insights into cognition, both human and manufactured, may be gained. Furthermore, in a rather naive sense, the notion that the neural substrate implements symbolic processing in the brain is an obvious and natural one. In this view, symbolic connectionism implements a form of combined bottom-up (connectionist) and top-down (symbolic) processing that compensate for the disadvantages of each (Minsky, 1991). Or more positively, this reinforces the procedural strengths of symbolic processing with the adaptiveness of connectionist processing. Structured neural networks resemble semantic networks in representing knowledge as structures with relations between them. The activity level of each node/neuron constitutes the amount of evidence for the symbol. There is a natural mapping between goal-driven symbolic representations and subsymbolic neural computations (Polk et al., 2002). Attractor networks possess attractors as stable discrete states in a distributed network. Production rules are asymmetric associations between symbols that map onto excitatory or inhibitory connections between attractors representing conjunctions between states, possible actions, and subgoals. This emulates the role of the dorsolateral prefrontal cortex in problem solving which represents subgoals.

Symbolic methods assume that meaning is implicit in the relations between abstract symbols. Such abstract symbols are ungrounded in that they are not associated with perception–action events in the world. In this view, abstract symbols such as words create meaning through the conjunction of relations to other abstract symbols. This may be quantified by a vector encoding the many co-occurrences of symbol pairs in k-dimensional space (nominally $k \sim 300$–400). Searle's Chinese room argument suggests that this is nonsense (Searle, 1980). Human cognition is fundamentally rooted in action-based behavior that is constrained and, indeed, dictated by the situation in the real world including the body of the agent (affordances). Furthermore, it has been shown experimentally that symbol grounding to referents in the real world must be implemented in principle (Glenberg and Robertson, 2000). Human cognition is consistent with meaning being derived from indexing arbitrary symbols (words) to real perception–action objects or events in the world (indexical hypothesis). The problem is how to discriminate between the variety of potential real-world referents in the world to which a symbol should be mapped. The only solution is to deny the utility of abstract symbols and replace them with perceptual symbols that are indexed directly to affordances. Meaning is inherent in perceptual experiences of the world and associated sets of bodily actions (affordances) applicable to the real-world situation. The relation between perceptions of the environment and actions in the environment may be modeled effectively through stimulus–response rules that may be learned neurally.

From these insights emerge symbolic connectionism. The chief advantage of symbolic connectionism is that it offers the prospect of combining a priori knowledge with new empirical knowledge.

11.2 It is a question of language

One of the earliest neural network models to demonstrate symbolic-type processing was NETtalk (Sejnowski and Rosenberg, 1987). It was a multilayer neural network system that was trained to convert English text into speech. It accepted strings of letters and spaces corresponding to English text as input and outputted a string of spoken words. The NETtalk architecture comprised 203 input neurons, 80 hidden neurons, and 26 output neurons. Text-to-speech requires transforming letter strings into phoneme strings. This process is complicated by the fact that English exhibits a high degree of irregular spelling. A seven-letter window was encoded into the input layer with each letter clustered into one of 29 input nodes. The central (fourth) letter yielded the desired phoneme output with the flanking letters providing context. Each one of the 26 output nodes encoded one phoneme associated with each letter. Text was fed into the input layer, while phonemes were extracted from the output layer. A backpropagation learning algorithm was used (the pocket algorithm that uses both positive and negative reinforcement may be used in place of the backpropagation algorithm.). It learned consonants and vowels from 1024 words after undergoing a phase of babbling similar to human infants. NETtalk formed internal representations distributed through groups of neurons. Many different combinations of weights yield the same performance indicating a high degree of redundancy, the basis of graceful degradation. NETtalk yielded an approximately 80% successful classification rate. NETtalk learned English as if it followed grammatical rules without the use of any grammatical rules.

This was enabled by the feature detection abilities of the hidden layer to extract such regularities (Tryon, 1993). More remarkably, it demonstrated some of the commonly observed errors in language learning in humans.

Connectionist systems have been used to learn the grammar of past tenses of English verbs including irregular ones and output the appropriate phonemic representations (Rummelhart and McClelland, 1986). Recurrent neural networks by virtue of their recurrent links are able to learn internal representations of temporal sequences (i.e., language) (Elman, 1990). Because of the nature of phonemes in language, a recurrent neural network can predict vowels from the preceding consonant but cannot reliably predict consonants from the preceding vowel. Words are not natural categories as there is no consistent distinction between words, compound words, and word phrases. This makes learning by example a natural approach in which the concept of "word" and their temporal sequences in sentences emerges through generalization. This overcomes a major limitation of symbolic approaches. However, the distinction between noun and verb is clear, and in many languages such as English, word order is constrained which may be defined in terms of relative frequency. Such generalizations may be encoded as internal representations over the hidden neurons, including nouns and verbs with nouns being followed by verbs. Discrete time-recurrent neural networks have been trained to classify strings of a regular language, and rules defining the learned grammar have been extracted from the network (Omlin and Giles, 1996; Wermter et al., 1996). Recurrent neural networks have been used to classify sequences of words into syntactic categories of noun, verb, adverb, adjective, preposition, determinant, or pronoun (Wermter, 2000). These findings suggest that linguistic rules are approximations to neural activation patterns that form the basis of causal processes in language. The synaptic weights reflect statistical properties of the training data similar to Bayesian inference.

Reactions to similar deployments of symbolic connectionism to language processing have been robustly defensive. Some responses have been emphatic that only symbol processing offers the appropriate representational structure for language processing (and indeed, for general reasoning and higher level cognition—this is the physical symbol system hypothesis (Newell, 1980; Pylyshyn, 1980)). Furthermore, symbol processing is characterized by its capacity for concatenation into compound expressions—this is the "language of thought" hypothesis. It was also contested that connectionist methods are limited in their capacity for language processing as they are capable only of stimulus–response associative modeling and symbolic rules are necessary for natural language (Pinker and Prince, 1988; Lachter and Bever, 1988). Criticisms based on the notion that connectionist systems cannot implement symbolic rules have been rendered invalid—simple neural networks can generate linguistic representations (Seidenberg, 1994). The fact remains that serial cognitive processes in human cognition are limited to around 100 steps at neural speeds. Furthermore, hidden Markov models have become dominant in language processing, particularly speech processing (Hinton, 1990). The connectionist architecture can represent probabilities and therefore implement hidden Markov models (Bengio and Frasconi, 1996; Trentin and Gori, 2003). The alpha-net is a recurrent neural network implementation of the hidden Markov model (Bridle, 1990). The forward (alpha) part of the Baum–Welch estimation maximization algorithm may be implemented as a recurrent neural network through nonlinear weighted summation. The alpha algorithm computes the sequences of states of a model, i.e., $\frac{\partial J}{\partial a_{ij}}$, where $J = \log P$, P = network output probability, and a_{ij} = forward weights. The backpropagation-through-time algorithm has a similar form to the backward (beta) pass of the Baum–Welch algorithm. The beta algorithm computes observation likelihood functions given the model, i.e., $\frac{\partial J}{\partial b_{ij}}$, where b_{ij} = backward weights. Furthermore, symbolic Markov sequences can be modeled by recurrent neural networks trained by an extended Kalman filter that provides continuous learning (Tino et al., 2004). These examples indicate that connectionist systems are capable of implementing language processing, that epitome of symbolicism. More generally, the universal Turing machine has been shown to be implementable on recurrent neural nets of sigmoid neurons (Siegelmann and Sontag, 1995). More precisely, any recursively computable partial function computable by a Turing machine can be implemented by such a network of 886 neurons. This essentially proves that the neural network can implement any program including any logic program like Prolog implementations of symbolic AI.

11.3 Localist symbolic connectionism

Localist representations correlate one concept with a specific individual or group of neurons (Feldman et al., 1988). The number of hidden nodes should equal or exceed the number of concepts to be stored. An example of a localist connectionist inference system is the connectionist realization of a structured semantic memory network (Shastri, 1988). Simple neuron-like elements encode concepts and their properties that are interconnected through inheritance relationships. The semantic network encodes a hierarchy of concepts through "is-a" links in which lower nodes inherit properties from higher nodes. Rapid inferencing is based on spreading activation to perform partial and best matching computations. An example of a semantic network-type system is the artificial non-monotonic neural network comprising a semantic network of "is-a" inheritance links and a neural network (Boutsinas and Vrahatis, 2001). The semantic network nodes comprised sets of positive and negative examples. After training the neural network, the system behaves as if it follows rules. Furthermore, after training, a refined set of rules can be extracted. Extracting logic rules from hidden and output neurons requires analysis of the weights of each neuron: antecedent-consequent rules are expressed locally to the neuron and then aggregated. The rule extraction algorithm converts neurons and connection weights into semantic network nodes and inheritance links with positive and negative relations. A dual system of structured neural networks—short-term semantic network memory and long-term neural memory—capable of high-level inferencing with frames or scripts may be modeled by symbolic connectionism (Dyer, 1990). Each frame possesses a number of roles which may be bound to fillers. The frames are stored in a neural network of nodes. Relations between the concepts are represented by weighted connections between nodes. Connection weights were encoded as the probability that the two nodes are active. Variable binding was handled by using unique signature association patterns to bind to concepts (Lange and Dyer, 1989). Each concept had a signature node that outputs its signature in terms of its activity. The symbols began as random patterns of activity. The signatures are integrated into the semantic network taking the role of symbolic backpointers. The symbols are recirculated through the network by learning the appropriate microfeatures (Dyer et al., 1992). Inferencing proceeds through spreading activation.

Rather than being constrained by the semantic network architecture, a typical expert system comprises a working memory, a knowledge base of rules, and an inference engine. Neural networks on the other hand represent knowledge in a distributed fashion (Pao and Sobajic, 1991). Neural expert systems combine both (Sima, 1995). MACIE is a connectionist expert system that used positive weights for reinforcement and negative weights for inhibition trained to generate simple if-then-else rules (Gallant, 1988). Each node had a confidence value to determine its truth value dependent on the weights, thereby establishing a mapping mechanism between the neural network and the symbolic rules:

$$p(y_i) = \frac{\sum_k w_{ik} p(y_i)}{\sum_k |w_{ik}|} \tag{11.1}$$

where y_i = neuron output.

KBANN (knowledge-based artificial neural network) and KCNN (knowledge-based conceptual neural network) are similar neural networks from which rules may be extracted (Fu, 1995; Towell and Shavlik, 1994). They constitute an initial knowledge base of hierarchically structured domain-specific PROLOG-like Horn clauses of the form: "if p_x and p_y and $\sim p_u$ and $\sim p_v$... then q (or $\sim q$)" where p = condition and q = conclusion. This constitutes prior knowledge. This hierarchical set of rules determines the topology and weights of the neural network. It is thus a localist network in which input neurons represent antecedents and output neurons represent consequents, sandwiching hidden neurons that represent conjunctions. The output responses of the neurons are initialized either to +1 or −1 determined by the Boolean logic of the rules—this is implemented through the sigmoid function with a steep near-signum response. Given the binary output alphabet, this describes a finite-state machine. Conjunctive rules are imported into the network with the consequent neuron bias adjusted to $\varphi = \left(n - \frac{1}{2}\right)w$, where n = number of positive antecedents and w = initial equal weight on each positive antecedent ($-w$ for all negated antecedents). Disjunctive rules are split into multiple rules with the same consequent and handled similarly. Any connection that is not involved in the rule set is initialized to zero, $w_{ij} = 0$. The neural network is then trained using a set of examples and a standard neural learning algorithm such as backpropagation or a variant such as the temporal backpropagation algorithm (Civelek-Aplasalan and Swigger, 1996) to refine the rules. The neural logic network performed logical inferencing through supervised clustering and matching (SCM) rather than gradient descent (Tan and Teow, 1997). Competitive activation of SCM resembles the adaptive resonance theory (ART) model. INSS is an alternative that used the cascade-correlation learning algorithm to add hidden neurons

(Osorio and Amy, 1999). TopGen is an extension to KBANN that dynamically adds hidden OR-node neurons to permit additional new antecedent-consequent rules to reduce false negatives (Opitz and Shavlik, 1995).

Rule extraction involves attempting to map a neural network to a set of rules (Tickle et al., 1998). There are two approaches to rule extraction from neural networks: decompositional and pedagogical (Andrews et al., 1995). The decompositional approach attempts to find expressions for hidden and output neurons with respect to their inputs. This involves discretization and pruning of the network followed by a search on the inputs to all neurons. The rules are not in general exact as the network's behavior can only be approximated by rules. The pedagogical approach constructs rules by sampling the trained neural network's responses to different inputs. This generates examples for a symbolic learning algorithm. An early example of such a symbolic learning system involved searching a hypothesis (version) space subject to constraints imposed by the training examples (Mitchell, 1982). Although the pedagogical approach is computationally more tractable than the decompositional approach, the rules generated are even more approximate. Connectionist inductive learning and logic programming (CIL^2P) algorithm is an example of a pedagogical approach combined with pruning of inputs rather than weights to reduce the size of the search space (D'Avila Garcez et al., 2001). One of the simplest decompositional rule extraction algorithms is the subset method that adopts a breadth-first search for subsets of weights exceeding the bias of a neuron. If the weights exceed the threshold to fire the neuron, a rule is written. For example, consider inputs B, C, D, and E feeding weights of 0.3, 0.3, 0.3, and −0.3 into a hidden node A with a bias of 0.5. The extracted rules would then be:

If B, C and $\sim E$ then A
If B, D and $\sim E$ then A
If C, D and $\sim E$ then A
If B, C and D then A

The exhaustive subset rule is limited to small networks, but branch-and-bound versions exist. The rules created however are generally inferior in performance to the underlying trained neural network.

RuleNet is a three-layer neural network with an input, hidden, and output layer that learns string-to-string mappings. The weights from the input to hidden units encode the condition part of the rule. The connectionist scientist game induces hypotheses from observations until a hypothesis explains the observations correctly. RULEX is another algorithm for rule extraction from a trained neural network (Andrews and Geva, 2002). The knowledgetron (KT) algorithm derives production rules from knowledge-based neural nets with concept attributes that are distinguished into positive attributes (pos-atts that are necessary) with positive weights and negative attributes (neg-atts that must not be present) with negative weights (Fu, 1992, 1994, 1999). For each hidden and output neuron, KT searches for combinations of pos-atts whose summed weight exceeds the threshold; for each combination of pos-atts, KT forms a confirming rule q coupled with neg-atts to strengthen the combination. To form a disconfirming rule $\sim q$, KT searches for combinations of neg-atts and then uses negated pos-atts to strengthen the combination. The *M*-of-*N* rule extracts rules from the neural network by searching for antecedents of the form "if (*M* of the following *N* antecedents are true) then..." (Towell and Shavlik, 1993; Setiono, 2000). If $N = M$, purely conjunctive rules result, and if $M = 1$, disjunctive rules result. For example, the XOR rule can be expressed as "If (exactly 1 of the 2 inputs is true) then odd parity, else even parity." Rule extraction algorithms can be applied to recurrent neural networks (Giles and Omlin, 1994; Jacobsson, 2005). Alternatively, a self-organizing map has been used to extract natural language knowledge from a recurrent neural network (Bianco et al., 2000). Clustering of the outputs of the recurrent neurons was achieved so that each of the recurrent network outputs was presented as input to the self-organizing map. It competitively clustered patterns with similar characteristics from positive and negative examples.

Once rules have been extracted, a clustering algorithm such as the *k*-means algorithm selects groups of links that have similar weights, averages them, and assigns that average to all weights of that class. The DOLCE (dynamic online clustering and state extraction) algorithm involves using an adaptive clustering algorithm (such as a Gaussian mixture model) to partition and model the hidden states of a trained recurrent neural network (Das and Mozer, 1998). Low link weights are then eliminated through pruning. One such pruning algorithm is the optimal brain damage algorithm, which shrinks neural networks into more compact form. Full pruning involves iteratively removing the lowest weighted links and retraining as long as the network performance deteriorates within an acceptable level. Once pruned, the backpropagation algorithm is then applied to retrain the thresholds of the hidden and output neurons while freezing the weights. Rules are created by translating the bias and incoming weights of all hidden and output neurons into a rule with weighted antecedents. Although the learned rules are more complex than the original rules, they are superior in performance. They may be simplified by analyzing the possible combinations of antecedents that can exceed the threshold, resulting in more but simpler rules. *M*-of-*N* rule extraction yields superior rules to the C4.5 symbolic learning method (successor to ID3 decision tree learning algorithm (Quinlan, 1986)).

The REANN (rule extraction from artificial neural networks) is a more recent method (Kamruzzaman and Islam, 2006; Kamruzzaman and Sarkar, 2011). While training the neural network architecture using the backpropagation algorithm, it uses a constructive algorithm to determine the number of hidden nodes required. The backpropagation algorithm is used to train the initial network with one hidden node until the error is near constant. If the error is too large, another hidden node is added and the process repeated until the constant error becomes sufficiently small. This is followed by pruning of the network to remove redundant nodes. Pruning algorithms are applied to neural networks that are larger than necessary for the task (Reed, 1993). It prevents overfitting that occurs when the number of weights exceeds the number of training examples by removing unnecessary links. The brute force method is to set a weight to zero and observe the error. If the error is too great, the weight is restored, but if it is acceptable, it is eliminated. This is repeated for every weight and every training pattern imposing a computational complexity $O(mw^2)$, where m = number of training patterns and w = number of weights. Alternatively, it is possible to add a penalty cost or weight decay term (such as the sum of squared weights) to the error function so that the backpropagation algorithm drives weights to zero during training. This ensures that unnecessary connections with low weights are eliminated. The network is then retrained. The outputs of the hidden nodes are then discretized. A clustering algorithm is used to group similar hidden nodes whose outputs are changing, while constant output hidden nodes are frozen. Finally, the input–output rules are extracted from the input–output response of the hidden nodes using the REx algorithm. This algorithm extracts the rules, clusters them, and prunes them to remove redundant or more specific rules.

It has been suggested that discretization of networks to extract rules impairs their generalization capability (Taha and Ghosh, 1999). In fact, an approach for deriving antecedent-consequent rule strength p_{ij} from network weights has been proffered (Yoon et al., 1994):

$$p_{ij} = \frac{\sum_{k=0}^{n} w_{ik} w_{jk}}{\sum_{i=0}^{m} \left| \sum_{k=0}^{n} w_{ik} w_{jk} \right|} \tag{11.2}$$

where w_{ik} = input-hidden node weights and w_{jk} = hidden-output node weights.

KBANN has a fixed network topology: it is possible to add further knowledge to prior knowledge through a constructive technique by searching for hyperplanes (Fletcher and Obradovic, 1993). KT, subset, *M*-of-*N*, and REx extraction will only work on knowledge-based networks created from symbolic rules and cannot work on classical neural networks. Furthermore, there is no provision for handling uncertainty. However, a nonmonotonic reasoning framework implemented directly in symmetric connectionist networks (such as Hopfield and Boltzmann networks) has been demonstrated (Pinkas, 1995). Symmetric networks implement search for their minimum energy states. They learn representations of logic propositions from examples. The extended logic can accommodate uncertainty by employing assumptions about beliefs that are quantified with strength measures (penalties). Nonmonotonic reasoning can jump to conclusions based on evidence but later retract those conclusions if new contradictory evidence is forthcoming. The key mapping mechanism between connectionist energy and logical inferencing is through ranking functions—these ranking functions are computed by summing penalties for the assumptions of each logical assertion. Genetic algorithms have also been applied to rule extraction (Markowska-Kaczmar and Wnuk-Lipinski, 2004). In GenPar, each if-then rule is hierarchically encoded into a genetic algorithm similar to a classifier. They are evolved through crossover and mutation operators according to a fitness function that incorporates accuracy and complexity measures to encourage fidelity and comprehensibility.

There have been attempts to allow neural networks to learn from fewer examples by exploiting previously encoded knowledge (Mitchell and Thrun, 1992). The new exemplar is explained in terms of prior knowledge forming an explanation-based neural network (EBNN) using extracted symbolic rules. Inductive learning of an evaluation function $Q(s,a)$ estimates the expected cumulative rewards R for an action from a the initial state of the world s. Analytical learning reduces the training set (s,a) by estimating the slope of the Q-function for each (s,a) using a prior trained action model $M{:}s \rightarrow s'$:

$$\nabla Q(s,a) = \nabla R = \frac{\partial M(s)}{\partial s} \tag{11.3}$$

A discrete symbols layer may be regarded as characteristic of conscious planning emerging from a continuous underlying unconscious neural process layer—such an architecture has been modeled through PATON (Omori et al., 1999). An attention system generates a sequence of attention vectors that control inputs to the neural layer generating neural patterns and their corresponding symbols. Similarity coding between two neural excitation patterns corresponding to two different events in the outside world is accomplished by a distance measure between the two vectors. Logical inferencing can emerge from the information dynamics of neural processing in which the neural associations implement a form of nonmonotonic inferencing (Balkenius and Gardenfors, 1991). Symbolic connectionist systems can implement sensorimotor schemas of stereotypical motor behaviors (Shastri et al., 1997a, 1997b). These reactive schemas can be combined to represent complex behaviors. Schemas can also represent state space searches for path planning between initial and final states as spreading activation (Garagnani et al., 2002). A schema is a nonmonotonic inference mechanism defined by a vector $(\alpha_1, \ldots, \alpha_n)$ that is generated by a neural activity pattern $(x_1, \ldots, x_n)$ (Gardenfors, 2005; Blutner, 2004). Schemas (frames or scripts) may represent objects or scenarios with default assumptions constructed from microfeatures. A schema encodes an initial state (conditions), an action, and a goal state (consequences), representing episodic memory of past events. These constitute e-facts which are specific instances of t-facts, representing a statistical culmination of past events (prior probabilities). The focal clusters of SHRUTI represent schemas with inferencing implemented as the synchronous firing activity between focal clusters. The links that propagate such rhythmic activity encode relational rules. Fast neural dynamics underlies the emergence of slow symbolic inferences. Furthermore, the conjunction of two schemas α and β is determined by temporal synchroneity of the two neural activity patterns. However, complement and disjunction require symbolic representation, indicating the importance of both levels of representation. Spiking neurons in biological brains exhibit dynamic temporal binding—despite slow neural propagation, neural inferencing is rapid. There is evidence of neural synchronization through temporally coincident oscillations in the cerebral cortex (Bostrom, 1996). For instance, representations for visual recognition of an object ("what" pathway in the temporal cortex) and visual localization of an object ("where" pathway in the parietal cortex) for the same object must be associated with each other. Neural activity is defined by a fixed oscillation period ($\sim$10 ms in biological brains) and a pulse width (much less than the oscillation period). Phase-sensitive neurons allow the implementation of computation cycles in neural excitation (Shastri and Ajjaganadde, 1993). Variable binding is an essential feature for symbolic connectionist systems. Consider a production rule defining an antecedent and a consequent with a correspondence between the arguments of the predicate, e.g., (i) $\forall x,y,z[\text{give}(x,y,z) \rightarrow \text{own}(y,z)]$;

(ii) $\forall u,v[\text{own}(u,v) \rightarrow \text{can-sell}(u,v)]$; and (iii) $\forall x,y[\text{buy}(x,y) \rightarrow \text{own}(x,y)]$, where x = giver, y = recipient, z = object, u = seller, and v = object. The predicates form "is-a" relationships between themselves and may be implemented in neural networks. In SHRUTI, each concept C in the "is-a" hierarchy is encoded by a cluster of neurons. A "give" link is established between the arguments "recipient" and "object," while an "own" link is established between arguments "owner" and "object." Rules are then interconnection patterns that direct the propagation of rhythmic neural activity. Transient propagation of such rhythmic activity occurs between focal clusters with synchronous firing instigating dynamic binding. This synchronous firing of variable neurons with constant neurons corresponds to temporal dynamic binding between them (Bader and Hitzler, 2005). Thus, a variable x of the predicate give(x) is bound to an entity d if the nodes representing them fire during the same time period T when predicate p is active. In this fashion, neural activity patterns can be bound reflecting their symbolic representations.

11.4 Distributed symbolic connectionism

Localist connectionist representations are limited in capacity—they are the equivalent of the "grandmother" neuron that is physiologically implausible. Distributed representations offer advantages including requiring fewer neurons and much less memory than localist representations by virtue of network compression through the hidden nodes (Sharkey, 1991). Furthermore, localist connectionist systems are subject to the criticism that they are merely implementations of symbolic approaches. It has been questioned whether indeed the human brain has any true modularity at all as local brain damage can yield global if subtle effects, particularly with respect to "downstream" processing (Farah, 1994). Apparent modularity may result from differential weighting of different sensorimotor modality-specific knowledge rather than functionally modular-specific knowledge. In any case, the local connectionist approach is not biologically plausible. In a distributed representation, each neuron is used in multiple concepts, and multiple neurons are used to represent a single concept.

Touretsky's BoltzCONS system is a distributed connectionist system that creates and manipulates symbol structures dynamically (Touretsky, 1990). The symbol structures comprised linked lists, which can implement trees and stacks (such as parse trees) but implemented in a distributed network acting as an associative memory without the need for memory addresses. Associative memories store patterns in such a fashion that stored fragments are distributed through the network and can be reconstructed with partial inputs. The BoltzCONS architecture comprises a central memory containing sets of triples to encode graph structures. Triples of symbols are adopted to serve as cells of a linked list. Triples are often used to encode semantic networks such that triple (A R C) encodes a link of type R from symbol A to symbol C. A production rule may be constructed from two triples comprising the antecedent that is matched to working memory, with consequents comprising commands to add or delete triples from working memory. Variable binding is essential to human cognition, e.g., dog(*X*) →hairy(*X*) & barks(*X*), but they are a major source of difficulty in symbolic neural nets (Touretsky and Hinton, 1988; Browne and Sun, 2001). This may be illustrated by two simple example production rule triples:

Rule 1: $(F\ A\ B)\ (F\ C\ D) \rightarrow +(G\ A\ B) + (P\ D\ Q) - (F\ C\ B)$

If triples $(F\,A\,B)$ and $(F\,C\,D)$ are present in the antecedent, then add triples $(G\,A\,B)$ and $(P\ D\ Q)$ deleting $(F\ C\ D)$.

Rule 2: $({*x}\ A\ B)\ ({*x}\ C\ D) \rightarrow +(G\ {*x}\ P) - ({*x}\ R\ {*x})$

Variable $*x$ must be bound appropriately, so if triples $(F\ A\ B)$ and $(F\ C\ D)$ are present, $*x$ is bound to F, so triple $(G\ F\ P)$ is added and $(F\ R\ F)$ deleted. Larger tuples may be employed for more complex trees. Transitions between states can be represented through associations that can naturally represent stimulus–response rules. Associative memory was implemented on a Boltzmann machine that searches for matching rules using simulated annealing. Associated vector pairs may be learned using Hebb's rule, allowing subsequent retrieval based on a similarity measure between vectors x and x' combining correlation and Hamming distance as (Wichert, 2005):

$$s(x, x'_i) = a\sum_{i=1}^{n} x_j x'_j - b|x' - x| \tag{11.4}$$

Smolensky's (1990) tensor product binding method addresses the problem of structured representations and value/variable bindings. Structured objects such as frames S may be reduced to a number of roles R that may be filled with values F—these form sets of pairs. Value/variable pairs (F/R) are represented as neuronal activity that computes a product of a feature of a variable and a feature of its value. Neural activity states form the elements of a vector that may be regarded as a symbol. Thus, the connectionist representation of symbol structures is a mapping onto a vector space. This allows representation of conjunctions of symbols as vectors bound to other vectors through additive superposition. Fillers are bound to roles by forming the tensor product of their vectors. An n-dimensional vector representing an item f may be bound to an m-dimensional vector representing a role r through the outer product, the nm-dimensional vector $b = f.r$. This constitutes a tensor of rank 2, generating a square matrix of activations. It thus combines lexical symbols with their syntactic roles through an outer product learning mechanism. The network's neuron performs variable binding through the tensor product of the weighted inputs I:

$$b_{ij} = \sum_j w_j \sum_i I_{ji} \tag{11.5}$$

The binding units learn through the Hebb or Widrow–Hoff rule by correlating between a pair of role and filler neurons. This approach can be extended to recursive representations through higher order tensors—rank 3 representing a cube of activation $(u.v.w)$, rank 4 representing a hypercube of activation $(t.u.v.w)$, etc. The primary problem is that deep embedding causes rapid tensor product growth.

Plate's (1995) holographic reduced representations encode tree-structured objects into vectors. Circular convolution was used to associate symbols or frames represented by vectors. Pairs of associated vectors are stored in convolution–correlation memories. The two vectors are encoded into a memory trace matrix $I \times I \rightarrow T$, representing a generalized multiplication operation. Encoding is a circular convolution with the trace representing the sum of convolved pairs. Frames may be represented through convolution encoding. The frame comprises a label and a set of roles, each represented by a vector. The sum of the label of the frame and its roles may be convolved with their fillers to implement variable binding. Convolution encoding can also represent hierarchical structures. The most effective means for computing convolution is the fast Fourier transform. Convolution may be implemented in a neural network.

Pollack's (1990) RAAM (recursive autoassociative memory) is a fully distributed approach to symbolic connectionist representation. It has the same architecture as a standard three-layer feedforward network with two layers of interconnecting weights, one input to and the other output from the hidden layer. It employs the standard backpropagation algorithm for learning a compact representation encoded within the hidden nodes. It can encode/decode sequential data structures such as symbolic trees in fixed width patterns using a sequential stack with PUSH and POP functions. Trees are represented in the single layer of hidden nodes and are decoded cyclically at the output. The difference between RAAM and other neural nets lies in modes of presentation of input patterns and the decoding. For example, consider a binary tree: ((A B) (C D)). The input space is partitioned into n sections with k units per partition, where n = tree valency (=2 in this example). The output vector is identical to the input vector both with nk neurons, where k = number of hidden neurons forming a nk–k–nk network. First, A and B are presented in the two vector partitions at the input and autoassociated at the output using the backpropagation algorithm. The hidden neuron states are stored on a stack as $R1$. Secondly, C and D are presented at the input and similarly autoassociated at the output. The hidden neuron states are popped onto the stack as $R2$. $R1$ and $R2$ are then presented as input and autoassociated similarly. The resulting hidden neuron state $R3$ thus represents the total tree that can be decoded by presenting it directly into the hidden units—it will output $R1$ and $R2$. These are then presented to decode the original outputs. Thus, RAAM can encode and decode recursive structures. It was developed to compress and store words encoded in syntactic parse trees—RAAM has been used to construct distributed representations of syntactically structured sentence trees (Chalmers, 1990). The tree is recursively encoded from its terminal elements. This approach clearly demonstrates that symbolic tree structures can be encoded in a distributed fashion within a neural network.

11.5 Symbolic connectionism in biological models

CONSYDERR combines local and distributed architectures, whereby a localist representation is adopted for the first level (CL) and then a distributed architecture is used for the second level (CD) (Sun, 1993). The first level represents concepts as condition–action declarative rules in the form of an acyclic directed graph connecting nodes. These concepts are mapped to the distributed microfeatures of a neural network in the second level, representing procedural knowledge. They form distributed rules and are also represented by an acyclic directed graph. The first-level rules are executed first, which activates features in the second level. Then, the distributed rules are executed, which activate rule concepts of the first level with different strengths. CONSYDERR has similarities to case-based reasoning (Sun, 1992). Neurules is another approach that integrates case-based rules with the adaline neuron (Hatzilygeroudis and Prentzas, 2004a,b). The two-layer CLARION architecture is a further development on CONSYDDER that includes Q-learning implemented through backpropagation on the neural network (Sun and Peterson, 1998). The Q-learning algorithm is given by (Sun et al., 2007):

$$e(t) = \eta(r - Q(x, a)) \tag{11.6}$$

where η = learning rate and r = reward. It has been claimed that CLARION exhibits some of the characteristics of human consciousness (Sun, 1997). Symbolic declarative knowledge is accessible to consciousness, while procedural knowledge (motor skills) is not, illustrated in the tragic disease of Korsakoff's syndrome in which episodic memory (from which semantic memory is derived, both comprising declarative memory with similar encoding) may be impaired but motor memory is unaffected.

Motor skill encoding has long been of interest in robotics. A rule-based system may be employed to train cerebellar model articulation controller (CMAC) neural networks how to accomplish tasks such as controlling a robotic manipulator by observing rule-based task execution (Handelman et al., 1990). An execution monitor continually monitored the neural network performance and reengaged the expert system when it deviated from the desired behavior. The expert system implemented rule following, while the neural network offered generalization capabilities in a hierarchical configuration. This emulates human motor skill learning: it evolves from declarative mechanisms that require cognitive effort to reflexive mechanisms that are automatic once the skills are learned. This models associative learning of input–output vector pairs of sensorimotor skills.

11.6 Neurofuzzy systems

Fuzzy logic provides a natural bridge between first-order logic and neural networks, and indeed fuzzy-neural systems seem to have flourished perhaps more than other approaches to symbolic connectionism. There are several fuzzy variants on symbolic connectionism (Kasabov, 1996). Fuzzy logic is based on fuzzy if-then linguistic rules, representing prior knowledge that may be subject to modification through learning. The integration of fuzzy systems into neural networks offers some of the advantages of both by hybridizing subsymbolic and symbolic processing (Bezdek, 1993). Fuzzy logic offers a symbolic representation of syntactic rules, while neurons offer the ability to compute logical inferences with the numerical membership function providing the interface. The fuzzy rule defines in general a nonlinear mapping involving linguistic variables that encapsulate localized process knowledge. It has been shown that fuzzy inference systems and radial basis function networks are functionally equivalent (Jang and Sun, 1993). Fuzzy neural networks (FNNs) represent a generalization of the McCulloch–Pitts neuron. They may be classified into different types (Buckley and Hayashi, 1994): (i) FNN1 has real inputs but fuzzy weights; (ii) FNN2 has fuzzy inputs but real weights; and (iii) FNN3 has both fuzzy inputs and fuzzy weights.

Fuzzy sets are also often used in neural networks—neurofuzzy networks—in which the first layer represents normal input variables, the last layer represents normal output variables, and the hidden layers represent fuzzy rules. The connection weights are fuzzy. The antecedent and consequent of a fuzzy rule are encoded directly into the initial weight of the neural network. Each neuron represents a fuzzy membership function, while each link represents the weight of the fuzzy rule. Membership functions express the prior linguistic rules and may be of any shape. If the membership function is a Gaussian, it may have the same variance as a receptive field unit:

$$y = \mu(x) = e^{-\left((x-c)^2/2\sigma^2\right)} \tag{11.7}$$

where c = center (mean) of membership function and σ = width (variance) of membership function.

The set of fuzzy rules and their membership functions constitute a knowledge base. The fuzzy sets are converted as fuzzy connection weights with learning implemented by the neural network. Once the shape of the membership function is fixed, a neural network can optimize the parameters by gradient descent based on the network's predictions (though learning the membership function is possible requiring only the number of fuzzy rules to be encoded (Figueiredo and Gomide, 1999)). The neural network uses gradient descent to tune the membership function parameters that define its shape (width and central position); that is, it alters the fuzzy symbolic representation. The FNN may be defined by the function:

$$y_i = f(W, g, x) = \sum_{j=1}^{n} w_{ij} g\left(\sum_{k=1}^{m} w_{jk}x_k + w_{j0}\right) + w_{i0} \tag{11.8}$$

where W = weight vector of weights connecting jth hidden unit to inputs and ith output to hidden units, $g(\cdot)$ = sigmoidal transfer function, and x_k = inputs. The fuzzy inference system with a Gaussian membership function is a universal approximator according to the Stone–Weierstrass theorem (Wang and Mendel, 1992). The radial basis function network uses n local receptive fields to perform network mapping between inputs and outputs:

$$R_i(x) = R_i\left(|x - c_i|/\sigma_i^2\right) \tag{11.9}$$

The receptive field function is typically a Gaussian function with maximum response at the center of the receptive field of width σ:

$$R_i(x) = \mathrm{e}^{-|x-c_i|^2/\sigma_i^2} \tag{11.10}$$

The output is the sum of weighted input values of each receptive field function:

$$y = f(x) = \sum_{i=1}^{n} w_i R_i(x) \tag{11.11}$$

This is similar to an AND-OR fuzzy operation. Weight update is given by:

$$w_i(t) = w_i(t-1) + \eta_i(x(t) - w_i(t-1)) \tag{11.12}$$

To minimize the error between the desired output and the network output, self-organization can find c_i and σ_i and adaline or least means squares can find f_i. The Kohonen self-organizing map algorithm, which adopts the winner-takes-all algorithm, may be used to tune the membership function parameters, namely width and center. The function center is determined by:

$$|x - W_i| = \min|x - W_j| \tag{11.13}$$

where W_j = winner's weight vector defining the function center.

Weight update is given by:

$$W_i(t+1) = W_i(t) + \eta_i(t)h_{ij}(t)(x(t) - W_i(t)) \tag{11.14}$$

where $h_{ij}(t) = \exp\left(-\frac{d_{ij}^2}{\sigma^2(t)}\right)$ = neighborhood function, $d_{ij}(t) = |W_i - W_j|$ = distance between nodes i and j, $\sigma(t)$ = decreasing width, and $\eta_i(t)$ = decreasing learning parameter. The width of the membership function may be found using the N-nearest neighbors algorithm by minimizing the objective function:

$$E = \frac{1}{2}\sum_{i=1}^{n}\left(\left(\frac{d_{ij}}{\sigma_i}\right)^2 - r\right)^2 \tag{11.15}$$

where r = overlap parameter.

The Kohonen map suffers from two disadvantages: it is not incremental and its global dimensionality must be designed in. A fuzzy clustering algorithm that partitions the input–output space represents an alternative approach (Kukolj, 2002). The firing strength of the rule (weight) indicates the correlation strength between the input and output variables—it is defined as the T-norm or minimum (multiplication) operator of the membership function:

$$w_i = \mu_A(x_1)\mu_B(x_2) = \min(\mu_A(x_1), \mu_B(x_2)) \tag{11.16}$$

The overall output is the weighted sum of each rule's output:

$$f(x) = \sum_{i=1}^{n} w_i f_i \tag{11.17}$$

where n = number of fuzzy if-then rules.

The number of fuzzy if-then rules equates to the number of receptive field units. The membership function may be expressed as:

$$\mu_A(x_1) = k_1 \exp\left(-\frac{(x_1 - c_A)^2}{\sigma_1^2}\right) \text{ and } \mu_B(x_2) = k_2 \exp\left(-\frac{(x_2 - c_B)^2}{\sigma_1^2}\right) \tag{11.18}$$

The firing strength (weight) of rule i is given by:

$$w_i(x_1, x_2) = \mu_A(x_1)\mu_B(x_2) = \exp\left(-\frac{|x - c_i|^2}{\sigma_1^2}\right) = R_i(x) \tag{11.19}$$

The neurofuzzy system uses a set of fuzzy rules to approximate a mapping function represented as a three- to five-layered feedforward neural network (Chao et al., 1996). Neurofuzzy inferencing systems permit the use of sigmoid functions to generate bell-shaped membership functions on input data (Chokri, 2006).

The first (fuzzification) layer comprises the input variable (input layer); the second (hidden) layer comprises the membership function (Gaussian or a variant of that) of the input variables of the fuzzy rules; the third (hidden) layer performs matching of the preconditions of the fuzzy rules which outputs an AND operation on activated rules; the fourth (hidden) layer performs a fuzzy OR operation (weighted sum) to integrate the fuzzy rules; and the fifth (defuzzification) layer computes the output variables (center of gravity). FNN is trained using sample data in which input data is compared with the membership function of the premise part of the fuzzy rules. Fuzzy inference rules may be extracted from a four-layer neural network (Abe and Lan, 1995).

Many neural network architectures have been fuzzified such as fuzzified CMAC associative networks (Nie and Linkens, 1993; Peng and Woo, 2002). An FNN based on the multilayer perceptron using the backpropagation algorithm has been used to fuzzily classify patterns (Pal and Mitra, 1992). Fuzzy ARTMAP is a hybridization of the ART neural network with fuzzy logic (Carpenter et al., 1992; Carpenter and Grossberg, 1992). A hybrid neural network based on integrating the fuzzy ARTMAP and a rectangular basis function network has been shown to be able to learn and extract fuzzy rules (Tan et al., 2007). Fuzzy rules may be derived from the fuzzy ARTMAP following pruning of excess weights and discretization of continuous weights (Carpenter and Tan, 1995). It offers similar performance to the M-of-N algorithm. It is assumed that the fuzzy ARTMAP has been initially trained. The Cascade ARTMAP employs symbolic knowledge incorporated into the ARTMAP neural network as a generalization of the fuzzy ARTMAP with many similarities to other symbolic connectionist approaches (Tan, 1997). The fuzzy inference neural network (FINN) is a two-layer Kohonen network which uses three learning phases—self-organization, rule extraction, and supervised learning (Nishina and Hagiwara, 1997). ANFIS (adaptive network-based fuzzy inference system) is a multilayer feedforward network that implements Takagi–Sugeno fuzzy rules and uses backpropagation learning of the membership function parameters and least squares estimation $E(t)$ to learn other parameters (Jang, 1993; Jang and Sun, 1995). Weight update may be achieved through the fuzzy backpropagation algorithm (Gupta et al., 2006):

$$w_i(t+1) = \text{sat}(w_i(t) + \Delta w_i(t)) \tag{11.20}$$

where

$$\text{sat}(x) = \begin{cases} 1 & \text{if } x > 1 \\ x & \text{if } 0 \le x \le 1 \\ 0 & \text{if } x < 0 \end{cases}, \ \Delta w_i = -\eta \frac{\partial E}{\partial w_i}, \ E(t) = \frac{1}{2}\sum_j^n \left(y_j^d(t) - y_j(t)\right)^2 = \frac{1}{2}\sum_{j=1}^n e_j^2(t)$$

A Kalman filter was used to identify the system parameters by minimizing the mean square error between the desired and actual outputs in ANFIS (Sun, 1994a, 1994b). Neurofuzzy systems have been used to initialize a Kalman filter estimator to reduce divergence problems (Harris et al., 1999).

Causal connections between events define events as causes (necessary events) and other subsequent events as effects subject to certain secondary conditions (enabling possible events). This may be described in terms of modal logics with the fundamental necessary operator $\Box$ and the auxiliary possibility operator $\Diamond$ subject to the logical equivalence of $\Box a = \sim\Diamond \sim a$. It has been suggested that such modal operators may be fuzzified such that differentiation between the two functions is not usually certain—this may be encoded in a fuzzy evidential logic, which is readily implemented into a neural network of fuzzy rules (Sun, 1994a, 1994b). A logic-based neural network implements OR and AND neurons through the max and min fuzzy operation which define possibility and necessity measures, respectively. This formalism provides a connection between neural networks and rule-based logical reasoning. Case-based reasoning can be implemented through FNNs based on fuzzy AND and fuzzy OR neurons (Liu and Yan, 1995). The AND neuron is implemented through a Min-Max cascade operation, while the OR neuron is implemented through a Max-Min cascade operation (Predrycz and Rocha, 1993). Neural-fuzzy systems are highly suited to control systems (Lin and Lee, 1991; Zengqi and Zhidong, 1996) including process control in material processing tasks (Arafeh et al., 1999). A fuzzy feedforward controller equivalent to a PI control system trained using an online fuzzy identification scheme has been demonstrated (Tan and Dexter, 2000).

11.7 Future trends

A host of rejoinders to the question whether connectionist symbol processing is active or not is given in Blank et al. (1999). Symbolic connectionism is not just a theoretical exploration for cognitive science expositions. A multilayer network expert system from which symbolic knowledge can be extracted has been applied to medical diagnosis (Saito and Nakano, 1988). Of greater interest is the application of x-schemas (dynamic "executable" schemas) within the SHRUTI framework for generating motor behaviors (Shastri et al., 1997a, 1997b). X-schemas are hierarchical and distributed schemas that can be (de)composed into complex motor behaviors, i.e., planning into sequential, concurrent, and recursive actions. Each schema is encoded neurally as neural focal clusters that may be synchronized, forming networks of rules (motor plans) controlled by feedback loops from sensors. This effectively grounds the schemas. The authors contend that linguistic concepts are rooted in physical actions, an interesting and powerful notion (Gantucci et al., 2006).

There are numerous applications to which soft computing methods are effectively barred because of their opacity. Space missions are premised on reliability and transparency and almost solely employ symbolic methods in extending autonomous capabilities into outer space, e.g., Remote Agent on the Deep Space-1 spacecraft (Muscettola et al., 1998). This is where symbolic connectionist approaches offer the transparency of logic with the adaptability of learning. If the underlying mechanism of the neural network is accessible through the extracted rules, it can be inspected and analyzed. However, in most of the systems outlined, incremental learning of new rules requires retraining with the entire knowledge base due to the batch nature of backpropagation-type algorithms. This is neither practical nor desirable, but the use of Kalman filter-based continuous learning in neural networks offers a potential solution (Ruck et al., 1992; Iiguni et al., 1997). Kalman filters (and its variants) are an implementation of a Bayesian approach of combining prior knowledge (in this case, a knowledge-based model) and new empirical evidence (in this case, sensory data in the form of training pairs).

A true test of symbolic connectionism would be if a knowledge-based system like CYC, ACT-R, and/or SOAR could be implemented in a neural network. A step in that direction has been undertaken with a connectionist implementation of the ACT-R production system (Lebiere and Anderson, 1993). In ACT-R, declarative knowledge stored as knowledge structures (chunks similar to frames) and procedural knowledge as production rules could be implemented in connectionist associative memory. Nevertheless, hybrid symbolic connectionist systems demonstrate that symbolic system can be implemented in neural architectures. The distributed representations of symbolic systems quite categorically demonstrate that connectionist approaches can exhibit compositionality in which simpler structures can be combined into more complex structures (van Gelder, 1990). However, as in neural network and GOFAI research, there is a multitude of approaches with little coherence, indicating that there is no "standard model" like that in physics, making a convincing demonstration of general cognition a challenge, but then this applies to the whole of AI in general.

The primary issue for many of these techniques regards scaling to larger systems. It would be desirable to develop rule extraction algorithms that can extract compact generalized symbolic rules incorporating a Bayesian treatment of uncertainty reliably from arbitrary neural networks. I have not addressed some promising alternative avenues of research ranging from Bayesian approaches to evolutionary neural networks to neuronal group selection. Bayesian networks bear some similarities to connectionist expert systems—indeed, the latter may be regarded as approximations to Bayesian networks in that both are dependency networks (Laskey, 1990). Bayesian networks are also hybrid systems that combine syntactic connectionism with semantic symbols characterized by degrees of uncertainty. It has been postulated that the brain is a Bayesian inferencing machine (Friston, 2002, 2003), a notion with which I am inclined to agree, but that would be the subject of another forum.

References

Abe, S., Lan, M.-S., 1995. Fuzzy rules extraction directly from numerical data for function approximation. IEEE Trans. Syst. Man Cybern. 25 (1), 119–129.

Andrews, R., Geva, S., 2002. Rule extraction from local cluster neural nets. Neurocomputing 67, 1–20.

Andrews, R., Diederich, J., Tickle, A., 1995. Survey and critique of techniques for extracting rules from trained artificial neural networks. Knowl.-Based Syst. 8 (6), 373–389.

Arafeh, L., Singh, H., Putatanda, S., 1999. Neuro fuzzy logic approach to material processing. IEEE Trans. Syst. Man Cybern. Part C Appl. Rev. 29 (3), 362–370.

Bader, S., Hitzler, P., 2005. Dimensions of neural-symbolic integration—a structured survey. In: Artëmov, S.N., Barringer, H., d'Avila Garcez, A.S., Lamb, L.C., Woods, J. (Eds.), We Will Show Them: Essays in Honour of Dov Gabbay. College Publications, London, pp. 167–194.

Balkenius, C., Gardenfors, P., 1991. Nonmonotonic inferences in neural networks. Lund Univ. Cogn. Stud. 3, 1101–8453.

Bengio, Y., Frasconi, P., 1996. Input-output HMM's for sequence processing. IEEE Trans. Neural Netw. 7 (5), 1231–1249.

Bezdek, J., 1993. Review of probabilistic, fuzzy and neural models for pattern recognition. J. Intell. Fuzzy Syst. 1 (1), 1–25.

Bianco, A., Deigado, M., Pegalajar, M., 2000. Extracting rules from a (fuzzy/crisp) recurrent neural network using a self-organising map. J. Intell. Fuzzy Syst. 15, 595–621.

Blank, D., et al., 1999. Connectionist symbol processing: dead or alive? Neural Comput. Surv. 2, 1–40.

Blutner, R., 2004. Nonmonotonic inferences and neural networks. Synthese 142, 143–174.

Bostrom, N., 1996. Cortical integration: possible solutions to the binding and linking problems in perception, reasoning and long term memory. http://www.hedweb.com/nickb/cortical.htm.

Boutsinas, B., Vrahatis, M., 2001. Artificial monotonic neural networks. Artif. Intell. 132, 1–38.

Bridle, J., 1990. Alpha-nets: a recurrent neural network architecture with a hidden Markov model interpretation. Speech Comm. 9, 83–92.

Browne, A., Sun, R., 2001. Connectionist inference models. Neural Netw. 14 (10), 1331–1355.

Buckley, J., Hayashi, Y., 1994. Fuzzy neural networks: a survey. Fuzzy Set. Syst. 66, 1–13.

Cariani, P., 2001. Symbols and dynamics in the brain. BioSystems 60, 59–83.
Carpenter, G., Grossberg, S., 1992. Self-organizing neural network for supervised learning, recognition and prediction. IEEE Commun. Mag. 30, 38–49.
Carpenter, G., Tan, A.-H., 1995. Rule extraction: from neural architecture to symbolic representation. Connect. Sci. 7 (1), 3–26.
Carpenter, G., Grossberg, S., Markuzon, N., Reynolds, J., Rosen, D., 1992. Fuzzy ARTMAP: a neural network architecture for incremental supervised learning of analog multidimensional maps. IEEE Trans. Neural Netw. 3 (5), 698–713.
Chalmers, D., 1990. Syntactic transformations on distributed representations. Connect. Sci. 2 (1/2), 53–62.
Chao, C., Chen, Y., Teng, C., 1996. Simplification of fuzzy-neural systems using similarity analysis. IEEE Trans. Syst. Man Cybern. B Cybern. 26 (2), 344–354.
Chokri, S., 2006. Neuro-fuzzy network based on extended Kalman filtering for financial time series. World Acad. Sci. Eng. Technol. 15, 134–139.
Civelek-Aplasalan, F., Swigger, K., 1996. Temporal neural network model for constructing connectionist expert system knowledge bases. J. Netw. Comput. Appl. 19, 119–133.
D'Avila Garcez, A., Broda, K., Gabbay, D., 2001. Symbolic knowledge extraction from trained networks: a sound approach. Artif. Intell. 125, 155–207.
Das, S., Mozer, M., 1998. Dynamic on-line clustering and state extraction: an approach to symbolic learning. Neural Netw. 11 (1), 53–64.
Dyer, M., 1990. Distributed symbol formation and processing in connectionist networks. J. Exp. Theor. Artif. Intell. 2 (3), 215–239.
Dyer, M., Flowers, M., Wang, Y., 1992. Distributed symbol discovery through symbol recirculation: toward natural language processing. http://www.cs.ucla.edu/~dyer/Papers/DistSymDisc/DistSymDisc92.html.
Elman, J., 1990. Finding structure in time. Cogn. Sci. 14, 179–211.
Farah, M., 1994. Neuropsychological inference with an interactive brain: a critique of the locality assumption. Behav. Brain Sci. 17 (1), 43–104.
Feldman, J., Ballard, D., 1982. Connectionist models and their properties. Cogn. Sci. 6, 205–254.
Feldman, J., Fanty, M., Goddard, N., 1988. Computing with structured neural networks. IEEE Comput. 21 (3), 91–103.
Figueiredo, M., Gomide, F., 1999. Design of fuzzy systems using neurofuzzy networks. IEEE Trans. Neural Netw. 10 (4), 815–827.
Fletcher, J., Obradovic, Z., 1993. Combining prior symbolic knowledge and constructive neural network learning. Connect. Sci. 5 (3/4), 365–375.
Fodor, J., Pylyshyn, Z., 1988. Connectionism and cognitive architecture: a critical analysis. Cognition 28 (1/2), 3–71.
Friston, K., 2002. Functional integration and inference in the brain. Prog. Neurobiol. 68, 113–143.
Friston, K., 2003. Learning and inference in the brain. Neural Netw. 16, 1325–1352.
Fu, L., 1992. Neural network model for learning rule-based systems. Proc. Int. Jt Conf. Neural Netw. 1, 343–348.
Fu, L., 1994. Rule generation from neural networks. IEEE Trans. Syst. Man Cybern. 24 (8), 1114–1124.
Fu, L., 1995. Introduction to knowledge-based neural networks. Knowl.-Based Syst. 8 (6), 299–300.
Fu, L., 1999. Knowledge discovery based on neural networks. Commun. ACM 42 (11), 47–50.
Gallant, S., 1988. Connectionist expert systems. Commun. ACM 31 (2), 152–169.

Gantucci, B., Fowler, C., Turvey, M., 2006. Motor theory of speech perception reviewed. Psychon. Bull. Rev. 13 (3), 261–377.

Garagnani, M., Shastri, L., Wendelken, C., 2002. Connectionist model of planning via back-chaining search, reprint. www.icsi.berkeley.edu/~shastri/psfiles/CogSci02Plan.pdf.

Gardenfors, P., 2005. How logic emerges from the dynamics of information. In: Dynamics of Thought Synthese Library, vol. 300, pp. 83–108.

Giles, C., Omlin, C., 1994. Pruning recurrent neural networks for improved generalisation performance. IEEE Trans. Neural Netw. 5 (5), 848–851.

Glenberg, A., Robertson, D., 2000. Symbol grounding and meaning: a comparison of high dimensional and embodied theories of meaning. J. Mem. Lang. 43, 379–401.

Gupta, M., Homma, N., Hou, Z.-G., 2006. Fuzzy neural networks. StudFuzz 207, 205–233.

Handelman, D., Lane, S., Gelfand, J., 1990. Integrating neural networks and knowledge-based systems for intelligent robotic control. IEEE Control. Syst. Mag. 10 (3), 77–87.

Harris, C., Wu, Z., Gan, Q., 1999. Neurofuzzy state estimators and their applications. Annu. Rev. Control. 23, 149–158.

Hatfield, G., 1990. Gibsonian representations and connectionist symbol processing. Psychol. Res. 52, 243–252.

Hatzilygeroudis, I., Prentzas, J., 2004a. Integrating (rules, neural networks) and cases for knowledge representation and reasoning in expert systems. Expert Syst. Appl. 27, 63–75.

Hatzilygeroudis, I., Prentzas, J., 2004b. Neuro-symbolic approaches for knowledge representation in expert systems. Int. J. Hybrid Intell. Syst. 1 (3/4), 111–126.

Hinton, G., 1990. Preface to the special issue on connectionist symbol processing. Artif. Intell. 46, 1–4.

Holyoak, K., Spellman, B., 1993. Thinking. Annu. Rev. Psychol. 44, 265–315.

Iiguni, Y., Sakai, H., Tokumaru, H., 1997. Real-time learning algorithm for a multilayered neural network based on the extended Kalman filter. IEEE Trans. Signal Process. 40 (4), 959–966.

Jacobsson, H., 2005. Rule extraction from recurrent neural networks: a taxonomy and review. Neural Comput. 17, 1223–1263.

Jang, J.-S., 1993. ANFIS: adaptive network based fuzzy inference system. IEEE Trans. Syst. Man Cybern. 23 (3), 665–685.

Jang, J.-S., Sun, C.-T., 1993. Functional equivalence between radial basis function networks and fuzzy inference systems. IEEE Trans. Neural Netw. 4 (1), 156–159.

Jang, J.-S., Sun, C.-T., 1995. Neuro-fuzzy modelling and control. Proc. IEEE 83 (3), 378–406.

Kamruzzaman, S., Islam, M., 2006. Algorithm to extract rules from artificial neural networks for medical diagnosis problems. Int. J. Inf. Technol. 12 (8), 41–89.

Kamruzzaman, S., Sarkar, A., 2011. New data mining scheme using artificial neural networks. Sensors 11, 4622–4647.

Kasabov, N., 1996. Adaptable neuro production systems. Neurocomputing 13, 95–117.

Komendantskaya, E., 2009. Neurons OR symbols: why does OR remain exclusive? In: Proceedings of the International Joint Conference on Computational Intelligence, pp. 502–507.

Kukolj, D., 2002. Design of adaptive Takagi-Sugeno-Kang fuzzy models. Appl. Soft Comput. 2, 89–103.

Lachter, J., Bever, T., 1988. Relation between linguistic structure and associative theories of language learning—a constructive critique of some connectionist learning models. Cognition 28, 195–247.

Lange, T., Dyer, M., 1989. High level inferencing in a connectionist network. Connect. Sci. 1 (2), 181–217.

Laskey, K., 1990. Adapting connectionist learning to Bayes networks. Int. J. Approx. Reason. 4, 261–282.
Lebiere, C., Anderson, J., 1993. Connectionist implementation of the ACT-R production system. In: Proceedings of the 15th Annual Conference of Cognitive Science Society, pp. 635–640.
Lin, C.-T., Lee, C., 1991. Neural network-based fuzzy logic control and decision making. IEEE Trans. Comput. 40 (12), 1320–1336.
Liu, Z.-Q., Yan, F., 1995. Case-based diagnostic system using fuzzy neural network. Proc. IEEE Int. Conf. Neural Netw. 6, 3107–3112.
Low, B., Lui, H., Tan, A., Teh, H., 1991. Connectionist expert systems with adaptive learning capability. IEEE Trans. Knowl. Data Eng. 3 (2), 200–207.
Markowska-Kaczmar, U., Wnuk-Lipinski, P., 2004. Rule extraction from neural network by genetic algorithm with Pareto optimisation. In: Artificial Intelligence & Soft Computing. In: Lecture Notes in Computer Science, vol. 3070, pp. 450–455.
Minsky, M., 1991. Logical versus analogical or symbolic versus connectionist or net versus scruffy. AI Mag. 12 (2), 34–51.
Mitchell, T., 1982. Generalisation as search. Artif. Intell. 18 (2), 203–226.
Mitchell, T., Thrun, S., 1992. Explanation-based neural network learning for robot control. In: Giles, C., Hanson, S., Cowan, J. (Eds.), Advances in Neural Information Processing Systems, vol. 5. Morgan Kaufmann, San Mateo, CA.
Muscettola, N., Nayak, P., Pell, B., Williams, B., 1998. Remote agent: to boldly go where no AI system has gone before. Artif. Intell. 103, 5–47.
Newell, A., 1980. Physical symbol systems. Cogn. Sci. 4, 135–183.
Nie, J., Linkens, D., 1993. Fuzzified CMAC self-learning controller. In: Proceedings of the second IEEE International Conference on Fuzzy Systems, pp. 500–505.
Nishina, T., Hagiwara, M., 1997. Fuzzy inference neural network. Neurocomputing 14, 223–239.
Omlin, C., Giles, C., 1996. Extraction of rules from discrete-time recurrent neural networks. Neural Netw. 9 (1), 41–52.
Omori, T., Mochizuki, A., Mizutani, K., Nishizaki, M., 1999. Emergence of symbolic behaviour from brain like memory with dynamic attention. Neural Netw. 12, 1157–1173.
Opitz, D., Shavlik, J., 1995. Dynamically adding symbolically meaningful nodes to knowledge-based networks. Knowl.-Based Syst. 8 (6), 301–311.
Osorio, F., Amy, B., 1999. INSS: a hybrid system for constructive machine learning. Neurocomputing 28, 191–205.
Pal, S., Mitra, S., 1992. Multilayer perceptron, fuzzy sets and classification. IEEE Trans. Neural Netw. 3 (5), 663–697.
Pao, Y., Sobajic, D., 1991. Neural networks and knowledge engineering. IEEE Trans. Knowl. Data Eng. 3 (2), 185–192.
Peng, L., Woo, P.-Y., 2002. Neural-fuzzy control system for robotic manipulators. IEEE Control. Syst. Mag. 22 (1), 53–63.
Pinkas, G., 1995. Reasoning, nonmonotonicity and learning in connectionist networks that capture propositional knowledge. Artif. Intell. 77, 203–247.
Pinker, S., Prince, A., 1988. On language and connectionism: analysis of a parallel distributed processing model of language acquisition. Cognition 28, 73–193.
Plate, T., 1995. Holographic reduced representations. IEEE Trans. Neural Netw. 6 (1), 623–641.
Polk, T., Simen, P., Lewis, R., Freedman, E., 2002. Computational approach to control in complex cognition. Cogn. Brain Res. 15, 71–83.
Pollack, J., 1990. Recursive distributed representations. Artif. Intell. 46, 77–105.
Predrycz, W., Rocha, A., 1993. Fuzzy set based models of neurons and knowledge-based networks. IEEE Trans. Fuzzy Syst. 1 (4), 254–266.

Pylyshyn, Z., 1980. Computation and cognition: issues in the foundations of cognitive science. Behav. Brain Sci. 3, 111–169.
Quinlan, J., 1986. Induction of decision trees. Mach. Learn. 1 (1), 81–106.
Reed, R., 1993. Pruning algorithms—a survey. IEEE Trans. Neural Netw. 4 (5), 740–747.
Ruck, D., Rogers, S., Kabrisky, M., Maybeck, P., Oxley, M., 1992. Comparative analysis of backpropagation and the extended Kalman filter for training multilayer perception. IEEE Trans. Pattern Anal. Mach. Intell. 14 (6), 686–691.
Rummelhart, D., McClelland, J., 1986. On learning the past tenses of English verbs. In: McClelland, J., Rumelhart, D. (Eds.), Parallel Distributed Processing: Experiments in the Microstructure of Cognition 2: Applications. MIT Press, Cambridge, MA, pp. 216–271.
Saito, K., Nakano, R., 1988. Medical diagnostic expert system based on PDP model. Proc. IEEE Int. Conf. Neural Netw. 1, 255–262.
Sankar, A., Mammone, R., 1993. Growing and pruning neural tree networks. IEEE Trans. Comput. 42 (3), 291–299.
Searle, J., 1980. Minds, brains and programs. Behav. Brain Sci. 3 (3), 417–457.
Seidenberg, M., 1994. Language and cognition: the developing interface. Cognition 5, 385–401.
Sejnowski, T., Rosenberg, C., 1987. Parallel networks that learn to pronounce English text. Complex Syst. 1, 145–168.
Setiono, R., 2000. Extracting M-of-N rules from trained neural networks. IEEE Trans. Neural Netw. 11 (2), 512–519.
Sharkey, N., 1991. Connectionist representation techniques. Artif. Intell. 5, 143–167.
Shastri, L., 1988. Connectionist approach to knowledge representation and limited inference. Cogn. Sci. 12, 331–391.
Shastri, L., Ajjaganadde, V., 1993. From simple associations to systematic reasoning: a connectionist representation of rules, variables and dynamic bindings using temporal synchrony. Behav. Brain Sci. 16 (3), 417–451.
Shastri, L., Grannes, D., Narayanan, S., Feldman, J., 1997a. Connectionist encoding of parametrised schemas and reactive plans. In: Kraetzschmar, G.K., Palm, G. (Eds.), Hybrid Information Processing in Adaptive Autonomous Vehicles. Springer-Verlag, Berlin.
Shastri, L., Grannes, D., Narayanan, S., Feldman, J., 1997b. Connectionist encoding of parametrized schemas and reactive plans. In: SMART Symposium on Hybrid Information Processing in Autonomous Vehicles, Gunzburg, Germany.
Siegelmann, H., Sontag, E., 1995. On the computational power of neural nets. J. Comput. Syst. Sci. 50, 132–150.
Sima, J., 1995. Neural expert system. Neural Netw. 8 (2), 261–271.
Smolensky, P., 1988. On the proper treatment of connectionism. Behav. Brain Sci. 11 (1), 1–23.
Smolensky, P., 1990. Tensor product variable binding and the representation of symbolic structures in connectionist systems. Artif. Intell. 46, 159–216.
Sun, R., 1992. Connectionist model for commonsense reasoning incorporating rules and similarities. Knowl. Acquis. 4 (3), 293–321.
Sun, R., 1993. Robust reasoning: integrating rule-based and similarity-based reasoning. Artif. Intell. 75, 241–295.
Sun, C.-T., 1994a. Rule-based structure identification in an adaptive network-based fuzzy inference system. IEEE Trans. Fuzzy Syst. 2 (1), 64–73.
Sun, R., 1994b. Neural network model of causality. IEEE Trans. Neural Netw. 5 (4), 601–611.
Sun, R., 1997. Learning, action and consciousness: a hybrid approach toward modelling consciousness. Neural Netw. 10 (7), 1317–1331.
Sun, R., Peterson, T., 1998. Autonomous learning of sequential tasks: experiments and analyses. IEEE Trans. Neural Netw. 9 (6), 1217–1234.

Sun, R., Zhang, X., Slusarz, P., Mathews, R., 2007. Interaction between learning, explicit hypothesis testing learning and implicit-to-explicit knowledge extraction. Neural Netw. 20, 34–47.
Taha, I., Ghosh, J., 1999. Symbolic interpretation of artificial neural networks. IEEE Trans. Knowl. Data Eng. 11 (3), 448–463.
Tan, A.-H., 1997. Cascade ARTMAP: integrating neural computation and symbolic knowledge processing. IEEE Trans. Neural Netw. 8 (2), 237–250.
Tan, W., Dexter, A., 2000. Self-learning fuzzy controller for embedded applications. Automatica 36, 1189–1198.
Tan, A.-H., Teow, L.-N., 1997. Inductive neural logic network and the SCM algorithm. Neurocomputing 14, 157–176.
Tan, S., Lim, C., Rao, M., 2007. Hybrid neural network model for rule generation and its application to process fault detection and diagnosis. Eng. Appl. Artif. Intell. 20, 203–213.
Tickle, A., Andrews, R., Golea, M., Diederich, J., 1998. The truth will come to light: directions and challenges in extracting the knowledge embedded within trained artificial neural networks. IEEE Trans. Neural Netw. 9 (6), 1057–1067.
Tino, P., Cernansky, M., Benuskova, L., 2004. Markovian architectural bias of recurrent neural networks. IEEE Trans. Neural Netw. 15 (1), 6–15.
Touretsky, D., 1990. BoltzCONS: dynamical symbol structures in a connectionist network. Artif. Intell. 46, 5–46.
Touretsky, D., Hinton, G., 1988. Distributed connectionist production system. Cogn. Sci. 12, 423–466.
Towell, G., Shavlik, J., 1993. Extracting refined rules from knowledge-based neural networks. Mach. Learn. 13, 71–101.
Towell, G., Shavlik, J., 1994. Knowledge-based artificial neural networks. Artif. Intell. 70, 119–165.
Trentin, E., Gori, M., 2003. Robust combination of neural networks and hidden Markov models for speech recognition. IEEE Trans. Neural Netw. 14 (6), 1519–1531.
Tryon, W., 1993. Neural networks: 1. Theoretical unification through connectionism. Clin. Psychol. Rev. 13, 341–352.
van Gelder, T., 1990. Compositionality: a connectionist variation on a classical theme. Cogn. Sci. 14, 355–384.
Wang, L.-X., Mendel, J., 1992. Fuzzy basis functions, universal approximation and orthogonal least squares learning. IEEE Trans. Neural Netw. 3 (5), 801–814.
Wermter, S., 2000. Knowledge extraction from transducer neural networks. J. Appl. Intell. 12, 27–44.
Wermter, S., Sun, R., 2000. Overview of hybrid neural systems. In: Wermter, S., Sun, R. (Eds.), Hybrid Neural Systems. In: Lecture Notes in Artificial Intelligence, vol. 1778. Springer-Verlag Publishing, Berlin, pp. 1–13.
Wermter, S., Riloff, E., Scheler, G., 1996. Learning approaches for natural language processing. In: Wermter, S., Riloff, E., Scheler, G. (Eds.), Connectionist, Statistical and Symbolic Approaches to Learning for Natural Language Processing. In: Lecture Notes in Computer Science, vol. 1040. Springer-Verlag Publishing, Berlin.
Wichert, A., 2005. Associative computer: a hybrid connectionistic production system. Cogn. Syst. Res. 6, 111–144.
Yoon, Y., Guinaraes, T., Swales, G., 1994. Integrating artificial neural networks with rule-based expert systems. Decis. Support. Syst. 11, 497–507.
Zengqi, S., Zhidong, D., 1996. Fuzzy neural network and its application to controls. Artif. Intell. Eng. 10, 311–315.

Implementation of biomimetic central pattern generators on field-programmable gate array

12

M. Ambroise, T. Levi, S. Saïghi

12.1 Introduction

12.1.1 Interest in central pattern generators

The study of life sciences is evolving and requires new tools to acquire more accurate knowledge. These tools include the hybrid technique, which consists of connecting an artificial system to biological cells (Le Masson et al., 2002). The hybrid technique, based on research into imitating living organisms, may lead to the development of neuroprostheses (Hochberg et al., 2006, 2012; Nicolelis and Lebedev, 2009).

Several international projects are working on developing neuroprostheses, including the European Brainbow project (Brainbow, 2012) and the French Hyrene project (Joucla et al., 2013), in which we are involved. Although these two projects have a common objective, the implants they are developing are intended for different locations and functions. Indeed, the neuroprosthesis in the Brainbow project is a neuromorphic system aimed at reproducing the functional organization of damaged parts of the brain. In contrast, the neuroprosthesis in the Hyrene project focuses on microstimulation of the spinal cord to restore movement in patients.

In the animal kingdom, movement (walking in salamanders (Ijspeert et al., 2007), swimming in tadpoles (Li et al., 2014) and lampreys (Cohen et al., 1992), flying in crickets (Stevenson and Kutsch, 1987)), and even heartbeats (Cymbalyuk et al., 2002; Hill et al., 2001) are controlled by neural networks known as "Central Pattern Generators" (CPGs). Indeed, CPGs are neural networks that produce electrical activity consisting of burst phases alternating with action potentials and silence. CPGs, therefore, autonomously produce a rhythmic activity, with a rhythm that depends on their topology. In the context of this project, we focused on biomimetic CPG (i.e., with spiking neurons), implemented on an FPGA (Field-Programmable Gate Array) platform containing tools for the detection and stimulation of biological network activity in order to interact with living things. To advance this project, it was necessary to study CPGs in more detail prior to implementing them on FPGA.

Ijspeert (2008) demonstrated that CPG implementations were divided into several levels of abstraction. These ranged from the biophysical approach of the Hodgkin–Huxley (HH) model (Hodgkin and Huxley, 1952), described in detail below, to the more abstract mathematical approach, based on coupled oscillators (Zielinska, 1995).

Between these two extremes was the "connectionist" approach, using simpler, pulsed-neuron models to study the mechanisms specific to CPGs (Ekeberg, 1993).

The aim of the biophysical approach is to achieve proximity (or even equivalence) between the biological system and the simulated model, making it possible to conduct hybrid experiments. This is why Hill et al. (2001) reported measurements made on the biological CPGs responsible for leech heartbeats (intraburst frequency and bursting periods) before using the HH to simulate the characteristic activity of this CPG. The HH formalism is a neuron model close to biophysical reality, using conductances. Indeed, it is possible to inject the appropriate biological conductance measurements into this model, resulting in behavior similar to that observed in biology. HH is a complex model similar to living systems, requiring calculation tools that are difficult to implement (due to excessive costs on resources) digitally on FPGA (particularly the sigmoid and exponential functions). In view of this difficulty, despite its biophysical realism (or biorealism), the pulsed neuron model was not retained for our application.

The abstract approach focuses mainly on the structures of CPG networks and their phase dynamics. Neurobotics uses CPGs to move and coordinate the movements of bipedal (Li et al., 2013), multipedal, (Barron-Zambrano and Torres-Huitzil, 2013) or swimming robots (Ijspeert et al., 2007). Neurobotic applications are implemented on microprocessors or microcontrollers (Crespi and Ijspeert, 2006), mainly using sinusoidal non-linear oscillators (Fitzhugh-Nagumo, Stein, Van der Pol). The dynamics described by these systems were studied using standard mathematical tools (Zielinska, 1995), and it was, therefore, easy to simulate the varied movements found in the animal kingdom (e.g., trotting, walking, and running (Barron-Zambrano and Torres-Huitzil, 2013)). Despite a possible implementation of the Van Der Pol (VDP) model on FPGA, as demonstrated by Barron-Zambrano and Torres-Huitzil (2013), the level of abstraction was too high to envisage any connection with living organisms.

An intermediate (connectionist) approach was, therefore, necessary to achieve our objective of implementing CPGs on FPGA via a small-area-pulsed neuron model, usable both for the hybrid technique and neurobotic applications. This led us to process various neuron models, before finally choosing the Izhikevich model (IZH) (Izhikevich, 2003). In order to implement a CPG, we first studied biological CPGs in the literature and then reviewed the state of the art of CPG implementations. We then discuss the problems related to parameters and digital calculations before describing our implementation. This discussion will start with the neuron model (IZH), followed by the synapse used (short-term plasticity (Izhikevich and Edelman, 2008)), and end with the full system. As our goal is to come as close as possible to living organisms, our study includes a comparison between the activity of our implementation and that measured in a biological environment. This chapter ends with a section entitled *Conclusions and Perspectives*.

12.2 State of the art on CPG implementation

Before going any further, we should note that the previous studies and experiments were not restricted to a simple mathematical analysis but resulted in a digital or analog hardware implementation.

Several authors (Torres-Huitzil and Girau, 2008; Rice et al., 2009; Serrano-Gotarredona et al., 2009; Barron-Zambrano et al., 2010; Barron-Zambrano and Torres-Huitzil, 2013) have reported CPG implementations on FPGA for robotic applications. These were based on simple mathematical models of neurons (or simple formalisms), finding inspiration in key biological principles to solve an engineering problem (bioinspired systems) rather than closely imitating biological organisms with a view to understanding their mechanisms in preparation for hybrid experiments (biomimetic systems). For example, Guerrero-Riberas et al. (2006) implemented Leaky Integrate and Fire (LIF) neurons, as described below.

The simplest neuron model is Integrate and Fire (IF), expressed in a single equation. This model was reworked and extended to add a timed memory to the neuron membranes, resulting in the development of LIF neurons. LIF is indeed a simple model, based on two equations, capable of reproducing two families of neurons (regular-spiking, RS, and fast-spiking, FS), as well as their action potential activity, in a simplistic way. The immediate advantage of this type of model is that it is resource-frugal (logic gates and memories within the FPGA platform), but its drawback is that it does not always match biological time. This means it cannot be used in any hybrid applications, i.e., artificial neurons interfaced with biological neurons.

One hardware implementation for event calculation (otherwise known as "by action potential") was presented by Merolla et al. (2014). It consisted of an analog-digital chip designed for image processing, capable of simulating a million neurons and 256 million synapses. Neural networks embedded in the chip provided real time, multiobject detection, and image classification. The neurons on this chip used the TrueNorth model, an extension of the IF model. Neuromorphic platforms designed for specific tasks use simple models so that they can model large numbers of neurons and synapses. Despite this advantage, we did not use this platform, as the synapses were too simple to build CPGs.

However, in robotics, neural networks without action potentials are used in networks based on the Amari-Hopfield (Amari, 1972) or even simpler models (Van der Pol, 1928). Indeed, the CPGs used in this case to coordinate the movements of multipedal robots were based on sinusoidal oscillations with variable frequencies and amplitudes, supported by several parameters. Analog implementations have also been achieved by several teams (Linares-Barranco et al., 1994; Still and Tilden, 1998, Lee et al., 2007; Lewis et al., 2001; Nakada, 2003; Wijekoon and Dudek, 2008). These various solutions were not applicable in our approach, as we preferred to use neural networks.

Finally, in robotics, two policies on CPG emulation are commonly applied: either bioinspired oscillators or the implementation of simple bioinspired neurons.

In contrast, some studies aimed at stimulating cardiac CPGs (Simoni et al., 2004; Simoni and DeWeerth, 2007) have been conducted using neurons on silicon (Indiveri, et al., 2011).

In addition, several teams (Jung et al., 2001; Le Masson et al., 2002; Vogelstein et al., 2006) have developed hybrid experiments combining an artificial hardware network and biological neurons. These hybrid experiments include work by Sorensen et al. (2004), who created a hybrid system with a cardiac neuron and an artificial neuron on silicon (hardware implementation). This artificial neuron on silicon, based on a version of the HH (Hodgkin and Huxley, 1952), is capable of carrying out real-time calculations close to biological time. Once again, the HH model is complex enough to reproduce the most complex activities very accurately, but is also complex to implement, thus restricting the number of neurons that can be implemented. This is why a single CPG was implemented in the previous study. Olypher et al. (2006) demonstrated a hybrid system with a pharmacologically isolated living neuron connected to a single, software-simulated neuron with artificial synapses.

This chapter, therefore, proposes a digital implementation starting from a similar result (an implemented CPG), which may be extended up to 500 CPG (on a Spartan 6 FPGA platform). Ijspeert (2001) demonstrated that 40 CPG were sufficient to reproduce swimming and walking in a salamander. This implementation is intended to form the basis of hybrid experiments and may be used in robotic applications. The advantage of using an FPGA platform for digital implementation is that it is possible to simulate a large number of neurons in real time, as well as including other functions to suit the user's needs and environment.

Furthermore, the ease of reconfiguring an FPGA platform made implementation more flexible. Prototyping on FPGA thus facilitated rapid production on a circuit (a few months). The aim of using an FPGA platform rather than a software implementation was to integrate it in an embedded system with limited resources.

12.3 Stakes and challenges

As presented above, implementing a CPG requires either bioinspired oscillators, thus ruling out the possibility of hybrid experiments, or a complex, biomimetic model, which restricts the maximum number of neurons that can be implemented. The proposed system is, therefore, also capable of reproducing the CPG network necessary for the swimming and walking activity of a salamander (Ijspeert, 2001), as well as being used in hybrid experiments (Le Masson et al, 2002), with a view to developing a neuroprosthesis (Brainbow, 2012; Joucla et al., 2013).

This study, therefore, proposes a digital CPG implementation on an FPGA platform, capable of reproducing the model presented in Hill et al. (2001). This implementation combines biorealism with frugal consumption of resources.

To achieve this, we studied the CPG and its activity, then the neuron and synapse model and their respective implementations, and concluded by comparing it with a simulated model and a biological activity to confirm its relevance.

12.3.1 CPG

12.3.1.1 Choice of the model

The simplest biomimetic CPG studied to date is the one responsible for the leech heartbeat (Hill et al., 2001; Figure 12.1). This CPG consists of two neurons, connected to each other via inhibitory synapses. As this is the most basic network, it is

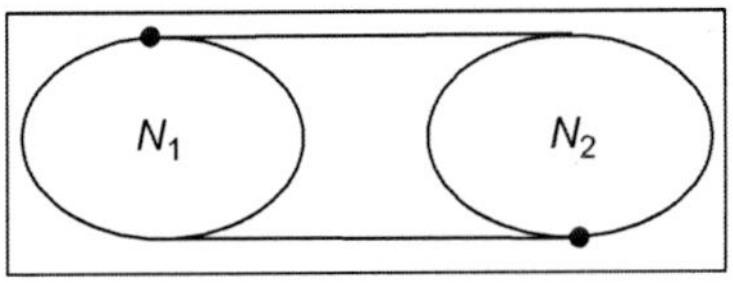

Figure 12.1 Architecture of elemental oscillator. Neuron cell bodies are represented by circles. Inhibitory synapses are represented by lines ending in black dots.

ideal for achieving a better understanding of the various phenomena that control its activity. This pair of neurons, also known as an elementary oscillator, is also the smallest network capable of generating oscillations under normal conditions. There are other structures for CPGs, each with a different number of synapses and neurons. In the context of our study, we also investigated a CPG with 8 neurons and 12 synapses (known as a segmental oscillator).

The reciprocally inhibitory synaptic interactions between the neurons within a CPG are caused by variations in the different ion currents as described by Angstadt and Calabrese (1991). Nadim et al. (1995) and Olsen et al. (1995) created a biophysical model of a pair of interneurons, connected to each other by inhibitory synapses. This model included ion current channels based on recorded voltage-clamp data (the voltage-clamp method is used by electrophysiologists to measure different ion currents by applying a voltage). The Hill model (Hill et al., 2001) was derived from a previous two-cell elementary oscillator model (Nadim et al., 1995), by adding a modification of the synaptic currents on the basis of biological data. A study of ion currents revealed that only the calcium ion current was involved in the CPG activity.

On the basis of these biological observations, only inhibitory synapses were used for this CPG and a few parameters were modified to change the CPG period.

In the HH formalism, each ion current within the synapses is the result of a conductance. Conductance synapses are complex and require a sigmoid function in the differential equations but, above all, timestamps of the different action potentials. Timestamping implies RAM storage of the action potential emission times, but RAM is a critical resource (much solicited by other applications) on an FPGA platform.

The next section describes the synapse model designed to function without conductances but still obtain similar results.

12.3.1.2 Architecture

Various studies have shown that this CPG triggers alternating activity and only requires a few neurons (2–10 neurons). Olsen and Calabrese (1996) proposed a new model, i.e., a segmental oscillator with behavior more similar to that of biological systems. Figure 12.2 shows a model of this system. The real-time, digital, segmental oscillator design was based on this architecture. In this study, we chose to reproduce both the elementary and segmental oscillators.

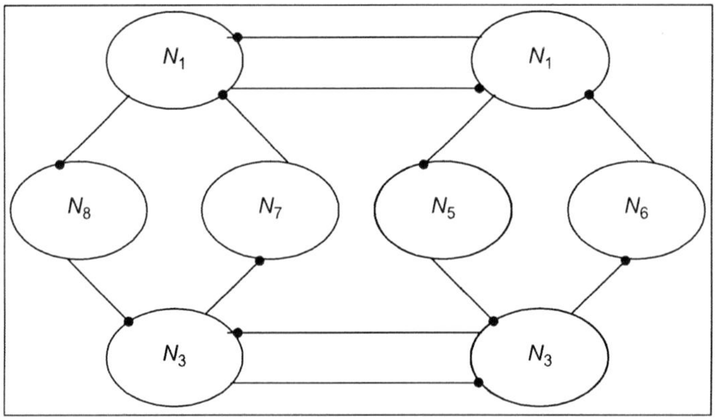

Figure 12.2 Architecture of a segmental oscillator. Neuron cell bodies are represented by circles. Inhibitory synapses are represented by lines ending in black dots.

12.3.1.3 Activity of the chosen CPG

According to several authors (Calabrese, 1995; Nadim et al., 1995; Olsen et al., 1995; Hill et al., 2001; Jezzini et al., 2004; Norris et al., 2007), the burst duration of an interneuron's action potentials are only dependent on regulating the activity of the interneuron itself and the opposing interneuron, which makes it easy to calibrate the different periods.

Neuron activity oscillates with a period of 10–12 s (Krahl and Zerbst-Boroffka, 1983; Calabrese et al., 1989; Olsen and Calabrese, 1996), also demonstrating that the neurons involved in a CPG are only connected by inhibitory synapses. Ijspeert (2001) reminded us that CPGs are autonomous networks. Despite this autonomy, the intervention of a sensory feedback improves control of both the CPG activity phase and the period. This aspect is not covered in this study.

12.3.2 Implementable model

12.3.2.1 Implementation issues

First of all, our FPGA platform, like digital systems in general, is subject to some limitations. The first concerns all the calculations to be carried out. We decided to use only fixed-point calculations in all cases. Although fixed-point calculations are less accurate than floating-point, this technique considerably simplified the implementation. Experimental results indicated that using 31 bits (1 sign bit, 11 for the whole number, and 19 for the decimals) made it possible to set the CPG with a period ranging from 1 to 30.5 s.

The second limitation was due to the fact that, in the long term, our system was not only intended to be embedded but also to support other functions embedded on the same platform, like detection and stimulation. Therefore, in this race toward a multipurpose system, the quantity of resources used was a critical element in the choice of the neuron and synapse models to be implemented. Indeed, the complexity of a model is directly linked to the quantity of resources (logic gates, RAM) required for it to function properly. Furthermore, as emphasized in the introduction, our system used a biologically realistic model.

A neuron model or formalism simply relies on differential equations to reproduce behavior (electrical activity) similar to that of biological cells. Our choice was based, therefore, on two criteria: the families of neurons that the model was capable of reproducing and the number of differential equations required to implement it. These criteria were used to compare models ranging from the simplest, LIF (Indiveri, 2007), to HH, including the IZH.

Hill et al. (2001) used the HH model to reproduce the leech cardiac system with eight neurons (Figure 12.2). The equations implemented for this model clearly revealed that the activity of interest could be produced using eight neurons of a single type, Regular Spiking (RS). This model consists of five currents, each with different conductances. In addition, the HH model reproduced all the families of neurons with a high level of accuracy in the form of the action potentials (spikes) generated. Its main drawback was the large number of parameters and equations involved. According to Grassia et al. (2011), the HH model requires the activation of 32 parameters to obtain an RS neuron and 26 for a Fast Spiking (FS) neuron. Furthermore, emulating an RS neuron requires four ion currents (reproducing the dynamics of potassium, slow potassium, sodium ions, and the theoretical leak channel, respectively). The LIF model, expressed in only two equations, is the exact opposite in terms of complexity but is only capable of simulating two families of neurons (RS and FS).

The IZH offers a good solution, as it is based on only two equations and is capable of reproducing different families of neurons by simply changing four parameters. Furthermore, according to Izhikevich (2004), this model is resource-frugal. This model was retained for its simplicity, the variability of the emulable families, and its ease of implementation.

12.3.2.2 Izhikevich model

The IZH model depends on four parameters to reproduce cortical neurons with behaviors ranging from simple spikes to bursts. From a mathematical standpoint, the model consists of a system of two-dimensional equations (Izhikevich, 2003):

$$\frac{\mathrm{d}v}{\mathrm{d}t} = 0.004v^2 + 5v - u + I_{\text{izh}} \tag{12.1}$$

$$\frac{\mathrm{d}u}{\mathrm{d}t} = a(bv - u) \tag{12.2}$$

$$\text{Si } v \geq 30\,\text{mV} => \begin{cases} v \leftarrow c \\ u \leftarrow u + d \end{cases} \tag{12.3}$$

The state variable, v, of these equations represents the membrane potential of a neuron, the u variable represents the regeneration of the membrane, taking into account the activation of the potassium channel and the inactivation of the sodium channel, and I_{izh} represents the input current to the neuron resulting from the activities of presynaptic neurons.

To make the neural network more realistic, the I_{izh} current is expressed as the sum of three currents—the polarization current, I_{bias}, the current combining all the inhibitions affecting a neuron, I_{inh}, and the current combining all the excitations affecting a neuron, I_{exc}. These currents and their roles are described in detail in the next subsection. As suggested in the publication by Cassidy and Andreou (2008), Equation (12.1) was multiplied by 0.78125 to facilitate its implementation on a digital platform (in particular, multiplications or divisions involving powers of 2 result in left or right shifts, respectively). These modifications led to Equation (12.4), where the coefficient for u was still 1, thanks to I_{bias}.

$$\frac{dv}{dt} = {}^{1}/_{32}v^2 + 4v + 109.375 - u + I_{bias} + I_{exc} + I_{inh} \qquad (12.4)$$

$$\frac{du}{dt} = a(bv - u) \qquad (12.5)$$

Each neuron was defined by a total of nine parameters—four Izhikevich parameters (a, b, c, and d), two state variables (u and v), and the three currents (I_{bias}, I_{exc}, and I_{inh}). Once the model had been chosen, it was necessary to examine the synapse model necessary to complete our spiking neural network.

12.3.2.3 Synapse model and synaptic short-term plasticity

All neural networks may be described simply by a set of neurons and synapses. The dynamics of an entire network can change completely, according to the synapses used. Synapse models, like neuron models, should also be biologically realistic and resource-frugal.

In biology, synapses provide connections between neurons and transmit inhibitory or excitatory synaptic currents, depending on their type and, of course, the activity of the presynaptic neuron. In compliance with Izhikevich (2003), every time a presynaptic neuron in our implementation emitted a spike, a synaptic weight (W_{syn}) was added to the synaptic current of the postsynaptic neuron.

When W_{syn} is positive, the synapse is excitatory, and when W_{syn} is negative, the synapse is inhibitory. AMPA is an excitatory neurotransmitter, which depolarizes the membrane of a neuron, while GABA is an inhibitory neurotransmitter with a hyperpolarizing effect. Depolarization or hyperpolarization is represented by a positive or a negative contribution to the synaptic currents. Thanks to the effects of AMPA and GABA, all the excitatory or inhibitory synaptic currents tend toward zero in an exponentially decreasing manner (Ben-Ari et al., 1997). To summarize, the I_{exc} current is always positive and the I_{inh} current is always negative. However, both of these synaptic currents obey the same law of exponential decrease (or increase). This gives, therefore, I_{syn}, a synaptic current such that:

$$I_{syn}(t) = -\tau_{syn} \cdot I'_{syn}(t) = -\tau_{syn} \cdot \frac{I_{syn}(t+T) - I_{syn}(t)}{T} \quad (12.6)$$

$$I_{syn}(t+T) = \left(1 - \frac{T}{\tau_{syn}}\right) \cdot I_{syn}(t) \quad (12.7)$$

With a calculation step, T, equal to 1 ms and τ_{syn} (in ms):

$$I_{syn}(t+1) = \left(1 - \frac{1}{\tau_{syn}}\right) \cdot I_{syn}(t) \quad (12.8)$$

Transposing (12.8) for digital implementation gives:

$$I_{syn}[n+1] = I_{syn}[n] - \frac{1}{\tau_{syn}} \cdot I_{syn}[n] \quad (12.9)$$

This law was one of two key elements for the successful implementation of our CPG. The second element required for successful implementation of the CPG was short-term plasticity, where W_s was the synaptic weight added to the synaptic currents, in turn dependent on W_{syn}.

As the synaptic behavior described in Hill et al. (2001) required too many resources to be implemented on an FPGA, the method chosen to mimic biological behavior was short-term plasticity (Tabak et al., 2000). The short-term plasticity of a synapse is a biological phenomenon by which the synaptic weight of a synapse decreases (or increases) after each presynaptic spike emitted.

According to Matsuoka (1987), there are four methods for maintaining stable activity in a network (regulating the intensity of the stimuli, changing the network input, adapting the stimuli, and changing the connection weights). Short-term plasticity is a phenomenon that changes and regulates the connection weights according to the activity of the network. This phenomenon was discovered in neurobiology and modeled by Izhikevich and Edelman (2008).

As previously described, each time a presynaptic neuron emitted a spike, the synapse added its weight, W_s, to the synaptic current of the postsynaptic neuron. At the same time, the scaling factor (x_{syn}), with an equilibrium value of 1, was multiplied by parameter P. If P is greater than 1, x_{syn} increases, thus describing short-term synaptic facilitation. In contrast, if P is less than 1, it results in synaptic depression. The x_{syn} factor varies between 0 and P and regulates synaptic weight, W_{syn}.

To summarize, when a spike is emitted, W_s is added to a single synaptic current:

$$I_{syn}[n+1] = I_{syn}[n] + W_s \quad (12.10)$$

$$\text{Avec } W_s[n] = x_{syn}[n] W_{syn} \quad (12.11)$$

At the same time, variations in the x_{syn} factor are observed after each spike, expressed as percentage P.

$$x_{syn}[n+1] = P \cdot x_{syn}[n] \tag{12.12}$$

As presented previously, the scaling factor x_{syn} has an equilibrium value of 1. This is achieved by applying Equation (12.13) when the presynaptic neuron does not emit any spikes according to a time constant τ_{syn}.

$$x_{syn}[n+1] = (1 - x_{syn})/\tau_{syn} \tag{12.13}$$

The key parameters are synaptic weight, W_{syn}, scaling factor, x_{syn}, and percentage, P. Each synapse is defined by these three parameters. These parameters are stored in the RAM of our host platform. The τ_{syn}, τ_{ampa}, and τ_{gaba} parameters are also stored in the RAM but are shared.

In addition, for the various exponential decreases, we chose not to divide by time constant τ, but to multiply by the inverse of the time constant. This operation is equivalent and explains why we also refer to the $1/\tau$ ratio in Section 12.3.4.

12.3.3 Implementation into hardware

12.3.3.1 Computations core

Instead of implementing N neurons on the FPGA platform to obtain a network of N neurons, a computation core dedicated to the neurons was implemented. Indeed, the state of a neuron is defined by nine parameters. Some of these parameters are recalculated and then saved to RAM for use in the next millisecond (1 ms is the time step for solving the Izhikevich equations). This reasoning is valid for each neuron in the network, leading to the observation that, by creating computation pipelines for the u and v variables and time-multiplexing the nine parameters, it was possible to calculate all the neurons in the network, one after the other.

The computation core dedicated to synapses was implemented on the same principle as the one dedicated to neurons (Ambroise et al., 2013).

The overall architecture is presented in Figure 12.3.

12.3.3.2 System blocks

Presenting the architecture in this way provides an overview of the way the entire system operates, on the basis of three blocks: the computation core dedicated to neurons, the one dedicated to synapses, and the RAM. The way each of these three blocks is connected is presented in Figure 12.3.

To summarize, the computation core dedicated to neurons updates the state variables for all the neurons (u and v) and applies the exponential decrease to each synaptic current. In our neural network, the role of the computation core dedicated to synapses is to update all the currents and connection weights. This computation core, therefore, behaves in two different ways, depending on whether it receives a spike or not.

Furthermore, the IZH model has a time step resolution of 1 ms, which must be applied. Consequently, all the "u" and "v" value updates, the exponential decrease

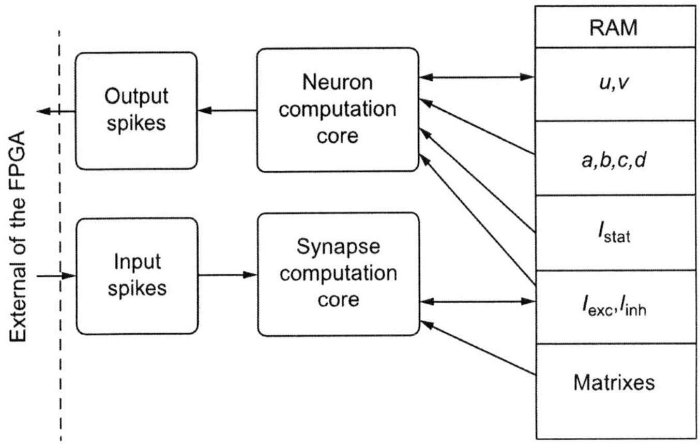

Figure 12.3 Global architecture of the spiking neural network.

in synaptic currents, and the synaptic value updates (currents and depression factor) must be completed during the same millisecond.

Our implementation consisted of a network of N_n neurons and N_s synapses. Each synapse was described by three parameters: a weight, W_{syn} (indicating whether the synapse was inhibitory or excitatory, depending on its sign), a scaling factor, x_{syn}, and a percentage, P. Consequently, three twin matrixes were stored in the RAM for these three parameters, in addition to a connectivity matrix (indicating the postsynaptic neurons connected to each presynaptic neuron).

To minimize the size of RAM, the matrixes were created with N_n lines. The ith line in the connectivity matrix thus corresponded to the connectivity of presynaptic neuron N_i with the other neurons. In this way, synapses were identified by the addresses of their postsynaptic neurons. To summarize, so that each neuron could have a different-sized connectivity list, each line in the connectivity matrix ended with the address of a virtual "end of list" neuron, N_{n+1}. This address, therefore, limited the connectivity list of each neuron and saved memory space.

This is not an optimal solution in cases where a neuron is connected to itself and all the others (the worst case) but saves memory in other cases. Furthermore, this worst case does not correspond to a biologically plausible network and this remains the best solution for a CPG implementation with few synapses. Indeed, according to Marom and Shahaf (2002) and Garofalo et al. (2009), each neuron in a network is connected to 10–30% of the other neurons in the same network.

The occurrences with the address N_{n+1} in the connectivity matrix are replaced by element 0 in the three other matrices. For example, if synapse 10 is the synapse connecting presynaptic neuron 2 to postsynaptic neuron 15 with a synaptic weight of 5, a scaling factor of 1, and a percentage of 0.1%, then address 10:

- in the connectivity matrix is address 15 (address of the postsynaptic neuron)
- in the synaptic weight matrix is 5 (synaptic weight value)
- in the percentage matrix is 0.1
- in the scaling factor matrix is 1

As RAM is also a precious resource, it was not used to store $N_n \times N_n$ matrices. Indeed, CPGs are only small neural networks (8 neurons and 12 synapses).

In the European Brainbow project, our platform hosted 100 neurons and 1200 (external and internal) synapses. Furthermore, a synaptic delay was added to our network for this project. A synaptic delay consists of delaying the arrival of an action potential for a time ranging from 1 to 51 ms. To achieve this, each synapse had a 6-bit delay value T_{delay} and a 50-bit vector capable of storing an action potential in the T_{delay} position. Every millisecond, the 50-bit vectors are shifted to the right and the current action potential is indicated by the least-significant bit.

Table 12.1 shows the resources required for the implementation, according to the number of options (delay and short-term plasticity) required.

12.3.4 Results

RS-type neurons were used in all our CPGs and had the following parameters: $a=0.002$, $b=0.2$, $c=-65$, and $d=8$.

12.3.4.1 Comparison between model and artificial CPG

Our first test consisted of comparing the activity of the artificial CPG and that of the CPG simulating an elementary oscillator. This latter was produced by the Neuron simulation software and used the HH described in Hill et al. (2001).

In our artificial CPG, an elementary oscillator was also used: it had identical inhibitory synapses with a synaptic weight, W_{syn}, of -4 and a percentage, P, equal to 10%. The time constants were: $\tau_{gaba}=2000$ ms and $\tau_{syn}=10{,}000$ ms.

The mechanism behind the activity of our artificial CPG was as follows. Neuron N_1 from the elementary oscillator inhibited a second neuron, N_2, via synapse S_1. The effect of short-term plasticity gradually reduced the inhibition of S_1 until it became

Table 12.1 Implementation on Spartan 6 LX 150 for 100 neurons and 1200 synapses

		Architecture fixed point on 31 bits			
Options of the SNN					
Delay		X	X		
Short-term plasticity		X		X	
Resources	Available total				
Slices FFs	184,304	2398	1981	2075	1720
Slice LUT	92,152	4219	3558	4034	3409
DSP48A1	180	36	28	36	28
RAMB16WER	268	40	22	20	8
RAMB8BWER	536	17	11	15	11
Total RAM	4824 kb				

negligible compared to the GABA effect. At the same time, the GABA effect eliminated the inhibition received. Therefore, at a given time, N_1 no longer inhibited neuron N_2 sufficiently, enabling it to restart its activity and inhibit neuron N_1 via synapse S_2. While it was inhibited, the scaling factor, x_{syn}, for the inactive synapse, S_1, increased until it reached 1 (equilibrium value), thus regenerating the synapse and ensuring it was ready for the precise moment when S_2 became exhausted.

The principle also made it possible to obtain a segmental oscillator. In Figure 12.2, N_1/N_2 and N_3/N_4 correspond to elementary oscillators and are coupled with coordination neurons N_5/N_6 and N_7/N_8. The connectivity between each of these neurons is as shown in Figure 12.2. The connection weights of the elementary oscillators were −4, with percentages of 1%. The output synapses from the elementary oscillator neurons to the coordination neurons had connection weights of −5.2 and a percentage of 1%. The coordination neuron synapses had connection weights of −1.5 and a percentage of 0.1%. The time constants were: $\tau_{gaba} = 1000$ ms and $\tau_{syn} = 5000$ ms.

Table 12.2 presents the results obtained using these parameters.

The average characteristics of the action potential bursts (burst period, duty cycle, and intraburst frequencies) are shown in a table published by Hill et al. (2001). This table was used to compare our digital CPGs with biological CPGs.

An initial examination of Table 12.2 revealed that the biological period and duty cycle were maintained.

The difference between our implementation and the biological system consisted of variations in the intraburst frequency.

Indeed, in the biological system, the frequency of the action potentials started at a low value (around 5 Hz), increased up to a maximum value (around 17 Hz), and then decreased to a low value (around 6 Hz). In contrast, in our implementation, the intraburst frequency varied in a similar way, starting at a low value (around 6 Hz), increasing to a plateau at a maximum value (around 10 Hz), and decreasing to a low frequency (around 8 Hz).

Our digital implementation simplified a biological phenomenon to emulate the required behavior, but was unable to duplicate all the mechanisms responsible for CPG and, consequently, did not reproduce all the details (particularly variations in intraburst frequency).

Table 12.2 Comparison of burst characteristics in the two digital implementations and the biological system

	Biological system	Digital elemental oscillator	Digital segmental oscillator
Mean period	11 ± 1 s	11.9 ± 0.1 s	11.5 ± 1 s
Mean duty cycle	57.2 ± 2.9%	49.2–50%	56.5 ± 4%
Mean spike frequency	11.9 ± 2.1 Hz	8.7 ± 2.7 Hz	9 ± 2 Hz
Initial spike frequency	4.3 ± 0.7 Hz	6.1 ± 0.2 Hz	6.7 ± 0.2 Hz
Peak spike frequency	17.5 ± 3.2 Hz	10 Hz	11 Hz
Final spike frequency	5.8 ± 1.0 Hz	8.3 ± 0.4 Hz	9.0 ± 0.5 Hz

Despite these approximations, we managed to reproduce the behavior of the leech heart CPG using a simple neuron model (IZH model) and a synapse with short-term plasticity (Izhikevich and Edelman, 2008). One future prospect for decreasing variations in the duty cycle, thus improving CPG stability, is described in Section 13.3.5.

12.3.4.2 Table of parameters

In general, it is possible to change the dynamics (activity) of a CPG by modifying the number of neurons and synapses. However, in our implementation, it was also possible to modify the CPG frequency and/or burst duration by changing only a single parameter in the same configuration (i.e. the same number of neurons and synapses).

Table 12.3 shows that multiplying τ_{syn} and τ_{gaba} resulted in a longer period.

According to Ijspeert (2001), CPGs used for neurobotic applications have varying periods and phases, in order to emulate different paces (walk, trot, and gallop) (Still et al., 2006). Using one table for each pace, it is possible to build a robot capable of several different paces.

The periods required for human walking are around 10 s (Joucla et al., 2013), whereas those required for neurobotic applications are shorter, around 1 s.

12.3.5 Conclusion and perspectives

It is possible to design an artificial, biomimetic CPG on an FPGA platform. The CPG used to produce the leech heartbeat was implemented with a minimum of resources without reducing its biorealism, on the basis of the various experiments reported in Section 12.3.4.

From a topological standpoint, the implementation of a calculation core dedicated to neurons (IZH model) and synapses (with short-term plasticity) initially made it possible to operate with frugal resources (see Table 12.4), while, at the same time,

Table 12.3 Variations in the mean period with different values for the parameter τ_{syn}

I_{bias}	w	p	τ_{syn}	τ_{gaba}	Mean period (s)
Parameters for CPG for hybrid experiment					
6.9	−5	0.01	0.0002	0.001	4.6
6.9	−5	0.01	0.0001	0.0005	13.6
6.9	−5	0.01	0.00005	0.00025	30.5
Parameters for neurobotics CPGs					
6.9	−5.4	0.01	0.0004	0.002	2.4
6.9	−6.2	0.01	0.0008	0.004	1.2
6.9	−9.1	0.01	0.0016	0.008	1

Table 12.4 Resources required to implement one network of 500 CPG on a Spartan 6 LX 150 board

Resources	Total available	Used for one segmental CPG	Used for 500 CPG
Slice FFs	184,304	2602	6665
Slice LUT	92,152	4253	21,119
DSP48A1	180	42	42
RAMB8BWER	536	10	492
Total RAM	4824 kb		

building a larger network. Indeed, this implementation is capable of hosting a 500 CPG network on the Spartan6 FPGA platform.

The short-term prospect is to continue investigating and learning to control CPGs, using a more stable neuron model, such as the one developed by Touboul (2009). Part of our team is focusing on this model, which is stabler than the one proposed by Izhikevich and also requires very few resources (Grassia et al., 2014).

One medium-term perspective would be to incorporate this system in hybrid movement experiments. For example, it is entirely possible to envisage stimulating a rat spinal cord by incorporating MEAs (Multi Electrode Array) and functions for detecting and processing action potentials into the experimental platform and using a commercial stimulator.

A variety of long-term objectives may be envisaged: designing ASIC or even neuroprostheses for hybrid experiments, including a robotic salamander capable of moving and even swimming. Indeed, our system is capable of hosting 500 CPGs, whereas only 40 are required to reproduce the swimming movement of a salamander.

References

Amari, S., 1972. Characteristic of the random nets of analog neuron-like elements. IEEE Trans. Syst. Man Cybern. 2, 643–657. http://dx.doi.org/10.1109/TSMC.1972. 4309193.

Ambroise, M., Levi, T., Joucla, S., Yvert, B., Saighi, S., 2013. Real time biomimetic central pattern generators in an FPGA for hybrid experiments. Front. Neurosci. 7, 215. http://dx.doi.org/10.3389/fnins.2013.00215.

Angstadt, J.D., Calabrese, R.L., 1991. Calcium currents and graded synaptic transmission between heart interneurons of the leech. J. Neurosci. 11, 746–759.

Barron-Zambrano, J.H., Torres-Huitzil, C., 2013. FPGA implementation of a configurable neuromorphic CPG-based locomotion controller. Neural Netw. 45, 50–61. http://dx.doi.org/10.1016/j.neunet.2013.04.005.

Barron-Zambrano, J.H., Torres-Huitzil, C., Girau, B., 2010. FPGA-based circuit for central pattern generator in quadruped locomotion. Aust. J. Intell. Inf. Process. Syst. 12, 24–29.

Ben-Ari, Y., Khazipov, R., Leinekugel, X., Caillard, O., Gaiarsa, J.L., 1997. GABAA, NMDA and AMPA receptors: a developmentally regulated 'ménage à trois. Trends Neurosci. 20, 523–529. http://dx.doi.org/10.1016/S0166-2236 (97)01147-8.

Brainbow, 2012. Brainbow Project European Union's Seventh Framework Programme (ICT-FETFP7/2007-2013, FET Young Explorers scheme) Under Grant Agreement no 284772. Available online at: www.brainbowproject.eu.

Calabrese, R.L., 1995. Half-center oscillators underlying rhythmic movements. In: Arbib, M.A. (Ed.), The Hand Book of Brain Theory and Neural Networks. MIT Press, Cambridge, MA, pp. 444–447.

Calabrese, R.L., Angstadt, J., Arbas, E., 1989. A neural oscillator based on reciprocal inhibition. Perspect. Neural Syst. Behav. 10, 33–50.

Cassidy, A., Andreou, A.G., 2008. Dynamical digital silicon neurons. In: IEEE Biomedical Circuits and Systems Conference, BioCAS 2008, pp. 289–292. http://dx.doi.org/10.1109/BIOCAS.2008.4696931.

Cohen, A.H., Ermentrout, G.B., Kiemel, T., Kopel, N., Sigvardt, K.A., Williams, T.L., 1992. Modelling of intersegmental coordination in the lamprey central pattern generator for locomotion. Trends Neurosci. 15, 434–438. http://dx.doi.org/10.1016/0166-2236(92)90006-T.

Crespi, A., Ijspeert, A.J., 2006. Amphibot II: An Amphibious snake robot that crawls and swims using a central pattern generator. In: Proceedings of the 9th International Conference on Climbing and walking robots, pp. 19–27.

Cymbalyuk, G.S., Gaudry, Q., Masino, M.A., Calabrese, R.L., 2002. Bursting in leech heart interneurons: cell-autonomous and network-based mechanisms. J. Neurosci. 22, 10580–10592.

Ekeberg, O., 1993. A combined neuronal and mechanical model of fish swimming. Biol. Cybern. 69, 363–374.

Garofalo, M., Nieus, T., Massobrio, P., Martinoia, S., 2009. Evaluation of the performance of information theory-based methods and cross-correlation to estimate the functional connectivity in cortical networks. PLoS One 4, e6482. http://dx.doi.org/10.1371/journal.pone.0006482.

Grassia, F., Buhry, L., Levi, T., Tomas, J., Destexhe, A., Saighi, S., 2011. Tunable neuromimetic integrated system for emulating cortical neuron models. Front. Neurosci. 5, 134. http://dx.doi.org/10.3389/fnins.2011.00134.

Grassia, F., Levi, T., Kohno, T., Saighi, S., 2014. Silicon neuron: digital hardware implementation of the quartic model. In: International Symposium on Artificial Life and Robotics.

Guerrero-Riberas, R., Morrison, A., Diesmann, M., Pearce, T., 2006. Programmable logic construction kits for hyper-real-time neuronal modeling. Neural Comput. 18, 2651–2679. http://dx.doi.org/10.1162/neco.2006.18.11.2651.

Hill, A.A., Lu, J., Masino, M.A., Olsen, O.H., Calabrese, R.L., 2001. A model of a segmental oscillator in the leech heartbeat neuronal network. J. Comput. Neurosci. 10, 281–302. http://dx.doi.org/10.1023/A:1011216131638.

Hochberg, L.R., Serruya, M.D., Friehs, G.M., Mukand, J.A., Saleh, M., Caplan, A., et al., 2006. Neuronal ensemble control of prosthetic devices by a human with tetraplegia. Nature 442, 164–171. http://dx.doi.org/10.1038/nature04970.

Hochberg, L.R., Bacher, D., Jarosiewicz, B., Masse, N.Y., Simeral, J.D., Vogel, J., et al., 2012. Reach and grasp by people with tetraplegia using a neutrally controlled robotic arm. Nature 485, 372–375. http://dx.doi.org/10.1038/nature11076.

Hodgkin, A.L., Huxley, A.F., 1952. A quantitative description of membrane current and its applications to conduction and excitation in nerve. J. Physiol. 117, 500–544.

Ijspeert, A., 2001. A connectionist central pattern generator for the aquatic and terrestrial gaits of a simulated salamander. Biol. Cybern. 84, 331–348. http://dx.doi.org/10.1007/s004220000211.

Ijspeert, A., 2008. Central pattern generators for locomotion control in animals and robots: a review. Neural Netw. 21, 642–653. http://dx.doi.org/10.1016/j.neunet.2008. 03.014.

Ijspeert, A., Crespi, A., Ryczko, D., Cabelguen, J., 2007. From swimming to walking with a salamander robot driven by a spinal cord model. Science 315, 1416–1420. http://dx.doi.org/10.1126/science.1138353.

Indiveri, G., 2007. Synaptic plasticity and spike-based computation in VLSI networks of integrate-and-fire neurons. Neural Inf. Process. Lett. Rev. 11, 135–146.

Indiveri, G., Linares-Barranco, B., Hamilton, T., Van Schaik, A., Etienne-Cummings, R., Delbruck, T., 2011. Neuromorphic silicon neuron circuits. Front. Neurosci. 5, 73. http://dx.doi.org/10.3389/fnins.2011.00073.

Izhikevich, E.M., 2003. Simple model of spiking neurons. IEEE Trans. Neural Netw. 14, 1569–1572. http://dx.doi.org/10.1109/TNN.2003.820440.

Izhikevich, E.M., 2004. Which model to use for cortical spiking neurons. IEEE Trans. Neural Netw. 15, 1063–1070. http://dx.doi.org/10.1109/TNN.2004.832719.

Izhikevich, E.M., Edelman, G.M., 2008. Large-scale model of mammalian thalamocortical systems. PNAS 105 (9), 3593–3598.

Jezzini, S., Hill, A.A., Kuzyk, P., Calabrese, R.L., 2004. Detailed model of intersegmental coordination in the timing network of the leech heartbeat central pattern generator. J. Neurophysiol. 91, 958–977. http://dx.doi.org/10.1152/jn.00656.2003.

Joucla, S., Ambroise, M., Levi, T., Lafon, T., Rousseau, L., Lissorgues, G., Lewis, N., Saighi, S., Renaud, S., Yvert, B., 2013. Generation of locomotor-like activity in the lesioned rat spinal cord driven by an artificial CPG. In: IEEE EMBS-NRE.

Jung, R., Brauer, E.J., Abbas, J.J., 2001. Real-time interaction between a neuromorphic electronic circuit and the spinal cord. IEEE Trans. Neural Syst. Rehabil. Eng. 9, 319–326. http://dx.doi.org/10.1109/7333.948461.

Krahl, B., Zerbst-Boroffka, I., 1983. Blood pressure in the leech. J. Exp. Biol. 107, 163–168.

Le Masson, S., Debay, D., Bal, T., 2002. Feedback inhibition controls spike transfer in hybrid thalamic circuits. Nature 417, 854–858. http://dx.doi.org/10.1038/nature00825.

Lee, Y.J., Lee, J., Kim, K.K., Kim, Y.B., Ayers, J., 2007. Low power CMOS electronic central pattern generator design for a biomimetic underwater robot. Neurocomputing 71, 284–296. http://dx.doi.org/10.1016/j.neucom.2006.12.013.

Lewis, M.A., Hartmann, M.J., Etienne-Cummings, R., Cohen, A.H., 2001. Control of a robot leg with an adaptive VLSI CPG chip. Neurocomputing 38–40, 1409–1421. http://dx.doi.org/10.1016/S0925-2312(01)00506-9.

Li, C., Lowe, R., Ziemke, T., 2013. Humanoids learning to walk: a natural CPG-actor-critic architecture. Front. Neurorob. 7. http://dx.doi.org/10.3389/fnbot.2013.00005, 5.

Li, W.-C., Merrison-Hort, R., Zhang, H.-Y., Borisyuk, R., 2014. The generation of antiphase oscillations and synchrony by a rebound-based vertebrate central pattern generator. J. Neurosci. 34 (17), 6065–6077.

Linares-Barranco, B., Sánchez-Sinencio, E., Rodríguez-Vázquez, A., Huertas, J.L., 1994. CMOS analog neural network systems based on oscillatory neurons. In: Zaghloul, M., Meador, J., Newcomb, R. (Eds.), Silicon Implementation of Pulse Coded Neural Networks. Kluwer Academic Publishers, Boston, pp. 199–247.

Marom, S., Shahaf, G., 2002. Development, learning and memory in large random networks of cortical neurons: lessons beyond anatomy. Q. Rev. Biophys. 35, 6387. http://dx.doi.org/10.1017/S0033583501003742.

Matsuoka, K., 1987. Mechanism of frequency and pattern control in the neural rhythm generators. Biol. Cybern. 56, 345–353. http://dx.doi.org/10.1007/BF00319514.

Merolla, P.A., Arthur, J.V., Alvarez-Icaza, R., Cassidy, A.S., Sawada, J., Akopyan, F., Jackson, B.L., Imam, N., Guo, C., Nakamura, Y., Brezzo, B., Vo, I., Esser, S.K., Appuswany, R., Taba, B., Amir, A., Flickner, M.D., Risk, W.P., Manohar, R.,

Modha, D.S., 2014. A million spiking-neuron integrated circuit with a scalable communication network and interface. Science 345, 668–673. http://dx.doi.org/10.1126/science.1254642.

Nadim, F., Olsen, O.H., De Schutter, E., Calabrese, R.L., 1995. Modeling the leech heartbeat elemental oscillator. J. Comput. Neurosci. 2, 215–235.

Nakada, K., 2003. An analog cmos central pattern generator for interlimb coordination in quadruped locomotion. IEEE Trans. Neural Netw. 14, 1356–1365. http://dx.doi.org/10.1109/TNN.2003.816381.

Nicolelis, M.A.L., Lebedev, M.A., 2009. Principles of neural ensemble physiology underlying the operation of brain-machine interfaces. Nat. Rev. Neurosci. 10, 530–540. http://dx.doi.org/10.1038/nrn2653.

Norris, B., Weaver, A., Wenning, A., Garcia, P., Calabrese, R.L., 2007. A central pattern generator producing alternative outputs: phase relations of leech heart motor neurons with respect of premotor synaptic input. J. Neurophysiol. 98, 2983–2991. http://dx.doi.org/10.1152/jn.00407.2007.

Olsen, O.H., Calabrese, R.L., 1996. Activation of intrinsic and synaptic currents in leech heart interneurons by realistic waveforms. J. Neurosci. 16, 4958–4970.

Olsen, O.H., Nadim, F., Calabrese, R.L., 1995. Modeling the leech heartbeat elemental oscillator: II. Exploring the parameter space. J. Comput. Neurosci. 2, 237–257. http://dx.doi.org/10.1007/BF00961436.

Olypher, A., Cymbalyuk, G., Calabrese, R.L., 2006. Hybrid systems analysis of the control of burst duration by low-voltage-activated calcium current in Leech heart interneurons. J. Neurophysiol. 96, 2857–2867. http://dx.doi.org/10.1152/jn.00582.2006.

Rice, K.L., Bhuiyan, P.A., Taha, T.M., Vutsinas, C.N., Smith, M.C., 2009. FPGA implementation of Izhikevich spiking neural network for character recognition. In: International Conference on Reconfigurable Computing and FPGAs (Cancun), pp. 451–456.

Serrano-Gotarredona, R., Oster, M., Lichtsteiner, P., Linares-Barranco, A., Paz-Vicente, R., Gómez-Rodríguez, F., et al., 2009. CAVIAR: A45k-Neuron, 5 M-Synapse, 12G-connects/sec AER hardware sensory-processing-learning- actuating system for high speed visual object recognition and tracking. IEEE Trans. Neural Netw. 20, 1417–1438. http://dx.doi.org/10.1109/TNN.2009.2023653.

Simoni, M., De Weerth, S., 2007. Sensory feedback in a half-center oscillator model. IEEE Trans. Biomed. Eng. 54, 193–204. http://dx.doi.org/10.1109/TBME. 2006.886868.

Simoni, M., Cymbalyuk, G., Sorensen, M., Calabrese, R., De Weerth, S., 2004. A multi-conductance silicon neuron with biologically matched conductances. IEEE Trans. Biomed. Eng. 51, 342–354. http://dx.doi.org/10.1109/TBME.2003.820390.

Sorensen, M., De Weerth, S., Cymbalyuk, G., Calabrese, R.L., 2004. Using a hybrid neural system to reveal regulation of neuronal network activity by an intrinsic current. J. Neurosci. 24, 5427–5438. http://dx.doi.org/10.1523/JNEUROSCI.4449- 03.2004.

Stevenson, P.A., Kutsch, W., 1987. A reconsideration of the central pattern generator concept for locust flight. J. Comp. Physiol. A. 161, 115–129.

Still, S., Tilden, M.W., 1998. Controller for a four legged walking machine. In: Smith, L.S., Hamilton, A. (Eds.), Neuromorphic Systems: Engineering Silicon from Neurobiology. World Scientific Publishing Co Pte Ltd, Singapore, pp. 138–148. http://dx.doi.org/10.1142/9789812816535_0012.

Still, S., Hepp, K., Douglas, R.J., 2006. Neuromorphic walking gait control. IEEE Trans. Neural Netw. 17, 496–508. http://dx.doi.org/10.1109/TNN.2005.863454.

Tabak, J., Senn, W., O'Donovan, M., Rinzel, J., 2000. Modeling of spontaneous activity in developing spinal cord using activity-dependent depression in an excitatory network. J. Neurosci. 20, 3041–3056.
Torres-Huitzil, C., Girau, B., 2008. Implementation of central pattern generator in an FPGA-based embedded system. In: 18th International Conference on Artificial Neural Networks, vol. 5164, pp. 179–187. http://dx.doi.org/10.1007/978-3-540- 87559-8_19.
Touboul, J., 2009. Importance of the cut off value in the quadratic adaptive integrate-and-fire model. Neural Comput. 21, 2114–2122. http://dx.doi.org/10.1162/neco. 2009.09-08-853.
Van Der Pol, B., 1928. The heartbeat considered as a relaxation oscillation, and an electrical model of the heart. Philos. Mag. 6, 763–775.
Vogelstein, R.J., Tenore, F., Etienne-Cummings, R., Lewis, M.A., Cohen, A.H., 2006. Dynamic control of the central pattern generator for locomotion. Biol. Cybern. 95, 555–566. http://dx.doi.org/10.1007/s00422-006-0119-z.
Wijekoon, J., Dudek, P., 2008. Compact silicon neuron circuit with spiking and bursting behavior. Neural Netw. 21, 524–534. http://dx.doi.org/10.1016/j.neunet.2007. 12.037.
Zielinska, T., 1995. Coupled oscillators utilized as gait rhythm generators of a two-legged walking machine. Biol. Cybern. 74, 263–273.

Bio-inspired multi-robot systems

13

B. Ranjbar-Sahraei, K. Tuyls, I. Caliskanelli, B. Broeker, D. Claes, S. Alers, G. Weiss

13.1 Introduction

Recent years have seen an increasing interest in nature-inspired modeling for solving complex computational problems in disciplines at the intersection of computer science, robotics, and economics. An interesting natural phenomenon is the coordination behavior that can be observed in colonies of social insects such as ants and bees. For instance, recent work shows a strong potential in creating artificial systems that mimic insect behavior for solving complex coordination tasks such as, e.g., routing on the internet, mobile *ad hoc* network routing, robotic tasks (Lemmens and Tuyls, 2012; Dressler and Akan, 2010; Floreano and Mattiussi, 2008). These insects have evolved over a long period of time and display remarkable behaviors that are highly suitable for addressing the complex tasks that they are facing. Swarm optimization algorithms, like ant colony optimization (ACO) (Dorigo et al., 2006b), rely on pheromone trails to mediate (indirect) communication between agents. Such insect-inspired multi-agent research has also opened the possibility of applying some of these techniques to robotic systems, i.e., swarm robotics (Dorigo and Roosevelt, 2004; Şahin, 2005). Swarm robotic systems are motivated by a wide range of application areas, such as for instance surveillance and patrolling, where mobile guarding robots are considered as an alternative and improvement over fixed security cameras and even humans. Other application areas include exploration and identification of hazardous environments (e.g., nuclear plants and fire detection), mobile sensor networks, wireless sensor and robot networks, space exploration, etc.

Though easy to simulate, artificial pheromones are hard to bring into real life robotic applications as pheromones need to be deployed and sensed by robots while they decay over time. Recently, non-pheromone-based algorithms were developed as well (Lemmens, 2011). Such algorithms are inspired by the foraging and nest-site selection behavior of (mainly) bees. Generally speaking, bees explore the environment in search for high-quality food sources, and once returned to the hive, they start to dance in order to communicate the location of the source. Using this dance, bees recruit other colony members for a specific food source. The more bees adopt a certain transportation path, the more bees will eventually perform the same dance. Since few dances will not attract enough bees, the best transportation path will eventually prevail.

We draw inspiration from these insect behaviors with the goal to create emergent intelligent systems for distributed coordination that can be deployed in real-world settings on physical platforms. One of the physical platforms we will consider in this chapter is the e-puck robot that has moderate resources such as limited sensing, computation, and actuation capabilities (Mondada et al., 2009). Another platform we will consider is the Turtlebot robot that has more extensive resources, contains advanced cameras and carries a general purpose computer (Willow Garage, 2014). We will overview some of our multi-robot swarm experiments in this chapter using simulations and the real robotic platforms, e-puck and Turtlebot robots. Finally, we will describe how the future trend of swarm robotics is moving toward heterogeneity among robots in a swarm.

The remainder of this chapter is structured as follows. Section 13.2 provides the required background on biological inspirations used in this chapter and reviews the related work in the areas of coordination in multi-robot systems. Section 13.3 describes the ant-inspired coordination principle, whereas Section 13.4 shows bee-inspired coordination principles and is split into two parts: (1) Section 13.4.1 covers the foraging behavior of honeybees and (2) Section 13.4.2 exploits pheromone signaling process in honeybees. Future trends of bio-inspired coordination on multi-robot platforms are presented in Section 13.5. The main conclusion of this research is presented in Section 13.6.

13.2 Background

This section provides the required background knowledge to understand the remainder of this chapter. It is divided into two main parts: Section 13.2.1 explains underlying biological inspirations of ant and bee colonies in detail, whereas Section 13.2.2 discusses related work on coordination and coverage in multi-robot and distributed network systems (e.g., sensor nets) based on bio-inspired principles.

13.2.1 Biological inspirations

This section provides the required background knowledge of three different biological inspirations used in this chapter. We start by introducing stigmergic behavior of ants, continue with foraging behaviors of honeybees, and end with the pheromone signaling mechanism for queen bee selection within honeybee colonies.

13.2.1.1 Stigmergic behavior of ants

Most of the research in swarm intelligence revolves around the behavior of ants (Dorigo and Stützle, 2004; Dorigo and Blumb, 2005; Dorigo et al., 2006b). The principle is simple yet elegant: ants deposit a pheromone trail on the path they take during travel. Using this trail, they are able to navigate toward their nest or food and communicate with their peers. More specifically, ants employ an indirect recruitment strategy by accumulating pheromone trails. When a trail gets strong enough, other ants are attracted to it and will follow this trail toward a food destination. The more ants follow a trail, the more pheromone is accumulated and, in turn, the trail becomes more attractive for being followed. This is known as the autocatalytic process. Since long paths take more time to traverse, it will require more ants to sustain a long path. As a consequence, short paths will eventually prevail (see Figure 13.1a). We explain the details of stigmergic coordination algorithm in Section 13.3.

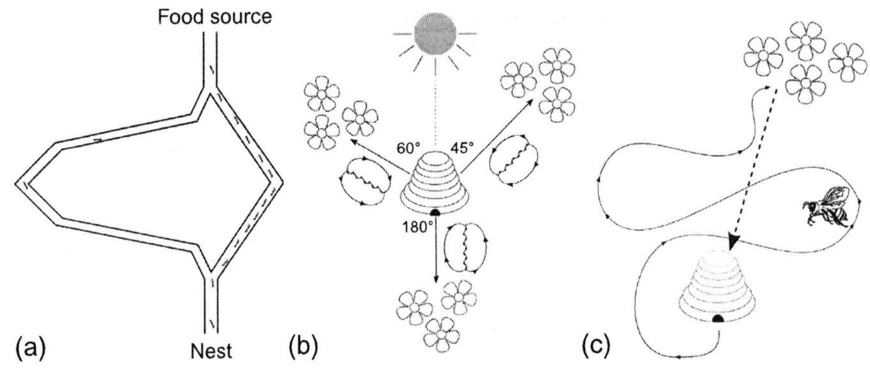

Figure 13.1 Biological inspiration (a) ants exploring two paths; the shortest path prevails. (b) Honeybee waggle dance communicating a PI vector. (c) Lévy flight and path integration.

13.2.1.2 Foraging behavior of honeybees

Foraging honeybees display two types of behavior, i.e., recruitment and navigation. In order to recruit other colony members for food sources, honeybees inform their nest mates of the distance and direction of these food sources by means of a waggling dance performed on the vertical combs in the hive. This dance (i.e., the bee language) consists of a series of alternating left-hand and right-hand loops, interspersed by a segment in which the bee waggles her abdomen from side to side. The duration of the waggle phase is a measure of the distance to the food. The angle between the sun and the axis of a bee's waggle segment on the vertical comb represents the azimuthal angle between the sun and a target location, i.e., the direction in which a recruit should fly (see Figure 13.1b and c). Other members of the colony can adopt the "advertisement" for a food source. The decision mechanism for adopting an "advertised" food-source location by a potential recruit is not completely understood. It is considered that the recruitment among bees is a function of the quality of the food source.

Different species of social insects, such as honeybees and desert ants, make use of non-pheromone-based navigation. Non-pheromone-based navigation mainly consists of Path Integration (PI), which is the continuous update of a vector by integrating all angles steered, and all distances covered (Collett et al., 1998). A PI vector represents the insect's knowledge of direction and distance toward its destination. To construct a PI vector, the insect does not use a mathematical vector summation, but employs a computationally simple approximation (Collett et al., 1998). Using this approximation, the insect is able to return to its destination directly. More precisely, when the path is unobstructed, the insect solves the problem optimally. However, when the path is obstructed, the insect has to fall back on other strategies such as exploration or landmark navigation (Cheng et al., 1987; Collett et al., 2002) to solve the problem. Obviously, bees are able to fly, i.e., when they encounter an obstacle, they can mostly choose to fly over it. However, even if the path is unobstructed, bees tend to navigate over the entire path using landmarks. The landmarks divide the entire path into segments and each landmark has a PI vector associated with it. This behavior decreases navigation errors and ensures robustness. We refer to a home-pointing PI vector as a Home Vector (HV). PI is used in both exploration and exploitation. During exploration, insects constantly update their HV. It is however not used as an exploration strategy. During exploitation, the insects update both their HV and the PI vectors indicating the food source and use these vectors as guidance to a destination. Section 13.4.1 defines foraging-inspired robot coordination algorithm in details.

13.2.1.3 Pheromone signaling behavior of honeybees

The queen bee selection mechanism in honeybee colonies is used to orchestrate the colony by assigning responsibilities to each individual. Roberts (1986) explains the process of larvae differentiation in beehives as an example of such orchestration. Bees have developed a special hormonal system to ensure every beehive has a queen, which maintains the stability of the colony and orchestrates the behavior of all other bees. Throughout its life, a queen bee stimulates a pheromone called Queen Mandibular Pheromone (QMP), which makes the worker bees aware of its presence as a queen. This hormonal mechanism works as follows: the worker bees lick the queen bee and pass the pheromone on to the others. If there is no pheromone passed through the worker bees anymore, this will be an indicator that the queen is dead or has disappeared. In that case, emergency queen cells will be created and workers will select a larva to be fed with large amounts of the royalactin protein (Roberts, 1986). That protein induces the differentiation of honeybee larvae into a new queen. If worker bees keep receiving the pheromone, they will be aware that there is a queen bee to orchestrate the colony and will take no action toward building emergency queen cells.

We describe our *BeePCo* algorithm in detail based on the analogy described in Table 13.1 (see Caliskanelli et al., 2014). Accordingly, the role of queen bee denotes a robot that is responsible for managing the execution of all service requests it receives. Throughout Section 13.4.2, we will refer to such a robot as Queen Robot (QR). They can dynamically differentiate from other robots to indicate their duties for redundancy control (by tuning the pheromone level parameter). However, for the *BeePCo* algorithm presented in this chapter, we allow all the robots to be QRs and we focus on using pheromones as a way of indicating covered arena area rather than role differentiation for redundancy control (unlike in our previous work on WSNs; Caliskanelli et al., 2012b).

Table 13.1 Correlation between bees' pheromone stimulation and multi-robot systems

Bee's pheromone stimulation	Multi-robot systems
Queen bee	Robot responsible for processing services
Worker bees	Robots
Pheromone level	Parameter used for queen robot selection
Lifetime of bee	Operation lifetime of the robot

13.2.2 Related work

This section gives an overview of relevant literature that has described, analyzed, and deployed bio-inspired coordination techniques for multi-robot systems. It is split into three main parts: we start with a generic definition of the multi-robot coverage problem and overview some examples, we continue by providing significant examples of ant inspired and bee-inspired techniques that are used to solve complex problems (i.e., MAC level routing, load balancing, task allocation and resource scheduling, network coverage, etc.) in the broad research area of autonomous, distributed, and networked systems.

13.2.2.1 Coordination and coverage techniques

The concept of coverage is a metric for evaluating robotic systems, which was first introduced by Gage (1992). He defined three basic types of coverage: blanket coverage, in which the objective is to achieve node formation, which maximizes the total detection area; barrier coverage, which aims to minimize the probability of undetected intrusion through the barrier; and sweep or repetitive coverage with the goal to cover all accessible interest points in a given environment over time, while maximizing the rate of visits over all points and minimizing the total distance traveled by all robots.

Blanket coverage is most common for the deployment of mobile sensor networks in an unknown environment; the sensor nodes are initially placed in a compact configuration, where the nodes are trying to spread out such that the area covered by the network is maximized. One example for such a use case is a hazardous material leak in a damaged structure. Mobile sensor nodes equipped with chemical sensors spread out from an initial position to gather information about location and concentration of the hazard. Due to the fact that the communication infrastructure could be damaged, the nodes have to insure their own network structure even if single nodes get lost or destroyed. Many approaches in this field are based on the potential field technique first introduced by Khatib (1985).

Barrier and repetitive coverage problems originate from the computational geometry *Art Gallery Problem* (El-Sherbeny, 2010) and its variant for mobile guard, the *Watchman Route Problem* (Packer, 2008).

In robotics, *repetitive-coverage* can be described as a problem where a team of robots has to visit multiple *points of interests* (POI) in a known environment frequently, to perform certain tasks. The goal of such algorithms is to keep the average visit frequency over all POIs high, while achieving a minimal total traveled distance and a balanced workload over all robots. Typical real-world use cases for such problems are patrolling, lawn mowing and chemical spill cleanup.

Another important form of multi-robot coverage is *terrain coverage* or multi-robot exploration. It can be defined as a problem where a robot tries to visit each and every location in a continuous bounded unknown environment by avoiding obstacles and perform defined tasks as proposed by Correll and Martinoli (2006), Gabriely and Rimon (2003), and Pirzadeh and Snyder (1990). A terrain coverage algorithm must generate a coverage path, which is a chain of motion steps for a robot; the optimal coverage path takes minimal time and guarantee to cover the entire terrain and perform the task efficiently.

13.2.2.2 Ant-inspired techniques

Ant-based multi-robot coverage is highly inspired by the notion of stigmergic communication introduced by Dorigo (1992). The basic idea underlying this form of communication is that pheromones are used as a medium for transmitting messages among artificial ants. During the past few years, variants of Dorigo's method, known as ant colony optimization, have been developed, and it has been shown that it allows for very efficient distributed control and optimization in a variety of problem domains (Dorigo et al., 2006a). Wagner et al. (1999) were the first, who invested stigmergic multi-robot coordination for covering/patrolling the environment. In their approach, the robots were supposed to be able to (1) deposit chemical odor traces and (2) evaluate the strength of smell at every point they reach. Based on these assumptions, they used robots to model an unmapped environment as a graph, and they proposed basic graph search algorithms (such as Depth-First-Search and Breadth-First-Search) for solving robotic coverage problems. Many other researchers used this graph-based modeling scheme in order to design solutions for multi-robot patrolling/covering problems, e.g., Elor and Bruckstein (2009, 2010), Glad et al. (2008, 2010), and Yanovski et al. (2003).

In contrast to the mentioned graph-based techniques, a geometrical framework can also be used for addressing the swarm robotic coverage problem. One of the most important geometric techniques is Voronoi-based coverage that has been introduced for solving robot coverage problems (e.g., see Cortes et al., 2004, 2005; Schwager et al., 2011, 2009). These Voronoi-based techniques aim at devising coverage algorithms, which work according to the following basic rule: *Each vehicle moves toward the center of its Voronoi region*. Based on this rule, many researchers have proposed modified covering approaches, which are adaptable to changes in the environment and are provably convergent (e.g., Schwager et al., 2009; Breitenmoser et al., 2010). However, all these geometrical algorithms require a group of robots with the capability of direct communication and in most of the cases also need very complex mathematical computations (e.g., calculating margins and center of mass for an individual Voronoi region), which limits their potential real-world usage. In Section 13.3, we show how robots can use stigmergic and Voronoi-like coverages with a very simple technique.

Another related research topic is focused on the "real" implementation of stigmergic communication in real-world experiments. For example, chemical substances such as ethanol (C_2H_5OH) are used instead of natural pheromones by Fujisawa et al. (2008). However, with recent developments in communication technology, electrical devices such as Radio Frequency Identification Devices (RFIDs) have gained much interest for such applications. Johansson and Saffiotti (2009) and Herianto et al. (2007) used RFIDs for mapping and exploring an unknown environment. Moreover, Ziparo et al. (2007) proposed a coordinated exploration and multi-robot SLAM for large teams of rescue robots by using RFIDs as environment features.

13.2.2.3 Bee-inspired techniques

Bee Colony Optimization (BCO) was introduced independently by Lemmens et al. (Lemmens et al., 2007a,b; Lemmens and Tuyls, 2012) and by Karaboga et al. (Karaboga, 2010; Karaboga and Basturk, 2008). Unlike ACO (which is only inspired from the notion of stigmergic communication), scientists are inspired by various behaviors of bees: foraging behavior in Lemmens et al. (Lemmens et al., 2011; Lemmens, 2011), Beehive protocol (Wedde et al., 2004), BeeSensor (Saleem and Farooq, 2007), bees mating procedure (Senthilkumar and Chandrasekaran, 2011; Sahoo et al., 2013), and pheromone signaling mechanism in PS (Caliskanelli et al., 2013).

Karaboga et al. (Karaboga, 2010; Karaboga and Basturk, 2008) introduced the Artificial Bee Colony (ABC) algorithm in which bees represent the search agents and their environment represents the potential solutions. In their work, the high-quality candidate solutions represent a pollen source which encourages further exploration of the region by additional bee agents. In the networking context, protocols have been developed in which network packets are treated as biologically inspired agents. Karaboga et al. improved their technique in Akay and Karaboga (2009) by tuning its parameters and modifying their initial work (Karaboga and Basturk, 2007). In the Beehive protocol (Wedde et al., 2004), packets search for efficient routes through an IP network in a process modeled after the foraging behavior of bees. Similar work targeted specifically at WSNs is BeeSensor (Saleem and Farooq, 2007) in which routing is performed via classes of packets following different types of bee behavior: for example as scouts and foragers. The redundancy introduced by BeeSensor is capable of increasing the proportion of delivered packets compared to AODV (Perkins and Royer, 1999), although it experiences increased latency due to the possibility for bee packets to select suboptimal routes during exploration. A general framework through which a set of biological agents can attempt to simultaneously satisfy multiple possibly conflicting objectives (such as latency, energy efficiency, and delivery success in a WSN) is provided in MONSOON (Boonma and Suzuki, 2008). Previous work has also mapped the bee colony model more directly to WSN hardware, with individual nodes representing individual bees, status within the hive corresponding to node responsibilities, and signaling chemicals corresponding to data packets.

Recent work has applied bee protocols specifically to WSN load balancing (Senthilkumar and Chandrasekaran, 2011), which is inspired by the bees mating procedure. This approach focuses on cluster set-up communication overheads by restricting the communications with bee mating election algorithm. Removing the redundant communications inside the cluster increases the successful delivery ratio while decreasing the latency.

Caliskanelli et al. explore the pheromone signaling mechanism in honeybee colonies in Caliskanelli et al. (2012a, 2013) to solve the load balancing (i.e., to distribute the network load among processing elements) and redundancy control issues in large-scale WSNs. Caliskanelli and Indrusiak improved their parameter-rich technique in Caliskanelli and Indrusiak (2013a) by tuning its parameters and modifying their initial work (Caliskanelli et al., 2013). Later on, they applied pheromone signaling process on WSRNs (Wireless Sensor Robot Networks) in Caliskanelli and Indrusiak (2014).

13.3 Ant-inspired multi-robot coordination

This section describes the concept of Ant-Inspired Multi Robot Coordination, *stigmergy*, and introduces an interesting case study called Stigmergic Coverage (StiCo), which is based on the principle of ants' pheromone-based communication. This case study includes the multi-robot coordination principle, simulations, experiments, and also the modeling of StiCo.

In stigmergic coordination, the environment is used as a medium to transfer information among agents: agents deposit traces in the environment in order to send different types of signals, encoded with the source location, to the other agents. The accumulation of traces in the environment provides a shared memory, which allows memoryless simple agents to coordinate easily, while agents might not have any self-awareness of other agents. Furthermore, the use of stigmergic communication allows for coordination among agents of different types, as well studied by Dorigo et al. (2012) in the Swarmanoid project and also adopted to explain the softly heterogeneous swarms by Ranjbar-Sahraei et al. (2013a). In short, the use of stigmergic communication results in high robustness and adaptability, an extremely easy implementation at the microscopic level and yet very efficient at the macroscopic level.

13.3.1 Case study

The StiCo approach follows the principle of indirect, stigmergic coordination to establish a simple but efficient coverage of the environment. In contrast to the classical stigmergic coordination in Ant System (AS), where (1) agents have a tendency to move straight with minor deviations and (2) traces act as sources of attraction, in StiCo robots orbit in circles, instead of moving straight, and the traces have repulsive characteristics instead of attracting the agents. These two differences turn the path-finding characteristic of AS into efficient area coverage of StiCo.

The robustness, scalability, and functional extensibility (see the work by Ranjbar-Sahraei et al., 2012a) make StiCo an interesting alternative to Voronoi-based and graph-based multi-robot coverage approaches, which currently are dominant in the field. Moreover, because of these features, StiCo has a broad application potential. The multi-robot coverage experiment can be used for various monitoring, rescue, and patrolling missions.

13.3.1.1 StiCo principle

In StiCo, robots are equipped with two simple sensors (in the front-left and front-right directions like an ant antenna), capable of detecting immediate traces. Each robot orbits in a circle with a predetermined radius. Based on the circling direction (CW or CCW), one sensor would be considered as the interior sensor and the other one as the exterior one. When the interior sensor detects pheromone, the robot changes its circling direction immediately as shown in Figure 13.2a–c. Otherwise, if exterior

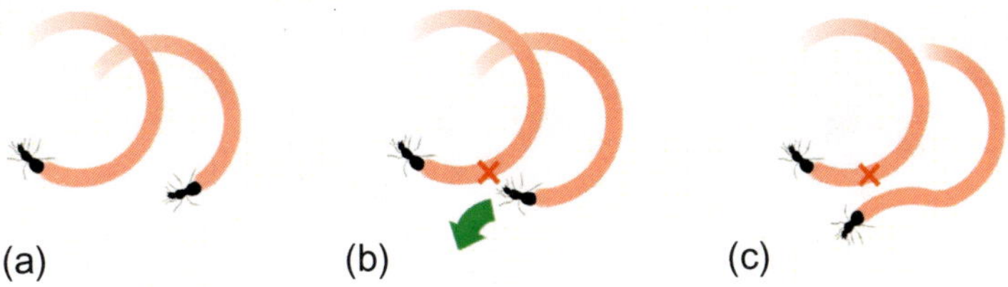

Figure 13.2 StiCo coordination principle: (a) Robots circle around. (b) The right robot detects pheromone. (c) The right robot changes circling direction.

sensor detects pheromone, the robot continues rotating in the same direction until it does not detect pheromone anymore. The amount of pheromone deposited by each robot can practically be adjusted based on pheromone evaporation rates, in a way that robots do not collide with their own pheromones. For further information on StiCo principle, see the work by Ranjbar-Sahraei et al. (2012c).

13.3.1.2 Simulation of StiCo

In order to demonstrate the performance of StiCo, first we translate the previously mentioned rules into an algorithm as shown in Algorithm 1.

The StiCo algorithm is simulated with identical robots in a 40 m × 40 m field. The linear velocity of each robot is 2 m/s, and the angular velocity is set to ± 1.0 rad/s. Further details of the simulation environment are provided by Ranjbar-Sahraei et al. (2012b). The coverage algorithm for 40 robots that move based on StiCo is illustrated in Figure 13.3.

In order to demonstrate potential capabilities of this simple algorithm, we consider a nonconvex unknown environment as shown in Figure 13.4a. This environment can

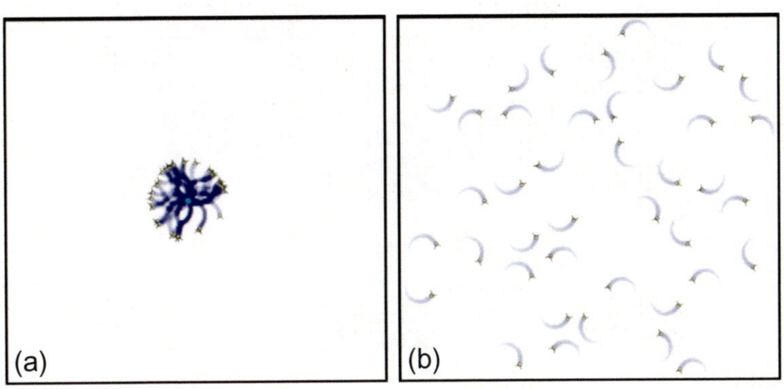

Figure 13.3 Evolution of StiCo in a simple environment (blue shadows are deposited traces). (a) Initial snapshot. (b) Final snapshot.

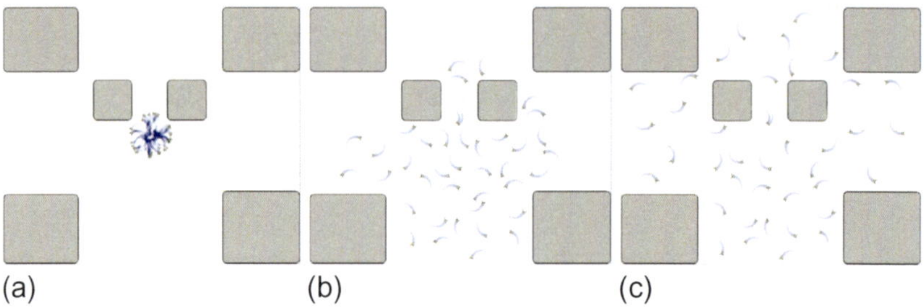

Figure 13.4 Evolution of StiCo in a complex environment. In this simulation, artificial pheromones are deposited on the margins of obstacles to make them detectable for robots. (a) Initial snapshot. (b) Intermediate snapshot. (c) Final snapshot.

represent a devastated area after earthquake or a street map in an emergency condition. Forty robots are initiated at the center of the environment. The coverage steps are illustrated in Figure 13.4a–c.

13.3.1.3 Experiments on StiCo

Motivated by the technique proposed by Kronemann and Hafner (2010), Ranjbar-Sahraei et al. (2013b) have designed a test bed as shown in Figure 13.5. This test bed provides the capability of stigmergic communication to the robots of a swarm.

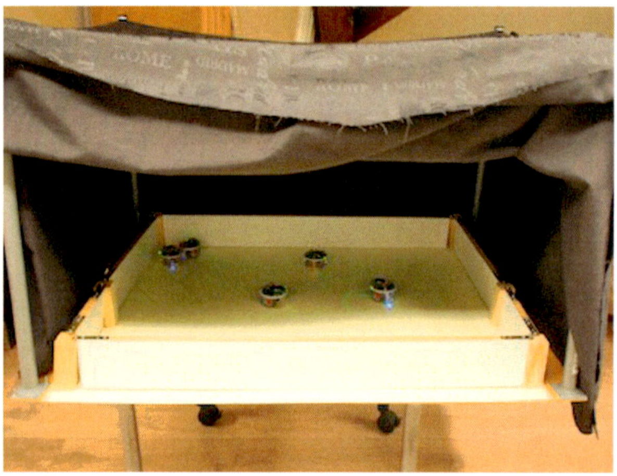

Figure 13.5 Darkroom with glow-in-the-dark floor, where the e-puck robots circle around and emit UV light onto the floor.

Algorithm 1 StiCo algorithm

```
Require: Each robot can deposit/detect pheromone trails
  Initialize: Choose circling direction (CW/CCW)
  loop
    while (no pheromone is detected) do
      Circle around
      deposit pheromone
    end while
    if (interior sensor detects pheromone) then
      Reverse the circling direction
    else
      while (pheromone is detected) do
        Rotate
      end while
    end if
  end loop
```

In this setting, the floor is covered by a glow-in-the-dark foil (i.e., a foil covered by phosphorescent material, which absorbs UV light and reemits the absorbed light at a lower intensity for up to several minutes after the original excitation), and robots are equipped with UV-LEDs pointing toward the floor. Therefore, as robots move around, they leave glowing trails behind themselves. Furthermore, for detection of these trails, in contrast to the simple method used by Kronemann and Hafner (2010), in which photosensors were used to detect glowing trails, the e-puck's on-board camera is used to detect the trails. By capturing an image and applying a green filter to it, the detailed pattern of green trails in the image are extracted and these patterns are used to measure the presence of trail and also its density over different locations.

Implementation of the StiCo coverage approach with real robots is shown in Figure 13.6a–f.

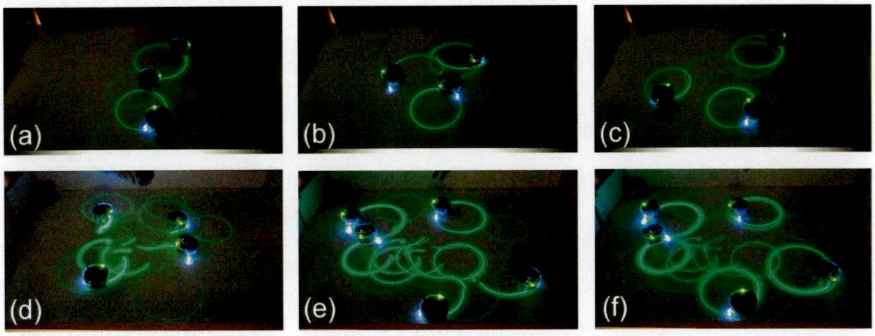

Figure 13.6 Vision-based stigmergic coverage using glowing trails. (a)–(c) Three robots converging into a stable configuration and forming three singular territories. (d)–(f) Five robots converging into a stable configuration and forming five singular territories.

13.3.1.4 Mathematical modeling of StiCo

Due to the simplicity of StiCo's rules for individual robots and the overall complex, yet efficient, behavior of the swarm, many of the classical modeling techniques such as the state-space representation (e.g., used by Ranjbar-Sahraei et al., 2014, to model behaviors in a social network) cannot be used. Instead, the probabilistic modeling techniques studied by Martinoli et al. (2004) and Lerman et al. (2005) are the best fit to such swarm robotic systems.

Ranjbar-Sahraei et al. (2013d) proposed to consider the number of singular robot territories (i.e., the circular region bounded with a single robot traces) as the performance criterion for StiCo. Let us define the state C^n, $n=1, 2, \ldots, M$ for the case that there are n singular territories in the environment. Then, we need a mathematical expression to compute the probability of transition from state C^{n1} to state C^{n2}, in one iteration. This probability is denoted by $P_{n1,n2}$. The first step for computing probability $P_{n1,n2}$ is to partition a general state C^n to all of its possible configurations (the word *partition* refers to a concept of number theory). The configuration $C^n_{T_{a1},T_{a2},\ldots,T_{ak}}$ denotes a configuration in state C^n, in which T_{ai} denotes existence of one ai-tuple in the configuration. If we define $Q^n(K)$ as the probability that a swarm be in state C^n in K-th iteration, then the discrete state transition model can be written as

$$\begin{bmatrix} Q^1(K+1) \\ Q^2(K+1) \\ \vdots \\ Q^M(K+1) \end{bmatrix} = \begin{bmatrix} P_{1,1} & \cdots & P_{M,1} \\ \vdots & \ddots & \vdots \\ P_{1,M} & \cdots & P_{M,M} \end{bmatrix} \begin{bmatrix} Q^1(K) \\ Q^2(K) \\ \vdots \\ Q^M(K) \end{bmatrix} \tag{13.1}$$

For computing $P_{n,n-1}$, which is the transition from C^n to C^{n-1}, the chance that a singular territory becomes a member of a double group should be computed. Let $L(M, n)$ be a function that computes number of possible configurations of M territories, in which exactly n of them are singular. Then, consider the t-th configuration of C^n as

$$C^n_{\underbrace{T_1,T_1,\ldots,T_1}_{n},\underbrace{T_2,T_2,\ldots,T_2}_{r_t},T_{a1_t},T_{a2_t},\ldots,T_{ak_t}} \tag{13.2}$$

The probability for transitions from the t-th configuration of C^n to one of the configurations of C^{n-1}, C^{n+1}, and C^{n+2} are computed as $P_{n,n-1}$, $P_{n,n+1}$, and $P_{n,n+2}$, respectively. Finally, if we ignore the probability for transition from C^n state to the states C^i, in which $i<n-1$ or $i>n+2$, then the probability for remaining in the same state is

$$P_{n,n} = 1 - P_{n,n+1} - P_{n,n+2} - P_{n,n-1} \tag{13.3}$$

In order to check the conditions of fundamental Ergodic Theorem for Markov chains on P matrix, these conditions are simply explained as: (1) P should be stochastic: The values of P must be within the range (0, 1) and each column (or row) sums to 1. (2) P should be irreducible: From each state of our system, it must be possible to get to any other state. (3) P should be aperiodic: The graph represented by P should not be

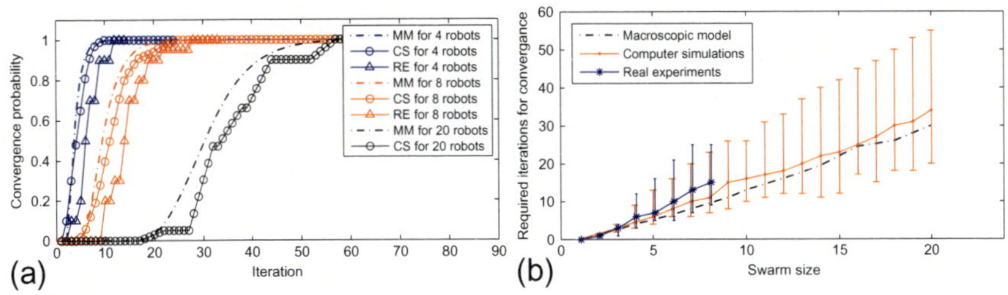

Figure 13.7 Model verification (a) convergence probability in different iterations (MM: Macroscopic Model, CS: Computer Simulations, RE: Real Experiments). (b) Effects of swarm size on convergence time.

bipartite. The first condition holds based on the fact that each probability is in the range of (0, 1), and Equation (13.3), which shows each column sums to 1. The two other conditions can be easily checked with constructing the graph represented by P. Therefore, P is a Markov chain, which can denote a stationary configuration $\prod = \lim_{i\to\infty} P^i \cdot Q(0)$, where $Q(0)$ can be any initial probability distribution for initial configuration.

13.3.1.5 Comparison of model, simulations, and experiments

Three groups of 4, 8, and 20 robots are initialized at the center of an environment. For each group, the probability of being in the final stationary configuration, $Q(\cdot)$, is first computed using the macroscopic model, then computed by using computer simulations, and finally by using real robot experiments. The results of computing the convergence probability are illustrated in Figure 13.7a. The presented results show that the macroscopic model can estimate the behavior of StiCo for robotic swarms of various sizes. As shown in Figure 13.7b, the convergence speed of StiCo increases linearly with growth of the swarm population.

13.4 Bee-inspired multi-robot coordination

This section describes our bee-inspired multi-robot coordination algorithms and is split into two parts. Section 13.4.1 presents foraging behavior-inspired approach, whereas Section 13.4.2 explains the pheromone signaling-inspired approach to solve multi-robot coordination problem.

13.4.1 Bee-inspired biomimicry foraging

In this section, we describe the bees foraging behavior-inspired algorithm, and we illustrate the direct usage of the principles of foraging inspired coordination in swarm intelligence on multi-robot systems. For this set of experiments, we use two types of robot systems: (1) robots with limited resources (e-pucks) and (2) robots with extended resources (Turtlebots). Furthermore, we present results of these two implementations on both robot platforms, discuss the use of sensors for robot localization, camera and video processing for object detection, and the means for having local communication between robots. For further details about our *foraging coordination* approach, please see Alers et al. (2011, 2013a,b, 2014b,c) and Lemmens et al. (2011).

13.4.1.1 Case study

In our approach, recruitment behavior is implemented in analogy with biological bees' dance behavior. Agents share information on previous search experience (i.e., the direction and distance toward a certain food source) only when they are in the hive. Agents in the hive can then decide whether to exploit previous search experience obtained from other agents in the hive, or to exploit their own search experience, if available. As mentioned earlier, bees use an unknown decision mechanism to decide whether to exploit another bee's experience.

The general structure of our bee-inspired algorithm is quite similar to that of algorithms in ASs. It implements both recruitment and navigation behavior and consists of three functions.

13.4.1.2 Bee-inspired algorithm

First, a procedure called ManageBeesActivity() handles agents' activity based on their internal state. Each agent is in one of six internal states. In each state, a specific behavior is performed. Agent state "AtHome" indicates that the agent is located at the hive. While in this state, the agent determines to which new state it will go. Agent state "StayAtHome" also indicates that the agent is located at the hive. However, while in this state it will remain there unless there is previous search experience available to exploit. Previous search experience is represented by a PI vector indicating a food source. If such experience is available, the agent will leave the hive to exploit the previous search experience. Agent state "Exploitation" indicates that the agent is exploiting previous search experience. An agent either exploits its own search experience or acquires a PI vector from other agents inside the hive. The agent determines which cell to move to in order to match the PI vector indicating the food source. Agent state "Exploration" indicates that the agent is exploring its environment in search for food. Agent state "HeadHome" indicates that the agent is heading home without carrying any food. The agent reaches home by following its Homing Vector (HV). The HV is a PI vector indicating the hive. From the moment an agent starts its foraging trip, this HV is continuously calculated for each agent. Agent state "CarryingFood" indicates that the agent has found food and that it is carrying the food back toward the hive. The agent's return path depends on the same HV as with agent state "HeadHome." Next come the experiments, which show how a group of real robots can coordinate using bee-inspired algorithm.

13.4.1.3 Experiments using robots with limited resources (e-pucks)

The bee foraging experiments show the effectiveness of the embodied foraging behavior in a swarm of e-pucks. In Figure 13.8, we present the stages that the experiment goes through. The goal of the experiment is to show that each separate behavior actually works in an embodied swarm. Therefore, the experiment starts with a swarm of e-pucks surrounding the hive (see Figure 13.8a). Figure 13.8b shows the stage in which a portion of the swarm starts foraging while others remain around the hive, waiting for the information to exploit. Figure 13.8c presents the situation in which an exploring e-puck finds food and returns to the hive by using its constructed PI vector. Once returned to the nest, the e-puck communicates its PI findings by means of a virtual dance. The hive collects these experiences and offers these to recruits. Finally, Figure 13.8d gives the situation in which other e-pucks communicated with the hive and have attained the PI vector toward the food source and are traveling to the food source guided by this PI vector. A demonstration movie can be found online.[1]

Experiments using robots with extended resources (Turtlebots)

In this set of experiments, we introduce the swarm robotics with extended resources. These swarms use general purpose computers, high quality and advanced video cameras, 3D sensors for mapping (e.g., laser range finders), accurate wheel encoders that make enhanced odometry possible, fused data of accelerometers, and a gyroscope.

The Turtlebot platform is a robot with extended resources. This robot is equipped with a laptop with core-i3 CPU for computation that is running the Robot Operating System[2] framework. As a main sensing unit, the Turtlebot is equipped with a Kinect sensor. The full RGBD information is used to detect and locate AR markers. For static obstacle detection, we only use the depth information of the sensor together with three

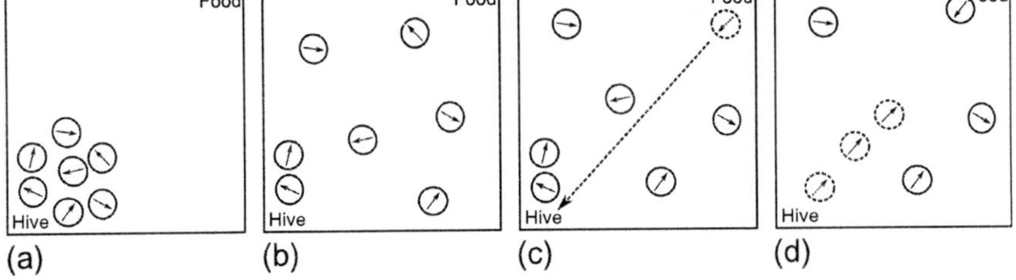

Figure 13.8 The four stages of Biomimicry Foraging. (a) All robots start at the nest location. (b) The robots randomly disperse through the environment looking for a food location. (c) A robot that has found food returns to the nest location by the shortest possible path. (d) The food location is communicated to other robots and they start to exploit this food source.

[1] http://swarmlab.unimaas.nl/papers/bnaic2011demo/.

[2] http://www.ros.org/.

bumpers that are located in the front half of the robot. Furthermore, the robot estimates its position by integrating the wheel odometry and gyro information. Hence, no map of the environment is built and the only known reference point is the target location marker. This can lead to the problem that if the odometry is faulty, the robot does not always find the target location back. As a solution, the robots fall back into a search mode, if this is the case. Another solution could be to implement a Northstar-like navigation system, by providing a fixed frame of reference, which is almost always visible from any location.

To enable visual robot-robot detection, we equipped every Turtlebot with six unique markers, which are oriented in a way that at least one marker is visible from any angle. To track and decode these markers, we make use of a toolkit called ALVAR; more specifically, we use the ROS wrapper[3] of this library. We use a customized bundle detection method to determine the center of the detected robot dependent on the decoded markers. Kalman filtering is applied to get better and more stable readings and consequently a more accurate estimate of the detected robot's position, heading, and speed. These parameters are used again for collision avoidance.

Communication is realized over Wi-Fi with a UDP connection to each Turtlebot using the LCM library.[4] Even though global communication would be possible, we limit the communication such that every robot listens only to its own channel. To simulate local communication, the robots can only communicate with another robot when it is in view and in close proximity, i.e., less than 1 m away.

In order to avoid robot to robot collisions, we rely on the marker detection to predict positions and speeds of the other robots. This information can be used to efficiently compute a noncolliding speed vector as we have developed previously in Claes et al. (2012). In contrast to this previous approach, in which the robot-robot detection was avoided by using a global reference frame and broadcasting the positions to all robots via Wi-Fi, solely the marker detection and the predictions using a Kalman filter are used. This means that a few collisions still might occur due to failure to detect the markers of the other robots and additionally, there are certain configurations in which the robots cannot see each other due to the field of view of the Kinect sensor, e.g., when two robots drive in a V-shape toward each other, the field of view of the Kinect is too narrow to detect the other robot.

As shown by Alers et al. (2014a), multiple Turtlebots perform a foraging task, i.e., starting at the Hive (H) location and randomly exploring the unknown environment for a specific Food (F) location. This is shown in Figure 13.9. Another way of locating a food location is by asking bypassing robots for a known food location, which is done by simulating local communication over Wi-Fi. When the source is found, the robot starts to exploit this source, i.e., driving from the food to the hive location until the food is depleted or a better source is found. A video showing this demonstration can be found in the online material.[5]

[3] http://wiki.ros.org/ar_track_alvar.

[4] https://code.google.com/p/lcm/.

[5] http://swarmlab.unimaas.nl/papers/aamas-2014-foraging.

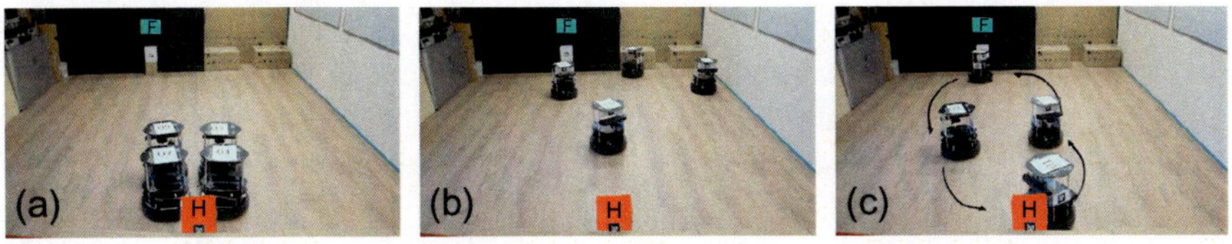

Figure 13.9 Multi-robot foraging using swarm robots with extended resources. (a) All robots start at the hive (H) location. (b) Robots are exploring the unknown environment randomly. The left two robots have found the food (F) location and are foraging between the hive and the food location. (c) All robots have converged to foraging behavior.

13.4.2 Bee-inspired pheromone signaling

In this section, we show some initial outcomes of the honeybee-inspired pheromone signaling method that allows a team of robots to maximize the total area covered in an environment in a distributed manner.

The same pheromone signaling method is applied to the multi-robot coverage problem as is introduced in Caliskanelli et al. (2014). The proposed coverage technique is inspired by the behavior described in Section 13.2. The role of queen bee denotes a robot that is responsible for managing the execution of all service requests it receives. Throughout this chapter, we will refer these robots as QR, and their responsibility (service) is to patrol in the field. The basic strategy of the algorithm is based on the periodic transmission of pheromones by QRs, and its retransmission by recipients to their neighbors. The pheromone level at each robot decays with time and with distance to the source. All robots accumulate pheromone received from other QRs and if at a particular time the pheromone level of a robot is below a given threshold, this robot will differentiate itself into a QR. To make it clear, the threshold we used for this work is 0 and as such all the robots are QRs at all times. Although we do not particularly benefit from robot differentiation in this work (unlike our previous research on WSNs Caliskanelli et al., 2012a, 2013), we still describe the differentiation process for the sake of completeness and to provide a base for our future work on multi-robot coverage. In the *BeePCo* technique, the level of pheromone indicates the resource usage and robot density in a particular area of the network. Areas in the robotic arena that have lower level of pheromone at a given time demonstrate less resource usage, and less robot density as opposed to other parts of the network. This means, areas with low pheromone level have either a low coverage or not covered at all. Some preliminary performance experiments are shown in the next sections.

13.4.2.1 Case study

To evaluate the performance of *BeePCo*, we have designed a three-tier system-level simulation model that represents the application layer (consisting of tasks), platform layer (consisting of robots), and the mapper (that maps the tasks from the application layer to the platform layer). Our system-level simulator, *Fast*, is written in Java, and it is an abstract simulator—trading accuracy for efficiency, scalability, and flexibility. For further details about *Fast*, please see Caliskanelli et al. (2012a, 2013).

The set of experiments in this section aims to show the area coverage and network connectivity of the proposed *BeePCo* technique. Area coverage in this study is referred to as maximization of the total area covered by the sensors of the involved robot(s), as defined by Gage (1992). On the other hand, network connectivity refers to the ability to transfer data between robots. As the proposed technique is more suitable for noncritical applications, we focus on participial network connectivity instead of full connectivity. The simulation setup consists of a system of 40 robots, each having a sensing and communication radius of 25 cm. The application arena size is set to 300 cm × 300 cm, where the robots are initially deployed randomly in the center of the arena, in a square region of size 5 cm × 5 cm. We examine two different scenarios:

- *BeePCo with network assurance* represents a case where the robots try to keep the wireless communication channels alive throughout the simulation. This restricts robots to move too far away from each other. The algorithm is forcing robots to move backward if a robot is not connected to at least one other robot in the arena. This scenario is developed to be used for applications where events are expected to be reported to the sink, such as patrolling.
- *BeePCo without network assurance* represents a case where a maximum spread of the robots on the arena is required in order to maximize area coverage.

Figure 13.10 shows the spread of 40 robots when network assurance is required from the *BeePCo* algorithm. Figure 13.10a–c represents the layout of the robots and their

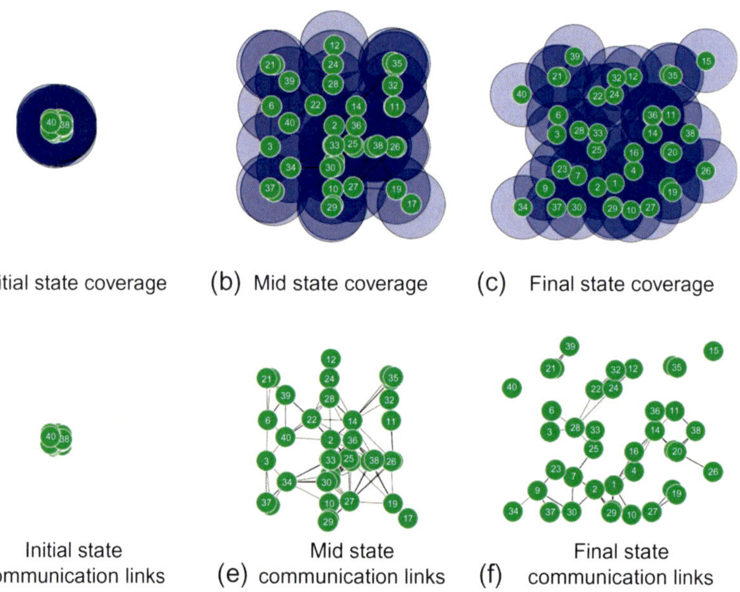

Figure 13.10 Spread of an MRS of 40 robots: (a)–(c) area coverage and (d)–(f) connectivity of the communication links when network connectivity is assured by *BeePCo*.

spread over the arena incrementally. The area that is covered by each robot is plotted by a blue circle indicating the transmission range of each robot, and is normalized with the surface of the arena. Figure 13.10d–f shows how the active wireless communication links between the robots evolve as time elapses. Robots are deployed in the middle of the arena in the initial stage as shown in Figure 13.10a and d. In the initial stage, coverage is very low, whereas connectivity is very high. As time passes by, robots start spreading in the arena as shown in Figure 13.10b and e; the area coverage increases where the network connectivity remains high. At the end of the simulation, robots spread out as much as they can while trying to keep the wireless communication channels active as shown in Figure 13.10c and f.

Figure 13.11 illustrates the spread of the robots when network connectivity is not assured. Similar to Figure 13.10, area coverage and connectivity are inspected on an arena with 40 robots. In this set of experiments, we use the same setup as shown in Figure 13.10. Figure 13.11a and d shows the initial stage of the robots after deployment. As can be seen from Figure 13.11a, the *BeePCo* algorithm without network assurance performs very similar to (Figure 13.10a and d) *BeePCo* algorithm with network assurance. Later on as the simulation evolves, Figure 13.11b and e starts spreading wider as opposed to Figure 13.10b and e. By the end of the simulation, robots are spread all along the arena where the area coverage gets very high as shown in Figure 13.11c. Unlike the area coverage, network connectivity is lost almost entirely.

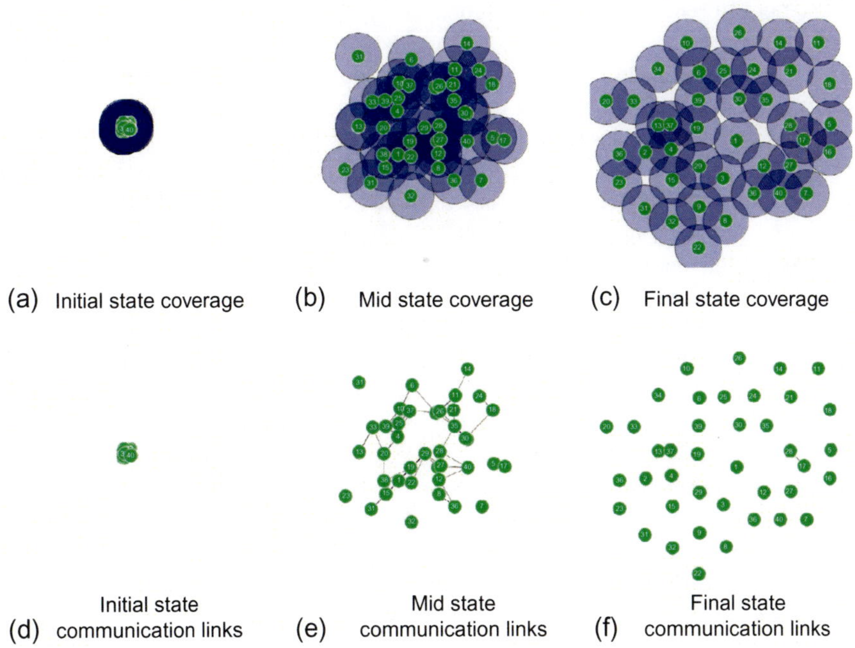

Figure 13.11 Spread of an MRS of 40 robots: (a)–(c) area coverage and (d)–(f) connectivity of the communication links when network connectivity is assured by *BeePCo*.

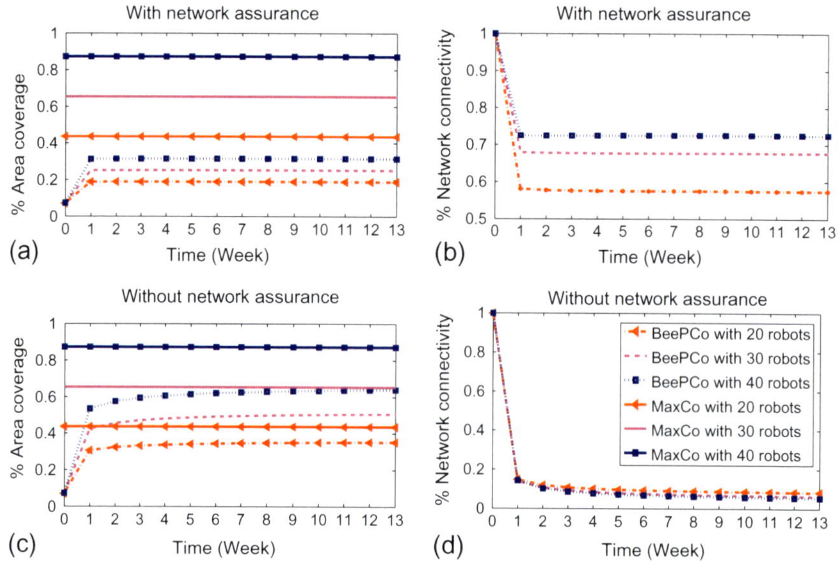

Figure 13.12 Experimental results: (a) and (c) % area coverage, (b) and (d) % network connectivity with different number of robots in an MRS.

Dramatic difference in the network connectivity is observed between Figures 13.10f and 13.11f.

The results shown in Figure 13.12 are based on 30 different runs over six different configurations (with and without network assurance each with the three alternatives for the number of robots in the environment), in a total of 180 simulation runs to ensure the statistical significance. Each run simulated the case study for 13 weeks, to illustrate the long-term effects of the spread of the *BeePCo* coverage algorithm based on bees' pheromone signaling process. MaxCo results are based on mathematical calculations based on the total transmission area over total area.

Figure 13.12 shows the percentage of the area coverage (a) and (c) and the percentage of network connectivity (b) and (d). *BeePCo* algorithm to illustrate the effects of the number of the robots on two different scenarios: with and without the network assurance. In addition to experiments shown in Figures 13.10 and 13.11, the number of robots is varied (with 20 and 30) and experiments are held while the simulation setup is kept the same. Our observations are as follows:

Independent from the network assurance, the area coverage increases as the number of the robots increase. This behavior is shown in Figure 13.12a and c on *BeePCo* algorithm and MaxCo; area coverage achieves highest percentage with 40 robots. Area coverage is approximately 10% more when network connectivity is not assured in all three ranges of number of robots. Network connectivity is very low when network is not assured as shown in Figure 13.12d and is irrelevant from the number of the robots. Figure 13.12a exhibits that *BeePCo* algorithm with network assurance increases network connectivity 50% more than *BeePCo* with no network assurance. This does not reflect on area coverage, which we believe is the benefit of *BeePCo* with network assurance. The performance difference in terms of area coverage between *BeePCo* with and without network assurance is less than 10% in a system with 20 robots. Although this difference increases up to 15% as the number of robots increases, we believe *BeePCo* with network assurance brings much more benefit (as opposed to *BeePCo* without network assurance) in terms of connectivity by 50%.

13.5 Future trends

Polymorphism is a known phenomenon in biological systems, meaning that various forms or types of individuals are seen among the members of a single species. This phenomenon can be seen in many different expressions in nature, ranging from polymorphic ants and birds (with differences in, e.g., size, color, and strength) to different blood types in humans. Natural polymorphism can be categorized into discrete variations (e.g., blood groups) and continuous ones (e.g., smooth height variations in human population).

Recently, heterogeneity of agents has attracted the attention of different research communities in computer science, artificial intelligence, and robotics. For example, Montes de Oca et al. (2009) have studied various types of heterogeneity that can be ascribed to particle swarm optimizers and have shown how this can improve the efficiency of computational techniques. Heterogeneity of complex networks has been also studied, e.g., by Moreno et al. (2002), where the dynamics of epidemics in complex heterogeneous architectures are investigated.

Recently, heterogeneity has found its way to swarm robotics as well. Dorigo et al. (2012) have introduced a distributed robotic swarm, namely *Swarmanoid*, which consists of three different robot types (eye-bots, hand-bots, and foot-bots). Such structures, in which different robots have different capabilities and different goals, refer to the hard heterogeneity in swarms. On the other hand, softly heterogeneous swarm robotics introduced by Ranjbar-Sahraei et al. (2013a) refer to the situation in which a group of similar robots all have the same goals but slightly different levels of capability. As an example of such systems, consider a scenario in which a group of simple robots try to uniformly disperse in an unknown environment. Each robot can simply compute its distance with the neighboring robots and after computing the borders of its own territory, moves toward the center of the territory. Gradually, all robots make a uniform coverage in the area (i.e., known as Voronoi coverage). This approach can be very efficient in convex environments. However, as soon as nonconvexities such as obstacles are added to the environment, this approach fails as robots get stuck behind the obstacles (i.e., reaching the local optimum in a coverage problem). For this specific problem, Staňková et al. (2013) and Ranjbar-Sahraei et al. (2013c) proposed and extended a coverage method, namely StaCo, based on the concept of Stackelberg game, which uses soft heterogeneity in a swarm to overcome the problem of local optima.

The concept of heterogeneity in robotic swarms suggests that these swarms can perform better than the long-established uniform swarms in various scenarios. For instance, they can perform both exploration and exploitation of an environment in a rescue mission, or can act highly flexibly in passing obstacles and nonconvexities in a flocking mission. In short, inspired by polymorphism in biological organisms, using this concept of heterogeneity in robotic swarms is a promising practice for overcoming the available limitations in swarm robotics.

13.6 Conclusions

Coordination is a key challenge when deploying teams of distributed multi-robot systems. Lightweight interactions among robots (i.e., wireless communications) are not only a desired feature for such platforms; they are a great need. Furthermore, simple yet effective algorithms that avoid complex heavy computations are desirable in multi-robot systems. Therefore, bio-inspired solutions for the challenging problem of multi-robot coordination are gaining more importance. In this chapter, we presented an overview of our work on ant- and bee-inspired coordination principles for coordination in multi-robot systems.

In Section 13.3, we described our ant-inspired StiCo approach and illustrate its effectiveness on a case study of deployed e-pucks. We illustrated the performance of the StiCo approach using a dark room that allows emission of UV light on the floor. The glowing trails of the robots are captured by on-board cameras of e-pucks. Experimental results showed that simple communication principle of ants can be used to address the multi-robot coordination problem.

In Section 13.4.1, we presented the bee-inspired foraging algorithm to solve the coordination problem of multi-robot systems. We showed the impact of the foraging algorithm on two different experimental setups: (1) a swarm of robots with limited resources (e-pucks) and (2) a swarm of robots with extended resources (Turtlebots). The experiments served as a proof of concept: First, we showed how the bee-inspired mechanism can be used in a real-life autonomous robotic swarm, which mimics the basic foraging behavior of bees. Second, by the direct deployment of bee-inspired algorithms onto a robot swarm, scalability, robustness, and efficiency on foraging tasks in more complex and dynamic environments were investigated.

In Section 13.4.2, we explained the bee-inspired pheromone signaling mechanism to address coordination in multi-robot systems. We explored its performance consequences on a case study using a system-level simulator, *Fast*. We illustrated the spread of a multi-robot system of 40 robots using the *BeePCo* algorithm with and without the network connectivity assurance. We report area coverage and communication links for both scenarios. Illustrations of both scenarios showed that the pheromone signaling algorithm can be used to address the coordination and coverage problem in multi-robot systems. We also showed that the *BeePCo* algorithm achieves larger coverage when the network connectivity is not assured (for one-shot applications, i.e., fast exploration of an unknown environment) as opposed to scenarios when the network connectivity is assured (where events are expected to be reported, i.e., long-term periodic patrolling).

References

Akay, B., Karaboga, D., 2009. Parameter tuning for the artificial bee colony algorithm. In: Proceedings of the 5th International Conference on Computational Collective Intelligence. Semantic Web, Social Networks and Multiagent Systems, Wroclaw, Poland. Springer-Verlag, Berlin, ISBN: 978-3-642-04440-3, pp. 608–619.

Alers, S., Bloembergen, D., Hennes, D., de Jong, S., Kaisers, M., Lemmens, N., Tuyls, K., Weiss, G., 2011. Bee-inspired foraging in an embodied swarm. In: Proceedings of the Tenth International Conference on Autonomous Agents and Multi-Agent Systems (AAMAS), pp. 1311–1312.

Alers, S., Ranjbar-Sahraei, B., May, S., Tuyls, K., Weiss, G., 2013a. An experimental framework for exploiting vision in swarm robotics. In: ADAPTIVE 2013, The Fifth International Conference on Adaptive and Self-Adaptive Systems and Applications, pp. 83–88.

Alers, S., Ranjbar-Sahraei, B., May, S., Tuyls, K., Weiss, G., 2013b. Evaluation of an experimental framework for exploiting vision in swarm robotics. In: Advances in Artificial Life, ECAL, vol. 12, pp. 775–782.

Alers, S., Claes, D., Tuyls, K., Weiss, G., 2014a. Biologically inspired multi-robot foraging. In: Proceedings of the 2014 International Conference on Autonomous Agents and Multi-Agent Systems (AAMAS). International Foundation for Autonomous Agents and Multiagent Systems, pp. 1683–1684.

Alers, S., Claes, D., Tuyls, K., Weiss, G., 2014b. Biologically inspired multi-robot foraging. In: Proceedings of the 2014 International Conference on Autonomous Agents and Multi-Agent Systems (AAMAS), pp. 1683–1684.

Alers, S., Tuyls, K., Ranjbar-Sahraei, B., Claes, D., Weiss, G., 2014c. Insect-inspired robot coordination: foraging and coverage. In: Artificial Life, vol. 14.

Boonma, P., Suzuki, J., 2008. MONSOON: a coevolutionary multiobjective adaptation framework for dynamic wireless sensor networks. In: Proceedings of the 41st Annual International Conference on System Sciences, January 2008, p. 497. http://dx.doi.org/10.1109/HICSS.2008.323.

Breitenmoser, A., Schwager, M., Metzger, J.C., Siegwart, R., Rus, D., 2010. Voronoi coverage of non-convex environments with a group of networked robots. In: Proceedings of the International Conference on Robotics and Automation (ICRA 10), May 2010, pp. 4982–4989.

Caliskanelli, I., Harbin, J., Indrusiak, F., Polack, L., Mitchell, P., Chesmore, D., 2012a. Runtime optimisation in wsns for load balancing using pheromone signalling. In: 3rd IEEE International Conference on NESEA, December 2012.

Caliskanelli, I., Harbin, J., Indrusiak, L.S., Mitchell, P., Chesmore, D., Polack, F., 2012b. Runtime optimisation in wsns for load balancing using pheromone signalling. In: 2012 IEEE 3rd International Conference on Networked Embedded Systems for Every Application (NESEA), pp. 1–8.

Caliskanelli, I., Harbin, J., Indrusiak, L.S., Mitchell, P., Polack, F., Chesmore, D., 2013. Bio-inspired load balancing in large-scale wsns using pheromone signalling. Int. J. Distrib. Sens. Netw. 2013, 1–14.

Caliskanelli, I., Indrusiak, L., 2013a. Search-based parameter tuning on application-level load balancing for distributed embedded systems. In: Proceedings of the 11th IEEE/IFIP International Conference on Embedded and Ubiquitous Computing (EUC 2013).

Caliskanelli, I., Indrusiak, L., 2014. Using mobile robotic agents to increase service availability and extend network lifetime on wireless sensor and robot networks. In: 12th IEEE International Conference on INDIN, July 2014.

Caliskanelli, I., Broecker, B., Tuyls, K., 2014. Multi-robot coverage: a bee pheromone signalling approach. In: Submitted to the International Conference on Artificial Life and Intelligent Agents (ALIA 14).
Cheng, K., Collett, T., Pickhard, A., Wehner, R., 1987. The use of visual landmarks by honeybees: bees weight landmarks according to their distance from the goal. J. Comp. Physiol. A. 161 (3), 469–475.
Claes, D., Hennes, D., Tuyls, K., Meeussen, W., 2012. Collision avoidance under bounded localization uncertainty. In: Proceedings of IEEE/RSJ International Conference on Intelligent Robots and Systems (IROS 2012), Vilamoura, Portugal, October 2012.
Collett, M., Collett, T.S., Bisch, S., Wehner, R., 1998. Local and global vectors in desert ant navigation. Nature 394 (6690), 269–272.
Collett, M., Harland, D., Collett, T.S., 2002. The use of landmarks and panoramic context in the performance of local vectors by navigating honeybees. J. Exp. Biol. 205, 807–814.
Correll, N., Martinoli, A., 2006. Collective inspection of regular structures using a swarm of miniature robots. In: Ang, J., Marcelo, H., Khatib, O. (Eds.), Experimental Robotics IX. In: Springer Tracts in Advanced Robotics, vol. 21. Springer, Berlin, Heidelberg, ISBN: 978-3-540-28816-9, pp. 375–386. http://dx.doi.org/10.1007/11552246_36.
Cortes, J., Martinez, S., Karatas, T., Bullo, F., 2004. Coverage control for mobile sensing networks. IEEE Trans. Robot. Autom. 20 (2), 243–255.
Cortes, J., Martinez, S., Bullo, F., 2005. Spatially-distributed coverage optimization and control with limited-range interactions. ESAIM Control. Optim. Calc. Var. 11, 691–719.
Dorigo, M., 1992. Optimization, learning and natural algorithms. Thesis report, Politecnico di Milano, Italy.
Dorigo, M., Blumb, C., 2005. Ant colony optimization theory: a survey. Theor. Comput. Sci. 344, 243–278.
Dorigo, M., Roosevelt, A.F., 2004. Swarm robotics. In: Special Issue: Autonomous Robots, Citeseer.
Dorigo, M., Stützle, T., 2004. Ant Colony Optimization. A Bradford Book. MIT Press, Cambridge.
Dorigo, M., Birattari, M., Stutzle, T., 2006a. Ant colony optimization. IEEE Comput. Intell. Mag. 1556-603X. 1 (4), 28–39. http://dx.doi.org/10.1109/MCI.2006.329691.
Dorigo, M., Birattari, M., Stutzle, T., 2006b. Ant colony optimization: artificial ants as a computational intelligence technique. IEEE Comput. Intell. Mag. 1 (4), 28–39.
Dorigo, M., Floreano, D., Gambardella, L.M., Mondada, F., Nolfi, S., Baaboura, T., Birattari, M., Bonani, M., Brambilla, M., Brutschy, A., et al., 2012. Swarmanoid: a novel concept for the study of heterogeneous robotic swarms. IEEE Robot. Autom. Mag. 20 (4), 60–71.
Dressler, F., Akan, O.B., 2010. A survey on bio-inspired networking. Comput. Netw. 54 (6), 881–900.
Elor, Y., Bruckstein, A.M., 2009. Multi-a(ge)nt graph patrolling and partitioning. In: Proceedings of the 2009 IEEE/WIC/ACM International Joint Conference on Web Intelligence and Intelligent Agent Technology—Volume 02, WI-IAT'09, Washington, DC, USA. IEEE Computer Society, Washington, DC, USA, ISBN: 978-0-7695-3801-3, pp. 52–57. http://dx.doi.org/10.1109/WI-IAT.2009.125.
Elor, Y., Bruckstein, A., 2010. Autonomous multi-agent cycle based patrolling. In: Swarm Intelligence. Lecture Notes in Computer Science, vol. 6234. Springer, Berlin, Heidelberg, ISBN: 978-3-642-15460-7, pp. 119–130.
El-Sherbeny, N.A., 2010. Vehicle routing with time windows: an overview of exact, heuristic and metaheuristic methods. J. King Saud Univ. Sci. 22 (3), 123–131. http://dx.doi.org/10.1016/j.jksus.2010.03.002.

Floreano, D., Mattiussi, C., 2008. Bio-inspired artificial intelligence: theories, methods, and technologies. The MIT Press, Cambridge, MA, USA.

Fujisawa, R., Imamura, H., Hashimoto, T., Matsuno, F., 2008. Communication using pheromone field for multiple robots. In: IEEE/RSJ International Conference on Intelligent Robots and Systems, 2008, IROS 2008, September 2008, pp. 1391–1396.

Gabriely, Y., Rimon, E., 2003. Competitive on-line coverage of grid environments by a mobile robot. Comput. Geom. 24 (3), 197–224. http://dx.doi.org/10.1016/S0925-7721(02)00110-4.

Gage, D.W., 1992. Command control for many-robot systems. In: 19th Annual AUVS Technical Symposium, pp. 22–24.

Glad, A., Simonin, O., Buffet, O., Charpillet, F., 2008. Theoretical study of ant-based algorithms for multi-agent patrolling. In: Proceeding of the 2008 Conference on ECAI 2008: 18th European Conference on Artificial Intelligence. IOS Press, Amsterdam, The Netherlands, ISBN: 978-158603-891-5, pp. 626–630. http://dl.acm.org/citation.cfm?id=1567281.1567417.

Glad, A., Simonin, O., Buffet, O., Charpillet, F., 2010. Influence of different execution models on patrolling ant behaviors: from agents to robots. In: Proceedings of the Ninth International Conference on Autonomous Agents and Multi-Agent Systems (AAMAS'10).

Herianto, Sakakibara, T., Kurabayashi, D., 2007. Artificial pheromone system using RFID for navigation of autonomous robots. J. Bionic Eng. 4 (4), 245–253.

Johansson, R., Saffiotti, A., 2009. Navigating by stigmergy: a realization on an RFID floor for minimalistic robots. In: IEEE International Conference on Robotics and Automation, 2009, ICRA'09, May 2009, pp. 245–252.

Karaboga, D., 2010. Artificial bee colony algorithm. Scholarpedia 5 (3), 6915.

Karaboga, D., Basturk, B., 2007. A powerful and efficient algorithm for numerical function optimization: artificial bee colony (ABC) algorithm. J. Glob. Optim. 39 (3), 459–471.

Karaboga, D., Basturk, B., 2008. On the performance of artificial bee colony (ABC) algorithm. Appl. Soft Comput. 8 (1), 687–697.

Khatib, O., 1985. Real-time obstacle avoidance for manipulators and mobile robots. In: Proceedings of the 1985 IEEE International Conference on Robotics and Automation, March 1985, vol. 2, pp. 500–505. http://dx.doi.org/10.1109/ROBOT.1985.1087247.

Kronemann, M.L., Hafner, V.V., 2010. Lumibots—making emergence graspable in a swarm of robots. In: The ACM Designing Interactive Systems Conference, pp. 408–411.

Lemmens, N., 2011. Bee-Inspired Distributed Optimization. Maastricht University, Netherlands.

Lemmens, N., Tuyls, K., 2012. Stigmergic landmark optimization. Adv. Complex Syst. 15 (8), 1150025.

Lemmens, N., de Jong, S., Tuyls, K., Nowé, A., 2007a. A bee algorithm for multi-agent systems: recruitment and navigation combined. In: ALAg 2007, AAMAS'07 Honolulu, Hawai.

Lemmens, N., de Jong, S., Tuyls, K., Nowé, A., 2007b. Bee behaviour in multi-agent systems. In: Adaptive Agents and Multi-Agent Systems III. Adaptation and Multi-Agent Learning, 5th, 6th, and 7th European Symposium, ALAMAS 2005-2007 on Adaptive and Learning Agents and Multi-Agent Systems, Revised Selected Papers, pp. 145–156.

Lemmens, N., Alers, S., Tuyls, K., 2011. Bee-inspired foraging in a real-life autonomous robot collective. In: Proceedings of the 23rd Benelux Conference on Artificial Intelligence (BNAIC), pp. 459–460.

Lerman, K., Martinoli, A., Galstyan, A., 2005. A review of probabilistic macroscopic models for swarm robotic systems. In: Swarm Robotics. Springer, Berlin, pp. 143–152.

Martinoli, A., Easton, K., Agassounon, W., 2004. Modeling swarm robotic systems: a case study in collaborative distributed manipulation. Int. J. Robot. Res. 23 (4–5), 415–436.

Mondada, F., Bonani, M., et al., 2009. The e-puck, a robot designed for education in engineering. In: 9th Conference on Autonomous Robot Systems and Competitions, vol. 1. IPCB: Instituto Politcnico de Castelo Branco, Castelo Branco, Portugal, pp. 59–65. http://www.est.ipcb.pt/robotica2009/.

Montes de Oca, M.A., Pena, J., Stutzle, T., Pinciroli, C., Dorigo, M., 2009. Heterogeneous particle swarm optimizers. In: IEEE Congress on Evolutionary Computation, 2009, CEC'09. IEEE, Piscataway, NJ, pp. 698–705.

Moreno, Y., Pastor-Satorras, R., Vespignani, A., 2002. Epidemic outbreaks in complex heterogeneous networks. Eur. Phys. J. B 26 (4), 521–529.

Packer, E., 2008. Robust geometric computing and optimal visibility coverage. PhD thesis, Stony Brook, New York, USA, AAI3338238.

Perkins, C., Royer, E., 1999. Ad-hoc on-demand distance vector routing. In: Proceedings of the 2nd IEEE Workshop on Mobile Computing Systems and Applications, February 1999, pp. 90–100. http://dx.doi.org/10.1109/MCSA.1999.749281.

Pirzadeh, A., Snyder, W., 1990. A unified solution to coverage and search in explored and unexplored terrains using indirect control. In: Proceedings of the IEEE International Conference on Robotics and Automation, May 1990, vol. 3, pp. 2113–2119. http://dx.doi.org/10.1109/ROBOT.1990.126317.

Ranjbar-Sahraei, B., Weiss, G., Nakisaee, A., 2012a. An adaptive stigmergic coverage approach for robot team. In: 24th Benelux Conference on Artificial Intelligence (BNAIC), pp. 210–217.

Ranjbar-Sahraei, B., Weiss, G., Nakisaee, A., 2012b. Stigmergic coverage algorithm for multirobot systems (demonstration). In: Proceedings of the Eleventh International Conference on Autonomous Agents and Multiagent Systems (AAMAS), vol. 3, pp. 1497–1498.

Ranjbar-Sahraei, B., Weiss, G., Nakisaee, A., 2012c. A multi-robot coverage approach based on stigmergic communication. In: Multiagent System Technologies. In: Lecture Notes in Computer Science, vol. 7598. Springer, Berlin, pp. 126–138, ISBN: 978-3-642-33689-8.

Ranjbar-Sahraei, B., Alers, S., Staňková, K., Tuyls, K., Weiss, G., 2013a. Towards soft heterogeneity in robotic swarms. In: Proceedings of the 25th Benelux Conference on Artificial Intelligence (BNAIC), pp. 384–385.

Ranjbar-Sahraei, B., Alers, S., Tuyls, K., Weiss, G., 2013b. Stico in action. In: Proceedings of the 2013 International Conference on Autonomous Agents and Multi-Agent Systems. International Foundation for Autonomous Agents and Multiagent Systems, St. Paul, MN, USA., pp. 1403–1404.

Ranjbar-Sahraei, B., Staňková, K., Tuyls, K., Weiss, G., 2013c. Stackelberg-based coverage approach in nonconvex environments. In: Proceedings of the 12th European Conference on Artificial Life, vol. 12, pp. 462–469.

Ranjbar-Sahraei, B., Weiss, G., Tuyls, K., 2013d. A macroscopic model for multi-robot stigmergic coverage. In: Proceedings of the 2013 International Conference on Autonomous Agents and Multi-Agent Systems. International Foundation for Autonomous Agents and Multiagent Systems, St. Paul, MN, USA., pp. 1233–1234.

Ranjbar-Sahraei, B., Bou-Ammar, H., Bloembergen, D., Tuyls, K., Weiss, G., 2014. Theory of cooperation in complex social networks. In: 28th AAAI Conference on Artificial Intelligence.

Roberts, M.B.V., 1986. Biology: A Functional Approach. Nelson, London, ISBN: 0174480199. http://www.worldcat.org/isbn/0174480199.

Şahin, E., 2005. Swarm robotics: from sources of inspiration to domains of application. In: Swarm Robotics. Springer, Berlin, pp. 10–20.

Sahoo, R.R., Singh, M., Sahoo, B.M., Majumder, K., Ray, S., Sarkar, S.K., 2013. A light weight trust based secure and energy efficient clustering in wireless sensor network: honey bee mating intelligence approach. In: Procedia Technology.In: First International Conference on Computational Intelligence: Modeling Techniques and Applications (CIMTA) 2013, vol. 10. pp. 515–523. http://dx.doi.org/10.1016/j.protcy.2013.12.390.http://www.sciencedirect.com/science/article/pii/S2212017313005525.

Saleem, M., Farooq, M., 2007. Beesensor: a bee-inspired power aware routing protocol for wireless sensor networks. In: Giacobini, M. (Ed.), Applications of Evolutionary Computing. In: Lecture Notes in Computer Science, vol. 4448. Springer, Berlin, Heidelberg, ISBN: 978-3-540-71804-8, pp. 81–90. http://dx.doi.org/10.1007/978-3-540-71805-5_9.

Schwager, M., Rus, D., Slotine, J.J., 2009. Decentralized, adaptive coverage control for networked robots. Int. J. Robot. Res. 28 (3), 357–375.

Schwager, M., Rus, D., Slotine, J.J., 2011. Unifying geometric, probabilistic, and potential field approaches to multi-robot deployment. Int. J. Robot. Res. 30 (3), 371–383. http://dx.doi.org/10.1177/0278364910383444.

Senthilkumar, J., Chandrasekaran, M., 2011. Improving the performance of wireless sensor network using bee's mating, intelligence. Eur. J. Sci. Res. 55, 452–465.

Staňková, K., Ranjbar-Sahraei, B., Weiss, G., Tuyls, K., 2013. Staco: Stackelberg-based coverage approach in robotic swarms. In: The Fifth International Conference on Adaptive and Self-Adaptive Systems and Applications (ADAPTIVE).

Wagner, I.A., Lindenbaum, M., Bruckstein, A.M., 1999. Distributed covering by ant-robots using evaporating traces. IEEE Trans. Robot. Autom. 15 (5), 918–933.

Wedde, H.F., Farooq, M., Zhang, Y., 2004. Beehive: an efficient fault-tolerant routing algorithm inspired by honey bee behavior. In: Dorigo, M., Birattari, M., Blum, C., Gambardella, L., Mondada, F., Stützle, T. (Eds.), Ant colony optimization and swarm intelligence. In: Lecture Notes in Computer Science, vol. 3172. Springer, Berlin, Heidelberg, pp. 83–94, ISBN: 978-3-540-22672-7. http://dx.doi.org/10.1007/978-3-540-28646-2_8.

Willow Garage, 2014. Turtlebot. https://www.willowgarage.com/turtlebot.

Yanovski, V., Wagner, I.A., Bruckstein, A.M., 2003. A distributed ant algorithm for efficiently patrolling a network. Algorithmica 37, 165–186.

Ziparo, V., Kleiner, A., Marchetti, L., Farinelli, A., Nardi, D., 2007. Cooperative exploration for USAR robots with indirect communication. In: Proceedings of the 6th IFAC Symposium on Intelligent Autonomous Vehicles (IAV'07).

Bio-inspired climbing robots

M. Tavakoli, C. Viegas

14

14.1 Introduction

Climbing robots are a special breed of service robots developed in the last three decades and used for many tasks including inspection, cleaning, and maintenance of tall structures, which involve safety risks to human operators. Until now, more than 200 prototypes of climbing robots have been reported (Chen et al., 2006), with a wide range of sizes and weights and employing many different technologies. While there are several ways to climb a wall using various methods not previously observed in nature like, for example, wheels for the mobility and magnetic force for the adhesion to the surface, in nature, climbing is performed by crawling, snaking, and more often in more complex intelligent natural systems, with a combination of legs and grippers (Tavakoli et al., 2010a).

In this chapter, we explore the novel bio-inspired mechanisms used in climbing robots for adhesion and locomotion.

Bio-inspired robotics is about learning from nature and highly complex and efficient biological systems, and developing similar mechanisms that may solve a specific problem in the engineering field. The designer should then try to simplify and enhance that mechanism for the particular task of interest. The developed robotic system may outperform its corresponding biological inspiration, for this specific task.

When designing climbing mechanisms, there are basically two sets of problems and questions that should be answered in the early stages of the design. In the conceptual design stage of a climbing mechanism for a specific purpose, one needs to address:

A. What kind of adhesion mechanism should be applied to hold the mechanism on the vertical surface?
B. What type of locomotion mechanism should be utilized for climbing the specific type of structure?

These two problems are closely interrelated. One cannot be answered without taking into consideration the other. The former problem, the adhesion mechanism is a critical part of the climbing mechanism and should be specifically designed and optimized for a particular case. A lightweight and simple adhesion mechanism results in an overall lighter robot; thus, less power consumption and more autonomy for the robot can be granted. Regarding the adhesion mechanism of a climbing robot, one of the aspects that a designer needs to evaluate is the existence of any specific feature in the vertical surfaces that the robot should climb, that the adhesion mechanism may rely on. Taking advantage of these specific features of the environment is very important for design of lightweight robots with high maneuverability. For instance, if the climbing surface is ferromagnetic, many times a magnetic adhesion unit is the best choice, since it provides a very high adhesion force to weight ratio. Relying on specific features of the surface can be seen also in climbing animals. For instance, squirrels rely on the surface irregularities to hang their claws. But some animals such as snails can climb from a wider range of surfaces, as they take advantage of chemical adhesion.

The locomotion mechanism of the climbing robots depends significantly on the adhesion unit. Adhesion units should support the weight and the resulting torque of the whole robot in static and dynamic modes. Higher adhesion force to weight ratio in the adhesion units leaves a bigger space for increasing the overall robot performance in terms of autonomy, maneuverability (i.e., adding more active degrees of freedom (DoF)), and lifting weight. In this chapter, we intend to give an overview of the bio-inspiration in climbing animals in terms of adhesion and locomotion.

The first section is dedicated to bio-inspired adhesion technologies, ranging from mechanical fit used by most large climbing animals to wet and dry adhesion techniques used by small insects and reptiles. We also study microsynthetic adhesives which mimic gecko hair, chemical adhesion of the snails, or adhesion by suction, used by limpets. Other particular concepts such as posture change and pruning robots are also addressed.

The second section addresses the biomechanics involved in the locomotion of the climbing robots. This section comprises recent developments on legged robots, snake robots, spider robots, pendulum robots, brachiating, and others. In this section, we also briefly explore the bio-inspired mechanisms such as tails, dynamic balancing platforms, gliding membranes, etc., that are used to improve the robot's locomotion and balance and to allow obstacle surpassing and planar transitions.

The final section discusses the current challenges and limitations that robot designers face and likely future trends in this field. Some useful sources for further information and most prominent research and interest groups to follow on this robotics research field are presented.

14.2 Bio-inspired adhesion technologies

Climbing robots can be classified according to the mechanisms they employ for adherence and locomotion. The correct choice and use of these mechanisms is the main challenge when developing a climbing robot. In this section, we discuss the main bio-inspired adhesion technologies employed in this field.

Adhesion principles can be mainly distinguished based on two criteria (Longo and Muscato, 2008):

- Physical principle generating the adhesion force (e.g., mechanical fit, suction, etc.);
- Energy needed for generating the adhesion force (passive or active).

14.2.1 Mechanical seizing

Some climbing robots' adhesion technologies draw inspiration from arboreal organisms. These animals display many specializations for dealing with the mechanical challenges of moving through their habitats. For instance, primates use frictional gripping relying upon hairless fingertips. This type of mechanical adhesion allows them to hold to tree branches by squeezing the branch between the fingertips, thus generating frictional force. However, this type of grip depends upon the angle of the frictional force. Larger branches result in reduced gripping ability. Animals other than primates that use mechanical gripping, or seizing, in climbing include the chameleon, which has mitten-like grasping feet, and many birds that grip branches in perching or moving about. 3D Climber (Tavakoli et al., 2010b; Tavakoli et al., 2005) is an example of a developed robot that is inspired by mechanical seizing and use a four DoF arm and seizing grippers to move through complex three-dimensional environments possessing several bends and branches, in a similar way to what primates do (Figure 14.1).

Another type of robots possesses special grippers designed to adapt to specific features on their environment, such as the vertical moving fire fighting robot (Amano et al., 2001), which is capable of gripping handrails and quickly climb balconies on high-rise condominiums.

14.2.2 Mechanical form fit/penetration

Another type of mechanical adhesion that relies on penetration on smooth surfaces is achieved by animals which possess sharp claws or similar mechanisms. They also allow reorientation of the direction of forces the animal applies. Squirrels are a good example of animals which use their claws to grab to and climb tree trunks, having evolved highly mobile ankle joints which permit rotating the foot into a "reversed" posture. This allows the claws to hook into the rough surface of the bark, opposing the force of gravity.

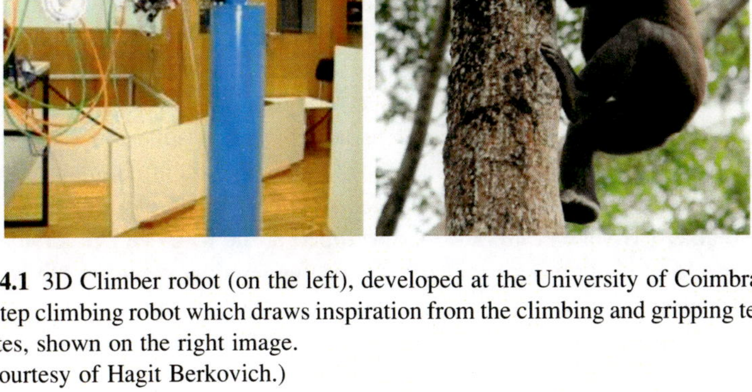

Figure 14.1 3D Climber robot (on the left), developed at the University of Coimbra, is a step-by-step climbing robot which draws inspiration from the climbing and gripping techniques of primates, shown on the right image.
(Image courtesy of Hagit Berkovich.)

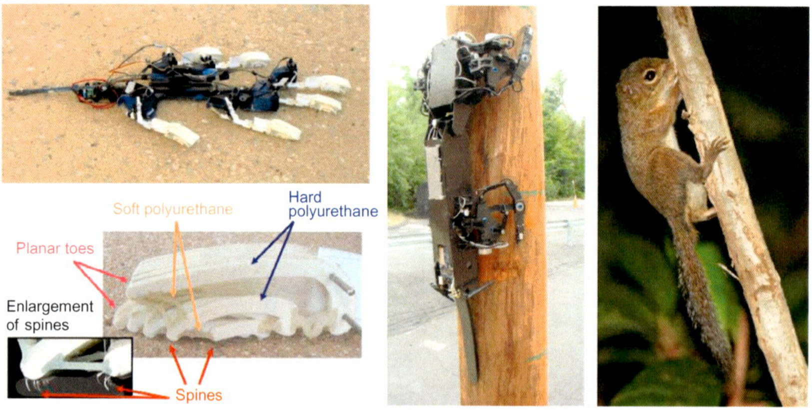

Figure 14.2 SpinyBot (on the left) developed at Stanford uses a novel patented technology that enables it to climb smooth, rough, uneven, porous, and dirty surfaces using arrays of small spines, which hook onto bumps and pits on the surface. In the center is the RiSE V3, another example of the use of micro spines for gripping the surface, just like squirrels, on the right, do with their claws.
(Image courtesy of Ben Twist.)

Spinybot from Stanford University (Kim et al., 2005; Asbeck et al., 2006) is a small climbing robot which uses several micro spines in its feet, which work just like claws, allowing it to adhere to the climbing surface. Another example of use of micro spines to penetrate the climbing surface is the RiSE V3 (Haynes et al., 2009), pole climbing robot. With a mass of 5.4 kg and employing several bio-inspired technologies, including flexible joints, complex leg motion, and balancing tail, this quadrupedal robot is capable of climbing wooden telephone poles with speeds up to 21 cm/s (Figure 14.2).

14.2.3 Wet adhesion and suction

Most of the small animals possess more complex adhesion mechanisms, including wet and dry adhesion, relying on van der Waals forces, fluid-mediated adhesive forces, and pneumatic and suction forces (Figure 14.3).

Wet adhesion, common in flies and beetles, functions either by suction or by capillary adhesion. Limpets use a combination of shell clamping, glue-like adhesion, and suction as adhesion mechanisms. Suction is mainly used when they need mobility, relying on stronger glue bonds (mean tenacity of glue-like adhesion is approximately equal to 0.23 MN/sq m and the mean tenacity of suction adhesion is approximately equal to 0.09 MN/sq m) and shell clamping rather than continuous muscular effort for long-term attachment (Smith, 1992; Smith, 1991; Ellem et al., 2002).

WallWalker (Miyake et al., 2007), developed at the Kagawa University in Japan, is an example of a climbing robot developed for window cleaning which uses wet adhesion and suction (Figure 14.4). Other robots which use suction for adhesion include the Roma (Balaguer et al., 2002; Balaguer et al., 1998), vortex-based suction robot (Bonaccorso et al., 2008), climbing robot with multiple suction chambers (Hillenbrand et al., 2008), among others.

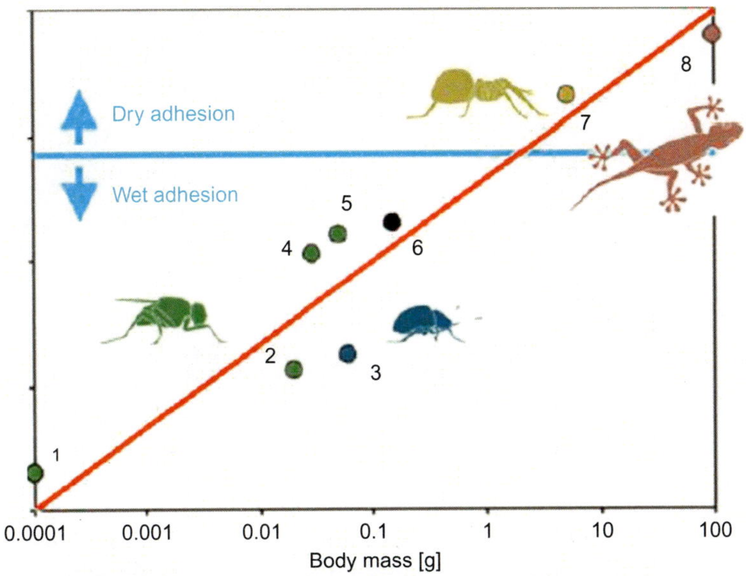

Figure 14.3 Adhesion mechanism according to body mass, for small animals. 1, 2, 4, 5: flies; 3: beetle; 6: bug; 7: spider; 8: geckonid lizards. Adapted from the book "Attachment Devices of Insect Cuticle" by Gorb (2001) and taken from Gorb et al. (2007) © IOP Publishing. Reproduced by permission of IOP Publishing. All rights reserved. The systems located above the blue line rely on van der Waals forces (dry adhesion), whereas the systems below the line rely mostly on capillary and viscous forces (wet adhesion).

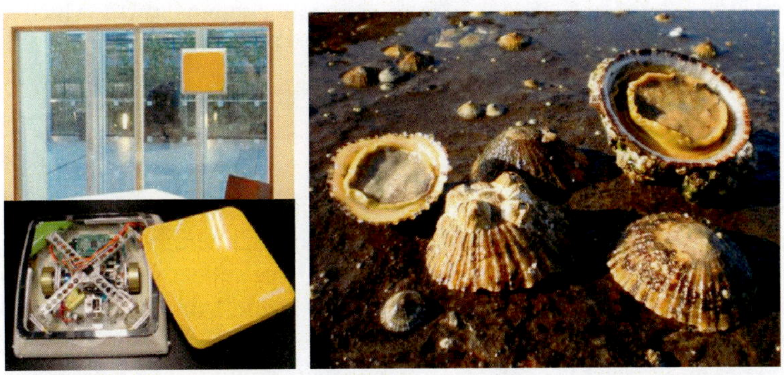

Figure 14.4 On the left, the WallWalker window cleaning climbing robot. On the right, an example of natural wet adhesion with suction used by limpets
(photo courtesy of Jay from Naturebum).

Contrary to one may think, the Madagascar's endemic sucker-footed bat (*Myzopoda aurita*) does not rely on suction for adhesion. In fact, it clings head-up to smooth leaves using specialized pads on its wrists and ankles (Riskin and Racey, 2010). This form of wet adhesion allows them to unpeel easily from the surface because of deformation of the pads, during crawling, but would also cause passive detachment if bats roosted

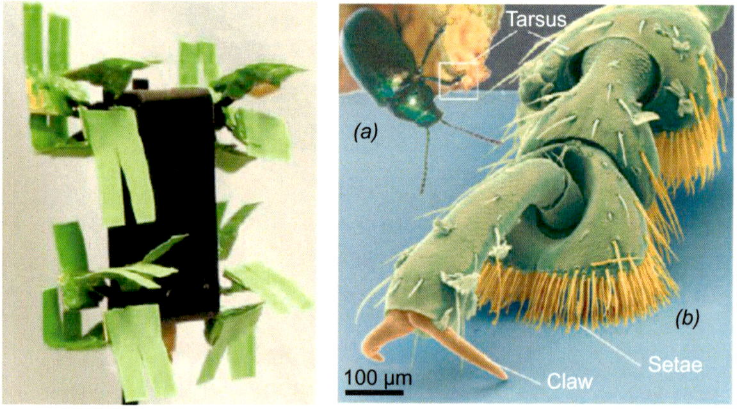

Figure 14.5 On the left, the Mini-Whegs™ wet adhesive pad climbing robot and on the right an example of the hairy attachment system (taken from Gorb et al. (2007) © IOP Publishing. Reproduced by permission of IOP Publishing. All rights reserved). Tarsus (b) of the chrysomelid beetle *Gastrophysa viridula* (a) attached to the smooth surface Gorb (2005) (colored scanning electron microscopy picture is the courtesy of Juergen Berger, MPI for Developmental Biology, Tubingen, Germany) and taken from Gorb et al. (2007) © IOP Publishing.
Reproduced by permission of IOP Publishing. All rights reserved.

head-down, like the vast majority of bats do, hanging by their toenails (Riskin et al., 2009). This provides an ecomorphological explanation to the head-up roosting behavior of these unique bats.

Mini-Whegs™ (Gorb et al., 2007) is a small climbing robot which uses wet adhesion through a patterned tape on four whegs (Figure 14.5).

14.2.4 Dry adhesion

Dry adhesion is best typified by the specialized toes of geckos. The gecko's trick to sticking to surfaces lies in the very fine hairs on its toes. Literally, billions of these tiny hairs make contact with the surface and create a huge collective surface area of contact. Each hair is made from multiple sections, a micro-hair which is roughly 5 μ in diameter, and atop each of these micro-hairs sit tens to hundreds of nano-hairs which are 200 nm in diameter (1/250th of a human hair) in a tree-like branching structure (Murphy and Sitti, 2009). This, in conjunction with van der Waals forces allows them to adhere to many substrates, even glass. Geckobot (Unver et al., 2006), StickyBot (Santos et al., 2008), and Waalbot (Murphy and Sitti, 2009) are gecko-inspired climbing robots which use elastomer adhesives on their fingers to adhere to the climbing surface (Figure 14.6). The Geckobot is a 100 g climbing robot with a body made of Delrin and adhesive polydimethylsiloxane elastomer surfaces on its four feet. To pull the adhesive surfaces from the surface during locomotion, it employs a peeling mechanism actuated by the leg motor and a compression spring. This allows for

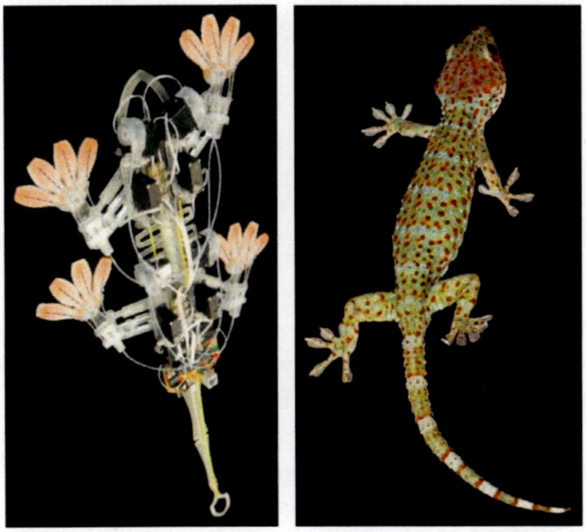

Figure 14.6 On the left is the StickyBot and on the right is an underside view of a Gecko showing the details of its fingers.

power-efficient detachment as seen in geckos. Its total length is 190 mm and width is 110 mm. It is capable of climbing with speeds up to 1 cm/s on inclined surfaces up to 85° (Unver et al., 2006). However, this is not an adhesion technology limitation. The StickyBot employs a synthetic adhesive patch termed directional polymer stalks on each of the four toes of each of the four feet. The limit surfaces, representing the friction and adhesion limits associated with a synthetic directional adhesive material, for individual patches are combined and linearized to produce a set of contact constraints for each foot of a climbing robot. The limit surfaces are convex and they intersect the origin in force space. These properties lead to efficient strategies for controlling internal forces between the feet to maximize the margin of stability with respect to disturbances and for attaching and detaching the feet smoothly, without unproductive energy expenditure. This feature allows the StickyBot to cling to surfaces with an overhang angle of at least 20° (Santos et al., 2008). Because the limit surfaces are asymmetric, foot orientation is also important. Observations of geckos reveal that they change the orientations of their feet, for example, when clinging to a ceiling or when running headfirst down a wall (Santos et al., 2008). This, however, is not yet used in any of these small gecko robots.

14.2.5 Chemical adhesion

Snails segregate a fluid which acts as glue to provide the necessary adhesion to the surface. The snail inspired wall climbing robot (Shapiro et al., 2005) works in a similar way by carrying hot-melt adhesive tubes which are heated and released as liquid into the robot tracks, as the robot moves, acting as a glue for the robot (Figure 14.7). Other similar robots using hot melt adhesives have been proposed by the Bio-Inspired Robotics Lab (BIRL) of ETH Zurich (Osswald and Iida, 2011; Wang et al., 2012; Wang et al., 2013). These robots combine high-payload capabilities with the ability to climb on various vertical terrains.

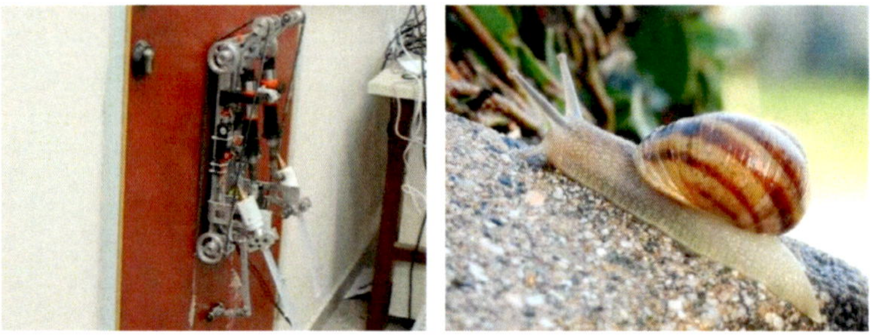

Figure 14.7 The snail-inspired wall climbing robot uses the same adhesion mechanism as a snail, by releasing a visa glue fluid which acts as glue.
(Snail photo by John D.)

However, similar to snails, these robots have the disadvantage of low climbing speeds, rating at 0.039 cm/s climbing speed, in the case of the small climbing turtle (Graber, 2012). This is mainly due to the time that they require to melt and solidify the glue. They are also extremely inefficient in terms of energy (Graber, 2012).

For arboreal animals, posture and balance are extremely important when climbing, due to the height of many branches and the potentially disastrous consequences of a fall. On horizontal and gently sloped branches, the primary problem is tipping to the side due to the narrow base of support. The narrower the branch, the greater the difficulty in balancing a given animal face. On steep and vertical branches, tipping becomes less of an issue, and pitching backward or slipping downward becomes the most likely failure (Cartmill, 1985). The same applies to climbing robots. However, most arboreal animals possess clever features which allow them to overcome such difficulties. Many arboreal species lower their center of mass to reduce pitching and toppling movement when climbing. This may be accomplished by postural changes, altered body proportions, or smaller size (Cartmill, 1985). The pruning robot developed by Kawasaki et al. (2008) and Ishigure and Kawasaki (2013) can stay on a tree without energy consumption by using its own weight using a two-DoF posture adjustment mechanism to keep the pruning robot in a horizontal posture (Figure 14.8).

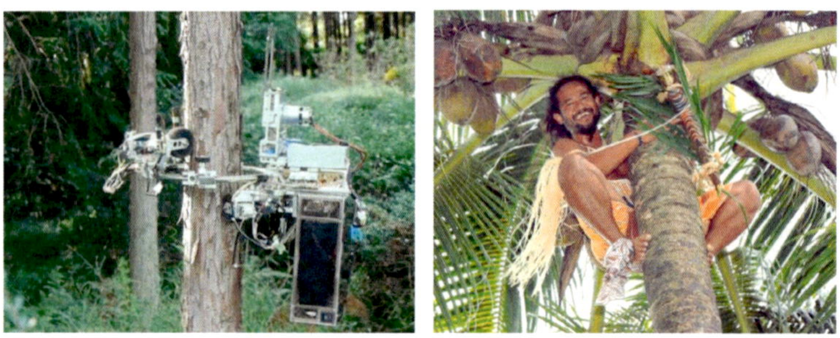

Figure 14.8 On the left, the pruning robot adjusts its posture to stay on the tree using only its weight. The same technique is used for centuries by coconut tree climbers.

14.3 Bio-inspired locomotion mechanisms

Climbing animals can be roughly divided into two groups: those animals which move steep, vertical, or overhanging surfaces (surface locomotion), and those who move among tall vegetation (arboreal locomotion). These two environments may produce quite different climbing methods. Anatomical specializations of arboreal locomotion animals include (Tavakoli et al., 2010a):

- Elongated limbs that assist them in crossing gaps, reaching fruit or other resources, testing the firmness of support ahead, and in some cases, brachiating.
- Prehensile tails, such as chameleons, spider monkeys, and possums, in order to grasp branches.

14.3.1 Brachiation

One of the most efficient locomotion mechanisms used by arboreal climbing animals is called Brachiation. This specialized form of locomotion is used by some primates (spider monkeys and gibbons, occasionally female orangutans) to move very rapidly while hanging beneath branches. It involves swinging with the arms from one handhold to another. Prehensile tails play a major role in this form of locomotion by acting as a gripper and by helping with balance. Gibbons are the experts of this mode of locomotion, swinging from branch to branch with distances up to 15 m, and traveling at speeds of as much as 56 km/h (Tavakoli et al., 2010a). While some pole climbing robots using grippers, such as the 3D Climber (Figure 14.1), may appear to follow this principle, they cannot be fully considered as brachiating robots since their locomotion is step by step and does not possess the dynamics of the brachiation.

A couple of works have been conducted on brachiating robots. Fukuda et al. (1991) proposed and simulated a brachiating robot design. Saito and Fukuda (1996) extended this work to create a three-dimensional robot closely resembling a siamang, called Brachiator-III. The robot consists of 12 DoF controlled by 14 motors, 2 of which are responsible for grasping. This robot is able to initiate brachiation from a stationary hanging position and continue moving beneath a horizontal series of ladder-like rungs. Kajima et al. (2003) constructed an even more complex robot consisting of 19 links and 20 actuators, called "Gorilla Robot II." It was designed to be able to walk bipedally or quadrupedally and brachiate, depending on the requirements set by the environment or task. It has the approximate proportions of a siamang and weights 20 kg (Bertram, 2004).

According to the studies (Usherwood et al., 2003; Usherwood and Bertram, 2003), the reason that the gibbons who weigh usually less than 10 kg, can brachiate on 56 km/h is that they do not generate torques on their shoulders and even the amount of torque on their handhold is surprisingly less than 2 N m (Chang et al., 2000). Gibbons use potential to kinetic energy conversions and vice versa for accelerating and decelerating. This method might be studied in order to reduce the amount of the necessary torque on joints, thus reducing the size of the motor and consequently reducing the total weight of the system. While passive walking has been extensively studied and applied, and there are also many interesting works on passive grasping, only until some years ago, researchers have started to study and model the interplay of passive locomotion, climbing, grasping, and body inertia management. Toshio Fukuda, director of the Micro-Nano Control and Bio-Robotics Laboratory at the Nagoya University in Japan, has been particularly active in this research topic (Kajima et al., 2004; Fukuda et al., 2006; Pchelkin et al., 2011).

14.3.2 Dragline locomotion

Recently, a novel bio-inspired locomotion mechanism has been developed by researchers from the Bio-inspired Robotics Lab at ETH of Zurich. Inspired by spiders producing draglines to assist locomotion, the dragline-forming mobile robot utilizes an alternative mobile technology where it achieves locomotion from a solid surface into a free space. The technology resembles the dragline production pathway in spiders to a technically feasible degree and enables robots to move with thermoplastic spinning of draglines (Figure 14.9). Thermoplastic adhesives are used as source material for the draglines. Experimental results show that a dragline diameter range of 1.17–5.27 mm was achievable by the 185 g mobile robot in descending locomotion from the solid surface of a hanging structure with a power consumption of 4.8 W and an average speed of 5.13 cm min^{-1} (Wang et al., 2014).

14.3.3 Limbless locomotion

Other different locomotion concepts observed in nature come from limbless animals, such as snakes or caterpillars. Many species of snakes are highly arboreal, and some have evolved specialized musculature for this habitat (Jayne, 1982). While moving in arboreal habitats, snakes move slowly along bare branches using a specialized form of

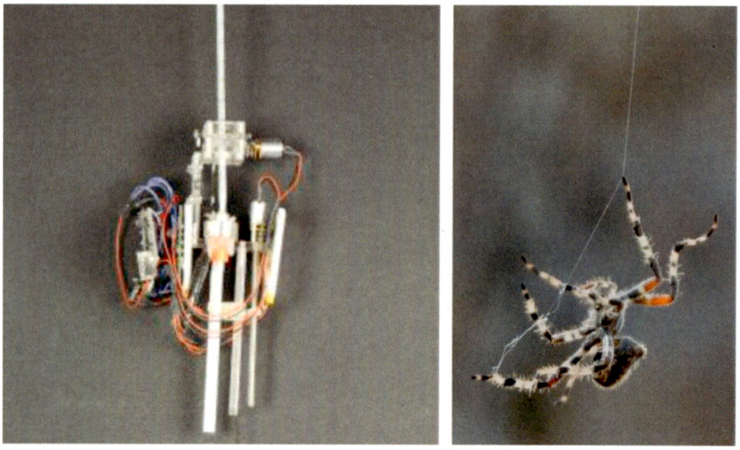

Figure 14.9 The ETH dragline-forming mobile robot, on the right, draws inspiration from spiders (spider photo credit: Stevie Benintende—www.whatsteviesees.com).

concertina locomotion (Astley and Jayne, 2007), but when secondary branches emerge from the branch being moved on, snakes use lateral undulation, a much faster mode. As a result, snakes perform best on small perches in cluttered environments, while limbed organisms seem to do best on large perches in uncluttered environments (Astley and Jayne, 2009).

Many robots which use this locomotion concept have been developed (Transeth et al., 2009; Yim et al., 2001; Wright et al., 2007a; Hopkins et al., 2009; Electric Power Research Institute, 2010). Their high number of DoFs and flexibility allows for easy obstacle surpassing and usability in any environment and surface type, making this concept of locomotion a specially promising one in the field of service climbing robots. Carnegie Mellon Biorobotics Lab researchers are especially active in developing several types of climbing and swimming inspection snake robots (Rollinson et al., 2013; McKenna et al., 2008; Wright et al., 2007b). Their 16 DoF, 2.9 kg climbing snake robot (Wright et al., 2012) is capable of climbing poles, trees, and branches just like snakes do (Figure 14.10).

Based on the vermicular motion of the pine caterpillar and inchworm, Wei Wang et al. proposed a two novel module climbing caterpillar robot with seven DoF (Wang et al., 2008). This small and lightweight climbing robot is capable of using two crawling principles of two typical caterpillars, pine caterpillar model and inchworm model, to climb vertical walls (Figure 14.11). The Softbot, developed at the Biomimetic

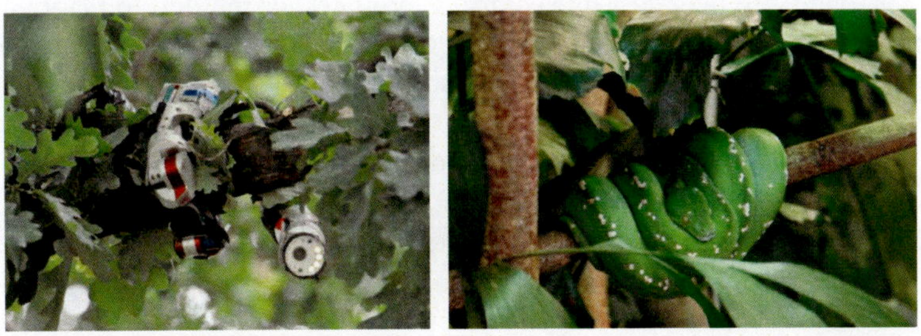

Figure 14.10 The CMU unified snake robot climbing a tree. This locomotion concept draws inspiration from snakes.

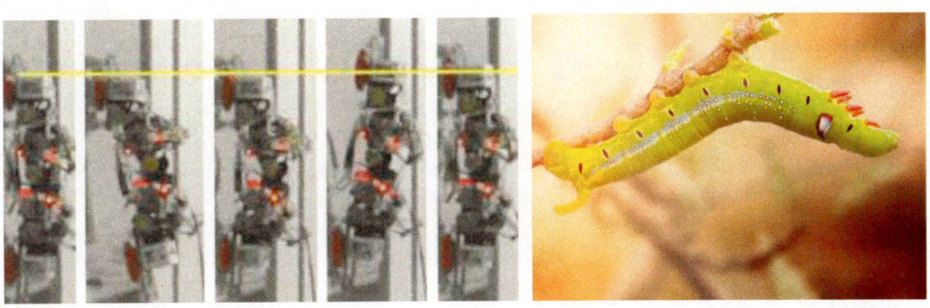

Figure 14.11 The caterpillar robot by Wei Wang et al., on the left, climbs walls using the crawling principles of caterpillars.

Devices Laboratory at Tufts University, is a soft robot which is continuously deformable and capable of collapsing and crumpling into small spaces. It is also based on the biomechanics and neural control system of a caterpillar (Trimmer et al., 2006).

14.3.4 Dynamic climbing

Other robots use climbing techniques inspired by climbing animals such as geckos and cockroaches, which rely on their own internal dynamic motions to gain height. The Dynamic Single Actuator Vertical Climbing Robot (Degani et al., 2007) benefits of its own internal dynamics that allows it to climb with only a single actuated DoF. By using a pendulum driven by an actuator, they manipulate the internal dynamics of the robot and the movement of its body, enabling it to move and climb while it rotates between two walls. Clark et al. also proposed a bio-inspired, two DoF vertical "running" robot assisted by springs. This robot also benefits from internal dynamic motions by employing the pendulous climbing model which shows remarkable similarities in dynamic wall-climbing behavior exhibited by many different animal species (Clark et al., 2007). Another small and lightweight climbing robot proposed by Dickson uses the Full-Goldman template for dynamic climbing and a single actuator to drive a miniature bipedal dynamic climbing platform, through the use of gears and springs (Figure 14.12; Dickson et al., 2013).

Other robots use tails, just like squirrels, primates, or reptiles, to manipulate their internal dynamic motions and enable them to climb. The ROCR: An Energy-Efficient Dynamic Wall-Climbing Robot (Provancher et al., 2011) is a pendular, two-link, serial chain robot that utilizes alternating handholds and an actuated tail to propel itself upward in a climbing style based on observation of human climbers and brachiating gibbons (Figure 14.13). Other already referenced climbing robots which use tails for balance include the Geckobot (Unver et al., 2006), StickyBot (Santos et al., 2008),

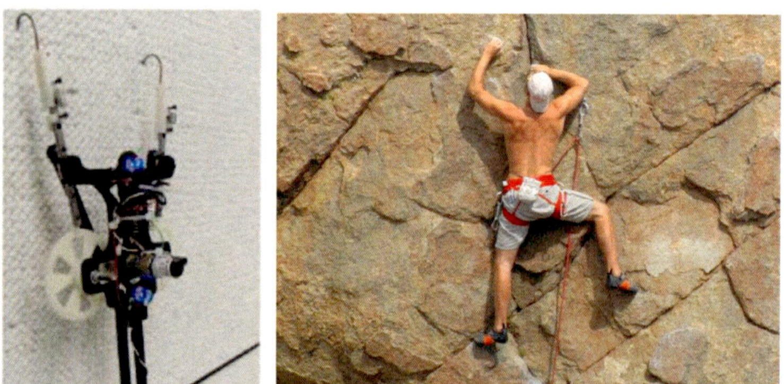

Figure 14.12 The miniature bipedal dynamic climbing platform, on the left, climbs walls with a single actuator taking advantage of its own internal dynamic motions, similar to the way animals and humans climb vertical walls.

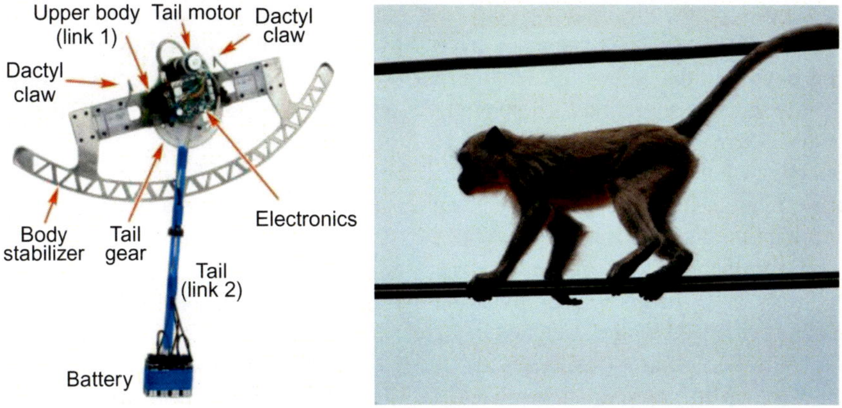

Figure 14.13 The ROCR robot on the right uses a tail to propel itself upward in a climbing style based on observation of brachiating gibbons.

and Waalbot (Murphy and Sitti, 2009). Some robots use their tails to climb steeper inclines without toppling, as is the case of the HELIOS Carrier (Guarnieri et al., 2009). Some climbing and jumping robots even use their tails for pitch control (Libby et al., 2012).

14.3.5 Multimodal locomotion

A type of locomotion which combines climbing and flying for a fast, agile, and efficient movement is the multimodal locomotion.

There are several examples of animals capable of multimodal locomotion. While climbing and gliding may not be necessarily more efficient than simply running (Byrnes et al., 2011), it is often used for overcoming obstacles, escaping predators, avoiding rough or complicated terrain, or simply quickly transit between tall vertical structures. A theory on the evolution of flight proposes a "top-down" approach (animals jumping from heights) with an intermediary gliding phase for arboreal climbing animals (Norberg, 1985).

The Draco genus of lizards, also referred to as "flying dragons," comprises more than 40 species of lizards, with body sizes ranging in mass between 3 and 20 g (McGuire and Dudley, 2011; McGuire and Dudley, 2005), which have developed the ability to glide and special physical adaptations to actively control their aerodynamic properties. Using elongated thoracic ribs and specialized musculature, they are able to actively control the aerodynamic properties of their gliding membrane, called patagium (McGuire and Dudley, 2011; Russell and Dijkstra, 2001). Draco lizards have also shown other physical adaptations along their necks, legs, and edges of their hind quarters that are used for maximizing the aerodynamic surface (McGuire and Dudley, 2011).

Other reptiles with radically different morphologies are also capable of gliding. Snakes in the genus Chrysopelea have shown the ability to glide using behavioral and physical adaptations to create an airfoil-shaped body to substantially decrease their descent accelerations. There are five species of "flying snakes" that flatten their bodies, increasing the surface area, and form a concave bottom surface creating an effective whole-body wing (Socha et al., 2010). The *Chrysopelea paradisi*, or the paradise tree snake, has even been shown to temporarily achieve a positive (upward) acceleration during flight (Socha et al., 2010).

But probably the most well-known examples of gliding animals are the flying squirrels. Like the above-mentioned reptiles, they also reveal special physical adaptations evidenced by the stretched patagial skin between their fore and aft limbs used for controlled gliding (Galvao et al., 2006). They have been observed to have glide ratios of up to approximately 3, e.g., a 30-m glide over a 10-m drop (Clark and Dickson, 2013). Some species of flying squirrel have shown the ability to modify the shape of their gliding membranes in flight using the abductor of the thumb. Due to this adaptation, small flying squirrels, in particular *Glaucomys Volans*, are extremely agile and maneuverable (Thorington et al., 1998). These animals have been reported to have glided durations of up to 15 s (Asari et al., 2007; Byrnes et al., 2008).

Researchers from Florida State University College of Engineering proposed the ICAROS platform which is capable of climbing prepared vertical surfaces and transitioning to a glide path with performance characteristics comparable to its biological counterparts (Clark and Dickson, 2013). Using the same iplatform, climbing platform proposed by Dickson et al. (2013), the ICAROS platform, with a mass of 350 g, is capable of climbing a carpet wall at 0.135 ± 0.01 m s^{-1}. When it reaches the top, it is able to glide thanks to its fixed-wing glider profile made of balsa wood, with a wing span of 72 cm, thus effectively combining these two forms of locomotion into a single platform. The ICAROS platform is capable of a glide ratio of approximately 2 m s^{-1} and a glide velocity of approximately 5.3 m s^{-1} on par with climbing and gliding animals. Same researchers are already working on the next generation of ARM2 S that utilizes a bio-inspired, flexible patagium for gliding flight similar to structures seen on flying squirrels and flying dragons. The platform will incorporate specialized, compliant feet for operation on numerous surfaces (Clark and Dickson, 2013).

14.4 Size and current technology constrains

While most small animals such as geckos and insects, as seen previously, rely on dry and wet adhesion, big animals such as gibbons and monkeys rely mostly on the dexterity of their body and use this dexterity to encircle and seize the object. They do not use specific adhesion techniques such as wet or dry adhesion. This is same for even heavier animals such as pandas and bears.

For climbing robots, if small robots are desired for applications such as video monitoring, bio-inspired adhesion, e.g., dry adhesion can contribute to the development of lightweight and fast robots. However, if the robot is required to carry bigger weights, such as inspection probes or cleaning and maintenance tools, the focus should be mainly on the locomotion mechanism. Arboreal animals take advantage of a complex and high dexterity locomotion mechanism with many DoFs. Due to the limitations in the current technologies, such as actuators (Tavakoli et al., 2010a), the bio-inspiration of the robot at this scale is still very limited. Reaching to the dexterity level of such animals is a challenging problem in terms of design, optimization, and implementation of the mechanical structure. It is also a challenging control problem. Researchers always tried to limit the number of DoFs of the climbing mechanism by scarifying the robot's maneuverability.

For example, a human arm alone has seven DoFs (not considering the fingers). According to Clauser et al. (1969), the average mass of the human arm is about 3.2 kg. Another analysis made with 44 male basketball players showed that the average value of their pick elbow torque on flexor is 103 N m and their shoulder joint is 160 N m. On the other hand, a single brushless motor equipped with a harmonic drive reduction (like the ones employed in the 3D Climber pole climbing robot (Tavakoli et al., 2010b)) can deliver about the same torque (160 N m) but weighs 4.2 kg. This simple example shows that with the current technology driving one DoF of an arm requires an actuator heavier than the total human arm. In another work, Tavakoli et al. analyzed the application of pneumatic muscles in robotic applications and climbing robots (Tavakoli et al., 2008) and concluded that application of pneumatic muscles would be even heavier than harmonic drive actuators.

After decades of investigation on humanoid robots by several research groups all over the world, now we can see humanoid robots that can walk, run, play football, dance, and climb the stairs. Yet humanoid robots cannot perform agile movements that are associated with impacts, such as jumping, because they cannot store kinetic energy.

The new developments of serially elastic actuators (SEAs) and, more recently, variable stiffness actuators (VSAs) are some important steps toward development of actuators that are tolerant to impact and are safe to be applied in robots that should interact with humans. New developments in soft and elastic robots are another recent and quickly growing area that can contribute in this field. Several types of soft robots are being developed in many research centers. In addition to being inherently safe, soft robots are generally more adaptive to their environment. Adapting to the environment is one of the key issues in the design and development of grasping and adhesion mechanisms for climbing robots. In summary, recent and continuing advances in new and lightweight actuators, SEAs and VSAs, soft robots such as soft articulated arms and adaptive grasping mechanisms, and finally in development of smart controllers that apply the biological control schemes, such as synergies, can contribute in the development of the next generation of bio-inspired climbing robots at a scale that can carry a reasonable payload for inspection, surveillance, and maintenance services.

14.5 Future trends

The continuous development of actuators with a higher power to weight ratio, the growth of 3D printing and manufacturing technologies, advances in the adhesion technologies, and soft and deformable robots will contribute in the development of future lightweight and agile miniature bio-inspired robots. At this scale, the effect of the robot mass and gravity will be less relevant, thus simplifying the robot mechanical structure, adhesion, and locomotion mechanisms, and reducing the amount of power needed to drive the robot. However, for bigger climbing robots that require carrying higher payloads, the problem is still to be addressed. At this scale, in addition to the adhesion problem, one of the biggest limitations for robotic designers comes from the actuator technology.

Scaling down on the size and complexity of drivers and actuators, in line with the development of more powerful processors and controllers, will allow researchers to explore complex locomotion concepts such as the snake motion, which possesses large potential in terms of climbing performance, adaptation to different environments and obstacles, speed, and maneuverability. Also, the theoretical study of the dynamical interplay of locomotion and gripping/grasping/clasping of under actuated legged climbing systems equipped with (rudimentary) hands has still to be performed. Moreover, the development of "frugal" control systems exploiting the robot "body" dynamics and managing the locomotion and grasping within a high-level holistic unified framework, as probably happens in nature, has yet to come.

Soft robotics (Lam and Xu, 2012) will also be an important future trend, exploring new areas of material sciences and mechanics to produce mechanisms capable of fully adapting to the environment and its surroundings, just like organisms do. With a soft structure and redundant DoFs, these robots can be used for delicate tasks in cluttered and/or unstructured environments, thus overcoming the most limitations of the current lab prototypes for service climbing and mobile robots.

Further information adhesion techniques in general may be found in the works of Longo and Muscato (2008). The widely accepted characterization of locomotion modes in the field of mobile robotics may be found in the work of Yim (1994).

References

Amano, H., Osuka, K., Tarn, T., 2001. Development of vertically moving robot with gripping handrails for fire fighting. In: IEEE/RSJ International Conference on Intelligent Robots and Systems (IROS), Maui (USA).

Asari, Y., Yanagawa, H., Oshida, T., 2007. Gliding ability of the Siberian flying squirrel Pteromys volans orii. Mamm. Study 32 (4), 151–154.

Asbeck, A.T., Kim, S., McClung, A., Parness, A., Cutkosky, M.R., 2006. Climbing walls with microspines. In: IEEE ICRA, Orlando, FL, USA.

Astley, H.C., Jayne, B.C., 2007. Effects of perch diameter and incline on the kinematics, performance and modes of arboreal locomotion of corn snakes (*Elaphe guttata*). J. Exp. Biol. 210, 3862–3872.

Astley, H.C., Jayne, B.C., 2009. Arboreal habitat structure affects the performance and modes of locomotion of corn snakes (*Elaphe guttata*). J. Exp. Zool. 311A, 207–216.

Balaguer, C., Pastor, J., Gimenez, A., Padron, V., Abderrahim, M., 1998. Roma: a multifunctional autonomous self-supported climbing robot for inspection application. In: Third IFAC Symposium on Intelligent Autonomous Vehicles, Madrid (Spain).

Balaguer, C., Giménez, A., Abderrahim, M., 2002. ROMA robots for inspection of steel based infrastructures. Ind. Robot 29 (3), 246–251.

Bertram, J., 2004. New perspectives on brachiation mechanics. Am. J. Phys. Anthropol 125 (S39), 100–117.

Bonaccorso, F., Bruno, C., Longo, D., Muscato, G., 2008. Structure and model identification of a vortex-based suction cup. In: Proceedings of the 11th International Conference on Climbing and Walking Robots and the Support Technologies for Mobile Machines (CLAWAR), Coimbra (Portugal).

Busko, K., Klossowski, M., 1998. Muscle torque of male basketball players playing at different floor positions. In ISBS-Conference Proceedings Archive, vol. 1, No. 1, Konstanz, Germany.

Byrnes, G., Lim, N.T.-L., Spence, A.J., 2008. Take-off and landing kinetics of a free-ranging gliding mammal, the Malayan colugo (*Galeopterus variegatus*). Proc. R. Soc. B 275, 1007–1013.

Byrnes, G., Libby, T., Lim, N.T., Spence, A.J., 2011. Gliding saves time but not energy in Malayan colugos. J. Exp. Biol. 214, 2690–2696.

Cartmill, M., 1985. Climbing. In: Functional Vertebrate Morphology. Belknap Press, Cambridge, pp. 73–88.

Chang, Y-.H., Bertram, J.E.A., Lee, D.V., 2000. The external forces and torques generated by the brachiating white-handed gibbon (Hylobates lar). Am. J. Phys. Anthropol. 113, 201–216.

Chen, S., Shang, J., Zhao, Z., Sattar, T., Bridge, B., 2006. Novel solutions to design problems of industrial climbing robots. In: Climbing and Walking Robots. Proceedings of the Eighth International Conference on Climbing and Walking Robots and the Support Technologies for Mobile Machines (CLAWAR 2005). Springer, Berlin, Heidelberg, pp. 139–146.

Clark, J.E., Dickson, J.D., 2013. Design of a multimodal climbing and gliding robotic platform. Trans. Mechatron. 18 (2), 494–505.

Clark, J., Goldman, D., Lin, P.-C., Lynch, G., Chen, T., Komsuoglu, H., Full, R., Koditschek, D., 2007. Design of a bio-inspired dynamical vertical climbing robot. In: Robotics: Science and Systems.

Clauser, C.E., McConville, J.T., Young, J.W., 1969. Weight, volume and center of mass of segments of the human body. Tech. Rep. AMRL TR 69–70, Wright Patterson Air Force Base, Ohio (NTIS No. AD-710 622).

Degani, A., Shapiro, A., Choset, H., Mason, M.T., 2007. A dynamic single actuator vertical climbing robot. In: IEEE/RSJ International Conference on Intelligent Robots and Systems, IROS 2007.

Dickson, J.D., Patel, J., Clark, J.E., 2013. Towards maneuverability in plane with a dynamic climbing platform. In: Robotics and Automation (ICRA), Karlsruhe, Germany.

Electric Power Research Institute, "Snake Robot," 2010. [Online]. Available: http://transsensorsrobots.epri.com/snake-robot.html. (accessed 01.06.13).

Ellem, G.K., Furst, J.E., Zimmerman, K.D., 2002. Shell clamping behaviour in the limpet *Cellana tramoserica*. J. Exp. Biol. 205, 539–547.

Fukuda, T., Hosokai, H., Kondo, Y., 1991. Brachiation type of mobile robot. In: Fifth International Conference on Advanced Robotics (ICAR 1991).

Fukuda, T., Doi, M., Hasegawa, Y., Kajima, H., 2006. Multi-locomotion control of biped locomotion and brachiation robot. In: Fast Motions in Biomechanics and Robotics.pp. 121–145.

Galvao, R., Song, A., Tian, X., Bishop, K., Swartz, S., Breuer, K., 2006. The aerodynamics of compliant membrane wings modeled on mammalian flight mechanics. In: American Institute Aeronautics Astronautics Meeting, San Francisco, CA.

Gorb, S., 2001. Attachment Devices of Insect Cuticle. Kluwer Academic Publishers, Dordrecht.

Gorb, S., 2005. Uncovering insect stickiness: structure and properties of hairy attachment devices. Am. Entomol, 31–35.

Gorb, S.N., Sinha, M., Peressadko, A., Daltorio, K.A., Quinn, R.D., 2007. Insects did it first: a micropatterned adhesive tape for robotic applications. Bioinspir. Biomim. 2, S117–S125, Biomimetic technologies: volume 1—materials and sensors.

Graber, L., 2012. Master Thesis—Self-Contained High Payload Robot for Climbing on Multiple Vertical Environments, Zurich.

Guarnieri, M., Debenest, P., Inoh, T., Takita, K., Masuda, H., Kurazume, R., Fukushima, E., Hirose, S., 2009. HELIOS carrier: tail-like mechanism and control algorithm for stable motion in unknown environments. In: IEEE International Conference on Robotics and Automation, ICRA 2009.

Haynes, G.C., Khripin, A., Lynch, G., Amory, J., Saunders, A., Rizzi, A.A., Koditschek, D.E., 2009. Rapid pole climbing with a quadrupedal robot. In: IEEE International Conference on Robotics and Automation (ICRA), Kobe, Japan.

Hillenbrand, C., Schmidt, D., Berns, K., 2008. CROMSCI—a climbing robot with multiple sucking chambers for inspection tasks. In: Proceedings of The 11th International Conference on Climbing and Walking Robots and the Support Technologies for Mobile Machines (CLAWAR), Coimbra (Portugal).

Hopkins, J.K., Spranklin, B.W., Gupta, S.K., 2009. A survey of snake-inspired robot designs. Bioinspir. Biomim. 4(2).

Ishigure, Y.H.K., Kawasaki, H., 2013. A pruning robot with a power-saving chainsaw drive. In: 2013 IEEE International Conference on Mechatronics and Automation (ICMA), Takamatsu.

Jayne, B.C., 1982. Comparative morphology of the semispinalis-spinalis muscle of snakes and correlations with locomotion and constriction. J. Morphol. 172, 83–96.

Kajima, H., Hasegawa, Y., Fukuda, T., 2003. Learning algorithm for a brachiating robot. Appl. Bionics Biomech. 1 (1), 57–66.

Kajima, H., Doi, M., Hasegawa, Y., Hasegawa, Y., 2004. A study on a brachiation controller for a multi-locomotion robot—realization of smooth, continuous brachiation. Adv. Robot. 18 (10), 1025–1038.

Kawasaki, H., Murakami, S., Kachi, H., Ueki, S., 2008. Novel climbing method of pruning robot. In: IEEE SICE Annual Conference 2008.

Kim, S., Asbeck, A., Cutkosky, M., Provancher, W., 2005. SpinybotII: climbing hard walls with compliant microspines. In: International Conference on Advanced Robotics, Washington (USA).

Lam, T.L., Xu, Y., 2012. State-of-the-art tree-climbing robots. In: Tree Climbing Robot, 78, Springer, Berlin, Heidelberg, pp. 5–8.

Libby, T., Moore, T.Y., Chang-Siu, E., Li, D., Cohen, D.J., Jusufi, A., Full, R.J., 2012. Tail-assisted pitch control in lizards, robots and dinosaurs. Nature 481, 181–184.

Longo, D., Muscato, G., 2008. Adhesion techniques for climbing robots: state of the art and experimental considerations. In: Plenary Talk at the 11th International Conference on Climbing and Walking Robots and the Support Technologies for Mobile Machines (CLAWAR), Coimbra (Portugal).

McGuire, J.A., Dudley, R., 2005. The cost of living large: comparative gliding performance in flying lizards (Agamidae: Draco). Am. Nat. 166, 93–106.

McGuire, J.A., Dudley, R., 2011. The biology of gliding in flying lizards (genus *Draco*) and their fossil and extant analogs. In: Biomechanics and Behavior Gliding Flight, Salt Lake City, UT.

McKenna, J.C., Anhalt, D.J., Bronson, F.M., Brown, H.B., Schwerin, M., Shammas, E., Choset, H., 2008. Toroidal skin drive for snake robot locomotion. In: 2008 IEEE International Conference on Robotics & Automation, Pasadena, California.

Miyake, T., Ishihara, H., Yoshimura, M., 2007. Basic studies on wet adhesion system for wall climbing robots. In: IEEE/RSJ International Conference on Intelligent Robots and Systems IROS 2007, San Diego, California, USA.

Murphy, M., Sitti, M., 2009. Waalbot: agile climbing with synthetic fibrillar dry adhesives. In: IEEE International Conference on Robotics and Automation (ICRA), Kobe (Japan).

Norberg, U., 1985. Evolution of vertebrate flight: an aerodynamic model for the transition from gliding to active flight. Am. Nat. 126, 303–327.

Osswald, M., Iida, F., 2011. A climbing robot based on hot melt adhesion. In: IEEE International Conference on Intelligent Robots and Systems (IROS 2011), San Francisco.

Pchelkin, S., Shiriaev, A.S., Mettin, U., Freidovich, L.B., Aoyama, T., Lu, Z., Fukuda, T., 2011. Shaping energetically efficient brachiation motion for a 24-DOF gorilla robot. In: 2011 IEEE/RSJ International Conference on Intelligent Robots and Systems (IROS), San Francisco, CA.

Provancher, W.R., Jensen-Segal, S.I., Fehlberg, M.A., 2011. ROCR: an energy-efficient dynamic wall-climbing robot. Trans. Mechatron. 16 (5), 897–906.

Riskin, D.K., Racey, P.A., 2010. How do sucker-footed bats hold on, and why do they roost head-up? Biol. J. Linn. Soc. 99, 233–240.

Riskin, D.K., Bahlman, J.W., Hubel, T.Y., Ratcliffe, J.M., Kunz, T.H., Swartz, S.M., 2009. Bats go head-under-heels: the biomechanics of landing on a ceiling. J. Exp. Biol. 212, 945–953.

Rollinson, D., Ford, S., Brown, B., Choset, H., 2013. Design and modeling of a series elastic element for snake robots. In: ASME Dynamic Systems and Controls Conference, Stanford, CA.

Russell, A.P., Dijkstra, L.D., 2001. Patagial morphology of *Draco volans* (Reptilia: Agamidae) and the origin of glissant locomotion in flying dragons. J. Zool. 253, 457–471.

Saito, F., Fukuda, T., 1996. A first result of the brachiator III—a new brachiation robot modeled on a siamang. In: Artificial Life V.

Santos, D., Heyneman, B., Sangbae, K., Esparza, N., Cutkosky, M.R., 2008. Gecko-inspired climbing behaviors on vertical and overhanging surfaces. In: IEEE International Conference on Robotics and Automation, ICRA 2008. Pasadena, CA, USA.

Shapiro, A., Mahpoda, I., Zuk, H., 2005. A snail inspired wall climbing robot for counter terrorism duty. In: The 30th Israeli Conference on Mechanical Engineering, Tel-Aviv Israel.

Smith, A.M., 1991. The role of suction in the adhesion of limpets. J. Exp. Biol. 161, 151–169.

Smith, A.M., 1992. Alternation between attachment mechanisms by limpets in the field. J. Exp. Mar. Biol. Ecol. 160 (2), 205–220.

Socha, J.J., Miklasz, K., Jafari, F., Vlachos, P.P., 2010. Non-equilibrium trajectory dynamics and the kinematics of gliding in a flying snake. Bioinspir. Biomim. 5, 1–12.

Tavakoli, M., Zakerzadeh, M., Vossoughi, G., Bagheri, S., 2005. Design and prototyping of a hybrid pole climbing and manipulating robot with minimum DOFs for construction and service applications. In: Climbing and Walking Robots: Proceedings of the Seventh International Conference Clawar 2004, Madrid (Spain).

Tavakoli, M., Marques, L., de Almeida, A.T., 2008. A comparison study on pneumatic muscles and electrical motors. In: IEEE International Conference on Robotics and Biomimetics ROBIO 08, Bangkok, Thailand.

Tavakoli, M., Marques, L., Bonsignorio, F., 2010a. Biomimetic inspiration in climbing robots. In: CLAWAR 2010.

Tavakoli, M., Marques, L., de Almeida, A.T., 2010b. Development of an industrial pipeline inspection robot. Ind. Robot. Int. J. 37 (3), 309–322.
Thorington, R.W., Darrow, K., Anderson, C.G., 1998. Wing tip anatomy and aerodynamics in flying squirrels. J. Mammal. 79, 245–250.
Transeth, A.A., Pettersen, K.Y., Liljebäck, P., 2009. A survey on snake robot modeling and locomotion. Robotica 27 (07), 999–1015.
Trimmer, B., Takesian, A., Sweet, B., Rogers, C., Hake, D., Rogers, D., 2006. Caterpillar locomotion: a new model for soft-bodied climbing and burrowing robots. In: Seventh International Symposium on Technology and the Mine Problem (vol. 1, pp. 1–10), Monterey, CA.
Unver, O., Uneri, A., Aydemir, A., Sitti, M., 2006. Geckobot: a gecko inspired climbing robot using elastomer adhesives. In: IEEE International Conference on Robotics and Automation, ICRA 2006, Orlando, Florida, USA.
Usherwood, J.R., Bertram, J.E.A., 2003. Understanding brachiation: insight from a collisional perspective. J. Exp. Biol. 206 (10), 1631–1642.
Usherwood, J.R., Larson, S.G., Bertram, J.E.A., 2003. Mechanisms of force and power production in unsteady ricochetal brachiation. Am. J. Phys. Anthropol. 120 (4), 364–372.
Wang, W., Wang, Y., Wang, K., Zhang, H., Zhang, J., 2008. Analysis of the kinematics of module climbing caterpillar robots. In: IEEE/ASME International Conference on Advanced Intelligent Mechatronics, AIM 2008, pp. 84–89.
Wang, L., Neuschaefer, F., Bernet, R., Iida, F., 2012. Design considerations for attachment and detachment in robot climbing with hot melt adhesives. In: IEEE International Conference on Robotics and Automation (ICRA 2012), St. Paul, USA.
Wang, L., Graber, L., Iida, F., 2013. Large-payload climbing in complex vertical environments using thermoplastic adhesive bonds. IEEE Trans. Robot. 29 (4), 863–874.
Wang, L., Culha, U., Iida, F., 2014. A dragline-forming mobile robot inspired by spiders. Bioinspir. Biomim. 9(1).
Wright, C., Johnson, A., Peck, A., McCord, Z., Naaktgeboren, A., Gianfortoni, P., Gonzalez-Rivero, M., Hatton, R., Choset, H., 2007a. Design of a modular snake robot. In: IEEE/RSJ International Conference on Intelligent Robots and Systems, IROS 2007, pp. 2609–2614.
Wright, C., Johnson, A., Peck, A., McCord, Z., Naaktgeboren, A., Gianfortoni, P., Gonzalez-Rivero, M., Hatton, R., Choset, H., 2007b. Design of a modular snake robot. In: 2007 IEEE/RSJ Intl. Conference on Intelligent Robots and Systems, San Diego, CA, USA.
Wright, C., Buchan, A., Brown, B., Geist, J., Schwerin, M., Rollinson, D., Tesch, M., Choset, H., 2012. Design and architecture of the unified modular snake robot. In: 2012 IEEE International Conference on Robotics and Automation, St. Paul, MN.
Yim, M., 1994. A taxonomy of locomotion. In: Chapter 3 of the PHD Thesis, Locomotion with a unit-modular reconfigurable robot, at the department of mechanical engineering of Stanford University.
Yim, M., Homans, S., Roufas, K., 2001. Climbing with snake-like robots. In: IFAC workshop on mobile robot technology, pp. 21–22.

Locomotion rhythm generation using pulse-type hardware neural networks for quadruped robots

15

K. Saito, Y. Ikeda, M. Takato, F. Uchikoba

15.1 Introduction

Recently, many types of multilegged robot had proposed because multilegged robot could easily locomote on uneven surface compared with crawler-type or wheel-type robot (Mcghh and Iswandhi, 1979; Raibert et al., 2008). Most of multilegged robots mimic the living organisms because living organisms realize the autonomous operation using excellent structure and active neural networks control by compact advanced systems. Therefore, some advanced studies have been done to realize the excellent functions of living organisms by using biomimetics technologies (Habib et al., 2007; Habib, 2011). To utilize the robot more effectively, robot control required more complicated and advanced systems. Programmed control by digital systems based on microcontroller has been the dominant system among the robot control (Mcghh and Iswandhi, 1979; Fujita and Kitano, 1998). However, it is difficult to program the complicate autonomous operation to the microcontroller because of memory capacity. Therefore, some studies about artificial neural networks have been paid attention for applying to the robot control (Kimura et al., 2001; Fukuoka et al., 2003).

Oscillatory patterns of electrical activity are a ubiquitous feature in neural networks. Living organisms use several oscillatory patterns to operate movement, swallowing, heart rhythms, etc. (Delcomyn, 1980; Michael, 2002). To clarify oscillatory patterns, coupled neural oscillators are drawing attention. Synchronization phenomena or bifurcation phenomena of coupled neural oscillators have been studied using the Hodgkin–Huxley model (Hodgkin and Huxley, 1952) or Bonhoeffer–van der Pol model (van der Pol, 1927), which is a Class II neuron. Therefore, the synchronization phenomena of the coupled neural oscillators using mathematical neuron models have become the focus for generating the oscillatory patterns of living organisms (Tsumoto et al., 2003, 2006; Tsuji et al., 2007). However, using the mathematical neuron models in large-scale artificial neural networks is difficult to process in continuous time because the computer simulation is limited by the computer's performance, such as the processing speed and memory capacity. In contrast, using the hardware neuron model is advantageous because even if a circuit scale becomes large, the nonlinear operation can perform at high speed and process in continuous time. Therefore, the construction of a hardware model that can generate oscillatory patterns is desired. The hardware ring coupled oscillators have already been studied as a system which can demonstrate the various oscillatory patterns and the synchronization phenomena (Endo and Mori, 1978; Kitajima et al., 2001). For this reason, the ring coupled oscillators are expected to be a structural element of the cellular neural networks. However, most of the hardware models contain the inductor in circuit architecture (Endo and Mori, 1978; Kitajima et al., 2001; Yamauchi et al., 1999, 2003). If the system contains the inductor on the circuit system, it is difficult to implement the system for integrated circuit.

We are studying about neural networks using pulse-type hardware neuron models (P-HNM) (Matsuoka et al., 2002; Nakabora et al., 2004; Saito et al., 2011, 2012). The P-HNM has the same basic features of biological neurons such as threshold, refractory period, and spatiotemporal summation characteristics and enables the generation of continuous action potentials. Furthermore, the P-HNM could oscillate without an inductor so it is easy to implement the system for integrated circuit.

Previously, we proposed the coupled neural oscillators using P-HNM for microrobot. It was constructed by cell body models and synaptic models which has excitatory and inhibitory synaptic connections. We described the oscillating phenomena in an autonomous system (Saito et al., 2011, 2012).

In this chapter, P-HNN which can generate the locomotion rhythms for quadruped robot was proposed. First, mechanical components of quadruped robot were shown. Second, we discuss about locomotion rhythm generation using P-HNN which is the electrical components. Finally, quadruped locomotion of the robot which was controlled by the P-HNN was shown. As a result, P-HNN could generate the locomotion rhythms of the quadruped robot without using any computer programs.

15.2 Quadruped robot system

We constructed the 100, 125, 80 mm, width, length, height in size-miniaturized quadruped robot system (see Figure 15.1). The weight of the robot system was 530 g. The quadruped robot system consisted of mechanical components and electrical components. The mechanical components of quadruped robot consist of a body frame, four servo motors, link mechanisms, and four legs. Four legs comprised the link mechanisms and each legs using exactly same parts.

The electrical components of quadruped robot consist of a control bode, P-HNN, and battery. The mechanical components and the electrical components are discussed in Sections 15.3 and 15.4, respectively.

15.3 Mechanical components of the quadruped robot

In this section, the basic mechanical components of the fabricated quadruped robot were shown. The mechanical components of quadruped robot consist of body frame, four servo motors, link mechanisms, and four legs.

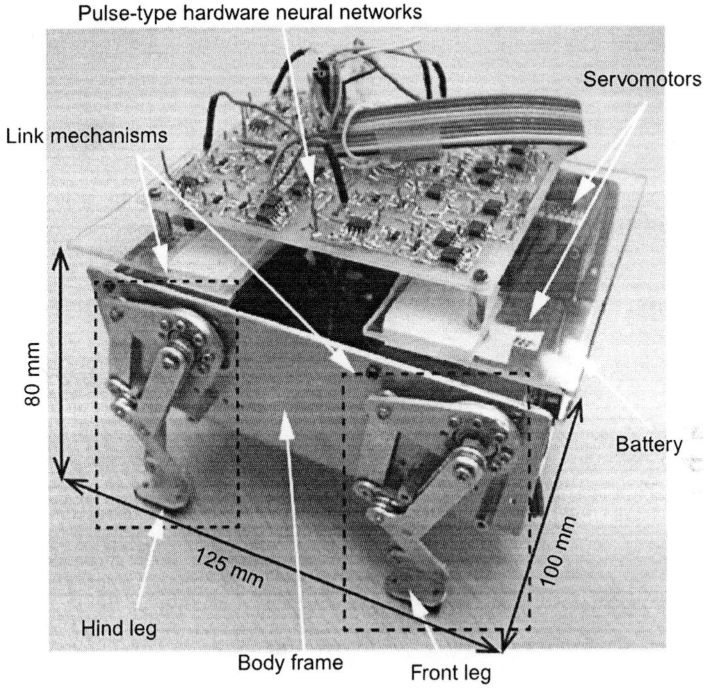

Figure 15.1 Constructed quadruped robot system.

15.3.1 Mechanical parts of the quadruped robot

Figure 15.2 shows the mechanical parts of the quadruped robot. Mechanical parts were made from aluminum base alloys 2017 and 5052 (Japanese Industrial Standards). We used the aluminum base alloy 5052 for body frame and aluminum base alloy 2017 for other mechanical parts. The mechanical parts were machined by the computerized numerical control machining system. Rods A, B, C, D, E, and F were components of link mechanisms which could assemble the single leg.

15.3.2 Link mechanisms of the quadruped robot

Quadruped robot system has only four servomotors to actuate four legs. Therefore, the movements to generate the locomotion of each leg were realized by using link mechanisms. In this chapter, we used the servomotor HSR-8498HB (Hitec Multiplex Japan) because the maximum torque was enough to actuate our quadruped robot system.

Figure 15.3 shows the link mechanism of the quadruped robot. Two sets of four-link mechanism are joined to realize the movement of the leg. Rod A, Rod B, and Rod C consist of the primary link where Rod D, Rod E, and Rod F comprise the secondary link, respectively.

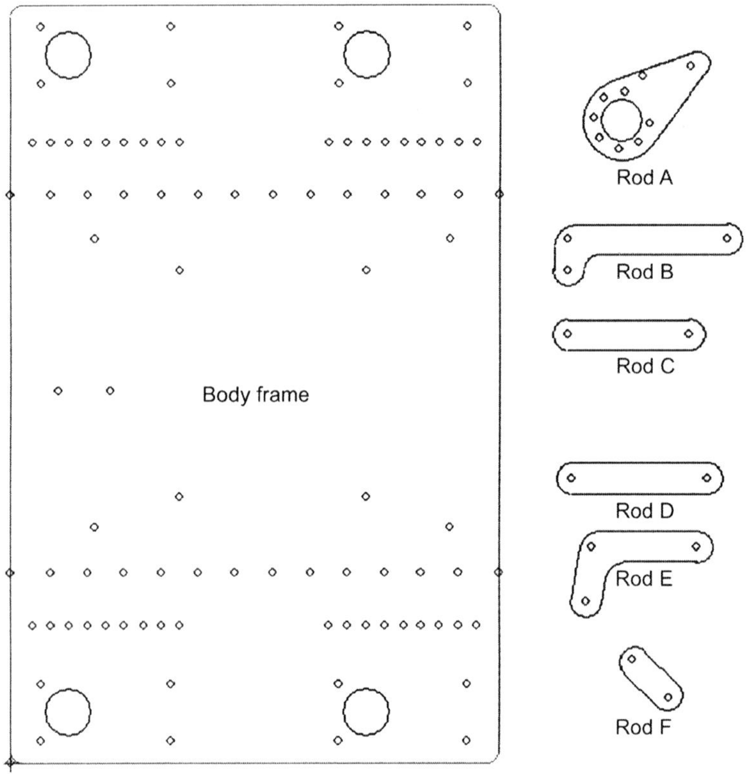

Figure 15.2 Mechanical parts of the quadruped robot.

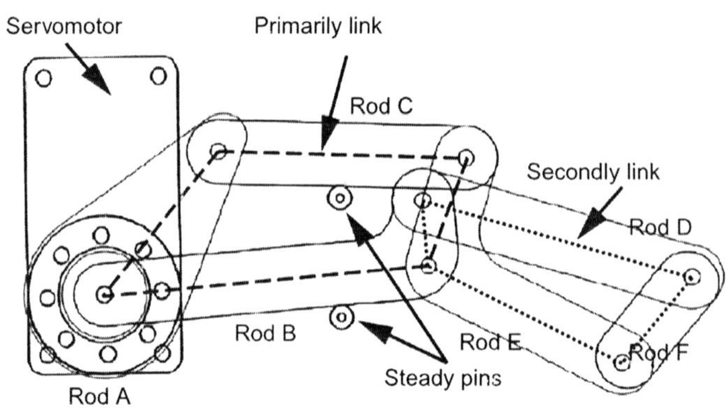

Figure 15.3 Link mechanism of the quadruped robot.

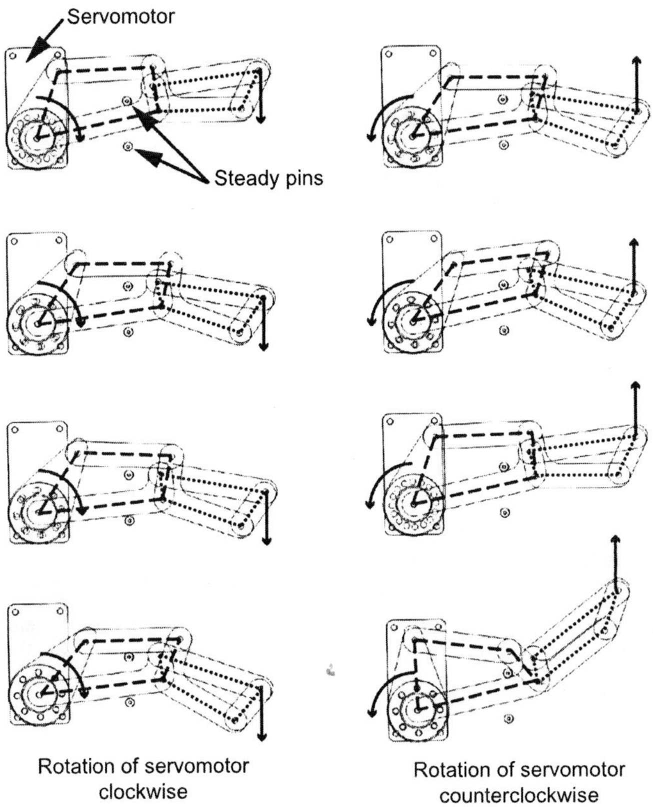

Figure 15.4 Example of the movements of link mechanism and leg.

Figure 15.4 shows the example of the movements of link mechanism and leg. In the case of clockwise rotation of servomotor, leg will move backward. On the other hand, in the case of counterclockwise rotation of servomotor, leg will move forward. Therefore, changing the rotation of servomotor, foot step of the legs could be realized. As a result, constructed quadruped robot needs only four servomotors to locomote by using link mechanism.

15.4 Electrical components of the quadruped robot

The electrical components of quadruped robot consist of a control bode, P-HNN, and battery. P-HNN consists of cell body models and synaptic models. In this section, we will show the circuit diagrams of cell body models and synaptic models.

15.4.1 Cell body model

Figure 15.5 shows the circuit diagram of the cell body model. The cell body model consists of a voltage control-type negative resistance, an equivalent inductance, resistors R_1, R_2, and membrane capacitor C_M. The voltage control-type negative resistance

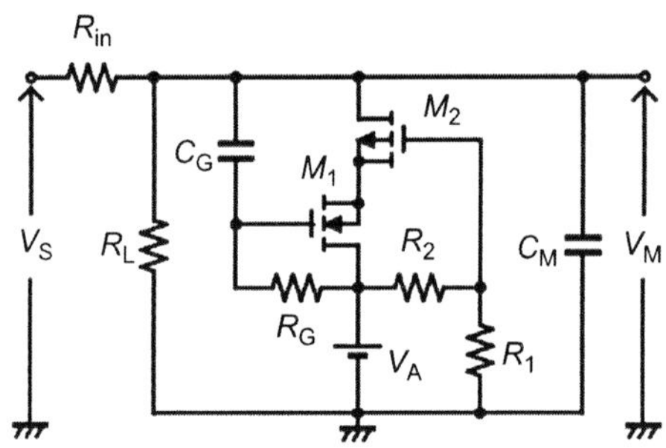

Figure 15.5 Circuit diagram of the cell body model.

circuit with equivalent inductance consists of n-channel MOSFET M_1, p-channel MOSFET M_2, voltage source v_A, leak resistor R_L, resistor R_G, and capacitor C_G. The cell body model has the negative resistance property which changes with time like a biological neuron and enables the generation of a continuous action potential v_M by a self-excited oscillation and a separately excited oscillation. Moreover, the cell body model can switch between both oscillations by changing v_A. The separately excited oscillation occurs by direct-current voltage stimulus or inputting the output voltage of synaptic model v_S.

15.4.2 Synaptic model

Figure 15.6 shows the circuit diagram of synaptic model. Figure 15.6a shows the excitatory synaptic model, and Figure 15.6b shows the inhibitory synaptic model. The synaptic model has the spatiotemporal summation characteristics similar to those of living organisms. Synaptic model outputs the output voltage v_S by spatiotemporal summate the output voltage of cell body model v_M. The spatial summation characteristics are realized by adder. Adder includes an inverting amplifier using an operational amplifier; the amplification factor of the inverting amplifier varies according to synaptic weight w,

$$w_E = R_{SE4}/R_{SE3} \tag{15.1}$$

$$w_I = R_{SI4}/R_{SI3} \tag{15.2}$$

where suffix E indicates excitatory and I indicates inhibitory synaptic models.

The temporal summation characteristics are realized by the operational amplifier RC integrator and the time constant t.

$$t_E = R_{SE1}C_{SE} \tag{15.3}$$

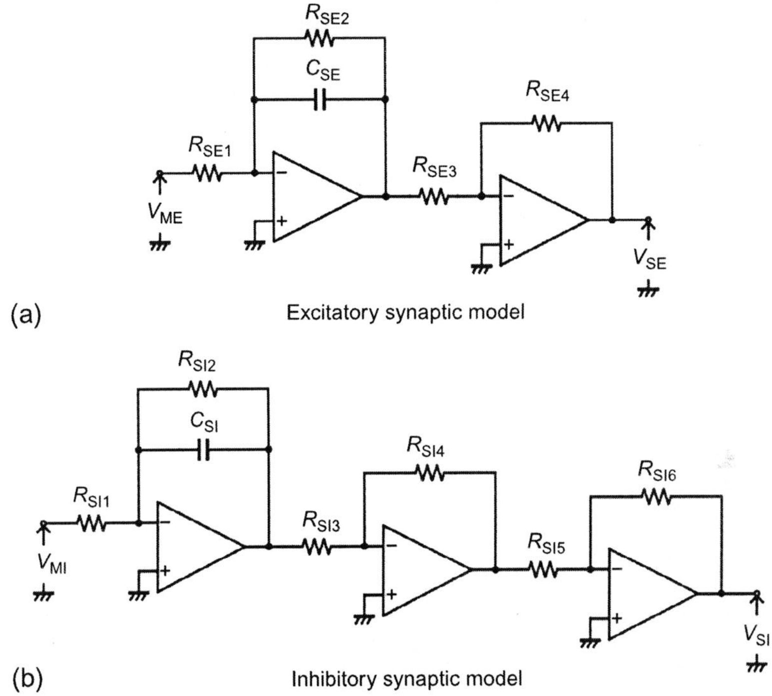

Figure 15.6 Circuit diagram of the synaptic model. (a) Excitatory synaptic model. (b) Inhibitory synaptic model.

$$t_I = R_{SI1}C_{SI} \tag{15.4}$$

The inhibitory synaptic model is obtained by reversing the output of the excitatory synaptic model. Figure 15.6 shows one input but in the P-HNN, we use multi-inputs including excitatory inputs and inhibitory inputs.

15.4.3 Excitatory inhibitory neuron pair model

In this section, excitatory inhibitory neuron pair model which consisted of two cell body models and two synaptic models was discussed. Excitatory inhibitory neuron pair model could output several oscillatory patterns using synchronization phenomena.

Figure 15.7 shows the circuit diagram of excitatory inhibitory neuron pair model. This figure shows that cell body models are coupled mutually by synaptic models. Excitatory synaptic model spatiotemporal summate the excitatory input (output voltage of cell body model v_{ME} and external input voltage v_{extinE}). Inhibitory synaptic model spatiotemporal summate the inhibitory input (output voltage of cell body model v_{MI} and external input voltage v_{extinI}). The circuit parameters of the two cell body model are same. (Please see Saito et al., 2011 for more details of synchronization phenomena and oscillatory patterns of mutual coupled excitatory inhibitory neuron pair model.)

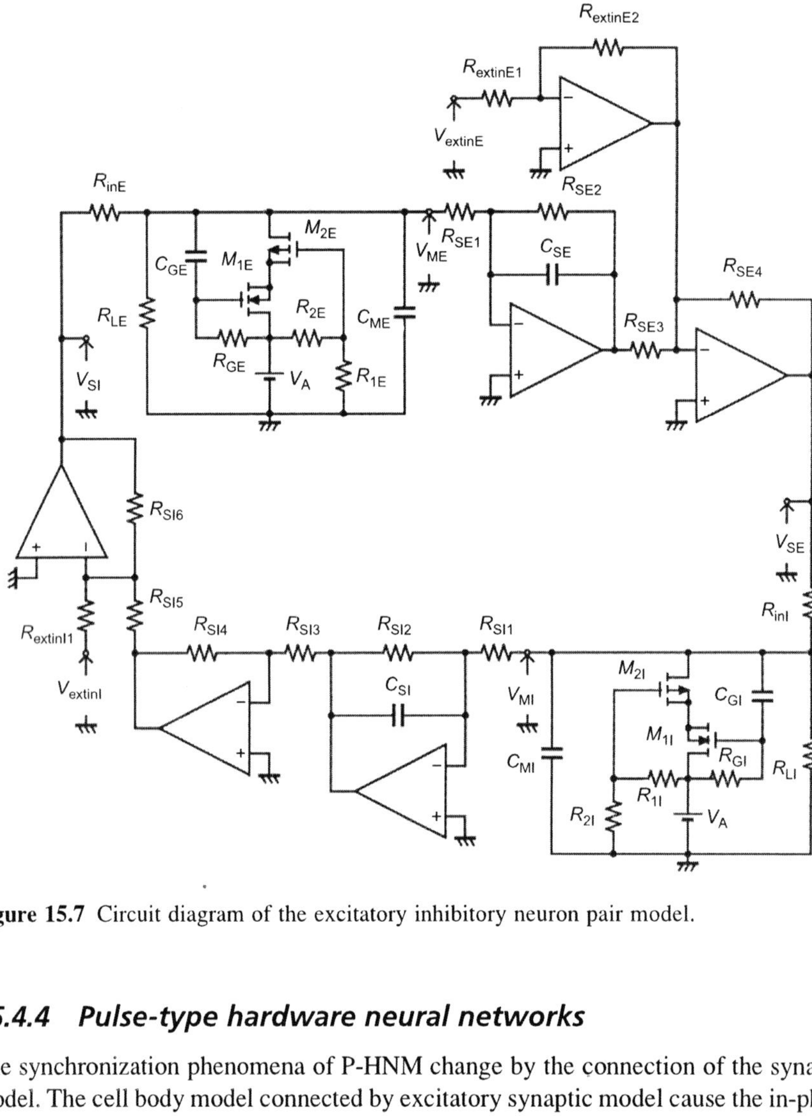

Figure 15.7 Circuit diagram of the excitatory inhibitory neuron pair model.

15.4.4 Pulse-type hardware neural networks

The synchronization phenomena of P-HNM change by the connection of the synaptic model. The cell body model connected by excitatory synaptic model cause the in-phase synchronization. The cell body model connected by inhibitory synaptic model causes the antiphase synchronization (for more detail, see Saito et al., 2011). In this chapter, we construct the P-HNN using excitatory inhibitory neuron pair models.

Figure 15.8 shows the connection diagram of the P-HNN. In Figure 15.8, big open circles indicate cell body model, small open circles indicate excitatory synaptic model, and small solid circles indicate inhibitory synaptic model. P-HNN consisted of four excitatory inhibitory neuron pair model coupled mutually by the 12 inhibitory synaptic models. Each excitatory inhibitory neuron pair model generates the locomotion rhythms of legs (left fore limb (LF), right fore limb (RF), the right hind limb (RH), and the left hind limb (LH)).

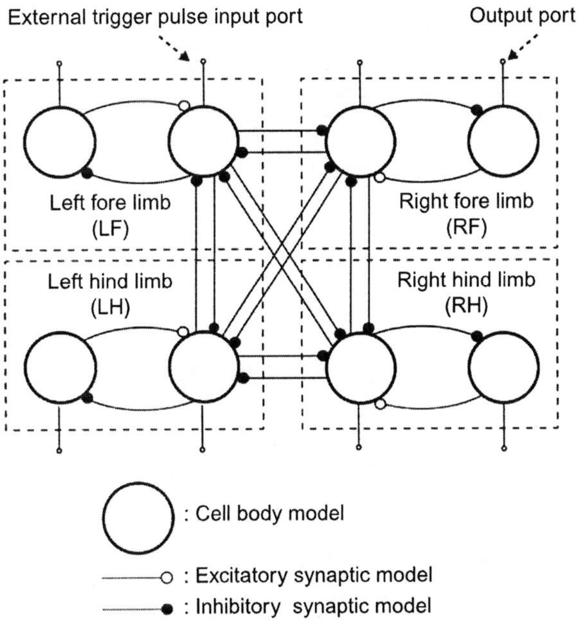

Figure 15.8 Connection diagram of the pulse-type hardware neural networks.

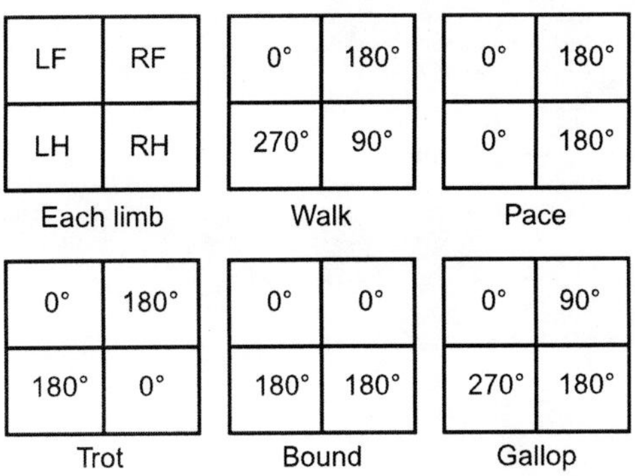

Figure 15.9 Relative phase difference of quadruped patterns with a typical example.

Figure 15.9 shows the relative phase difference of quadruped patterns with a typical example. In this figure, each limb indicates LF, RF, RH, and LH, respectively. In addition, the reference of relative phase difference is LF (0°). The quadruped locomotion patterns are regarded as different modes of coordination of the limb. Therefore, it is considered that quadruped locomotion pattern transitions arise from changing cooperation of the P-HNN that controls the inter-limb coordination.

Figure 15.10 shows the constructed P-HNN. P-HNN was mounted with the peripheral circuit to the flame retardant type 4 circuit board. Example of the generated locomotion rhythm using P-HNM was shown in Figure 15.11. The locomotion rhythm shown in Figure 15.11 is the basic locomotion rhythm of the quadruped robot.

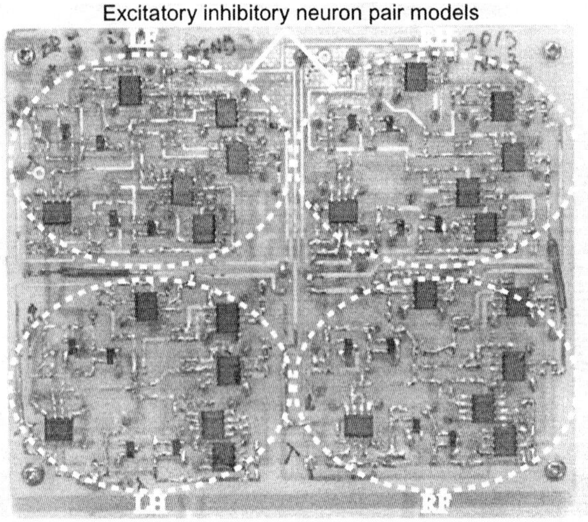

Figure 15.10 Constructed pulse-type hardware neural networks.

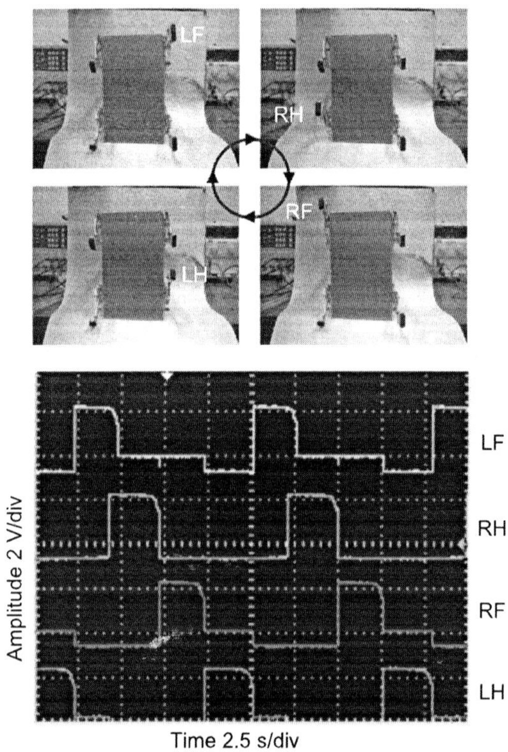

Figure 15.11 Example of the generated locomotion rhythm (walk).

As a result, constructed P-HNN could output various oscillatory patterns without using any computer programs.

15.5 Results

Using the constructed P-HNN, we generated the locomotion rhythms for quadruped robot.

Figure 15.12 shows the example of the locomotion of the quadruped robot. The locomotion rhythm generated by P-HNN was walk. This figure shows that constructed quadruped robot could locomote such as quadruped animal. As a result, quadruped robot could locomote by using the generated locomotion rhythms by using P-HNN.

Constructed P-HNN can change the locomotion rhythms by inputting the external trigger pulse. Figure 15.13 shows the example of changing the quadruped patterns of the quadruped robot. The external trigger pulse inputted to the external trigger pulse input port shown in Figure 15.8 by using waveform generator. P-HNN could memorize the inputted locomotion rhythm such as short memory. As a result, quadruped robot could switch the locomotion by inputting the external input to the P-HNN.

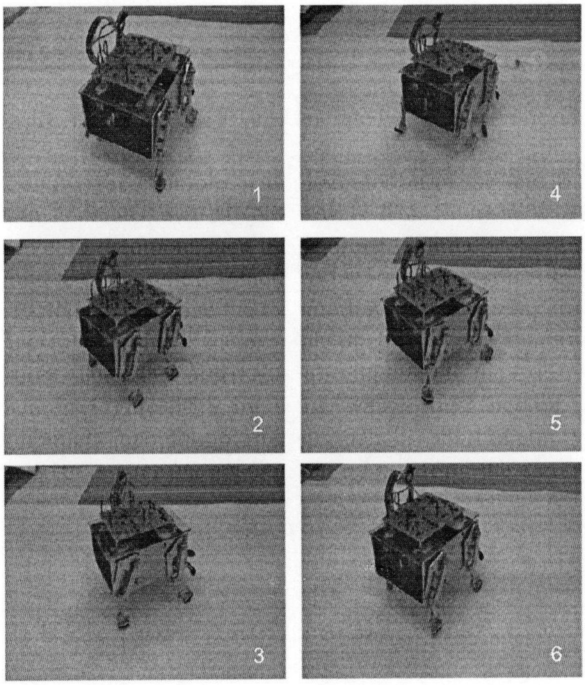

Figure 15.12 Example of the locomotion of the quadruped robot (walk).

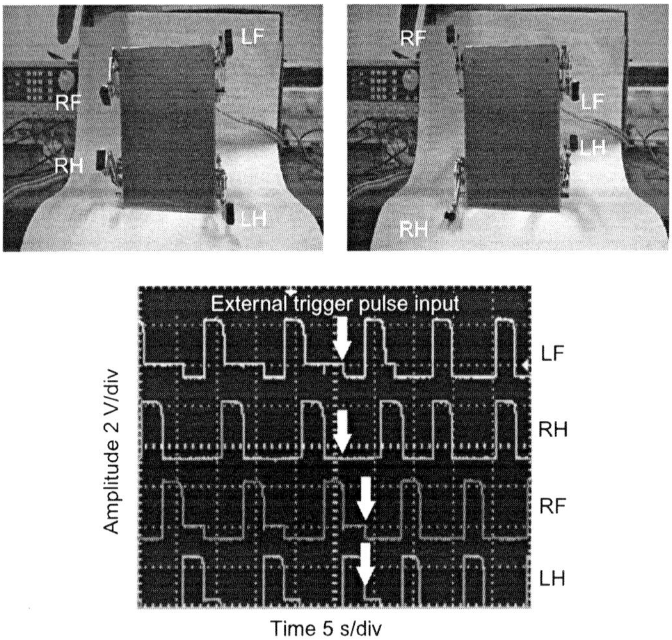

Figure 15.13 Example of changing the quadruped patterns (form walk to trot).

15.6 Conclusions

In this chapter, we have discussed about P-HNN which can generate the locomotion rhythms of quadruped robot. As a result, we developed the following conclusions.

1. Constructed quadruped robot needs only four servomotors to locomote by using link mechanism.
2. Constructed P-HNN could output various oscillatory patterns without using any computer programs.
3. Quadruped robot could locomote by using the generated locomotion rhythms by using P-HNN.
4. Quadruped robot could switch the locomotion by inputting the external input to the P-HNN.

In the future, we will construct the P-HNN by integrated circuit.

Acknowledgment

This study was supported by Nihon University College of Science and Technology Project Research, Nihon University Academic Research Grant (Total research, "14-002"). We appreciate the support.

References

Delcomyn, F., 1980. Neural basis of rhythmic behavior in animals. Science 210, 492–498.

Endo, T., Mori, S., 1978. Mode analysis of a ring of a large number of mutually coupled van der Pol oscillators. IEEE Trans. Circuits Syst. 25 (1), 7–18.

Fujita, M., Kitano, H., 1998. Development of an autonomous quadruped robot for robot entertainment. In: Autonomous Robots, vol. 5, Kluwer Academic Publishers, Boston, pp. 7–18.

Fukuoka, Y., Kimura, H., Cohen, A.H., 2003. Adaptive dynamic walking of a quadruped robot on irregular terrain based on biological concepts. Int. J. Robot. Res. 22 (3–4), 187–202.

Habib, M.K., 2011. Biomimetics: innovations and robotics. Int. J. Mechatron. Manuf. Syst. 4 (2), 113–134.

Habib, M.K., Watanabe, K., Izumi, K., 2007. Biomimetics robots: from bio-inspiration to implementation. In: Proceedings of the 33rd Annual Conference of the IEEE Industrial Electronics Society, pp. 143–148.

Hodgkin, A.L., Huxley, A.F., 1952. A quantitative description of membrane current and its application to conduction and excitation in nerve. J. Physiol. 117 (4), 500–544.

Kimura, H., Fukuoka, Y., Konaga, K., 2001. Adaptive dynamic walking of a quadruped robot using a neural system model. In: Advanced Robotics. Taylor & Francis, London, pp. 859–878.

Kitajima, H., Yoshinaga, T., Aihara, K., Kawakami, H., 2001. Burst firing and bifurcation in chaotic neural networks with ring structure. Int. J. Bifurcation Chaos 11 (6), 1631–1643.

Matsuoka, J., Sekine, Y., Saeki, K., Aihara, K., 2002. Analog hardware implementation of a mathematical model of an asynchronous chaotic neuron. IEICE Trans. Fundam. E85-A (2), 216–221.

Mcghh, R.B., Iswandhi, G.I., 1979. Adaptive locomotion of a multilegged robot over rough terrain. IEEE Trans. Syst. Man Cybern. 9 (2), 176–182.

Michael, A.A., 2002. The Handbook of Brain Theory and Neural Networks, second ed. MIT Press, Cambridge.

Nakabora, Y., Saeki, K., Sekine, Y., 2004. Synchronization of coupled oscillators using pulse-type hardware neuron models with mutual coupling. In: Proceedings of the 2004 International Technical Conference on Circuits/Systems, Computers and Communications, pp. 8D2L-3-1–8D2L-3-4.

Raibert, M., Blankespoor, K., Nelson, G., Playter, R., The BigDog Team, 2008. BigDog, the rough-terrain quadruped robot. In: Proceedings of the 17th World Congress the International Federation of Automatic Control, pp. 10822–10825.

Saito, K., Matsuda, A., Saeki, K., Uchikoba, F., Sekine, Y., 2011. Synchronization of coupled pulse-type hardware neuron models for CPG model. In: The Relevance of the Time Domain to Neural Network Models.Springer Series on Cognitive and Neural Systems, pp. 117–133.

Saito, K., Takato, M., Sekine, Y., Uchikoba, F., 2012. Biomimetics micro robot with active hardware neural networks locomotion control and insect-like switching behaviour. Int. J. Adv. Robot. Syst. 9 (226), 1–6.

Tsuji, S., Ueta, T., Kawakami, H., Aihara, K., 2007. Bifurcation analysis of current coupled BVP oscillators. Int. J. Bifurcation Chaos 17 (3), 837–850.

Tsumoto, K., Yoshinaga, T., Aihara, K., Kawakami, H., 2003. Bifurcations in synaptically coupled Hodgkin–Huxley neurons with a periodic input. Int. J. Bifurcation Chaos 13 (3), 653–666.

Tsumoto, K., Yoshinaga, T., Iida, H., Kawakami, H., Aihara, K., 2006. Bifurcations in a mathematical model for circadian oscillations of clock genes. J. Theor. Biol. 239 (1), 101–122.

van der Pol, B., 1927. On relaxation-oscillations. Lond. Edinb. Dubl. Philos. Mag. J. Sci. 2 (7), 978–992.
Yamauchi, M., Wada, M., Nishino, Y., Ushida, A., 1999. Wave propagation phenomena of phase states in oscillators coupled by inductors as a ladder. IEICE Trans. Fundam. E82-A (11), 2592–2598.
Yamauchi, M., Okuda, M., Nishino, Y., Ushida, A., 2003. Analysis of phase-inversion waves in coupled oscillators synchronizing at in-and-anti-phase. IEICE Trans. Fundam. E86-A (7), 1799–1806.

Biologically inspired antenna array design using Ormia modeling*,†,‡

16

M. Akcakaya, C. Muravchik, A. Nehorai

16.1 Introduction

For animals, source localization through directional hearing relies on the interaural acoustic cues: interaural time differences (ITDs), and interaural intensity differences (IIDs) of the incoming sound source (Popper and Fay, 2005). The ears of large animals are acoustically isolated from each other, i.e., the organs are located on opposite sides of the head or the body. For these animals, the distance between the hearing organs provides relatively large ITDs between the ipsilateral and contralateral ears (the ears closest to and furthest from the sound source, respectively). Moreover, a large body or head, with a size comparable to the incoming signal's wavelength (above one-tenth of the wavelength; Morse and Ingard, 1968), diffracts the incoming sound and increases the IIDs between received signals. Therefore, these big interaural differences can be detected by the hearing systems of large animals such as monkeys (Brown et al., 1978; Houben and Gourevitch, 1979), human beings (Masterton et al., 1969; Blauert, 1997), cats (Huang and May, 1996), horses (Heffner and Heffner, 1984), and pigs (Heffner and Heffner, 1989).

On the other hand, small animals may sense no diffractive effect in the incoming signal and hence have almost no IID between their two ears. Moreover, due to the closely spaced ears, the ITD drops below the level where it can be processed by the nervous systems of the animals. Therefore, many small animals develop a mechanism to improve these interaural differences (Michelsen, 1992). A pressure difference receiver is the most common mechanism employed by many animals in this category. In animals with pressure difference receivers, the ears are acoustically coupled to each other through internal air passages. Thus, the resulting force stimulating the eardrum is the difference between the internal and external acoustic pressures, and hence, the name

*The work of Dr. Arye Nehorai was funded by NSF grat CCF-0963742 and AFOSR Grant FA9550-11-1-0210.

†Based on Akcakaya and Nehorai (2010) and Akcakaya et al. (2011).

‡This chapter is based on the dissertation work completed by Dr. Murat Akcakaya when he was in Washington University in St. Louis.

pressure difference receiver (Popper and Fay, 2005). This structure amplifies the ITDs and IIDs and improves the directional hearing performances of many small animals (Fletcher and Thwaites, 1979; Michelsen et al., 1994; Palmer and Pinder, 1984; Eggermont, 1988; Narins et al., 1988; Knudsen, 1980).

We focus on the hearing system of a parasitoid fly *Ormia ochracea*. For reproduction, a female Ormia acoustically locates a male field cricket and deposits her larvae on or near the cricket (Cade, 1975). The localization occurs at night, relying on the cricket's mating call (Walker, 1986; Cade et al., 1996). The fly is very small and its ears are very closely separated, and physically connected to each other, resulting in ITDs as small as 4 ms (Robert et al., 1992, 1994). Moreover, there is a big incompatibility between the wavelength of the mating call (a relatively pure frequency peak around 5 KHz, with a resulting wavelength of 7 cm) and the size of the fly's hearing organ (around 1.5 mm), resulting in negligible IIDs (Morse and Ingard, 1968). It is theorized that these extremely small interaural differences cannot be processed by the nervous system of the Ormia. However, confounding the theory, the fly still locates the cricket very accurately, with as low as 2° of error in direction estimation (Mason et al., 2001; Akcakaya and Nehorai, 2008). Female Ormias have a mechanical structure (referred as intertympanal bridge) that connects their two ears, and it is this structure that amplifies the interaural differences to improve the localization accuracy (Miles et al., 1995; Robert et al., 1996, 1998). This mechanical coupling is unique to the female Ormia (Popper and Fay, 2005, Chapter 2); even the male Ormias do not have anything similar (Robert et al., 1994). From here on, by Ormia, we refer to the female *O. Ochracea*.

In this chapter, we propose to design biologically inspired small-sized compact antenna arrays to have high direction of arrival (DOA) estimation accuracy (Akcakaya et al., 2010, 2011a,b) and radiation performance (Akcakaya and Nehorai, 2010a,b). Our approach is inspired by the ears of the Ormia, which has a remarkable localization ability despite its small size (Mason et al., 2001; Akcakaya and Nehorai, 2008). In many civil and military applications, antenna arrays developed using the proposed approach would be valuable for sensing systems that are confined to small spaces demanding high resolution and DOA estimation accuracy from small-sized arrays (Bar-Shalom, 1987; Pavildis et al., 2001; Reddingt et al., 2005; Long, 2001; Brenner and Roessing, 2008; Nehorai and Paldi, 1994; Stoica and Sharman, 1990; Swindlehurst and Stoica, 1998).

16.2 Biologically inspired coupled antenna array for DOA estimation

Inspired by the Ormia's coupled ears, we develop a biologically inspired small-sized coupled passive antenna array with high DOA estimation performance. We realize the inspired coupling as a multi-input multi-output filter, which we call as biologically inspired coupling (BIC) filter, and accordingly employing this filter, we obtain the desired array response. In the following, by standard antenna array, we will refer to a system without the BIC. Note here that to simplify the analysis, we assume that we know the carrier frequency and the bandwidth of the incoming signal.

16.2.1 Antenna array model

We employ the following measurement model for a standard antenna array under the assumption of a narrow-band incoming signal (Stoica and Sharman, 1990). Then, the complex envelope of the measured signal is

$$\boldsymbol{x}(t) = \boldsymbol{A}(\boldsymbol{\phi})\boldsymbol{s}(t) + \boldsymbol{e}_{\mathrm{e}}(t), \qquad t = 1, \ldots, T \tag{16.1}$$

where

- $\boldsymbol{x}(t)$ is the $M \times 1$ output vector of the array with M antennas
- $\boldsymbol{s}(t) = [s_1(t), \ldots, s_Q(t)]$ is the $Q \times 1$ input signal vector with Q as the number of the sources
- $\boldsymbol{A}(\phi) = \left[\boldsymbol{a}(\phi_1), \ldots, \boldsymbol{a}\left(\phi_Q\right)\right]$ is the array response with ϕ_q as the DOA of the qth source
- $\boldsymbol{a}\left(\phi_q\right) = \left[1, \mathrm{e}^{-\left(\mathrm{j}\omega\Delta_q\right)}, \ldots, \mathrm{e}^{-\mathrm{j}\omega(M-1)\Delta_q}\right]$ for a uniform linear array (ULA)
- $\Delta_q = \frac{d \cos q(\phi_1)}{v}$ with d as the distance between each antenna, and v as the speed of signal propagation in the medium, and
- $\boldsymbol{e}_{\mathrm{e}}(t)$ is the additive environment noise.

Over the model described in Equation (16.1), we build the BIC as a filtering procedure and obtain the response of the proposed biologically inspired antenna array. As described below, we compute the BIC filter by converting the frequency response of the Ormia's ears to fit the desired radio frequencies.

16.2.2 Response of the Ormia's coupled ears

The coupled ears of the Ormia were modeled using a mechanical system composed of spring and dashpots as shown in Figure 16.1 (Miles et al., 1995). In this figure, the k_i's and c_i's, $i = 1,2,3$, are the spring and dashpot constants, respectively. In the proposed mechanical system, intertympanal bridge (the coupling structure between the two ears) is represented by two rigid bars connected at a pivot point through a coupling spring k_3 and a dashpot c_3. The system components at locations 1 and 2 are used to account for the dynamic properties of the tympanal membranes, bulbae acoustica (sensory organ), and surrounding structures (Miles et al., 1995). The governing differential equations for the mechanical system are written as

$$\begin{bmatrix} k_1 + k_3 & k_3 \\ k_3 & k_2 + k_3 \end{bmatrix} \begin{bmatrix} y_1 \\ y_2 \end{bmatrix} + \begin{bmatrix} c_1 + c_3 & c_3 \\ c_3 & c_2 + c_3 \end{bmatrix} \begin{bmatrix} \dot{y}_1 \\ \dot{y}_2 \end{bmatrix} + \begin{bmatrix} m_0 & 0 \\ 0 & m_0 \end{bmatrix} \begin{bmatrix} \ddot{y}_1 \\ \ddot{y}_2 \end{bmatrix} = \begin{bmatrix} x_1(t, \Delta) \\ x_2(t, \Delta) \end{bmatrix} \tag{16.2}$$

where

- $x_i(t, \Delta)$ and $i = 1, 2$ are the input signals
- $y_i(t)$ and $i = 1, 2$ are the displacements of each ear membrane, and
- m_0 is the effective mass assumed to be concentrated at the end of each rod.

Assuming zero initial values, we apply Laplace transform to Equation (16.2) and compute the transfer function

Figure 16.1 Mechanical model of the female *Ormia ochracea*'s ear (Miles et al., 1995).

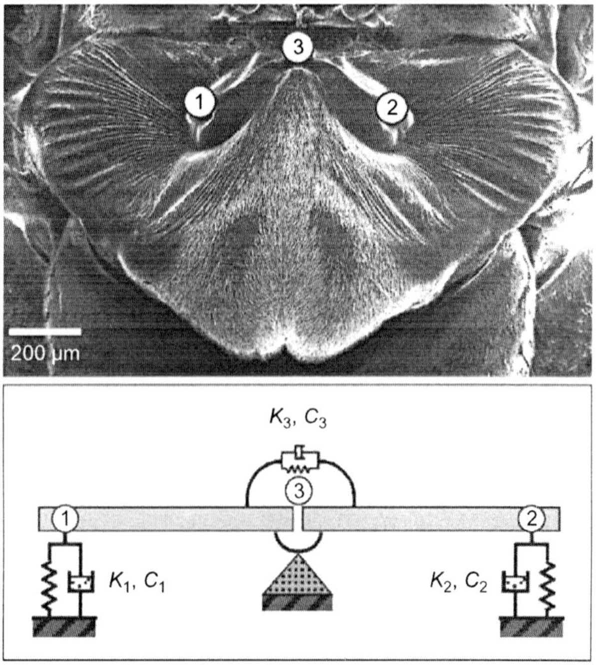

$$\begin{bmatrix} Y_1(s) \\ Y_2(s) \end{bmatrix} = 1/P(s)\begin{bmatrix} D_2(s) & -N(s) \\ -N(s) & D_1(s) \end{bmatrix}\begin{bmatrix} X_1(s) \\ X_2(s) \end{bmatrix} \tag{16.3}$$

where

- $Y_1(s)$ and $Y_2(s)$ and $X_1(s)$ and $X_2(s)$ are the Laplace transforms of $y_1(t)$ and $y_2(t)$ and $x_1(t)$ and $x_2(t)$, respectively
- $D_1(s) = m_0s^2 + (c_1 + c_3)s + k_1 + k_3$ and $D_2(s) = m_0s^2 + (c_2 + c_3)s + k_2 + k_3$ are the ear-specific responses in the presence of mechanical coupling
- $N(s) = c_3s + k_3$ is the coupling effect, and
- $P(s) = D_1(s)D_2(s) - N^2(s)$ is the characteristic function of the linear system.

Then, by substituting $x_1(t) = \delta(t) \leftrightarrow^{\mathrm{LT}} X_1(s)$ and $x_2(t) = x_1(t-\Delta) \leftrightarrow^{\mathrm{LT}} X_2(s) = \mathrm{e}^{-s\Delta}$, we compute the impulse responses of the Ormia's ears (here $\leftrightarrow^{\mathrm{LT}}$ is used to represent a Laplace transform pair)

$$\begin{aligned} H_1(s,\Delta) &= \left[D_2(s) - N(s)\mathrm{e}^{-s\Delta}\right]/P(s) \\ H_2(s,\Delta) &= \left[D_1(s)\mathrm{e}^{-s\Delta} - N(s)\right]/P(s) \end{aligned} \tag{16.4}$$

We present the amplitude and the phase responses of the Ormia's ears in Figures 16.2a and 16.3a, respectively. For comparison purposes, we also plot the amplitude and phase responses assuming zero coupling, $N(s) = 0$ in Figures 16.2b and 16.3b, respectively.

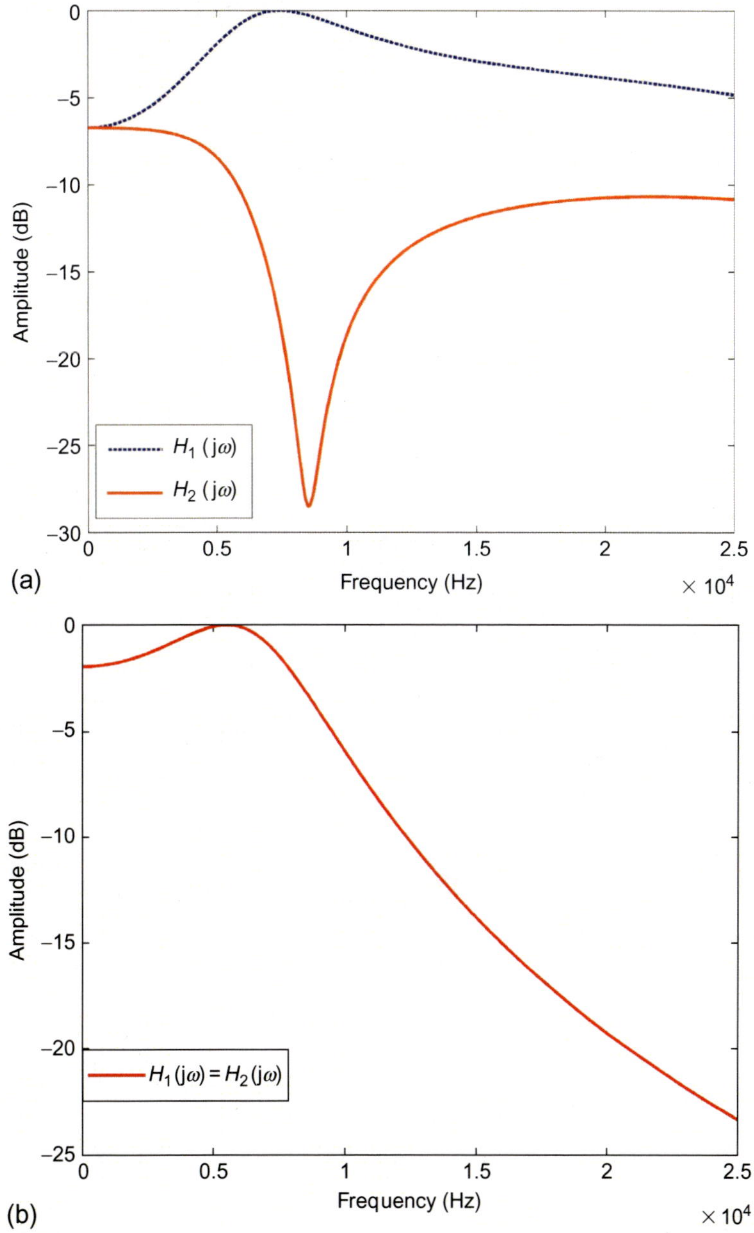

Figure 16.2 Amplitude responses of the *Ormia ochracea*'s two ears. (a) Coupled system. (b) Uncoupled system.

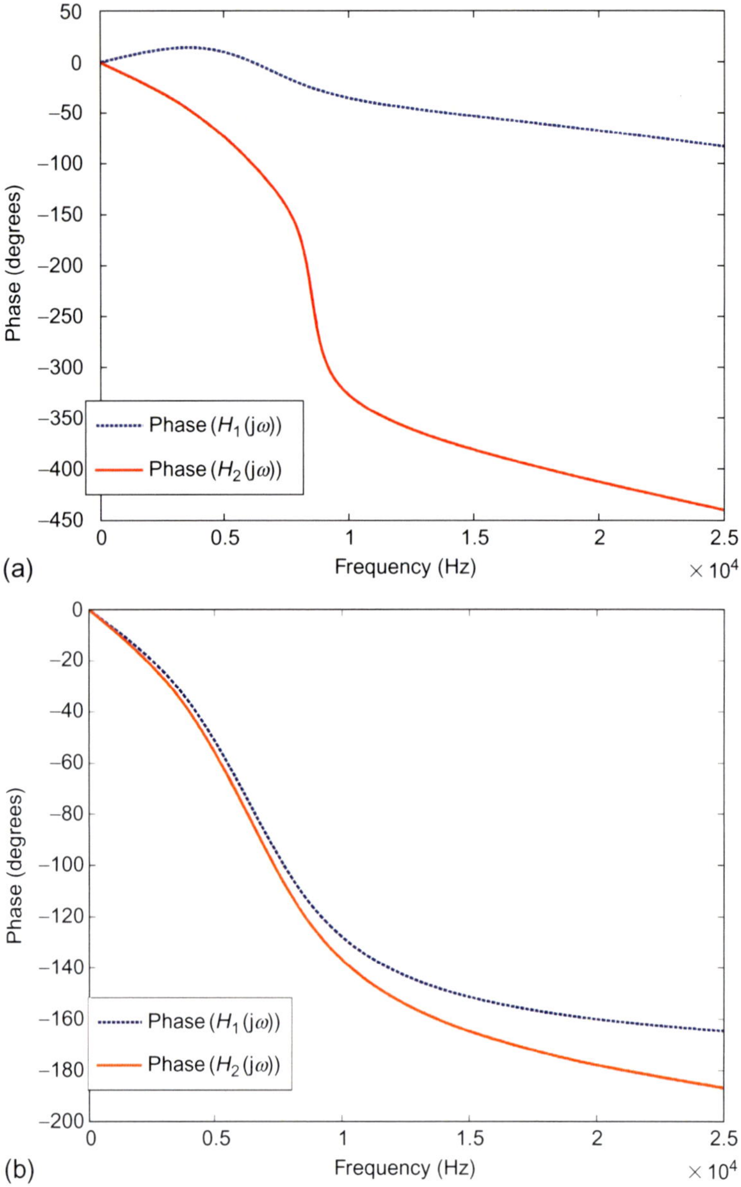

Figure 16.3 Phase responses of the *Ormia ochracea*'s two ears. (a) Coupled system. (b) Uncoupled system.

These responses are computed for 45° DOA using $s = j\omega = j2\pi f$ in Equation (16.4) and the effective mass, spring, and dashpot constants reported in Miles et al. (1995). Comparing the responses for coupled and uncoupled cases, we observe that the amplitude and the phase differences between the responses of the ears are amplified by the mechanical coupling. For further interpretation of the results, see Secti

16.2.3 Filter interpretation of the coupling

The mechanical coupling between the ears of the Ormia effectively creates larger distance between the ears resulting in a virtual array with a larger aperture (Akcakaya and Nehorai, 2008). Therefore, we observe amplification in the differences between the amplitude and the phase responses of different ears. Using Equation (16.4), we interpret, in Figure 16.4, the mechanical coupling as a two-input two-output filter that amplifies the differences between the responses of the Ormia's ears as shown in Figures 16.2 and 16.3. Inspired by this interpretation, we build a BIC filter first for two-antenna and then for multiple-antenna arrays. In the following, we show that BIC filter generates a virtual array with a larger aperture and hence improves the DOA estimation and radiation performance of an antenna array.

16.2.4 BIC array response design

We modify the two-input two-output system representing the Ormia's ears' responses illustrated in Figure 16.4 to fit the frequency response of the modified system into the range of desired radio frequencies. We achieve this conversion by reassigning the poles of the transfer function computed in Equation (16.3); that is, we choose the roots of the characteristic function $P(s) = D_1(s)D_2(s) - N^2(s)$ for frequencies of interest. Characteristic function has four complex roots with imaginary parts representing the resonance frequencies, f_1 and f_2 of the system. We change values of the mass, spring, and dashpot parameters as defined in the analogous mechanical system to shift these resonance frequencies to fit in the range of the frequencies that we desire the antenna array to operate. We keep the real parts of the roots as free variables, and later in Section 16.2.9, we illustrate how to use these variables to optimize the BIC filter.

For illustrative purposes, assuming a two-antenna array for a narrowband incoming signal with carrier frequency $f_c = 1$ GHz and bandwidth $B = 20$ MHz, we choose $f_1 = f_c - \frac{B}{2} = 0.99$ GHz and $f_2 = f_c + \frac{B}{2} = 1.01$ GHz as the desired resonance frequencies and show the resulting amplitude and phase responses of the modified two-input two-output system in Figure 16.5a and b. Recall that we substitute $s = j\omega = j2\pi f$ to calculate the amplitude and the phase responses. Similar to the system responses

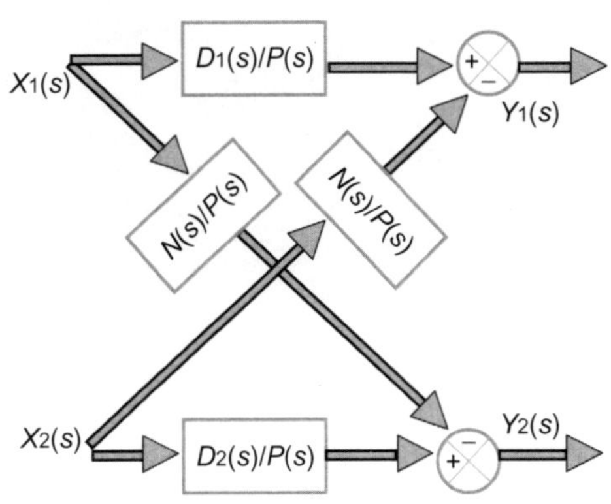

Figure 16.4 Two-input two-output filter representation of the Ormia's coupled ears' response.

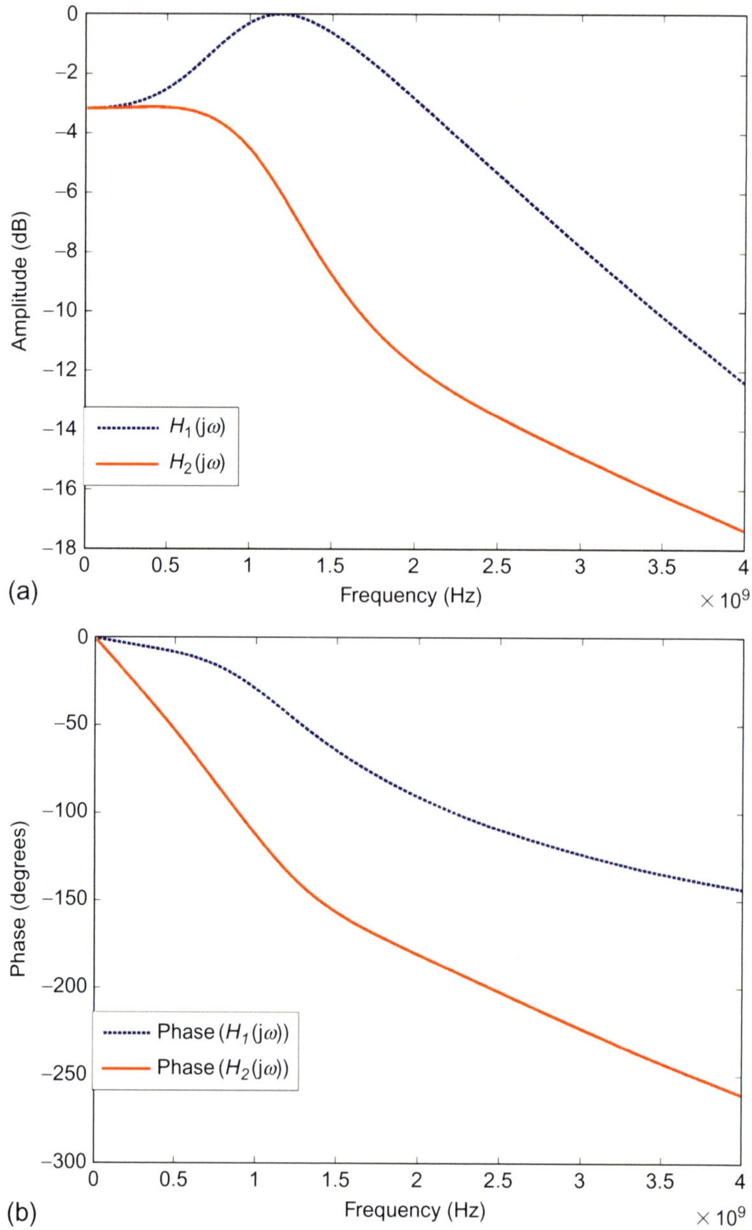

Figure 16.5 (a) Amplitude and (b) phase responses of the converted system.

presented in Figures 16.2 and 16.3, the designed system preserves a coupling structure to amplify the differences between the amplitude and phase responses of the system outputs.

16.2.5 Biologically inspired array processing

We illustrate the BIC antenna array design first for two-antenna arrays, and then we generalize the idea to multiple antennas. Assuming two identical antennas such that $D_1(\mathrm{j}\omega)=D_2(\mathrm{j}\omega)=D(\mathrm{j}\omega)$, and following the method proposed in Section 16.2.4, we design the BIC filter as

$$\boldsymbol{H}_\mathrm{I}(\mathrm{j}\omega)=\begin{bmatrix} D(\mathrm{j}\omega) & N(\mathrm{j}\omega) \\ N(\mathrm{j}\omega) & D(\mathrm{j}\omega) \end{bmatrix}^{-1} \tag{16.5}$$

Note here that we substitute $s=\mathrm{j}\omega=\mathrm{j}2\pi f$ to compute the frequency response of the filter from its system response. Then, applying this filter to the output of Equation (16.1) in the frequency domain, we obtain

$$\begin{bmatrix} Y_1(\mathrm{j}\omega) \\ Y_2(\mathrm{j}\omega) \end{bmatrix}=\boldsymbol{H}_I(\mathrm{j}\omega)\begin{bmatrix} X_1(\mathrm{j}\omega) \\ X_2(\mathrm{j}\omega) \end{bmatrix} \tag{16.6}$$

We assume that the incoming bandlimited signal is narrowband such that interelement spacing is much smaller than the reciprocal of the signal bandwidth (Dogandzic and Nehorai, 2001). We further assume that the incoming signal can be approximated as a summation of components which are almost pure in frequency such that $\boldsymbol{s}(t)=\sum_{n=1}^{N_\mathrm{F}} \boldsymbol{s}^n(t)$, where N_F is the number of such components. Note that the multiplication in Equation (16.6) corresponds to convolution in time domain. Due to the narrowband assumption, convolution of the BIC filter with each component of $\boldsymbol{s}(t)$ results in multiplication of the time domain incoming signal with the BIC filter computed at the corresponding frequencies of the components (Oppenheim et al., 1999; Ottersten et al., 1993; Krim and Viberg, 1996). Then under the abovementioned assumptions, we approximate the output of the BIC filter Equation (16.6) to the nth component as

$$\boldsymbol{y}^n(t)=\begin{bmatrix} y_1(t) \\ y_2(t) \end{bmatrix}^n=\boldsymbol{H}_I(\mathrm{j}\omega_n)\boldsymbol{A}^n(\phi)\boldsymbol{s}^n(t)+\tilde{\mathrm{e}}^n(t), \quad t=1,\ \ldots,T \tag{16.7}$$

where $\tilde{\boldsymbol{e}}^n(t)=\boldsymbol{e}^n_\mathrm{a}(t)+\boldsymbol{H}_I(\mathrm{j}\omega_n)\boldsymbol{e}^n_\mathrm{e}(t)$ such that only the environment noise is affected by the BIC filter. Here, $\boldsymbol{e}^n_\mathrm{a}(t)$ and $\boldsymbol{e}^n_\mathrm{e}(t)$ are the amplifier and environment noise components, respectively, and ω_f is the frequency of the component $\boldsymbol{s}^n(t)$. We collect the responses corresponding to all the components of $\boldsymbol{s}(t)$ as

$$\boldsymbol{y}(t)=\begin{bmatrix} \boldsymbol{y}^1 \\ \cdots \\ \boldsymbol{y}^{N_F} \end{bmatrix}=\boldsymbol{H}_I\boldsymbol{A}(\phi)\bar{\boldsymbol{s}}(t)+\tilde{\boldsymbol{e}}(t) \tag{16.8}$$

where

- $\boldsymbol{H}_{\mathrm{I}} = \mathrm{blkdiag}\,(\boldsymbol{H}_{\mathrm{I}}(\mathrm{j}\omega_1), \ldots, \boldsymbol{H}_{\mathrm{I}}(\mathrm{j}\omega_{N_{\mathrm{F}}}))$ is $2N_{\mathrm{F}} \times 2N_{\mathrm{F}}$ block diagonal matrix with $\boldsymbol{H}_{\mathrm{I}}(\mathrm{j}\omega_n)$ as the nth block diagonal entry.
- $\boldsymbol{A}(\boldsymbol{\phi}) = \mathrm{blkdiag}\left(\boldsymbol{A}^1(\boldsymbol{\phi}), \ldots, \boldsymbol{A}^{N_{\mathrm{F}}}(\boldsymbol{\phi})\right)$
- $\bar{\boldsymbol{s}}(t) = \left[(\boldsymbol{s}^1(t))^{\mathrm{T}}, \ldots, (\boldsymbol{s}^{N_{\mathrm{F}}}(t))^{\mathrm{T}}\right]$, and
- $\widetilde{\boldsymbol{e}}(t) = \left[(\widetilde{\boldsymbol{e}}^1(t))^{\mathrm{T}}, \ldots, (\widetilde{\boldsymbol{e}}^{N_{\mathrm{F}}}(t))^{\mathrm{T}}\right]$.

We next extend the model in Equation (16.8) to M identical antennas. We assume that each antenna is coupled to its immediate neighboring antennas in the array, i.e., each antenna (except for the first and the last antennas) is coupled to two antennas. Other array structures may also be possible; however, we focus on the linear arrays which are the most commonly used structures in antenna array processing. Consequently, for a linear antenna array with M identical antennas, we extend $\boldsymbol{H}_{\mathrm{I}}(\mathrm{j}\omega)$ defined in Equation (16.6) to an $M \times M$ tridiagonal form as

$$\boldsymbol{H}_{\mathrm{I}}(\mathrm{j}\omega)^{-1} = \begin{bmatrix} D(\mathrm{j}\omega) & N(\mathrm{j}\omega) & 0 & \ldots\ldots & 0 & \\ N(\mathrm{j}\omega) & D(\mathrm{j}\omega) & N(\mathrm{j}\omega) & 0 & \ldots & 0 \\ \ldots\ldots & \ldots\ldots & \ldots\ldots & \ldots\ldots & \ldots\ldots & \ldots\ldots \\ 0 & \ldots\ldots & & 0 & N(\mathrm{j}\omega) & D(\mathrm{j}\omega) \end{bmatrix} \tag{16.9}$$

16.2.6 Statistical assumptions

We assume in Equation (16.1) that

- $\boldsymbol{\phi} = \left[\phi_1, \ldots, \phi_Q\right]^T$ is the $Q \times 1$ vector f deterministic unknown DOA parameter
- $\bar{\boldsymbol{s}}(t)$ is a Gaussian input signal vector, $E[\bar{\boldsymbol{s}}(t)] = 0$, $E\left[\bar{\boldsymbol{s}}(t)\boldsymbol{s}(t')^{\mathrm{H}}\right] = \boldsymbol{P}\delta_{tt'}$, and $E\left[\bar{\boldsymbol{s}}(t)\boldsymbol{s}(t')^{\mathrm{H}}\right] = \boldsymbol{0}$ with $\boldsymbol{P}$ as the $QN_{\mathrm{F}} \times QN_{\mathrm{F}}$ unknown source covariance matrix, and for $t, t' = 1, \ldots, T$, $\delta_{tt'} = 1$ when $t = t'$ and zero otherwise
- $\widetilde{\boldsymbol{e}}(t)$ is Gaussian distributed and $E[\widetilde{\boldsymbol{e}}(t)] = 0$, $E\left[\widetilde{\boldsymbol{e}}(t)\widetilde{\boldsymbol{e}}(t')^{\mathrm{H}}\right] = (\sigma_{\mathrm{a}}^2\boldsymbol{I} + \sigma_{\mathrm{e}}^2\boldsymbol{H}_{\mathrm{I}}\boldsymbol{H}_{\mathrm{I}}^{\mathrm{H}})\delta_{tt'}$, and $E\left[\widetilde{\boldsymbol{e}}(t)\widetilde{\boldsymbol{e}}(t')^{\mathrm{T}}\right] = 0$ such that σ_{a}^2 and σ_{e}^2 are the unknown variances of amplifier and environment noise, respectively, and
- $\bar{\boldsymbol{s}}(t)$ and $\widetilde{\boldsymbol{e}}(t')$ are uncorrelated for all t and t'.

16.2.7 Maximum likelihood estimation

The maximum likelihood estimate (MLE) of the DOA is defined as the value that maximizes the likelihood function (see Equation (16.11)). It is asymptotically unbiased and it attains the Cramér–Rao bound (CRB) of minimum variance (Kay, 1993). In the following, we demonstrate the derivation of the MLE of DOA, and in Section 16.2.8, we compute the CRB on DOA estimation. First, following the statistical assumptions in Section 16.2.6, we write the probability density function of the measurements $\boldsymbol{y}(t)$ as

$$\prod_{t=1}^{T} p\left[y(t);\boldsymbol{\phi},\boldsymbol{P},\sigma_a^2,\sigma_e^2\right]=\prod_{t=1}^{T}\frac{1}{|\pi\boldsymbol{R}|}\exp\left[y(t)^{\mathrm{H}}\boldsymbol{R}^{-1}y(t)\right] \tag{16.10}$$

where $\boldsymbol{R}=E\left[y(t)y(t)^{\mathrm{H}}\right]=\widetilde{\boldsymbol{A}}(\boldsymbol{\phi})\boldsymbol{P}\widetilde{\boldsymbol{A}}(\boldsymbol{\phi})^{\mathrm{H}}+\sigma_e^2\boldsymbol{\Sigma}(\rho)$ with $\boldsymbol{\Sigma}(\rho)=\rho\boldsymbol{I}+\boldsymbol{H}_{\mathrm{I}}\boldsymbol{H}_{\mathrm{I}}^{\mathrm{H}}$, $\rho=\sigma_a^2/\sigma_e^2$, and $\widetilde{\boldsymbol{A}}(\boldsymbol{\phi})=\boldsymbol{H}_I\boldsymbol{A}(\boldsymbol{\phi})$. To whiten the noise, we compute $\boldsymbol{\Sigma}(\rho)^{-1/2}$ and define $\bar{y}(t)=\boldsymbol{\Sigma}(\rho)^{-\frac{1}{2}}y(t)$ and $\bar{\boldsymbol{A}}(\boldsymbol{\theta})=\boldsymbol{\Sigma}(\rho)^{-1/2}\widetilde{\boldsymbol{A}}(\boldsymbol{\phi})$, where $\boldsymbol{\theta}=[\rho,\boldsymbol{\phi}]^T$ is $(Q+1)\times 1$ vector of unknown parameters including the DOA, $\boldsymbol{\phi}$. Accordingly, the joint distribution of $\bar{y}(t)$ for $t=1,\ldots,T$ is

$$\prod_{t=1}^{T} p\left[\bar{y}(t);\phi,\rho,\boldsymbol{P},\sigma_e^2\right]=\prod_{t=1}^{T}\frac{1}{\left|\pi\widetilde{\boldsymbol{R}}\right|}\exp\left[\bar{y}(t)^{H}\widetilde{\boldsymbol{R}}^{-1}\bar{y}(t)\right] \tag{16.11}$$

where $\widetilde{\boldsymbol{R}}=E\left[\bar{y}(t)y(t)^{\mathrm{H}}\right]=\bar{\boldsymbol{A}}(\boldsymbol{\theta})\boldsymbol{P}\bar{\boldsymbol{A}}(\boldsymbol{\theta})^{\mathrm{H}}+\sigma_e^2\boldsymbol{I}$. We, then, follow the procedure explained in Stoica and Nehorai, (1995), first using Equation (16.11), we derive the MLEs of $\boldsymbol{P}$ and $\boldsymbol{\sigma}_e^2$ as a function of the unknown parameter vector $\boldsymbol{\theta}$, denoted by $\hat{\boldsymbol{P}}(\boldsymbol{\theta})$ and $\hat{\sigma}_e^2(\boldsymbol{\theta})$, respectively. We then concentrate the likelihood in Equation (16.11) using these MLEs, and accordingly find the MLE of $\boldsymbol{\theta}$ by solving the following optimization problem

$$\hat{\boldsymbol{\theta}}=\mathrm{argmin}_{\theta}\ \ln\left|\bar{\boldsymbol{A}}(\boldsymbol{\theta})\hat{\boldsymbol{P}}(\boldsymbol{\theta})\bar{\boldsymbol{A}}(\boldsymbol{\theta})^{\mathrm{H}}+\hat{\sigma}_e^2(\boldsymbol{\theta})\boldsymbol{I}\right| \tag{16.12}$$

where

- $\hat{\boldsymbol{P}}(\boldsymbol{\theta})=\bar{\boldsymbol{A}}(\boldsymbol{\theta})^{\dagger}\hat{\boldsymbol{R}}\left(\bar{\boldsymbol{A}}(\boldsymbol{\theta})^{\dagger}\right)^{\mathrm{H}}-\hat{\sigma}_e^2(\boldsymbol{\theta})\left(\bar{\boldsymbol{A}}(\boldsymbol{\theta})\bar{\boldsymbol{A}}(\boldsymbol{\theta})^{\mathrm{H}}\right)^{-1}$ is the MLE of $\boldsymbol{P}$ as a function of $\boldsymbol{\theta}$
- $\hat{\sigma}_e^2(\boldsymbol{\theta})=\frac{\mathrm{tr}\left(\boldsymbol{\Pi}^{\perp}\hat{\boldsymbol{R}}\right)}{M-Q}$ is the MLE of σ_e^2 as a function of $\boldsymbol{\theta}$
- $\hat{\boldsymbol{R}}=\sum_{t=1}^{T}y(t)y(t)^{\mathrm{H}}$ is the sample covariance
- $\bar{\boldsymbol{A}}(\boldsymbol{\theta})^{\dagger}=\left[\bar{\boldsymbol{A}}(\boldsymbol{\theta})^{H}\bar{\boldsymbol{A}}(\boldsymbol{\theta})\right]^{-1}\bar{\boldsymbol{A}}(\boldsymbol{\theta})^{\mathrm{H}}$
- $\boldsymbol{\Pi}^{\perp}=\boldsymbol{I}-\bar{\boldsymbol{A}}(\boldsymbol{\theta})\bar{\boldsymbol{A}}(\boldsymbol{\theta})^{\dagger}$.

16.2.8 Performance analysis

We analyze the array's statistical performance, i.e., accuracy in estimating the source direction, by computing the CRB. The CRB is the lower bound on estimation error for any unbiased estimator. We concentrate the likelihood function in Equation (16.11) with respect to $\boldsymbol{P}$ and σ_e^2 and compute the CRB on the covariance matrix of any unbiased estimator of $\boldsymbol{\theta}$. Using the results in Stoica and Nehorai (1990) and Nehorai and Paldi (1994),

$$\mathrm{CRB}(\boldsymbol{\theta})=\frac{\sigma_e^2}{2T}\left\{\mathrm{Re}\left(\mathrm{btr}\left[(1\otimes\boldsymbol{U})\,\square\,\left(\boldsymbol{D}^{H}\boldsymbol{\Pi}^{\perp}\boldsymbol{D}\right)^{\mathrm{bT}}\right]\right)\right\}^{-1} \tag{16.13}$$

where

- $\mathbf{1}$ is a $Q+1 \times Q+1$ matrix of ones
- $\boldsymbol{U}=\boldsymbol{P}\left[\bar{\boldsymbol{A}}(\boldsymbol{\theta})^H\bar{\boldsymbol{A}}(\boldsymbol{\theta})\boldsymbol{P}+\sigma_e^2\boldsymbol{I}\right]^{-1}\bar{\boldsymbol{A}}(\boldsymbol{\theta})^H\bar{\boldsymbol{A}}(\boldsymbol{\theta})\boldsymbol{P}$
- $\boldsymbol{D}=\left[\boldsymbol{D}_1\ldots\boldsymbol{D}_{Q+1}\right]$ with $\boldsymbol{D}_i=\frac{\partial\bar{\boldsymbol{A}}(\boldsymbol{\theta})}{\partial\theta_i}$
- btr and bT are block trace and transpose operators, respectively
- $\otimes$ is the Kronecker product, and
- $\boxdot$ is the block Schur–Hadamard product.

Note: see Appendix A for the definition of the block matrix operators.

16.2.9 Optimization of the BIC

In this section, we develop a method to maximize the localization performance of the antenna array by optimizing the CRB on DOA estimation with respect to the BIC parameters. We first introduce the optimization parameters and then formulate a cost function employing the CRB on DOA estimation for optimum performance. Note here that we optimize the value of the BIC for the antenna array structures (linear) and coupling configurations (coupling with adjacent antennas) as discussed in Section 16.2.5. Other array structures and different coupling configurations are also possible.

As explained in Section 16.2.4, to fit the frequency response of the modified BIC system into the range of desired radio frequencies, we change the imaginary parts of the poles of the characteristic function to shift the resonance frequencies of the system response while we keep the real parts as free variables. Therefore, under the constraints that we explain below, we have the freedom of choosing the real parts for optimum coupling design. As defined in (16.2) and as described in Section 16.2.4, we compute the poles of the system as functions of system parameters (k, c and m_0). As stated in Section 16.2.5, we assume identical antennas ($D_1(s)=D_2(s)=D(s)$ and hence $k_1=k_2=k$, $c_1=c_2=c$) and write the characteristic function $P(s)$ as

$$P(s)=D(s)^2-N(s)^2=m_0^2\left[\left(s^2+b_1s+a_1\right)-\left(b_2s+a_2\right)^2\right] \tag{16.14}$$

where $a_1=\frac{(k+k_3)}{m_0}$, $a_2=\frac{k_3}{m_0}$, $b_1=\frac{(c+c_3)}{m_0}$, and $b_2=\frac{c_3}{m_0}$ with the assumption that a_1, a_2, b_1, and b_2 are all positive. Then accordingly, we compute the poles of the characteristic function $P(s)$ as

$$\begin{aligned} p_{1,2} &= -r_1 \pm \sqrt{i_1} \\ p_{3,4} &= -r_2 \pm \sqrt{i_2} \end{aligned} \tag{16.15}$$

where $r_1=\frac{1}{2}(b_1+b_2)$, $r_2=\frac{1}{2}(b_1-b_2)$, $i_1=\frac{1}{4}\left[(b_1+b_2)^2-4(a_1+a_2)\right]$, and $i_2=\frac{1}{4}\left[(b_1-b_2)^2-4(a_1-a_2)\right]$. As explained in Section 16.2.4, to fit the frequency response of the modified BIC system into the range of desired radio frequencies, we change the imaginary parts. Note here that the real parameters, r_1 and r_2 are free parameters and we have the freedom to control them as long as due to the positivity assumption on a_1, a_2, b_1, and b_2. From Equations (16.9), (16.11), and (16.13)–(16.15), we observe that CRB is also a function of the real parts of the poles of the characteristics function. Accordingly, we propose to choose r_1 and r_2 by minimizing the CRB on DOA estimation. This is a reasonable choice since minimizing the CRB minimizes the lower bound on the error of the MLE of DOA. Defining $\boldsymbol{r} = [r_1, r_2]^{\mathrm{T}}$, we design the optimum BIC by solving the following constrained optimization problem

$$\operatorname{argmin}_{\boldsymbol{r}} \operatorname{tr}[\mathrm{CRB}(\boldsymbol{\theta}, \boldsymbol{r})] \quad \text{s.t.} \quad r_1 - r_2 > 0 \tag{16.16}$$

where by taking the trace of the $\mathrm{CRB}(\boldsymbol{\theta}, \boldsymbol{r})$, we minimize the sum of the variance of the errors on the DOA, $\boldsymbol{\phi}$, and noise-to-interference ratio (NIR) estimation. We define the numerical value of NIR as $\rho = \sigma_{\mathrm{a}}^2 / \sigma_{\mathrm{e}}^2$.

16.3 Biologically inspired coupled antenna beam pattern design

In this section, inspired by the female Ormia's coupled ears, we show that applying BIC among antennas is beneficial to achieve high radiation performance. Our goal is to demonstrate the effect of the BIC on the radiation performance. We would like to note that our approach, namely, employing BIC, might be also used to complement the existing superdirective (super gain) array design methods that overcome issues; for example, the effect of the undesired coupling on individual antenna impedance (Tucker, 1967; Newman et al., 1978; Popovic et al., 1999; Lee and Wang, 2008).

16.3.1 Biologically inspired coupled array factor

In this section, we compute the array factor of the proposed biologically inspired ULA. We start with the array factor of a standard ULA, positioned without loss of generality along the z-axis (see Figure 16.6). Since we focus on systems confined in small spaces, we also consider the undesired electromagnetic coupling between the array elements.

Under the far-field radiation and narrow-band signal assumption, we modify the ULA factor to include the undesired coupling between the elements (see also Allen and Diamond, 1966):

$$\mathrm{AF}(\theta) = \sum_{m=1}^{M} p_m \exp(-\mathrm{j}\,(m-1)(\omega\Delta + \beta)) \tag{16.17}$$

where

- $\mathrm{AF}(\theta)$ is the radiation pattern (desired amplitude and phase in each direction) of M-element array assuming isotropic antennas, which depends on the positions and excitations of the sensing elements in the system
- $\boldsymbol{p} = (p_1, \ldots, p_M)^{\mathrm{T}} = \boldsymbol{C}\boldsymbol{v}_{\mathrm{g}}$ is the vector of the currents on the antennas
- $\boldsymbol{v}_{\mathrm{g}} = [v_1, \ldots, v_M]$ is the vector of generator (excitation) voltages at the input of the antennas
- $\boldsymbol{C}$ is the undesired electromagnetic coupling between the array elements, (a transformation matrix, transforming generator voltages to the induced currents on each antenna)

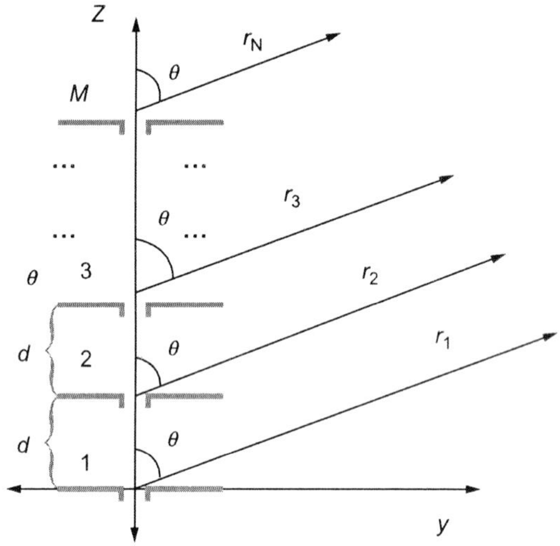

Figure 16.6 Far-field radiation geometry of M-element antenna array.

- As also defined earlier, $\Delta = \frac{d\cos\theta}{v}$ is the interelement time difference
- θ is the elevation angle (see Figure 16.6), and
- β is the excitation phase.

We compute $\boldsymbol{C}$ similar to Allen and Diamond (1966) as a function of self and mutual impedances between the antennas (see also discussions in Gupta and Ksienski (1983) and Svantesson (1998)). We summarize the computation of $\boldsymbol{C}$ in Appendix B. When the mutual impedances are zero, when there is no electromagnetic coupling, $\boldsymbol{C}$ reduces to a diagonal matrix. We compute the self and mutual impedances, assuming finite-length dipole antennas as the elements of the array, as explained in Balanis (1982), Chapter 8. Note that the standard literature often ignores $\boldsymbol{C}$, which is reasonable for sufficiently large interelemental distances.

The usual goal of the array-factor design is to select the excitation voltages, v_g, and phase, β, to obtain a desired radiation pattern. Our goal is to include the BIC in the array factor for fixed $\boldsymbol{v}_g$ and β values and demonstrate the improvement in the directivity gain, half-power beamwidth (HPBW), and side lobe level (SLL) of the radiation pattern.

Next, we generalize Equation (16.19) to include also the coupling biologically inspired by the Ormia's coupled ears. We follow the discussions in Sections 16.2.4 and 16.2.5 to obtain the frequency responses of the converted system and generalize Equation (16.17) employing

$$\begin{aligned} \mathrm{AF_I}(\theta) &= \sum_{m=1}^{M} p_m \left(\frac{H_2(w, \Delta, \beta)}{H_1(\omega, \Delta, \beta)} \right)^{m-1} \\ &= \sum_{m=1}^{M} p_m \left(\frac{D(\mathrm{j}\omega)\exp(-\mathrm{j}\,(\omega\Delta+\beta)) - N(\mathrm{j}\omega)}{D(\mathrm{j}\omega) - N(\mathrm{j}\omega)\exp(-\mathrm{j}\,(\omega\Delta+\beta))} \right)^{m-1} \end{aligned} \tag{16.18}$$

where $\frac{H_2(w, \Delta, \beta)}{H_1(\omega, \Delta, \beta)}$ is the ratio between the responses of two consecutive antennas in the BIC antenna array. These responses follow the same structure as the responses of Ormia's ears as defined in Equation (16.4), but operate in a different frequency range. This ratio generalizes the exponential terms in Equation (16.17) to include the BIC between antennas. In this setup, every antenna is coupled with its immediate neighbor antennas. In Equation (16.18), we also assume identical antennas such that $D_1(\mathrm{j}\omega) = D_2(\mathrm{j}\omega) = D(\mathrm{j}\omega)$. Note here that $N(\mathrm{j}\omega)$ represents the BIC and when there is no coupling ($N(\mathrm{j}\omega) = 0$), $\mathrm{AF_I}(\theta)$ reduces to $\mathrm{AF}(\theta)$.

16.3.2 Performance measures

In this section, we describe our measures that we employ to analyze the radiation performance. First, taking into account the antenna factor (element factor) and the BIC, we compute the radiation intensity of the antenna array in a given direction (Balanis, 1982)

$$U_{\mathrm{I}}(\theta, \phi) = [\mathrm{EF}(\theta, \phi)]_n^2 [\mathrm{EF}(\theta, \phi)]_n^2 [\mathrm{AF_I}(\theta)]_n^2 \tag{16.19}$$

where

- $[\mathrm{EF}(\theta, \phi)]_n^2$ is the normalized element factor, far-zone electric field of a single element (in our work we assume that the array is formed with finite-length dipoles, see also Section 16.4.2)
- $[\mathrm{AF_I}(\theta)]_n^2$ is the normalized array factor, and
- $U_{\mathrm{I}}(\theta, \phi)$, the radiation intensity in a given direction, is the power radiated from an antenna array per unit solid angle.

Hence, the radiated power P_{rad} is

$$P_{\mathrm{rad}} = = \int_0^{2\pi} \int_0^{\pi} U_{\mathrm{I}}(\theta, \phi) \sin\theta \, \mathrm{d}\theta \, \mathrm{d}\phi \tag{16.20}$$

where θ and ϕ are the elevation and azimuth angles, respectively, and $\sin\theta \, \mathrm{d}\theta \, \mathrm{d}\phi$ is the unit solid angle.

Using the radiation intensity, we consider the following measures to analyze the performance of the beam pattern design:

- Directivity, $D_{\mathrm{I}}(\theta, \phi)$, is the ratio of the radiation intensity in a given direction to the average radiation intensity

$$D_{\mathrm{I}}(\theta, \phi) = \frac{4\pi U_{\mathrm{I}}(\theta, \phi)}{P_{\mathrm{rad}}} \tag{16.21}$$

  where $\frac{P_{\mathrm{rad}}}{4\pi}$ is the average radiation intensity over all angles. In our work, for comparison purposes, we consider the directivity gain in a desired direction.
- HPBW, in terms of the elevation angle, θ, for a fixed azimuth angle, ϕ. HPBW is defined as the angle between two half-power directions (Balanis, 1982).

- Sidelobe level (SLL) defined as the maximum value of the radiation pattern in any direction other than the desired one.

The directivity gain, HPBW, and SLL measure how effectively the power is directed (steered) in a given direction. For a good performance, it is desirable to have large $D_I(\theta, \phi)$, small SLL, and narrow HPBW in a desired direction.

16.3.3 Optimization of the BIC

In this section, we develop a method to maximize the radiation performance by optimizing the BIC. We formulate the optimization problem to improve the radiation performance. For an antenna array, we choose the directivity gain in a desired direction as the utility function to be maximized. This is a reasonable choice since the directivity gain is also related to the SLL and the HPBW of the radiation pattern. Generally, it is true that the patterns with smaller SLL and HPBW values have larger directivity gain. Following the discussions from Section 16.2.9, using Equations (16.4), (16.14), (16.15), and (16.18)–(16.21), we observe that directivity is also a function of the real parts of the poles of the characteristics function. Accordingly, to optimize the BIC for maximum directivity, we propose to choose r_1 and r_2 by solving the following constrained optimization problem in the desired direction of transmission with elevation θ and azimuth ϕ

$$\max_{\boldsymbol{r}} D_I(\theta, \phi, \boldsymbol{r}) \quad \text{s.t.} \quad r_1 - r_2 > 0 \tag{16.22}$$

16.4 Numerical results

In this section, we present numerical simulation results for the comparison of radiation and localization performances of biologically inspired coupled and standard antenna arrays. In the following, by BIC and standard arrays, we refer to the systems with and without the BIC.

16.4.1 BIC antenna array for DOA estimation

We compare the localization performances of the BIC and standard multiple-antenna arrays using Monte Carlo simulations. In these examples, we focus on the optimally designed BIC as described in Section 16.2.9. We follow the statistical assumptions stated in Section 16.2.6.

We compare the BIC array with the multichannel cross-correlation method. Under our statistical assumptions, multichannel cross-correlation method asymptotically reduces to the ML estimation of DOA using a standard antenna array (Chen et al., 2003). Therefore, for comparison, we demonstrate the results of the ML estimation of the DOA and compute the corresponding CRB using the standard antenna array and the antenna array with BIC. We focus on the small-sized compact arrays that are very important for civil and military purposes to be used in tactical and mobile applications which are confined in small spaces. We use the following scenarios for the multiple-antenna array.

- ULA: Five identical dipole antennas, $d = 0.1\lambda$ and $d = 0.2$ interelement distances
- $f_c = 1$ GHz is the carrier frequency; $f_1 = 0.99$ GHz and $f_2 = 1.1$ GHz are the resonant frequencies which are employed as in Section 16.2.4; $\rho = \sigma_a^2/\sigma_e^2$ is the NIR as defined in Section 16.2.9; signal-to-noise ratio is $\mathrm{SNR} = \frac{\mathrm{tr}\left[\widetilde{\boldsymbol{A}}(\boldsymbol{\phi})\boldsymbol{P}\widetilde{\boldsymbol{A}}(\boldsymbol{\phi})^H(\boldsymbol{\phi})\right]}{\sigma_e^2 \mathrm{tr}[\boldsymbol{\Sigma}(\rho)]}$; root-mean-square error is $\mathrm{RMSE} = \sqrt{\frac{1}{\mathrm{MC}} \sum_{i=1}^{\mathrm{MC}} \left(\hat{\phi}_i - \phi_0\right)^2}$, where MC is the number of Monte Carlo simulations; ϕ_0 is the true value of the DOA; and $\hat{\phi}_i$ is the estimate of DOA at the ith simulation; and $\mathrm{MC} = 1000$.

We demonstrate our results on DOA estimation performance in Figures 16.7–16.11. In Figure 16.7a and b for a fixed SNR = − 10 dB and the true value of the azimuth of DOA, $\phi_0 = 55°$, we plot the RMSE for the maximum likelihood estimation of DOA, and CRB of DOA estimation for the standard and BIC arrays with $d = 0.1\lambda$ and $d = 0.2\lambda$ interelement spacings, respectively. Since BIC creates a virtual array with larger aperture, we observe that the CRB on DOA estimation error and RMSE of MLE are smaller for the BIC array, meaning a decrease in estimation error and an improvement in the localization performance. Moreover, the MLE algorithm attains the bound asymptotically. BIC array outperforms the standard array in ML estimation of DOA accuracy. Therefore, asymptotically BIC array is better than the multichannel cross-correlation method, which is asymptotically the ML estimation of DOA using standard array.

In Figure 16.8, for $N = 10$ time samples and $\phi_0 = 55°$, we plot the CRB on DOA estimation for the standard and BIC ULAs for different SNR values and demonstrate the decrease in the minimum bound on the estimation error due to the BIC. Figures 16.7 and 16.8 confirm that the BIC decreases the minimum bound on estimation error and improves the performance of DOA estimation. The BIC works as a multi-input multi-output filter creating a virtual array with a larger aperture.

In Figure 16.9, we illustrate the CRB on the error of the DOA estimation as a function of the azimuth values of the DOA for fixed $N = 10$ time samples and SNR = − 10 dB. We observe that the BIC array always outperforms the standard array, and as the azimuth increases the estimation accuracy increases.

In Figure 16.10, for fixed $N = 10$ time samples and SNR = − 10 dB, we demonstrate the CRB on the error of DOA estimation as a function of the interelement spacing of the antennas d. We observe that the improvement due to the BIC decreases as d increases. For $d = 0.5\lambda$, the performances of the standard and the BIC array are the same. We conclude that for the antenna systems that have interelement spacing lower than 0.5λ, the BIC provides an improvement in the localization performance. From a practical standpoint, this comparison favors even more BIC over standard arrays. Indeed, it is very hard to implement a standard array with small d due to the unwanted

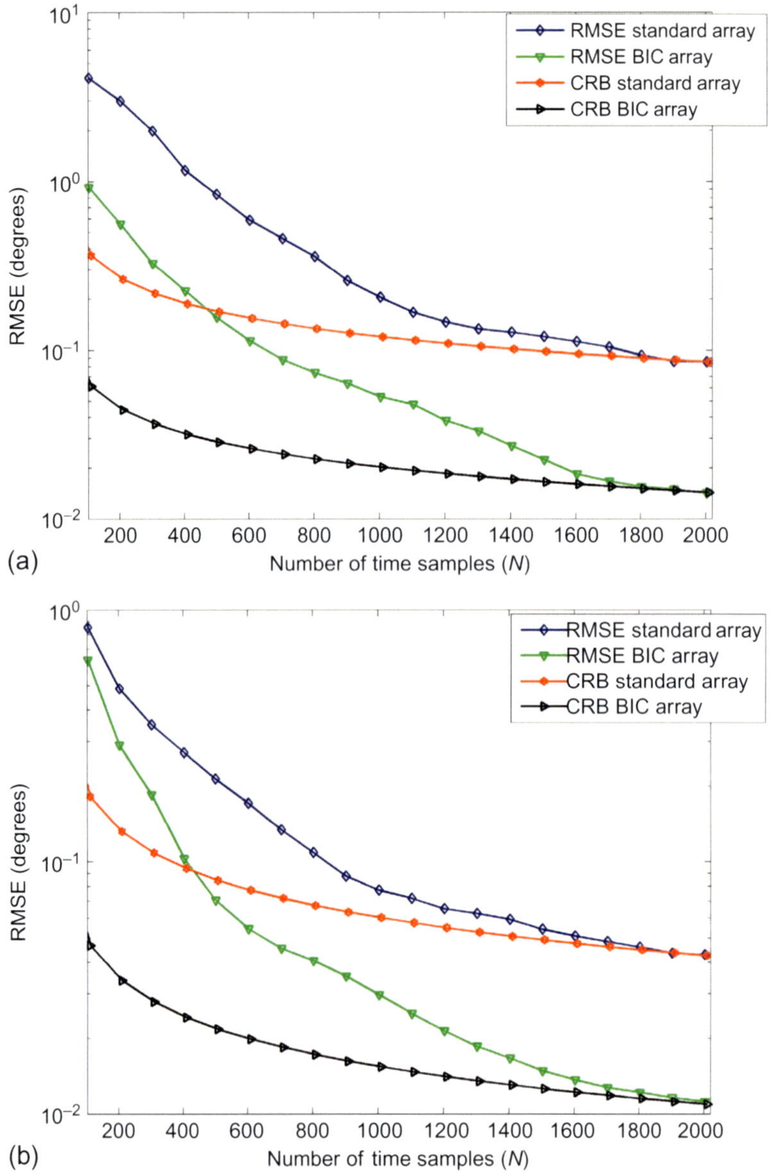

Figure 16.7 Square root of the mean-square error in the direction estimation and corresponding Cramér–Rao bounds versus number of time samples for the standard and BIC uniform linear arrays with different interelement spacings, d, and SNR = − 10 dB. (a) $d = 0.1\lambda$. (b) 0.2λ.

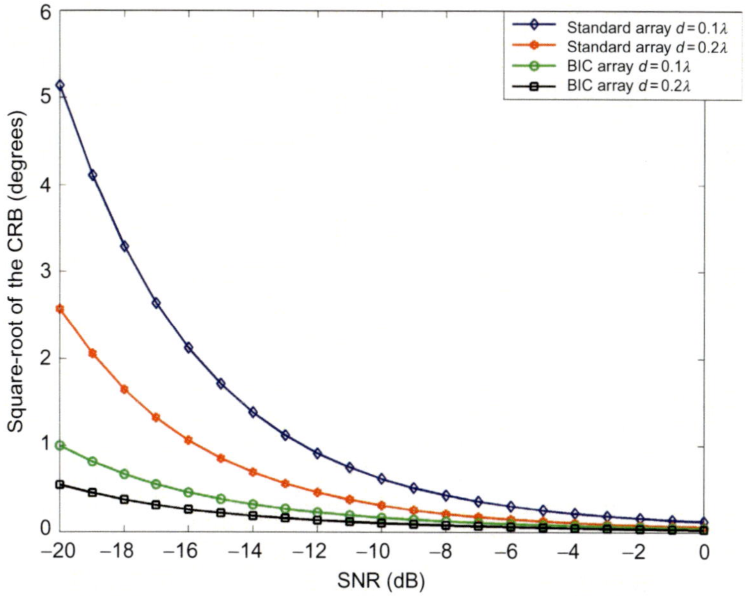

Figure 16.8 Square root of the Cramér–Rao bound on direction of arrival estimation versus SNR for standard, and BIC uniform linear arrays with different interelement spacings, $d = 0.1\lambda$ and $d = 0.2\lambda$, and $N = 10$ time samples.

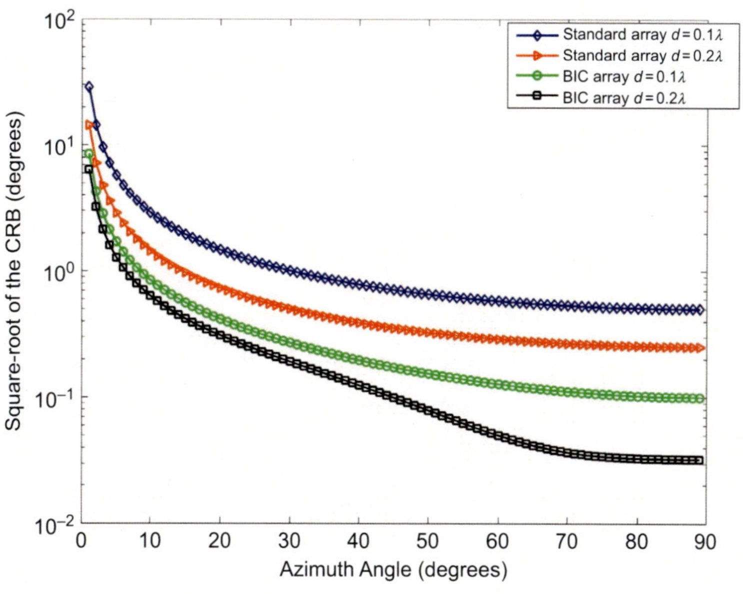

Figure 16.9 Square root of the Cramér–Rao bound on direction of arrival estimation versus direction of arrival (azimuth) for standard, and BIC uniform linear arrays with different interelement spacings, $d = 0.1\lambda$ and $d = 0.2\lambda$, $N = 10$ time samples, and SNR $= -10$ dB.

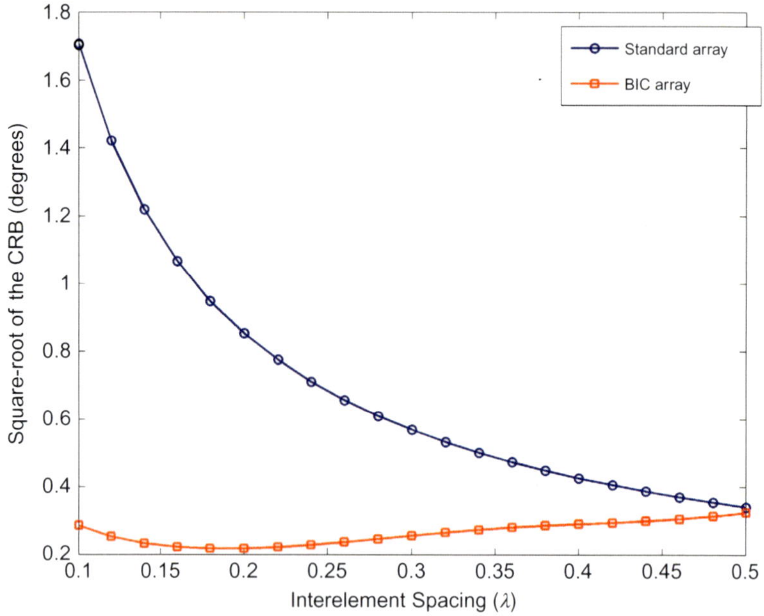

Figure 16.10 Square root of the Cramér–Rao bound on direction of arrival estimation versus inter-element spacing, d, for standard, and BIC uniform linear arrays, $N = 10$ time samples, and SNR = − 10 dB.

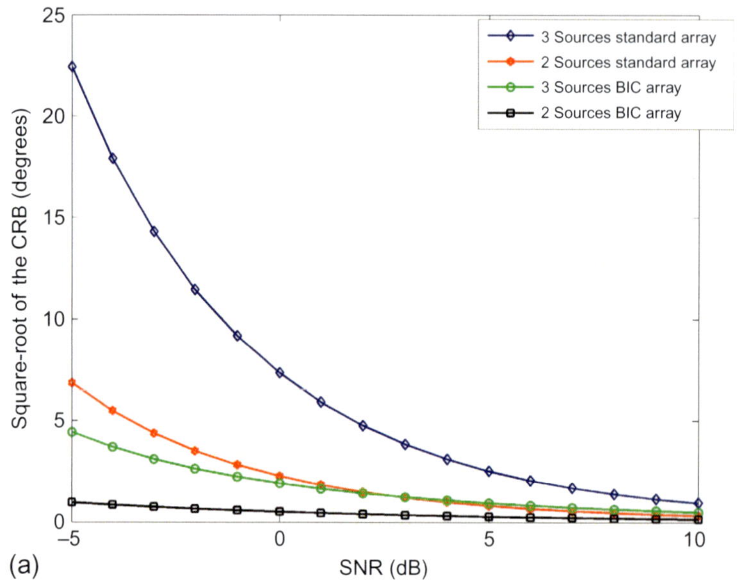

Figure 16.11 Square root of the Cramér–Rao bound on direction of arrival estimation versus SNR for standard, and BIC uniform linear arrays with different number of sources, Q, $N = 10$ time samples. (a) $Q = 2$, 3.

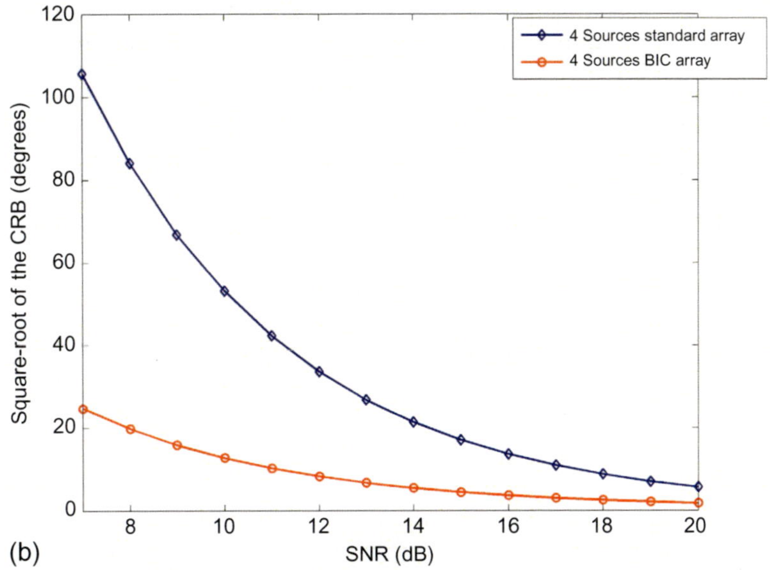

Figure 16.11, cont'd (b) $Q=4$.

coupling among close elements. However, a BIC array may be designed to absorb, to a certain extent, the unwanted coupling. This will be the subject of further work.

In Figure 16.11, we show the performances of the BIC and standard linear arrays for multiple incoming sources. In this example, the interelement distance is $d=0.2\,\lambda$. Since we use $M=5$ antennas for our examples, we assume the maximum number of the incoming sources is $Q=4$ (in order to have a well-posed problem.) Well-posedness is a necessary condition for the Fisher information matrix to be nonsingular (see Hochwald and Nehorai, 1996, for details). We choose 55°, 10°, 45°, and 85° as the azimuths of the true DOA of the incoming sources 1, 2, 3, and 4, respectively. In this figure, we plot the CRB on the estimation of the DOA of the first source as a function of the SNR in the presence of other sources. For $Q=2$, we use the sources 1 and 2, for $Q=3$, we use sources 1, 2, 3, etc. We observe that the BIC array has better localization performance than the standard array in the presence of multiple sources.

16.4.2 BIC for antenna beam pattern design

In this section, we compare the radiation performances of the BIC and standard antenna arrays. For comparison, we plot the radiation pattern and compare the directivity gain, HPBWs, and sidelobe attenuation of these systems. BIC parameters are optimally designed using the algorithm described in Section 16.3.3. We use the following system setup for illustration purposes.

- We consider uniform (uniform excitation voltages) ordinary and binomial (binomial expansion coefficients as the excitation voltage values) end-fire arrays with 20 identical dipole antennas (Balanis, 1982; Chapter 8), maximum at $\theta = 0°$ and $\beta = -w\Delta$.
- We assume the radiation frequency is $f = 1$ GHz.
- The undesired coupling matrices, $\boldsymbol{C}$ for 0.5λ-wavelength antenna system with different inter-element distances ($d = 0.25\lambda$ and $d = 0.1\lambda$) are calculated according to Balanis (1982) for finite-length thin-dipole antennas.
- The antennas are located on the z-axis parallel to y-axis, then assuming azimuth $\phi = 90°$ (on the y–z plane, see Figure 16.6), we compute the element factor for a finite-length dipole antenna as $\mathrm{EF}(\theta, 90°) = \left[\dfrac{\cos\left(\dfrac{kl}{2}\sin\theta\right) - \cos\left(\dfrac{kl}{2}\right)}{\cos\theta}\right]$ with $k = \frac{2\pi}{\lambda}$, λ as the wavelength of the radiated signal, and l as the length of each antenna.

We demonstrate our results in Figures 16.12 and 16.13 and summarize the calculated directivity gains and HPBW values in Tables 16.1 and 16.2, respectively. We observe that the BIC array with uniform excitation voltages outperforms the uniform standard array in terms of sidelobe suppression, directivity, and HPBW (see Figure 16.12, and Tables 16.1 and 16.2). For binomial array, in Figure 16.13, we observe that neither the standard nor the BIC array has sidelobes, but the BIC array has much narrower HPBW and hence better directivity gain (see also Tables 16.1 and 16.2). The physical reason of the improvement in the radiation performance is the BIC that works as a multi-input multi-output filter, magnifying the amplitude and phase differences (time differences) between the outputs of the successive antennas and creating a virtual array with a larger aperture. In the beam pattern design, the virtual array with larger aperture creates a radiation pattern with higher directivity and sidelobe suppression, and lower HPBW. Note also that in these examples the effect of the BIC increases as the distance between the antennas, d, decreases.

16.5 Summary

We designed a small-sized multiple-antenna array with couplings biologically inspired by the mechanically coupled ears of *O. ochracea*. First, we obtained the response of the mechanical model representing the coupling between the Ormia's ears. We then converted this response to the desired radio frequencies. Assuming uniform linear antenna array, we implemented the BIC using the converted system as a multi-input multi-output filter and obtained a passive antenna system with BIC. For the resulting system, we derived the maximum likelihood estimates of the DOA and computed the Cramér–Rao lower bound on estimation error as a performance measure. We later developed an active transmitting antenna array with BIC. For the resulting system, we computed the directivity gain, HPBW, and SLL as radiation performance measures. For both passive and active antenna arrays, we proposed an algorithm to optimally choose the BIC for maximum localization and radiation

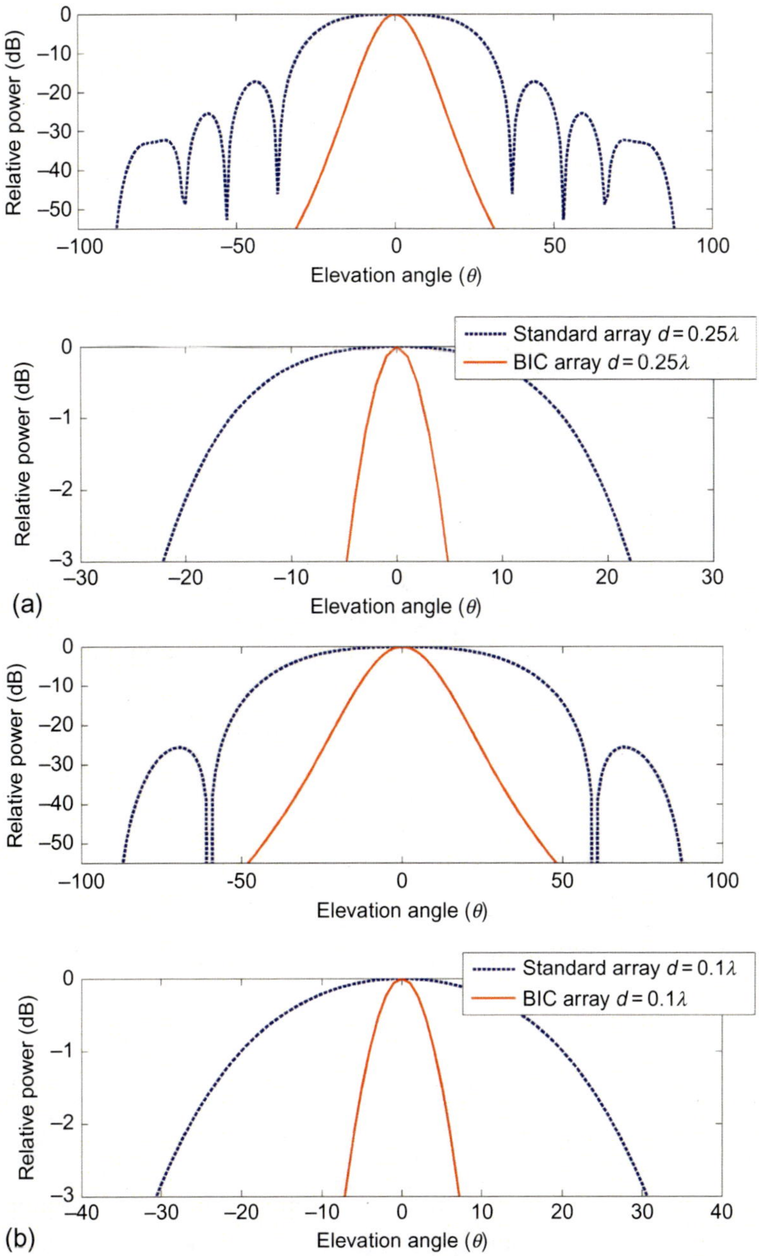

Figure 16.12 Power patterns of the uniform ordinary end-fire antenna arrays using standard approach, and BIC for (a) $d = 0.25\lambda$, (b) $d = 0.1\lambda$ interelement spacings. The bottom halves of the figures present the half-power beamwidth.

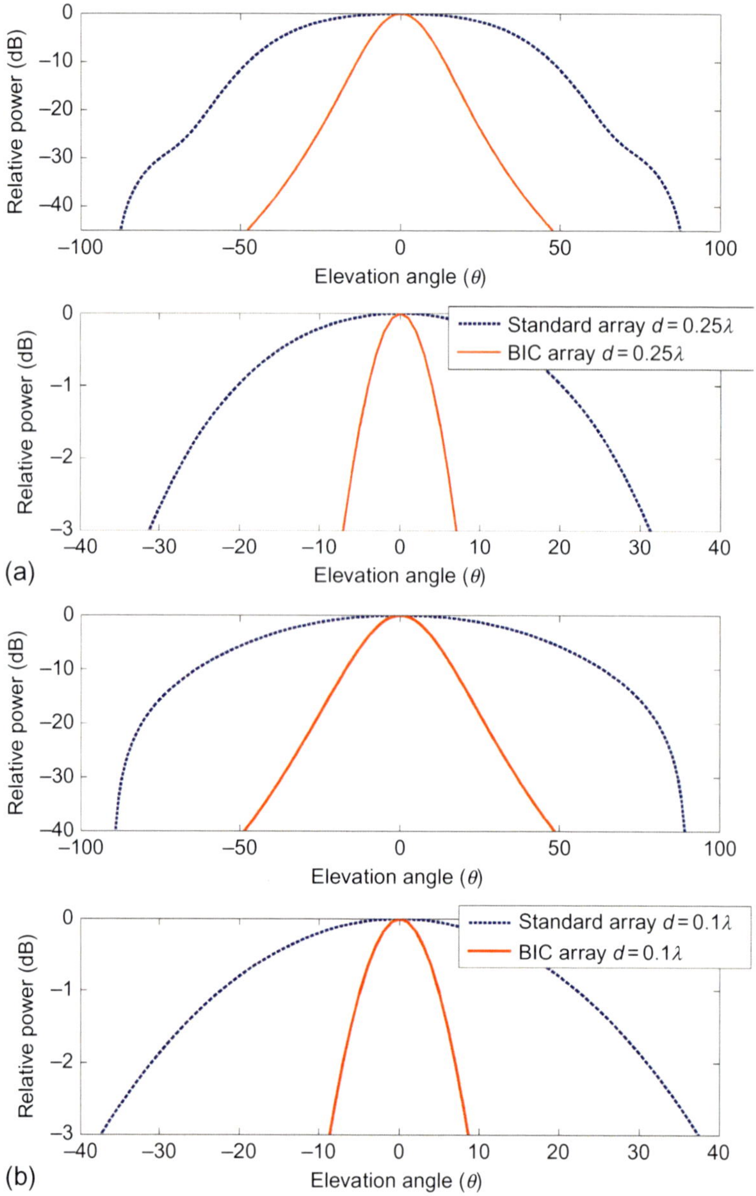

Figure 16.13 Power patterns of the binomial end-fire antenna arrays using standard approach, and BIC for (a) $d=0.25\lambda$, (b) $d=0.1\lambda$ interelement spacings. The bottom halves of the figures present the half-power beamwidth.

Table 16.1 Directivity gains of the antenna arrays in the desired direction $\theta = 0°$ and $\phi = 90°$ (in dB)

	Uniform		Binomial	
	$d = 0.25\lambda$	$d = 0.1\lambda$	$d = 0.25\lambda$	$d = 0.1\lambda$
Standard array	13.96 dB	10.77 dB	10.81 dB	8.08 dB
BIC array	25.62 dB	22.16 dB	22.75 dB	20.35 dB

Table 16.2 Half-power beamwidths of the antenna arrays (degrees)

	Uniform		Binomial	
	$d = 0.25\lambda$	$d = 0.1\lambda$	$d = 0.25\lambda$	$d = 0.1\lambda$
Standard array	45°	62°	63°	76°
BIC array	9.8°	14.6°	14.2°	17.4°

performance. With numerical examples, we demonstrated the improvement in localization and radiation performance due to the BIC.

Future directions include extension of the BIC to different array configurations, specifically optimization of the array configuration for the maximum biologically coupling effect. Also, it is of interest to investigate the deterioration in performance due to the undesired coupling. In this context, it will be interesting to compute the maximum likelihood estimation algorithm and corresponding CRB for finding the source directions as well as the unknown, undesired mutual coupling parameters (calibration). The sensitivity of the BIC system to calibration error will also be analyzed. The next logical step will be to add polarimetry vector sensors and to demonstrate the improvement in the source identifiability capacity and angular resolution of the system. Different polarizations could also provide additional degrees of freedom for optimum beam pattern design.

Appendix A Definition of block matrix operators

In this appendix, similar to Nehorai and Paldi (1994), we define several block matrix operators used in Section 16.2. We employ the following notation for a block-wise partitioned matrix A of size $m\mu \times n\nu$

$$A = \begin{bmatrix} A_{<11>} & \cdots & A_{<1n>} \\ \vdots & \ddots & \vdots \\ A_{<m1>} & \cdots & A_{<mn>} \end{bmatrix} \tag{16.23}$$

where $A_{<ij>}$ is a $\mu \times \nu$ size matrix.

Definition A.1 Block Schur–Hadamard product
Similar to $\boldsymbol{A}$ a matrix $\boldsymbol{B}$ of size $mv \times n\eta$ has blocks $\boldsymbol{B}_{<ij>}$ of dimension $v \times \eta$ (equal size). Then the block Schur–Hadamard product $\boldsymbol{A} \boxdot \boldsymbol{B}$ is an $m\mu \times n\eta$ block-wise partitioned matrix with the following entries.

$$\left(\boldsymbol{A} \boxdot \boldsymbol{B}\right)_{<ij>} = \boldsymbol{A}_{<ij>}\boldsymbol{B}_{<ij>} \tag{16.24}$$

such that each block entry is an $\mu \times \eta$ matrix.

Definition A.2 Block transpose
The block-transposed matrix $\boldsymbol{A}^{\mathrm{bT}}$ is an $n\mu \times mv$ sized matrix with the following block entries

$$\left(\boldsymbol{A}^{\mathrm{bT}}\right)_{<ij>} = \boldsymbol{A}_{<ij>} \tag{16.25}$$

Definition A.3 Block trace operator
Assume $\boldsymbol{A}$ of (16.23) has $\mu = v$. Then the block trace operator btr $[\boldsymbol{A}]$ is an $m \times n$ sized matrix with entries

$$(\mathrm{btr}[\boldsymbol{A}])_{<ij>} = \mathrm{tr}\left(\boldsymbol{A}_{<ij>}\right) \tag{16.26}$$

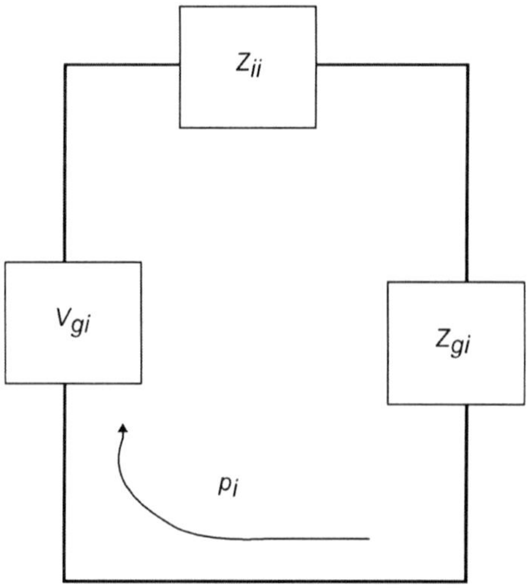

Figure 16.14 Circuit model of the ith antenna element in transmitting mode.

Appendix B Computation of the electromagnetic coupling matrix *C*

An antenna in the transmitting mode can be modeled as in Figure 16.14. Assuming M element antenna array, and considering the mutual effect of the other antennas in the array, the induced current on the ith antenna can be computed through (see also Balanis, 1982, and Allen and Diamond, 1966)

$$p_i\left(Z_{ii}+Z_g\right)=v_{gi}-\sum_{k\neq 1}^{M}p_kZ_{ik} \tag{16.27}$$

where

- p_j for $j=1,\ldots,M$ is the induced current on the jth antenna
- Z_{jj} is the self-impedance of the jth antenna
- Z_g is the generator impedance
- v_{gj} is the generator voltage applied to the jth antenna
- Z_{jk} is the mutual impedance between the jth and kth antennas.

Assuming identical antennas and generators (identical self and generator impedances), from Equation (16.27) we can write

$$\begin{bmatrix} Z_{11}+Z_g & Z_{12} & \cdots & Z_{1M} \\ Z_{21} & Z_{22}+Z_g & \cdots & Z_{2M} \\ \cdots & \cdots & \cdots & \cdots \\ Z_{M1} & Z_{M2} & \cdots & Z_{MM}+Z_g \end{bmatrix}\begin{bmatrix} p_1 \\ \vdots \\ p_M \end{bmatrix}=\begin{bmatrix} v_{g1} \\ \vdots \\ v_{gM} \end{bmatrix} \tag{16.28}$$

Then since $\boldsymbol{p}=\boldsymbol{C}\boldsymbol{v}$, we have

$$\boldsymbol{C}=\begin{bmatrix} Z_{11}+Z_g & Z_{12} & \cdots & Z_{1M} \\ Z_{21} & Z_{22}+Z_g & \cdots & Z_{2M} \\ \cdots & \cdots & \cdots & \cdots \\ Z_{M1} & Z_{M2} & \ldots & Z_{MM}+Z_g \end{bmatrix}^{-1} \tag{16.29}$$

References

Akcakaya, M., Muravchik, C., Nehorai, A., 2010. Biologically inspired coupled antenna array for direction of arrival estimation. In: Proceedings of the 44th Asilomar Conference on Signals, Systems and Computers, Pacific Groove, CA, USA.

Akcakaya, M., Muravchik, C., Nehorai, A., 2011a. Biologically inspired coupled antenna array for direction of arrival estimation. IEEE Trans. Signal. Process. 59 (10), 4795–4808.

Akcakaya, M., Muravchik, C., Nehorai, A., 2011b. Performance analysis of biologically inspired coupled circular antenna array. In: Proceedings of the IEEE Antennas and

Propagation Society International Symposium (APSURSI)', Spokane, WA, USA, pp. 1530–1533.
Akcakaya, M., Nehorai, A., 2008. Performance analysis of Ormia ochracea's coupled ears. J. Acoust. Soc. Am. 124 (4), 2100–2105.
Akcakaya, M., Nehorai, A., 2010a. Biologically inspired coupled antenna beam pattern design. Bioinspir. Biomim. 5 (4), 046003.
Akcakaya, M., Nehorai, A., 2010b. Biologically inspired coupled beam pattern design. In: Proceedings of the IEEE 5th International Waveform Diversity and Design Conference, Niagara Falls, ON, Canada, pp. 48–52.
Allen, J., Diamond, B., 1966. Mutual coupling in array antennas. Technical Report 424MIT Lincoln Laboratory, Lexington, MA.
Balanis, C., 1982. Antenna Theory: Analysis and Design. John Wiley and sons, New York.
Bar-Shalom, Y., 1987. Tracking and Data Association. Academic Press Professional, San Diego, CA, USA.
Blauert, J., 1997. Spatial Hearing, The Psychophysics of Human Sound Localization. MIT Press, Cambridge, MA.
Brenner, A.R., Roessing, L., 2008. Radar imaging of urban areas by means of very high-resolution SAR and interferometric SAR. IEEE Trans. Geosci. Remote Sens. 46, 2971–2982.
Brown, C., Beecher, M., Moody, D., Stebbins, W., 1978. Localization of primate calls by Old World monkeys. Science 201, 753–754.
Cade, W., 1975. Acoustically orienting parasitoids: fly phonotaxis to cricket song. Science 190, 1312–1313.
Cade, W., Ciceran, M., Murray, A., 1996. Temporal patterns of parasitoid fly (Ormia ochracea) attraction to filed cricket song (Gryllus integer). Can. J. Zool. 74, 393–395.
Chen, J., Benesty, J., Huang, Y., 2003. Robust time delay estimation exploiting redundancy among multiple microphones. IEEE Trans. Speech Audio Process. 11 (6), 549–557.
Dogandzic, A., Nehorai, A., 2001. Cramer-Rao bounds for estimating range, velocity, and direction with an active array. IEEE Trans. Signal Process. 49 (6), 1122–1137.
Eggermont, J., 1988. Mechanism of sound localization in anurans. In: Fritzsch, B., Ryan, M., Wilczynski, W., Hetherington, T., Walkowiak, W. (Eds.), The Evolution of the Amphibian Auditory System. John Wiley, New York, NY.
Fletcher, N.H., Thwaites, S., 1979. Acoustical analysis of the auditory system of the cricket Teleogryllus commodus (walker). J. Acoust. Soc. Am. 66 (2), 350–357.
Gupta, I., Ksienski, A., 1983. Effect of mutual coupling on the performance of adaptive arrays. IEEE Trans. Antennas Propag. 31 (5), 785–791.
Heffner, H., Heffner, R., 1984. Sound localization in large mammals: localization of complex sounds by horses. Behav. Neurosci. 98, 541–555.
Heffner, R., Heffner, H., 1989. Sound localization, use of binaural cues, and the superior olivary complex in pigs. Brain Behav. Evol. 33, 248–258.
Hochwald, B., Nehorai, A., 1996. Identifiability in array processing models with vector-sensor applications. IEEE Trans. Signal Process. 44 (1), 83–95.
Houben, D., Gourevitch, G., 1979. Auditory localization in monkeys: an examination of two cues serving directional hearing. J. Acoust. Soc. Am. 66, 1057–1063.
Huang, A., May, B., 1996. Spectral cues for sound localization in cats: effects of frequency domain on minimum audible angles in the median and horizontal planes. J. Acoust. Soc. Am. 100, 2341–2348.
Kay, S.M., 1993. Fundamentals of Statistical Signal Processing, Volume 1: Estimation Theory. Prentice Hall PTR, Upper Saddle River, NJ.
Knudsen, E., 1980. Sound localization in birds. In: Popper, A., Fay, R. (Eds.), Comparative Studies of Hearing in Vertebrates. Springer, New York, NY.

Krim, H., Viberg, M., 1996. Two decades of array signal processing research: the parametric approach. IEEE Signal Process Mag. 13 (4), 67–94.
Lee, T., Wang, Y.E., 2008. Mode-based information channels in closely coupled dipole pairs. IEEE Trans. Antennas Propag. 56, 3804–3811.
Long, M.W., 2001. Radar Reflectivity of Land and Sea. Artech House, Dedham, MA.
Mason, A.C., Oshinsky, M.L., Hoy, R.R., 2001. Hyperacute directional hearing in a microscale auditory system. Nature 410, 686–690.
Masterton, B., Heffner, H., Ravizza, R., 1969. The evolution of human hearing. J. Acoust. Soc. Am. 45, 966–985.
Michelsen, A., 1992. Hearing and sound communication in small animals: evolutionary adaptations to the laws of physics. In: Webster, D., Fay, R., Popper, A. (Eds.), The Evolutionary Biology of Hearing. Springer-Verlag, New York, NY.
Michelsen, A., Popov, A.V., Lewis, B., 1994. Physics of directional hearing in the cricket Gryllus bimaculatus. J. Comp. Soc. Physiol. A 175 (2), 153–164.
Miles, R.N., Robert, D., Hoy, R.R., 1995. Mechanically coupled ears for directional hearing in the parasitoid fly Ormia ochracea. J. Acoust. Soc. Am. 98 (6), 3059–3070.
Morse, P., Ingard, K., 1968. Theoretical Acoustics. McGraw-Hill, New York, NY.
Narins, P., Ehret, G., Tautz, J., 1988. Accessory pathway for sound transfer in a neotropical frog. Proc. Natl. Acad. Sci. USA 1508–1512.
Nehorai, A., Paldi, E., 1994. Vector-sensor array processing for electromagnetic source localization. IEEE Trans. Signal Process. 42 (2), 376–398.
Newman, E., Richmond, J., Walter, C., 1978. Superdirective receiving arrays. IEEE Trans. Antennas Propag. 26 (5), 629–635.
Oppenheim, A.V., Schafer, R.W., Buck, J.R., 1999. Discrete-Time Signal Processing, second ed. Prentice Hall PTR, Upper Saddle River, NJ.
Ottersten, B., Viberg, M., Stoica, P., Nehorai, A., 1993. Exact and large sample approximations of maximum likelihood techniques for parameter estimation and detection in array processing. In: Haykin, S., Litva, J., Shepherd, T. (Eds.), Radar Array Processing. Springer-Verlag, Berlin, pp. 99–151.
Palmer, A.R., Pinder, A., 1984. The directionality of the frog ear described by a mechanical model. J. Theor. Biol. 110 (2), 205–215.
Pavildis, I., Morellas, V., TsiamyrTzis, P., Harp, S., 2001. Urban surveillance systems: from the laboratory to the commercial world. Proc. IEEE 89, 1478–1497.
Popovic, B., Notaros, B., Popovic, Z., 1999. Supergain antennas: a novel philosophy of synthesis and design. In: Proceedings of the 26th URSI General Assembly, Toronto, Ontario, Canada, p. 7675.
Popper, A., Fay, R. (Eds.), 2005. Sound Source Localization, Vol. 22 of Handbook of Auditory Research. In: Springer, New York, NY.
Reddingt, N.J., Bootht, D.M., Jonest, R., 2005. Urban video surveillance from airborne and ground-based platforms. In: IEE International Symposium on Imaging for Crime Detection and Prevention (ICDP), Australia.
Robert, D., Amoroso, M.J., Hoy, R.R., 1992. The evolutionary convergence of hearing in a parasitoid fly and its cricket host. Science 258 (5085), 1135–1137.
Robert, D., Miles, R.N., Hoy, R.R., 1996. Directional hearing by mechanical coupling in the parasitoid fly Ormia ochracea. J. Comp. Physiol. A 179 (1), 29–44.
Robert, D., Miles, R.N., Hoy, R.R., 1998. Tympanal mechanics in the parasitoid fly Ormia ochracea: intertympanal coupling during mechanical vibration. J. Comp. Physiol. A 183 (4), 443–452.
Robert, D., Read, M.P., Hoy, R.R., 1994. The tympanal hearing organ of the parasitoid fly Ormia ochracea (diptera, tachinidae, ormiini). Cell Tissue Res. 275 (1), 63–78.

Stoica, P., Nehorai, A., 1990. Performance study of conditional and unconditional direction-of-arrival estimation. IEEE Trans. Acoust. Speech Signal Process. 38 (10), 1783–1795.

Stoica, P., Nehorai, A., 1995. On the concentrated stochastic likelihood function in array signal processing. Circuits Syst. Signal Process. 14 (5), 669–674.

Stoica, P., Sharman, K., 1990. Maximum likelihood methods for direction-of-arrival estimation. IEEE Trans. Acoust. Speech Signal Process. 38 (7), 1132–1143.

Svantesson, T., 1998. The effects of mutual coupling using a linear array of thin dipoles of finite length. In: Proceedings of the Ninth IEEE SP Workshop on Statistical Signal and Array Processing, pp. 232–235.

Swindlehurst, A., Stoica, P., 1998. Maximum likelihood methods in radar array signal processing. Proc. IEEE 86 (2), 421–441.

Tucker, D., 1967. Superdirective arrays: the use of decoupling between elements to ease design and increase bandwidth. Radio Electron. Eng. 34 (4), 251–256.

Walker, T., 1986. Monitoring the flight of filed crickets (Gryllus spp.) and a tachinid fly (euphasiopterix ochracea) in north Florida. Fla. Entomol. 69, 678–685.

Index

Note: Page numbers followed by *f* indicate figures and *t* indicate tables.